Dear Prospective Doctor;

Students differ both in their needs and in their styles of learning. Some students may choose to pursue, in addition to this book, an MCAT preparatory *course*. For those who do, the authors recommend The Princeton Review.

The Princeton Review offers the fastest-growing and most comprehensive MCAT preparatory course in the nation. They specialize in teaching MCAT science conceptually and in training students to use good testing strategy to succeed on the MCAT. In addition, The Princeton Review recently joined forces with California-based MCAT preparatory group Hyperlearning, whose intense methods and comprehensive materials have proven very effective in preparing students for the MCAT in California. The Princeton Review / Hyperlearning combination creates the most complete, the most exhaustive, the most extensive MCAT preparatory course ever.

Students who take the Princeton Review MCAT course must be prepared for, and committed to, an intense preparatory experience. For weeks on end they will eat, sleep, and breathe just one thing—*the MCAT*. Together with trained, highly-skilled teachers who understand how the MCAT is designed and how its questions are built, the student will work through the most comprehensive course materials available, course materials whose pages number in the thousands.

- Princeton Review students thoroughly review every aspect of physics, inorganic chemistry, organic chemistry, biology, and verbal reasoning, *precisely as it is tested on the MCAT.*

- Our students master dozens of techniques and strategies custom-designed to crack the most challenging MCAT questions.

- Our students receive thousands of exercises and drills on which to practice these techniques and solidify his/her grasp of the concepts.

- Our students sit for eleven full-length simulated MCAT tests, administered under conditions similar to those they will be confronted with on the day of the real test.

- Computerized scoring, individual review with teachers, and extra help are included in the <u>most</u> complete MCAT preparatory course available.

For those students who feel they would benefit from an MCAT course, The Princeton Review's course is clearly the best choice. It is for this reason that we chose to publish this book in association with The Princeton Review.

Wishing you much success in your medical endeavors.

James L. Flowers, MD
Dr. James L. Flowers, MD

Ted Sil
Dr. Theodore Silver, MD

For more information call 1 - 800 2 REVIEW

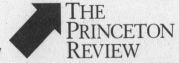

THE PRINCETON REVIEW

FLOWERS & SILVER
MCAT

1998-99 EDITION

THE PRINCETON REVIEW

FLOWERS & SILVER

MCAT

1998-99 EDITION

JAMES L. FLOWERS, M.D., M.P.H.
THEODORE SILVER, M.D.

RANDOM HOUSE, INC., NEW YORK 1998

ISBN 0-375-75003-7

Editor: Rachel Warren
Production Editor: Amy Bryant
Production Coordinator: Carmine Raspaolo

Manufactured in the United States of America on recycled paper.

9 8 7 6 5 4 3 2 1

1998-99 Edition

ACKNOWLEDGMENTS

The authors wish to thank the following people: Kyle Alexander, Daniel Silver, Jonathan Silver, Linda Tarleton, Doug McMullen, Jr., Deborah Guest, Valerie Knapp, Martha Link, M.D., Lynne Christensen, James T. Morgan, Eric Payne, John Sun, Ken Howard, Ken Riley, and Kim Magloire.

And many thanks to the production staff who's great patience and hard work made this all possible: Christine Lee, Chris Thomas, Glen Pannell, Illeny Maaza, John Pak, Matthew Covey, Meher Khambata, Robert McCormack, and especially Carmine Raspaolo.

Contents

CHAPTER 4

CHAPTER 5

CHAPTER 13

ATOMS, ELEMENTS, AND THE PERIODIC TABLE 231

CHAPTER 14

BONDING AND MOLECULAR FORMATION 249

CHAPTER 15

CHEMICAL REACTIONS I: FUNDAMENTAL PHENOMENA 265

CHAPTER 16

CHEMICAL REACTIONS II: EQUILIBRIUM DYNAMICS 285

CHAPTER 24

THE GENETIC MATERIAL: DEOXYRIBONUCLEIC ACID

CHAPTER 25

PERPETUATION OF THE SPECIES—THE BIOLOGY OF REPRODUCTION

CHAPTER 29

HUMAN PHYSIOLOGY I: GAS EXCHANGE, CIRCULATION, DIGESTION, AND MUSCULOSKELETAL FUNCTION 549

CHAPTER 30

HUMAN PHYSIOLOGY II:
THE RENAL, ENDOCRINE, AND NERVOUS SYSTEMS,
AND THE SENSORY ORGANS AND SKIN 591

CHAPTER 31

CHAPTER 32

CHAPTER 42

MASTERING VERBAL REASONING 837

CHAPTER 43

VERBAL REASONING DISTRACTERS 851

CHAPTER 44

SYSTEMATIC IDENTIFICATION OF CORRECT ANSWERS 861

CHAPTER 45

NINE SAMPLE VERBAL REASONING PASSAGES 869

CHAPTER 46

UNDERSTANDING THE MCAT ESSAY 909

CHAPTER 47

SIX ESSAY EXERCISES 917

APPENDIX

CHAPTER 1

UNDERSTANDING THE MCAT AND THE FLOWERS MCAT BOOK

1.1 THE MCAT

1.1.1 CREATION AND ADMINISTRATION OF THE TEST

The Medical College Admissions Test (MCAT) is produced, administered, and scored under the auspices of the Association of American Medical Colleges (AAMC), 2450 N Street NW, Washington, D.C., 20037-1123. Pursuant to a contract with AAMC, the test is created and administered by American College Testing (ACT) of Iowa City, Iowa, which for this purpose has created an office:

MCAT Program Office • P.O. Box 4056
Iowa City • Iowa 52243 • (319) 337-1357

The student obtains registration materials from the MCAT Program Office at this address. If, for some reason, one wishes to communicate with the MCAT Program Office by private courier (Federal Express, UPS, etc.), the address to use is:

MCAT Program Office • Tyler Building
2255 North Dubuque Road • Iowa City, Iowa 52243

1.1.2 TEST DESIGN AND SCORING

The MCAT has four components:

(1) Verbal Reasoning

(2) Scientific Reasoning: The Physical Sciences

(3) Writing Sample

(4) Scientific Reasoning: The Biological Sciences

The test and the 7-hour test day are structured in the following way:

Component	Number of Questions	Time (minutes)
Verbal Reasoning	65	85
Break		10
Physical Sciences	77	100
Lunch		60
Writing Sample	2	60
Break		10
Biological Sciences	77	100

The test-taker receives 4 scores, one for each component. The verbal reasoning component and the two scientific reasoning components (biological sciences and physical sciences) are scored on a scale of 1–15 where 1 is low and 15 is high. The writing sample component is scored on a scale of J–T where J is low and T is high.

1.1.2.1 Verbal Reasoning

The MCAT's verbal reasoning section largely resembles the "reading comprehension" components of other standardized tests. There are approximately 10 reading passages each of which may pertain to the humanities, the social sciences, or the natural sciences. Every passage is followed by 6–8 multiple choice questions. The section includes 65 questions in total and the student is allowed 85 minutes to answer them. While the number of passages is approximately 10, and the number of questions per passage approximately 7, the total number of questions is exactly 65.

Verbal reasoning questions (Chapters 42–45) test the student's ability to (a) recognize statements that paraphrase the passage's text (b) draw logical inferences on the basis of information presented in the passage, (c) characterize themes on which the passage is built, and (d) follow the lines of reasoning on which the passage or any of its portions might rest.

1.1.2.2 Scientific Reasoning: The Physical Sciences

The MCAT's physical sciences component (Chapters 4–22) is also structured, principally, on passages and questions. It presents approximately 10 reading passages relevant to physics and inorganic chemistry. Each passage is followed by approximately 7 multiple-choice questions that in some way pertain to (a) the passage or (b) matters tangentially related to it.

Frequently, the passage is accompanied by diagrams, graphs, and charts. These also form the bases of questions.

As is shown in the table above, the physical sciences component allows the student 100 minutes to address all passages and questions. The number of passages is approximately 10, and the number of questions per passage is approximately 7. The total number of questions per component, however, is exactly 77. Fifteen of the 77 do not pertain to passages. They stand apart, in 3 sets of 5.

1.1.2.3 Writing Sample

The MCAT's writing sample (Chapters 46 and 47) requires that you write 2 essays, each one within 30 minutes. For each essay you are (a) given a short statement that sets forth a philosophy or point of view, and (b) asked to comment on the statement's meaning and application.

1.1.2.4 Scientific Reasoning: The Biological Sciences

The MCAT's fourth section, biological sciences (Chapters 23–42), is structured just like the physical sciences section. It features (a) approximately 10 passages bearing on biology and organic chemistry, each followed by approximately 7 multiple-choice questions, and (b) 15 multiple-choice questions that stand on their own.

Like physical sciences passages, biological science passages frequently include diagrams, graphs, and charts. The number of passages is approximately 10, and the number of questions per passage approximately 7. The total number of questions is exactly 77, and the student is given 100 minutes to answer these questions.

1.2 THE FLOWERS & SILVER MCAT BOOK

This book offers a thorough program of review and preparation for the MCAT candidate. With respect to the biological and physical sciences (Chapters 3–42), it:

- Presents systematic reviews of all topics on which the MCAT draws

- Provides drills to reinforce knowledge and mastery

- Presents simulated MCAT passages and questions resembling those on the MCAT

With respect to the verbal reasoning (Chapters 42–45), and the writing sample (Chapters 46 and 47), this book:

- Teaches you how to systematically approach MCAT questions and exercises

- Gives you repeated opportunities for self-testing with simulated passages, questions, and exercises

1.2.1 ORGANIZATION

Each chapter features several sections organized and numbered according to a multiple decimal system. The first digit of each section represents the chapter number. It is followed by a decimal point and a second digit. The second digit represents the principal heading. It too is usually followed by a decimal point and a digit. This third digit represents a subheading. It too, may be followed by a decimal point and a fourth digit which represents a subheading within the first subheading. Additional decimal points and numbers are sometimes added when the material demands the introduction of additional subheadings.

The section in which this paragraph falls, for example, is numbered **1.2.1**. The first digit (1) means that it belongs to Chapter 1. The second digit (2) means that it belongs to the second principal heading within Chapter 1. The third digit (1) means that it belongs to the first subheading within the second principal heading of Chapter 1.

The next section is numbered **1.2.1.1** which designates a first subheading within the subheading **1.2.1**. The ease and logic of this organizational system is best understood through an examination of the table of contents.

1.2.1.1 Chapters Relating to Science

Chapters 4–12 address substantive physics. Chapters 13–22 concern inorganic chemistry. Chapters 23–32 relate to biology, and chapters 33–42 pertain to organic chemistry. Each chapter features a first principal section called **Mastery Achieved**, a second entitled **Mastery Applied**, and a third called **Mastery Verified**.

Typically the section entitled **Mastery Achieved** has a great many subsections, and subsections *within* subsections. It reviews the material germane to the chapter's title primarily with text but also with questions, problems, and exercises that enable you to test and master the material *as you work*. Answers and explanations follow these questions directly, so that the student, after arriving at an answer, immediately understands and corrects any errors that have been made.

The section entitled **Mastery Applied** provides a simulated MCAT passage relating to the subject of the chapter. Here you have the opportunity to apply your mastery to questions resembling those on the MCAT.

The section called **Mastery Verified** provides answers and explanations for the simulated MCAT passage.

1.2.1.2 Chapters Relating to Verbal Reasoning

Chapters 42–45 comprehensively prepare you for the MCAT's verbal reasoning section by revealing with repeated drill and practice (a) the manner in which *passages* are constructed, (b) the design on which *questions* are built, and (c) the logical and orderly system through which passages and questions should be addressed. Chapter 45 provides 10 simulated MCAT verbal reasoning sets (passage and questions) followed by answers and explanations.

1.2.1.3 Chapters Relating to Writing Sample

Chapter 46 explains the nature of the MCAT's writing sample component and teaches you how to systematically construct the essays.

Chapter 47 presents you with 10 simulated MCAT writing exercises, each followed by a model response. Together with chapter 46, it fully prepares you for the MCAT's writing sample component.

1.3 ADDITIONAL PREPARATION AND MATERIALS

1.3.1 AAMC MATERIALS

Many students will find that this book fully meets their needs for MCAT preparation. Some may also wish to have the practice tests and practice questions sold by the AAMC:

- The MCAT Student Manual (which includes Practice Test 1)

- Practice Test 2, together with Practice Items

- Practice Test 3

The entire set of documents just described (including shipping and handling) costs $54. Those who wish to purchase the set should request it from:

Association of American Medical Colleges, Publications
Department 66 • Washington, D.C. 20055

Enclose a check for $54 and ask to receive the MCAT student manual, Practice Test 2, Practice Items, and Practice Test 3.

To order by telephone (with Visa or MasterCard), call: 202-828-0416.

1.3.2 COURSES

Students differ both in their needs and in their styles of learning. Some of you may want to pursue, in addition to this book, an MCAT preparatory *course*. Among the courses available, the authors recommend the course offered by The Princeton Review (1-800-2-REVIEW).

CHAPTER 2

INSIGHTS INTO MCAT SCIENCE COMPONENTS

Before we move to a comprehensive review of MCAT-related science, let's briefly discuss the nature of MCAT science passages and questions and talk about the way you should approach and prepare for MCAT science passages.

2.1 MCAT SCIENCE PASSAGES AND QUESTIONS

This book reviews *all* of the science tested on the MCAT—and then some. Understanding science means understanding that its principles, laws, and concepts apply to limitless numbers of situations and phenomena; the very purpose of learning science is to be able to apply it in unfamiliar contexts.

Many MCAT passages are deliberately designed to present you with information that seems, at first, to be entirely *foreign*—no matter how thorough the student's preparation. The MCAT's writers have unlimited contexts in which to set passages and problems. An MCAT passage might, for example, offer a relatively detailed description of the devices and mechanisms associated with the operation of an electrical power plant, or the physics of aeroflight. The passage might feature unfamiliar terms like "feed water," "bus structure," "yawing moment," "induced drag," and "angle of attack." It might present equations and charts concerning seemingly foreign phenomena, such as "lagging current," "corona," "the Reynolds number," "lift coefficient," "airscrew efficiency," and "manifold pressure." The passages will often feature illustrations, graphs, and charts that might cause you to conclude that the passage and its questions are beyond your knowledge and ability. This is not true!

MCAT passages are deliberately designed to test your ability to see beyond unfamiliar subject matter and recognize that the *questions* asked are readily answerable with (a) a knowledge of basic science (as found in this book), (b) the capacity to interpret an illustration, graph, or table, and (c) the ability to read carefully and process unfamiliar scientific information.

2.1.1 ILLUSTRATION: THE BIOLOGICAL SCIENCES

No *premedical* student is expected to come to the MCAT with an understanding of the diseases and conditions that he will study as a *medical* student. Nevertheless, MCAT passages frequently do concern medical syndromes and diseases and there is no predicting what syndromes or diseases they might address.

Consider, for example, this excerpt from a simulated MCAT biological science passage:

Passage

Seizures involve uncontrolled and excessive activity of some or all of the central nervous system. Epilepsy is a disorder of the central nervous system in which the patient is prone to seizures. The disorder shows increased frequency among the families of afflicted individuals, but it does not show genotypes or heritability associated with classic Mendelian patterns.

Seizures can be categorized as focal or generalized. The generalized forms give rise to three recognized types: *petit mal*, *grand mal*, and *psychomotor*. Each type yields a fairly characteristic electroencephalogram, as shown in Figure 1. Figure 2 shows the alpha, beta, theta, and delta waves associated with a normal electroencephalogram.

An epileptic who is subject to grand mal seizures is thought to have an intrinsic, ongoing overexcitability of the affected neurons of the brain. The actual seizure might be generated by a variety of external stimuli. The seizure is probably brought to an end through feedback mechanisms in which inhibitory cerebral centers are stimulated.

Seizures do arise from conditions other than epilepsy. For example, excessive quantities of carbon dioxide in the blood (hypercapnia) are known to produce seizures, as do a variety of cerebral disorders, including brain tumor. Young children from infancy to approximately 7 years of age are sometimes prone to experience seizures when body temperature is markedly elevated. The manifestation of such febrile seizures on one or more occasions during childhood does not in itself suggest a diagnosis of epilepsy.

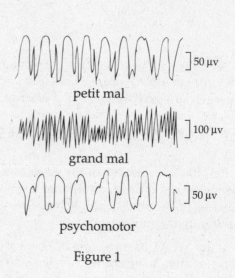

Figure 1

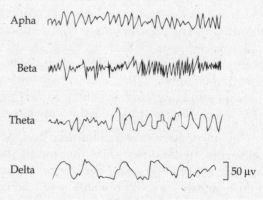

Figure 2

The MCAT writers know very well that seizures and epilepsy do not belong to the premedical syllabus; they do not expect you to have any background in the subject, so the appearance of a passage that relates to epilepsy and associated electroencephalographic data should not make you anxious. The *questions* that follow the passage should be answerable with your knowledge of premedical biology (Chapters 23-32). Consider these questions (which could follow a passage like the one just presented):

1. According to the passage, which one of the following would most likely give rise to a seizure?

 A. Excessive feedback inhibition within cerebral circuitry
 B. Failure of blood constituents to move metabolic byproducts from tissue to pulmonary alveoli
 C. Increased threshold of neuronal response within the brain and spinal cord
 D. Reduced number of action potentials within the brain and spinal cord

B is the correct answer. The test writers know that in conceptual substance, this question is truly unrelated to the subject of seizures. You could answer this question by noting that, according to the passage's last paragraph, "seizures may be caused by excessive quantities of carbon dioxide in the blood..." Once you have studied Chapter 29, you will know that elevated quantities of carbon dioxide in the blood result from a failure of blood constituents to carry metabolic waste products from the tissues to the pulmonary alveoli.

2. Which, among the following, is NOT characteristic of epilepsy?

 A. Increased excitability of central nervous system neurons
 B. Seizures induced by external stimuli
 C. Seizures of several identifiable patterns
 D. Identifiable homozygous and heterozygous states

D is the correct answer. Like question 1, this question is answerable from (a) what is presented in the passage and (b) what you know through your study of basic biology. According to the passage, epilepsy "does not show genotypes or heritability associated with classic Mendelian patterns." The fundamental principles of inheritance (Chapter 31) dictate that the absence of classic Mendelian genotypes and inheritance means the absence of identifiable homozygous and heterozygous states.

3. Among the following, the voltage difference between electroencephalographic peaks and troughs is greatest for:

 A. grand mal seizures
 B. petit mal seizures
 C. psychomotor seizures
 D. normal theta waves

A is the correct answer. You are not expected to be familiar with electroencephalograms, but you *are* expected to answer this question by examining Figures 1 and 2 calmly and logically. In Figure 1, the bracket to the right of the grand mal seizure wave is labeled 100 microvolts.

All other waves on both Figures 1 and 2 are associated with a similarly sized bracket labeled 50 microvolts. Logic dictates that the peaks and troughs associated with the grand mal wave carry a greater voltage difference than do those of any of the other waves mentioned in the passage.

4. A therapeutic agent with which of the following effects would most merit a trial for prevention of grand mal seizures?

A. Increasing the threshold for action potential within the central nervous system
B. Decreasing the threshold for action potential within the peripheral nervous system
C. Increasing the axon length for neurons within the central nervous system
D. Increasing the growth of connective tissue within the central nervous system

A is the correct answer. The passage attributes grand mal seizures to an "intrinsic, ongoing overexcitability of the affected neurons of the brain." On the basis of a fundamental knowledge of nerve function (Chapter 30) you know that excitability pertains to the threshold potential, which, for any given cell, induces an action potential. In order to prevent grand mal seizures, one would therefore want to decrease excitability, which would in turn require an increase of neuronal threshold potential.

2.1.2 ILLUSTRATION: THE PHYSICAL SCIENCES

The MCAT's physical science passages frequently involve subject matter and phenomena that you may not be familiar with. As in the case of the biological passages, all of the *questions* are answerable on the basis of logical thought, careful reading, and a basic knowledge of the science taught in Chapters 3-22. Consider, for example, this excerpt from a simulated MCAT physical science passage:

Passage

In the operation of a turbojet, the heat and pressure associated with a working fluid is harnessed to produce physical movement. Heated gas under high pressure is allowed to escape through a nozzle, which causes a reduction in the gas's temperature and pressure, and a concomitant increase in rearward velocity and momentum. If, and only if, the initial pressure of the working fluid is no greater than twice that of the surrounding pressure, a converging nozzle is employed as shown in Figure 1. Where the subscripts 1 and 2 refer, respectively, to sections 1 and 2 of the nozzle, the mass flow, m, is given by the equation:

$$m = A_2\rho\sqrt{2gJC_\rho T_t}\sqrt{\left(\frac{p_2}{p_1}\right)^{2/\gamma} - \left(\frac{p_2}{p_1}\right)^{(\gamma+1)/\gamma}}$$

$$v_2 = \sqrt{2gJC_p T}\sqrt{1-\left(\frac{p_2}{p_1}\right)^{(\gamma-1)/\gamma}}$$

m = mass flow
A = cross-sectional area
ρ = density
g = specific constant
J = work equivalent of heat
T_t = total temperature
C_p = specific heat at constant pressure
γ = specific heats
p = static pressure
v = velocity

Maximum flow corresponds to the attainment of critical pressure, which is the pressure at which fluid in the nozzle's throat is equal to the local velocity of sound. For most combustible gases used in turbojets surrounded by air, critical pressure = approximately $(0.5p_1)$

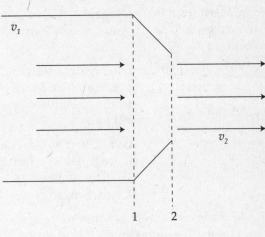

Figure 1

The usual premedical physics syllabus does *not* include any of the material just presented. Nevertheless, the questions that follow are answerable if you combine your knowledge of physical science with a logical and thorough reading of the passage.

1. If gas moving through the nozzle shown in Figure 1 undergoes ideal flow, which of the following is true?

   A. The velocity at section 1 is equal to pressure at section 1.
   B. The pressure at section 2 exceeds pressure at section 1.
   C. The velocity at section 1 exceeds velocity at section 2.
   D. The velocity at section 2 exceeds velocity at section 1.

D is correct. This question requires that you examine Figure 1 and consider it as you would any pipe or vessel of varying diameter. The laws of ideal flow (Chapter 7) say that for a fluid moving through a cylindrical vessel of varying size, increased diameter increases pressure and decreases velocity. Decreased diameter increases velocity and decreases pressure, and when you learn from the passage that the nozzle depicted in Figure 1 represents a vessel through which gas is flowing, you can conclude that the velocity at section 2 exceeds the velocity at section 1.

2. If, in Figure 1, the cross-sectional area of section 2 is increased by a factor of 3 and the density of the fluid is reduced by a factor of 4, mass flow will be:

   A. reduced by a factor of 0.75.
   B. reduced by a factor of 12.
   C. increased by a factor of 1.25.
   D. unchanged.

A is correct. The question tests your ability to apply algebraic logic to a seemingly complex equation. The equation plainly indicates that mass volume (m) is directly proportional to:

(cross-sectional area at section 2) × (density) = $A_2 p$

If A_2 is multiplied by 3 and p_1 is divided by 4, then the overall quantity $A_2 p$ is multiplied by a factor of $3/4 = 0.75$. Since m is proportional to $A_2 p$, the value of m is reduced by a factor of 0.75.

3. The emission of the fluid jet involves the conversion of:

   A. work to power.
   B. power to work.
   C. kinetic energy to potential energy.
   D. potential energy to kinetic energy.

D is correct. After studying energy conversions (Chapter 6), you will be able to answer this question by noting the relevant information in the passage's first paragraph: "...the heat and pressure associated with a working fluid is harnessed to produce physical movement." The system is one in which potential energy (inherent in the heat and pressure of the gas) is converted to kinetic energy (inherent in the motion of the gas). Moreover, you will know that options A and B are incorrect because work is never *converted* to power, or power to work.

4. Under which of the following conditions would a turbojet NOT employ a converging nozzle?

   A. When pressure and volume are inversely proportional
   B. When temperature and pressure are directly proportional
   C. When the working fluid is 1.5 times the pressure of the ambient pressure
   D. When ambient pressure is three times the pressure of the ambient pressure

D is correct. Again, in the passage's first paragraph you read: "If, and only if, the initial pressure of the working fluid is no greater than twice that of the surrounding pressure, a converging nozzle is employed." It logically follows that if the pressure of the working fluid is more than twice that of the surroundings (ambient pressure), a converging nozzle is *not* used.

2.2 READING, MATHEMATICS, AND MEMORIZATION

2.2.1 READING THE PASSAGE

Success on the MCAT's science sections requires that you read scientific text efficiently. In each chapter, you will encounter a simulated MCAT exercise that appears under the subheading **Mastery Applied**, and as you go through the exercise, you will see that in most cases, the answer to a question derives partly from the passage and partly from your knowledge of basic science.

On the other hand, (1) MCAT passages are frequently arcane and complex, and (2) no set of questions will draw on *all* of the information presented in the associated passage. You should first approach an MCAT science passage without attempting *fully* to comprehend all of its subject matter, or the workings of its illustrations, graphs, and tables. Instead, you should examine the passage and take note of its subject matter and organization, then examine the questions and for each one, return to the passage to find the necessary information.

If you are accustomed to reading material carefully and thoroughly, start to break yourself of this habit, because this will cost you time that you cannot afford. Reading with scrupulous attention to detail is undoubtedly an asset in *medical school* but it may, at times, be a handicap on the MCAT.

2.2.2 MATHEMATICS

Success on the MCAT requires a working knowledge of algebra, geometry, and trigonometry. For those who might have lost touch with these subjects, we offer a thorough review in the appendix to this book. If, in solving the many problems set forth in the chapters that follow, you stumble over mathematics, you should consult the appendix.

2.2.2.1 Formulas and Laws

The memorization of mathematical formulas plays a smaller role in answering MCAT questions than most students think. Our review of physics and inorganic chemistry involves many formulas and physical laws, but in each case we are careful to note which *aspects* of a formula or law require your attention.

For example, many of the mathematical formulas relevant to the MCAT are more important for the *proportions* they establish than for the equivalencies they create. Studying Coulomb's law (Chapter 8), you should recognize that force is (a) directly proportional to the charge of each object under consideration, and (b) inversely proportional to the square of the distance between the objects; this will serve you better than mechanically memorizing the formula. In connection with ideal gases (Chapter 19), if you understand that pressure and volume are inversely proportional and that temperature is directly proportional to each, you will fare better than one who has mechanically memorized $PV = nRT$ and the value of R (the ideal gas constant).

Throughout Chapters 4-23, we suggest that you place greater and lesser degrees of emphasis on various aspects of formulas and equations, according to the degree to which they are represented on the MCAT.

CHAPTER 3

PHYSICS AND THE MCAT: CONCEPTUAL PREMISES

3.1 MASTERY ACHIEVED

3.1.1 MASTERING UNITS

3.1.1.1 SI Units

Modern science expresses measurements according to the International System of Units, or SI. SI recognizes seven basic units, each of which measures fundamental quantity. Five of the seven are significant for the MCAT student:

	Measured Quantity	SI Unit	Symbol
1.	Distance/Displacement	meter	m
2.	Time	second	s
3.	Mass	kilogram	Kg
4.	Current	ampere	A
5.	Temperature	degrees kelvin	K

Table 3.1

SI also includes more complex units that are drawn from the basic ones. **Velocity**, for example, represents change in displacement over change in time and is expressed in meters per second (m/s). **Acceleration** represents change in velocity over change in time and is expressed in meters per second—per second (m/s^2).

Some complex quantities are normally expressed not as combinations of basic units, but in **derivative** units bearing their own names and symbols, for instance, the quantity of force is typically thought of as:

$$(mass) \times (acceleration)$$

which can also be written as:

$$(mass) \times (displacement\ per\ time—per\ time).$$

In basic units force can be expressed in kg • m/s^2, but for convenience it is normally measured in the derivative unit **newton (N)**, where $1N = 1kg • m/s^2$.

All derivative units that are significant to the MCAT are thoroughly discussed as they arise in chapters to follow, so you need not memorize them now. However, for now, take a brief look at Table 3.2:

Measured Quantity	SI Unit	Mathematical Derivation/Definition
1. Force	newton (N)	$1\,N = 1\,kg\ m/s^2$
2. Energy	joule (J)	$1\,J = 1\,N \bullet m$
3. Power	watt (W)	$1\,W = 1\,J/s$
4. Charge	coulomb (C)	$1\,C = 1\,A \bullet s$
5. Potential	volt (V)	$1\,V = 1\,J/C$
6. Resistance	ohm (Ω)	$1\,\Omega = 1\,V/A$
7. Capacitance	farad (F)	$1\,F = 1\,C/V$
8. Magnetic Field Strength	tesla (T)	$1\,T = 1\,N/A \bullet m$

Table 3.2

3.1.1.2 Dimensional Consistency

Calculations must be *dimensionally consistent*; units must be logically related, so that assessing dimensional consistency generally serves as a test for correctness. For example, if time is multiplied by acceleration using the units m/s^2, the result *must* be velocity, expressed in meters per second (m/s).

$$(\text{time}) \times (\text{acceleration}) = \text{velocity}$$

$$[(s) \bullet (m/s^2)] = [(m)(s)/s^2] = [\,(m)(s)/1 \bullet 1/(s)(s)] = (m)(s)/(s)(s) = m/s$$

If the result is in units other than m/s, then there is an error and you must redo your calculations. Similarly, if work is divided by displacement in SI units, the result must be force, expressed in newtons (N).

$$\text{work} \div \text{displacement} = \text{force}$$

$$J/m = (N \bullet m)/m = N$$

A result in units other than newtons (N) indicates an error; as you can see, this is one simple way to determine a calculation error.

Please solve this problem:

- Power is measured in the SI unit of watts (W) and represents work/time. "Work" represents force × distance. Force represents mass × acceleration. Which of the following expresses the quantity of 1 watt in terms of the *five basic* SI units?

  A. $kg \bullet m^2/s$
  B. $kg \bullet m^2/s^3$
  C. $kg^2/m^3 \bullet s$
  D. $kg/m^3 \bullet s^3$

Problem solved:

B is the correct answer.

From Table 3.2 we can see that Watts can be written as J/s. Joules can be broken down further to N•m, which can be broken down further to kg•m/s². Thus:

$$W = J/s = \frac{N \bullet m}{s} = \frac{Kg \frac{m}{s^2} \bullet m}{s} = \frac{Kg \bullet m^2}{s^3}$$

3.1.2 MASTERING GRAPHS

3.1.2.1 The Cartesian Coordinate System (CCS)

The MCAT candidate should understand graphs and the **cartesian coordinate system (CCS)**. In three dimensions, cartesian coordinates look like this:

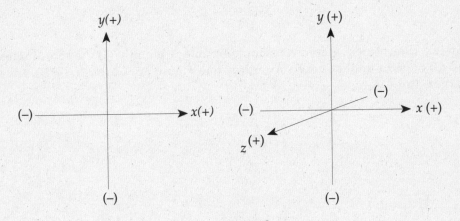

NOTE :
—Three perpendicular axes: x, y, and z.
—The arrow indicates the positive direction

Figure 3.1

The cartesian coordinate system allows for three dimensions, but MCAT graphs will almost always be two-dimensional, making use of the x- and y-axes only (not the z-axis). A plane defined by the x- and y- cartesian coordinates is called a **cartesian plane**.

3.1.2.2 CCS on the MCAT

The MCAT will usually present **straight-line graphs** as shown in Figure 3.2 (A) and (B), and **curvilinear graphs** as shown in Figure 3.2 (C).

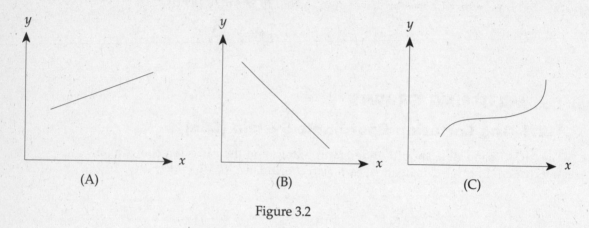

Figure 3.2

For any two-dimensional graph, you should be able to identify (1) the **coordinates**, (2) the **slope**, and (3) the **area under a curve**. As redrawn in Figure 3.3, Graphs (A), (B), and (C) highlight these three features.

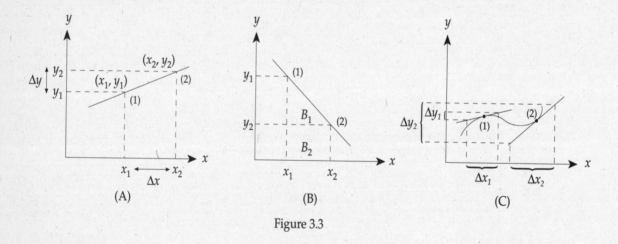

Figure 3.3

Coordinates

For any straight-line graph, coordinates describe a single point by identifying its location along each axis, vertical and horizontal. On Figure 3.3, Graph (A), point 1 has coordinates x_1 and y_1, meaning it is located x_1 units "along" the x-axis and y_1 units "up" the y-axis.

Slope

For any straight-line segment on a linear graph, slope is equal to $\dfrac{\Delta Y}{\Delta X}$. For points 1 and 2 on the line:

$$\Delta Y = Y_2 - Y_1$$

and

$$\Delta X = X_2 - X_1$$

(The quantity $\Delta Y = Y_2 - Y_1$ is called the Y component of the line segment between points 1 and 2, and $\Delta X = X_2 - X_1$ is the X component of the line segment between points 1 and 2.)

For a *straight-line* graph, the slope is equal at all positions and is found by reference to the values ΔY and ΔX for any two points. For Graph (A), Figure 3.3, the slope at all points is equal to the slope of the line segment: point 1 – point 2. For Graph (B), Figure 3.3, the slope at all points is equal to the slope of the line segment point 1 – point 2:

$$\frac{\Delta Y}{\Delta X} = \frac{Y_2 - Y_1}{X_2 - X_1}$$

The slope of Graph (B) is *negative*, since $Y_2 < Y_1$ and $X_1 < X_2$. Confirm that the slope is negative by noting that the line on Graph (B) runs downward to the right, which is characteristic of a negative slope. The line on Graph (A) runs upward to the right, which is characteristic of a positive slope.

Any equation of the form $y = mx + b$ will generate a straight-line graph with slope = m and y intercept = b. Therefore, the equation $y = 3x + 5$ generates a straight line with slope = 3 and y intercept = 5.

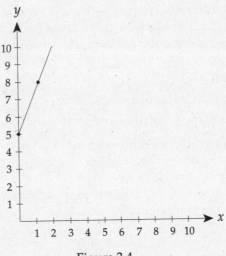

Figure 3.4

For a *curvilinear* graph, the slope at one point is *not* necessarily equal to the slope at any other point. For curvilinear graphs, therefore, the slope is equal to the slope of a line *tangent* to the curve at that point, measured by the value $\dfrac{\Delta Y}{\Delta X}$ for the tangent line.

On Graph (C), Figure 3.3, the slope at point 1 differs from the slope at point 2. As shown, the slope at point $1 = \dfrac{\Delta Y_1}{\Delta X_1}$. The slope at point $2 = \dfrac{\Delta Y_2}{\Delta X_2}$.

Because slope represents the ratio:

Y component : X component

it frequently represents quantities that are derived directly from the quantities depicted on the x and y axes. For example, if a graph plots time (x-axis) vs. displacement (y-axis), its slope is:

$$\frac{\Delta Y}{\Delta X} = \text{velocity}$$

If a graph plots time (x-axis) vs. velocity (y-axis), its slope is:

$$\frac{\Delta Y}{\Delta X} = \text{acceleration}$$

Area Under a Curve

The *area under* a given portion of a curve may be found by visualizing the area in terms of familiar geometric figures. In graph (B) of Figure 3.3, for example, the area under the curve between points 1 and 2 can be determined by partitioning the area into a triangle (B_1) and a rectangle (B_2). The area of the triangle ($\frac{1}{2}$ base × height) is added to the area of the rectangle (side × side) and this sum represents the total area.

Like the slope, the area under the curve may represent a quantity derived from values plotted on the x- and y-axes. If, for example, a graph should plot velocity (y-axis) vs. time (x-axis), the area under any segment of the curve represents displacement.

Please solve this problem:

- The slope of a curvilinear graph set forth on a cartesian plane is equal at any given point to:
    A. the slope of the graph at all other points.
    B. the area under the curvilinear graph, at that point.
    C. the slope of a line tangent to the curvilinear graph at that point.
    D. infinity.

Problem solved:

C is the correct answer. The question refers directly to section **3.1.2.2**, where it is explained that for a curvilinear graph, the slope at any point is equal to that of a hypothetical line tangent to the curve at that point.

3.1.3 REVIEW OF TRIGONOMETRY

3.1.3.1 Measuring Angles in Degrees and Radians

An angle (θ) may be described in degrees or in **radians**. A radian is the measure of a circle's radius as it is applied to the circle's circumference. That is, if a circle's radius is 2 cm, then one radian represents that portion of the circle corresponding to 2 cm of its circumference. Because the circumference of a circle = $2\pi r$, there are 2π radians in a circle. A radian is (a) that portion of the circle that corresponds in circumference to one radius, and also (b) the arc subtended by that portion of a circle. Therefore, you can say that the full 360° of a circle is equivalent to 2π radians. Since π = approx. 3.14, 360° = approx. 6.28 radians. Conversion between degrees and radians is a matter of simple proportion.

Remembering that 360° = 2π radians = 6.28 radians enables you to (1) express an angle in degrees if you know its value in radians, and (2) express an angle in radians if you know its value in degrees.

Please solve this problem:

- Express 267 degrees in radians.

Problem solved:

1. $267° \times$ _____ = _____ radians

2. $267° \times \dfrac{6.28 \text{ radians}}{360°}$ = _____ radians (*radians in the numerator!*)

3. $267° \times \dfrac{6.28 \text{ radians}}{360°}$ = 4.66 radians

3.1.3.2 Pythagorean Theorem

The **pythagorean theorem** describes the relationship among the three sides of any right triangle:

$$c^2 = a^2 + b^2$$

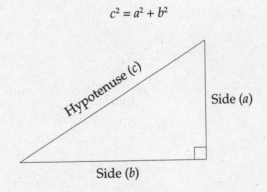

Side (b)

Figure 3.5

3.1.3.3 Trigonometric Functions

The three trigonometric functions **sine** (sin), **cosine** (cos), and **tangent** (tan) relate to the right triangle according to the mnemonic SOH CAH TOA.

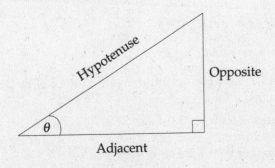

Figure 3.6

The three trigonometric functions relate graphically to the angles 90°, 180°, 270°, and 360°:

Sine

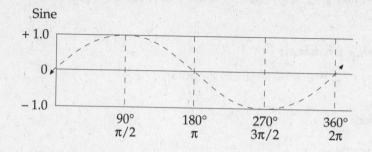

Cosine

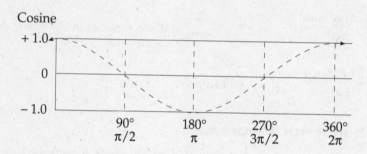

Tangent

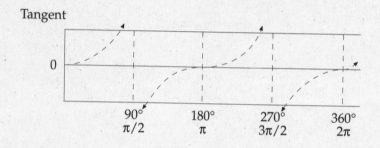

Figure 3.7

Be familiar with the terms **arcsin**, **arccos**, and **arctan**:

arcsin x means the angle whose sine = x

arccos x means the angle whose cosine = x

arctan x means the angle whose tangent = x

For example:

the sine of 30° = 0.5, so arcsin 0.5 = 30°

the tangent of 45° = 1, so arctan 1 = 45°

For any *small* angle (<15°) sine, cosine, and tangent may be *closely estimated* without reference to a table:

sin θ = θ (*expressed in radians!*)

tan θ = θ (*expressed in radians!*)

cos θ = 1

3.1.3.4 Three Right Triangles of Special Significance

Three right triangles have special importance for the MCAT and for trigonometry generally. They are:

1. The 30°, 60°, 90° right triangle. Its sides always bear the ratio:

$$a : 2a : a\sqrt{3}$$

- the 2 multiple represents the hypotenuse;

- the $\sqrt{3}$ multiple represents the side opposite the 60° angle;

- a represents the side opposite the 30° angle.

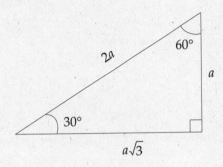

Figure 3.8

2. The 45°, 45°, 90° right triangle. Its sides always bear the ratio:

$$a : a : a\sqrt{2}$$

- the $\sqrt{2}$ multiple is associated with the hypotenuse;

- a is the length of each leg.

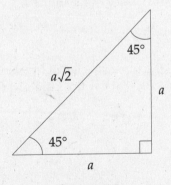

Figure 3.9

3. The right triangle with sides of 3:4:5. If in any right triangle the hypotenuse bears a ratio of 5:4 to any other side, then to the third side it bears the ratio 5:3. Similarly, if in any right triangle the hypotenuse bears a ratio of 5:3 to any other side, then to the third side it bears the ratio 5:4. If the legs of a right triangle bear a 3:4 ratio, then the hypotenuse will be 5.

Furthermore, the angle situated between the 3 and 5 sides is approximately 53° and the angle situated between the 5 and 4 sides is approximately 37°.

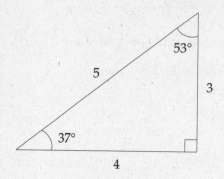

Figure 3.10

Of course, all three of these right triangles conform to the pythagorean theorem.

1. $1^2 + (\sqrt{3})^2 = 2^2$

2. $1^2 + 1^2 = (\sqrt{2})^2$

3. $3^2 + 4^2 = 5^2$

Familiarity with the ratios that apply to these three particular triangles will save you the time it would otherwise take to apply the pythagorean theorem.

Please solve this problem:

- A right triangle has sides 4 cm, 8 cm, and $\sqrt{48}$ cm. What are the values of its angles?

Problem solved:

The triangle conforms to one of the three special right triangles recently discussed. Notice immediately that two of the sides, 4 and 8, bear the ratio of 1:2:

$$4(1) = 4 \qquad 4(2) = 8$$

Therefore the other side is equal to $4\sqrt{3}$.

A triangle with sides in the ratio of $1:2:\sqrt{3}$ always has angles of 30°, 60°, and 90°.

Please solve this problem:

- A right triangle has an angle equal to 45° and a hypotenuse with length equal to $\sqrt{18}$ m. Find the lengths of the two remaining sides.

Problem solved:

Since all right triangles have one angle = 90° and this right triangle has one angle = 45°, the third angle must also = 45°, since $(180° - (90° + 45°)) = 45°$. Hence the problem involves a 45°, 45°, 90° right triangle. Its sides must bear the ratio $1:1:\sqrt{2}$, with the length of the hypotenuse being equal to $(a\sqrt{2})$, where a = the length of a side opposite one of the 45° angles.

Consider the number $\sqrt{18}$, and express it as $a\sqrt{2}$.

$$\sqrt{18} = a\sqrt{2}$$
$$a = \frac{\sqrt{18}}{\sqrt{2}}$$
$$a = \sqrt{9}$$
$$a = 3$$
$$\sqrt{18} = 3\sqrt{2}$$

In order for the triangle's sides to bear the ratio $1:1:\sqrt{2}$ the other two sides must be equal to $3(1) = 3$. The triangle's sides have lengths:

$$3 \text{ m, } 3 \text{ m, and } 3\sqrt{2} \text{ m.}$$

Please solve this problem:

- A right triangle has a hypotenuse with length of 36 cm and a leg with length of 21.6 cm. Find the length of the third side.

Problem solved:

Consider the two numbers 36 and 21.6. Do they reveal any of the ratios that pertain to the three special right triangles?

Examination reveals that:

$$(7.2)(5) = 36, \text{ and } (7.2)(3) = 21.6$$

The hypotenuse of 36 cm and side of 21.6 cm bear a ratio of 5:3. This must then be a 3:4:5 triangle, with each side multiplied by a coefficient of 7.2. The third side, therefore, must equal $(7.2)(4)$ cm = 28.8 cm.

Please solve this problem:

- A right triangle has two 45° angles. A side opposite one of them has a value of 13. What is the value of the hypotenuse?

Problem solved:

Among the three right triangles of special significance, one is the 45°, 45°, 90° right triangle for which the sides always bear the *ratio* $1:1:\sqrt{2}$. The two legs of a 45°, 45°, 90° right triangle are equal to each other and the hypotenuse is equal to (leg) $\times (\sqrt{2})$. Since we deal here with a right triangle of which one angle is 45°, it must be a 45°, 45°, 90° right triangle. The length of the legs is 13, and the length of the hypotenuse therefore is $13\sqrt{2}$.

CHAPTER 4

TRANSLATIONAL MOTION

4.1 MASTERY ACHIEVED

4.1.1 VECTORS

4.1.1.1 Scalar Quantities vs. Vector Quantities

A **scalar quantity** has magnitude but no direction. **Speed**, for example, is a scalar quantity. To state that an object travels at a speed of 450 m/s says nothing about the object's direction; it could be traveling north, south, east, west, or even along an irregular, non-linear path.

Distance is also a scalar quantity. To state that an object has traveled 300 meters gives no information about its ultimate position relative to its starting point. If the object starts at a point P, moves 150 meters to the west, and returns 150 meters to the east, then it has covered a *distance* of 300 meters, although it has come to rest at its starting point, P.

A **vector quantity** has magnitude *and* direction. It is symbolized by a line segment with an arrowed tip.

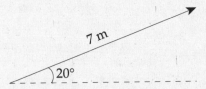

Length indicates magnitude, and orientation indicates direction. The figure above depicts a vector with a magnitude of 7 meters and a direction of 20° above the horizontal.

Velocity is a vector quantity. The designation "820 m/s to the left" describes a velocity; it has both magnitude and direction. The designation "820 m/s" does not. (It describes only speed, a scalar quantity). **Displacement** is another vector quantity. To state that an object has moved "760 cm to the north" is to describe the object's displacement. *Do not confuse distance and displacement.*

4.1.1.2 Vector Addition and Subtraction

When asked to *add* one vector to another:

1. Recognize that each vector may be freely "moved" about the page so long as its length and orientation are not disturbed.

2. Place the tail of either vector at the head of the other.

The line segment that runs from the free tail to the free head represents the vector sum, also known as the *resultant* vector.

Please solve this problem:

- Draw a vector, $\vec{C}$, that represents the sum of vectors $\vec{A}$ and $\vec{B}$ below.

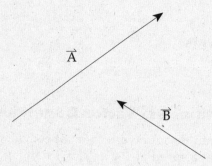

Problem solved:

Move the vectors so that the head of one touches the tail of the other (without changing either of their sizes, or orientations).

For example, you might proceed by placing the head of $\vec{B}$ at the tail of $\vec{A}$, like this:

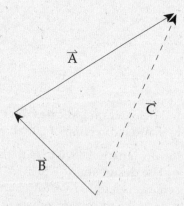

or by placing the head of $\vec{A}$ at the tail of $\vec{B}$, like this:

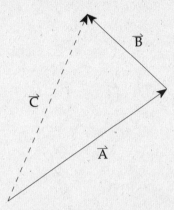

In either case, the resultant vector, $\vec{C}$, has the same magnitude and direction.

When adding vectors, be sure to place the head of one at the tail of the other. Do *not* place them tail to tail or head to head: The line segment that follows from that method does *not* constitute the resultant vector.

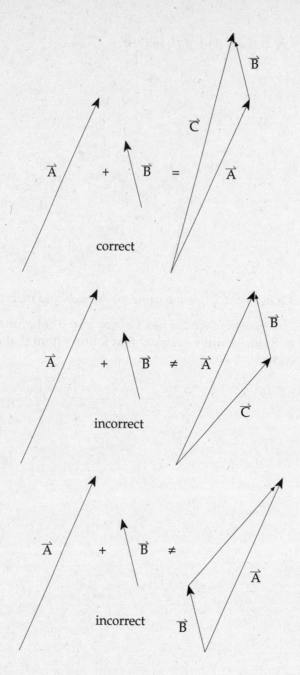

When asked to *subtract* one vector from another:

Add the *opposite* of one vector to the other vector.

$$\text{vector } \vec{A} - \text{vector } \vec{B} = \text{vector } \vec{A} + (-) \text{ vector } \vec{B}$$

To find the opposite (–) of a vector, keep its magnitude, but reverse its orientation by 180°. For example, $\vec{V}_1$ and $\vec{V}_2$ are vectors:

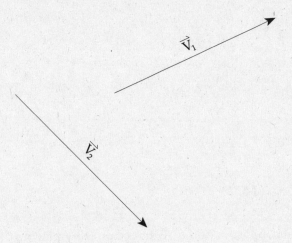

These are the vectors opposite to $\vec{V}_1$ and $\vec{V}_2$:

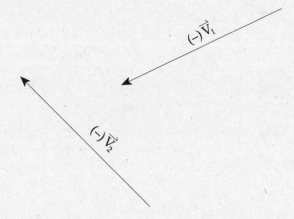

Please solve this problem:

- Draw a vector, $\vec{F}$, that represents $\vec{D}$ minus $\vec{E}$.

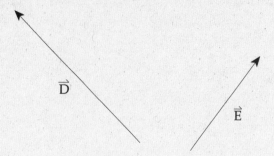

Problem Solved:

Convert vector $\vec{E}$ to its opposite. Add $(-)\vec{E}$ to vector $\vec{D}$ by placing the head of one at the tail of the other.

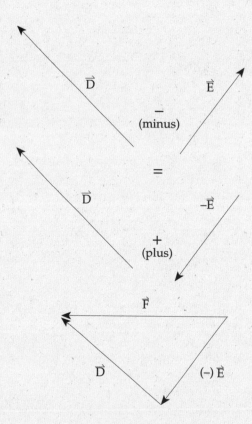

The diagram shows that the head of $(-)\vec{E}$ has been placed at the tail of $\vec{D}$. The line segment linking the tail of $(-)\vec{E}$ to the head of $\vec{D}$ represents the resultant vector, $\vec{F}$.

4.1.1.3 Component Vectors

On the MCAT, you may be asked to resolve a vector into its two **component vectors** and determine various parts of the system, such as the magnitude of the components, the angles between them, or the magnitude of the principal vector.

Given a principal vector $\vec{Z}$, the component vectors, $\vec{Z}_1$ and $\vec{Z}_2$, are vectors that:

- when added, using vector addition, result in the principal vector.

- are the legs of a right triangle, with a 90° angle between $\vec{Z}_1$ and $\vec{Z}_2$, and with the hypotenuse equal to the principal vector $\vec{Z}$.

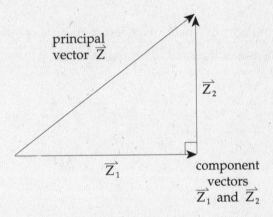

To resolve any principal vector $\vec{A}$ into its components, $\vec{A}_1$ and $\vec{A}_2$:

- Start by drawing the principal vector $\vec{A}$.

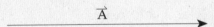

- Draw a right triangle with $\vec{A}$ as the hypotenuse and with a 90° angle between the two legs.

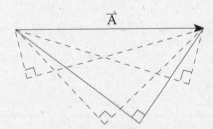

Notice that there are an infinite number of combinations of component vectors that can be drawn to these specifications. The two components that you choose to solve a given problem may either be specified by the problem itself or it may be left up to you to find the most convenient combination.

Find two component vectors, $\vec{A_1}$ and $\vec{A_2}$, such that

- the tail of component vector $\vec{A_1}$ meets the tail of principal vector $\vec{A}$, and the head of component vector $\vec{A_1}$ is at the 90° angle.

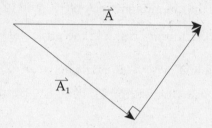

- the tail of component vector $\vec{A_2}$ meets the head of component vector $\vec{A_1}$, and the head of component vector $\vec{A_2}$ meets the head of principal vector $\vec{A}$.

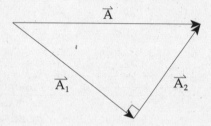

Having found two component vectors, we can now start to solve problems by setting up trigonometric relationships.

Please solve this problem:

- principal vector $\vec{A}$ = 10 meters,

    angle $\theta = 30°$

    $\cos \theta = 0.87$

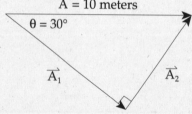

Find the magnitude of component vector $\vec{A_1}$.

Problem solved:

1. Recognizing the trigonometric relationship:

$$\cos 30° = \frac{[\vec{A}_1]}{[\vec{A}]}$$

where $[\vec{A}_1]$ is the magnitude of $\vec{A}_1$, and $[\vec{A}]$ is the magnitude of $\vec{A}$, we can rearrange the equation to read:

$$\vec{A}_1 = \vec{A} \cos 30°$$

2. Given the value of $\cos 30° = 0.87$, we set up the following:

$$\vec{A}_1 = (10 \text{ meters})(0.87)$$

3. Solving the equation, we see that $\vec{A}_1 = 8.7$ meters.

Please solve this problem:

- principal vector $\vec{A}$ = 10 meters

  angle θ = 30°

  $\sin \theta$ = 0.5

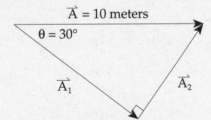

Find the magnitude of vector $\vec{A}_2$.

Problem solved:

1. Recognizing the trigonometric relationship:

$$\sin 30° = \frac{\vec{A}_2}{\vec{A}}$$

we can rearrange the equation to read:

$$\vec{A}_2 = \vec{A} \sin 30°$$

2. Given the value of $\sin 30° = 0.5$, we set up the following:

$$\vec{A}_2 = (10 \text{ meters})(0.5)$$

3. Solving the equation, we see that $\vec{A}_2 = 5$ meters.

Please solve this problem:

- principal vector $\vec{A}$ = 40 meters

  component vector $\vec{A_2}$ = 20 meters

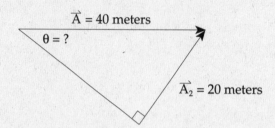

$\vec{A}$ = 40 meters

$\theta = ?$

$\vec{A_2}$ = 20 meters

Find the angle between the principal vector $\vec{A}$ and component vector $\vec{A_1}$.

Problem solved:

1. Recognizing the trigonometric relationship:

$$\sin\theta = \frac{\vec{A_2}}{\vec{A}}$$

we can find θ using the following formula:

$$\theta = \sin^{-1}\frac{\vec{A_2}}{\vec{A}}$$

2. Substituting into the equation,

$$\theta = \sin^{-1}\left(\frac{20}{40}\right)$$
$$\theta = \sin^{-1}(0.5)$$

3. Solving the equation, $\theta = 30°$.

4.1.1.4 Vectors on the Cartesian Coordinate System

A vector can easely be studied on a cartesian plane. Consider vector $\vec{A}$ in Figure 4.1.

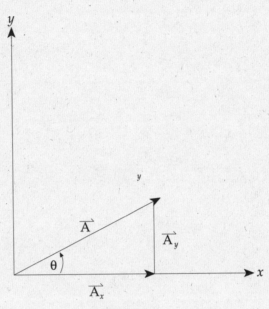

Figure 4.1

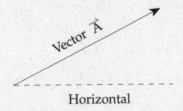

Horizontal

The *lengths* of $\vec{A}_x$ and $\vec{A}_y$ represent the coordinates of vector $\vec{A}$ on the x and y axes. The angle between the x axis and vector $\vec{A}$ (measured counterclockwise) is represented by θ. The following points should be noted:

1. $\vec{A}_x$ and $\vec{A}_y$ may themselves be viewed as component vectors of $\vec{A}$, because when they are added, the resultant vector is $\vec{A}$.

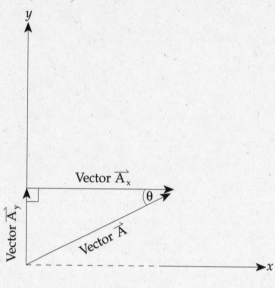

Figure 4.2

Figure 4.2 shows that the magnitude of vector $\vec{A}$ may be calculated via the pythagorean theorem when the magnitudes of $\vec{A}_x$ and $\vec{A}_y$ are known:

$$[\vec{A}]^2 = [\vec{A}_x]^2 + [\vec{A}_y]^2$$

2. If θ is known, the magnitude of vector $\vec{A}$ can be determined by simple trigonometry:

$$\cos\theta = \frac{[\vec{A}_x]}{[\vec{A}]} \qquad [\vec{A}] = \frac{[\vec{A}_x]}{\cos\theta}$$

$$\sin\theta = \frac{[\vec{A}_y]}{[\vec{A}]} \qquad [\vec{A}] = \frac{[\vec{A}_y]}{\sin\theta}$$

3. Strategic visualization of a line segment parallel and equal to $\vec{A}_y$ demonstrates that:

$$\tan\theta = \frac{[\vec{A}_y]}{[\vec{A}_x]}$$

$$\theta = \arctan\frac{[\vec{A}_y]}{[\vec{A}_x]}$$

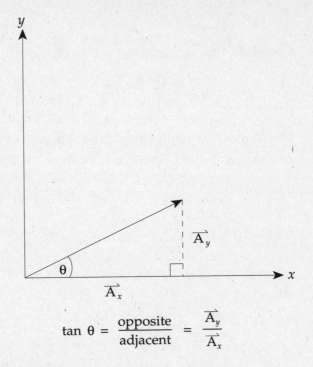

$$\tan \theta = \frac{\text{opposite}}{\text{adjacent}} = \frac{\vec{A}_y}{\vec{A}_x}$$

Please solve this problem:

- Determine the length and direction of vector $\vec{B}$ shown below.

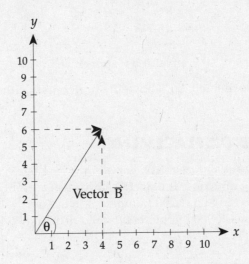

Vector $\vec{B}$

Problem solved:

1. Identify the magnitudes of $\vec{B}_x$ and $\vec{B}_y$:

$$[\vec{B}_x] = 4$$

$$[\vec{B}_y] = 6$$

With $\vec{B}_x$ and $\vec{B}_y$ now known, you may apply one of several procedures to identify the magnitude and direction of vector $\vec{B}$.

2. Determine the magnitude of $\vec{B}$:

$$[\vec{B}] = \sqrt{[\vec{B}_x]^2 + [\vec{B}_y]^2} = \sqrt{52} = \text{approx. } 7.21$$

3. Identify θ:

$$\cos\theta = \frac{[\vec{B}_x]}{[\vec{B}]} = \frac{4}{7.21} = 0.55$$

$$\theta = \arccos 0.55 = \text{approx. } 56°$$

or

$$\tan\theta = \frac{[\vec{B}_y]}{[\vec{B}]} = \frac{6}{4} = 1.5$$

$$\theta = \arctan 1.5 = \text{approx. } 56°$$

Vector $\vec{B}$ is directed approximately 56° above the horizontal, with a magnitude of approximately 7.21.

4.1.2 DISTANCE AND DISPLACEMENT

As we've said, distance is a scalar quantity. For any moving body, distance expresses the length of travel, regardless of direction. If object O starting at a point, P, moves 500 kilometers to the west, 700 kilometers to the east, 1,200 kilometers to the north, 1,500 kilometers to the south, 100 kilometers to the west, 300 kilometers to the north and 75 kilometers to the west, it moves a distance of:

$$500 \text{ km} + 700 \text{ km} + 1,200 \text{ km} + 1,500 \text{ km} + 100 \text{ km} + 300 \text{ km} + 75 \text{ km} = 4,375 \text{ km}$$

Displacement is a vector quantity. For any moving body, displacement describes *net* change in position, regardless of distance and regardless of path. Consider the displacement of object O, as described above:

$$\text{northward movement: } 1,200 \text{ km} + 300 \text{ km} = 1,500 \text{ km}$$

$$\text{southward movement: } 1,500 \text{ km}$$

Net movement in the north/south direction: 1,500 km – 1,500 km = 0

eastward movement: 700 km

westward movement: 500 km + 100 km + 75 km = 675 km

Net movement in the east/west direction: 25 km to the east

Object O followed a path a distance of 4,375 km. Its path and distance, however, are not reflected in its displacement. For object O, displacement equals 25 km to the east.

Please solve this problem:

- Which of the following statements correctly describes the motion of a body that travels a total *displacement* of 400 meters North?

  A. From its starting point, the body travels 200 meters due east and then 600 meters due west.

  B. From its starting point, the body travels 600 meters due west and then 200 meters due east.

  C. From its starting point, the body travels 200 meters due east and then 200 meters due west.

  D. From its starting point, the body travels 100 meters due east, 100 meters due west and 400 meters due north.

Problem solved:

D is the correct answer. The question requires that you understand displacement as a vector quantity. A vector takes into account the direction or the net distance between starting point and final resting point. The body described by D moves 100 meters east and then returns to its starting point by moving 100 meters west. It then moves 400 meters north to its final position. This is 400 meters north of its initial position and thus its displacement is 400 meters north.

4.1.3 SPEED AND VELOCITY

4.1.3.1 Speed

For any body moving at a constant speed, speed is equal to distance traveled/time elapsed.

$$Speed = d/t$$

If a body is not moving at a constant speed then its average speed between any two points will still be equal to distance traveled divided by time elapsed, but its instantaneous speed at any given instant will vary.

Because distance is a scalar and does not specify direction and because speed is derived using distance, speed is also a scalar.

When distance is plotted as a function of time on a Cartesian plane, the instantaneous speed at any point on the resulting curve is equal to the slope of the line tangent to that curve at that point.

4.1.3.2 Velocity

For any moving body **velocity** represents at any instant,

$$\frac{\text{displacement}}{\text{time}}$$

"Displacement" refers to instantaneous change in displacement, and is represented by ΔD. "Time" refers to an instantaneous change in time, Δt, so that in mathematical symbols:

$$\text{velocity} = \frac{\Delta D}{\Delta t}$$

Because displacement is expressed in units of length, velocity is expressed in units of $\frac{\text{length}}{\text{time}}$, creating the SI unit $\frac{\text{meter}}{\text{second}}$ (m/s), the same unit that expresses speed. However, because the numerator, D, represents displacement, a vector quantity, $\frac{\Delta D}{\Delta t}$ has direction, and *velocity is a vector quantity*.

Velocity can be represented on the cartesian plane in a manner that's very similar to that of speed. When displacement is plotted as a function of time, the velocity at any point on the resulting curve is equal to the slope at that point. If the point sits on a linear portion of the plot, velocity is equal to the slope of the line segment. If the point sits on a curvilinear portion of the plot, velocity is equal to the slope of a line segment *tangent* to the point.

Average velocity is analogous to average speed. It refers to the relationship $\frac{\text{displacement}}{\text{time}}$ over a prolonged period of time. If an object moves for a period of 1,200 seconds, during which it experiences displacement of 700 meters to the west, its average velocity is

$$\frac{700 \text{ m}}{1,200 \text{ s}} = 0.58 \text{ m/s, to the west}$$

4.1.3.3 Relative Velocity

For any moving object, **relative velocity** refers to a velocity of one object that's calculated with respect to some *other* object. If two objects, A and B, are in motion, and each has a velocity relative to the earth of v_a and v_b respectively, then the velocity of A relative to the velocity of B is simply the difference:

$$v_a - v_b$$

If object A has a velocity of 80 m/s east and object B has a velocity of 30 m/s east, the velocity of object A relative to that of object B is:

$$80 \text{ m/s} - 30 \text{ m/s} = 50 \text{ m/s}$$

$$v_a - v_b$$

Recall that a vector difference $v_a - v_b$ is equal to the vector sum: $v_a + (-)v_b$ (**4.1.1.2**).

Please solve this problem:

- As an automobile travels due west at 50 mi/hr, a bird flies over it at a velocity of 10 mi/hr in a direction 25° west of north. Draw a vector diagram that depicts the velocity of the automobile relative to that of the bird at the moment the bird is directly over the automobile (ignore the difference in height).

Problem solved:

The velocity v_a of the automobile relative to v_b, the velocity of the bird, is the difference between the vectors:

$$v_a - v_b = v_a + (-)v_b$$

As shown below, v_b is inverted by 180° to obtain $(-)v_b$. Vector v_a is then added to $(-)v_b$ by positioning the tail of $(-)v_b$ at the head of v_a. The line segment that joins the tail of v_a and the head of $(-)v_b$ gives the resultant vector $v_a - v_b$, which represents the velocity of the automobile relative to that of the bird.

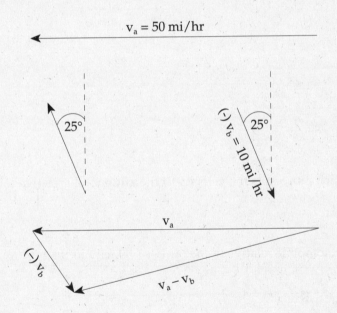

    With reference to relative velocity, the diagram drawn above depicts the following phenomena:

    If an object A is in motion relative to object B, and object B is in motion relative to object C, then the velocity of A relative to C is equal to the sum:

$$V_{ac} = V_{ab} + V_{bc}$$

where:

$$V_{ac} = \text{the velocity of A relative to C}$$
$$V_{ab} = \text{the velocity of A relative to B}$$
$$V_{bc} = \text{the velocity of B relative to C}$$

Refer to the previous problem (concerning the automobile and bird) and let:

        object A = the automobile
        object B = the bird
        object C = the earth

Relabeling the diagram to apply these designations, V_{ac}, V_{ab}, and V_{bc}, we draw:

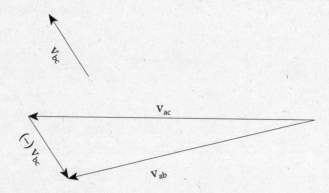

    Note that V_{ac}, which represents the velocity of the automobile relative to the earth, is equal to the sum:

$$V_{ac} = V_{ab} + V_{bc} =$$

(velocity of the automobile relative to the bird) + (velocity of the bird relative to the earth)

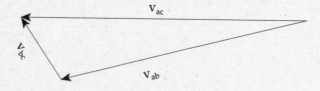

Please solve this problem:

- Two children are playing catch aboard a train that moves due south at 35 m/s. At a certain moment the ball is moving *relative to the train*, in a direction 30° to the east of south with magnitude of 7 m/s. Depict the velocity of the ball relative to the ground with a vector diagram bearing these labels:

V_{bg} = the velocity of the ball relative to the ground

V_{bt} = the velocity of the ball relative to the train

V_{tg} = the velocity of the train relative to the ground

Problem Solved:

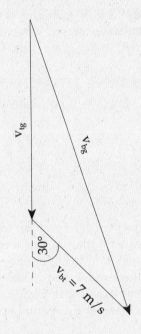

4.1.4 ACCELERATION

For any moving body, **acceleration** represents

$$\frac{\text{change in velocity}}{\text{time}}$$

Change in velocity is represented conceptually by the notion (final velocity – initial velocity), or $(v_f - v_i)$, expressed generally as Δv. "Time" is expressed as Δt.

This can be written:

$$\text{acceleration} = \left(\frac{\Delta v}{\Delta t}\right)$$

Because velocity v is a vector quantity, $\frac{\Delta v}{\Delta t}$ has direction; *acceleration is a vector quantity.*

4.1.4.1 Units of Acceleration

Acceleration represents *the rate at which velocity changes*. If, at a given time, an object's velocity has magnitude of 10 m/s and 1 second later it has magnitude of 17 m/s, then the object has increased its velocity by 7 m/s *in* 1 second. It has accelerated at 7 meters per second per second. Since velocity itself is expressed in units of $\dfrac{length}{time}$, and acceleration represents $\dfrac{\Delta \, velocity}{\Delta \, time}$, acceleration is measured in units of:

$$\frac{\dfrac{length}{time}}{time}$$

The SI unit for acceleration is "meters per second per second," or m/s/s.

If, at second 1, the velocity of object X is 30 m/s and at second 2 it has a velocity of 80 m/s in the same direction, then the object has increased its velocity by 50 m/s in 1 second, in that direction. This means it has accelerated in the same direction at a rate of:

$$50 \text{ meters per second per second} = 50 \text{ m/s/s}$$

Simple algebra demonstrates that 1 m/s/s is equivalent to:

$$m/s/s = \frac{m}{s} \div s = \left(\frac{m}{s}\right)\left(\frac{1}{s}\right) = \frac{m}{s^2}$$

The preferred SI unit for acceleration is m/s^2, which is *stated* "meters per second squared," and *means* "meters per second per second."

Acceleration may be negative (–) or positive (+). If an object's velocity increases with time, its acceleration is positive. If it decreases with time, its acceleration is negative. (An object with negative acceleration is sometimes said to experience *de*celeration.) If at second 0 the velocity of object Z is 120 m/s and at second 4 it has a velocity of 40 m/s in the same direction, then the object has *de*creased its velocity by 80 m/s in 4 seconds, in that direction. This means that it has accelerated in that same direction at a rate of (–)20 meters per second, per second (–20 m/s²).

4.1.4.2 Acceleration on the Cartesian Coordinate System

4.1.4.2.1 VELOCITY VS. TIME

Figure 4.5 depicts the motion of an object, Q, on a cartesian plane. The x-axis represents time and the y-axis represents velocity. Points E, F, and G are arbitrarily chosen as positions at which acceleration will be evaluated.

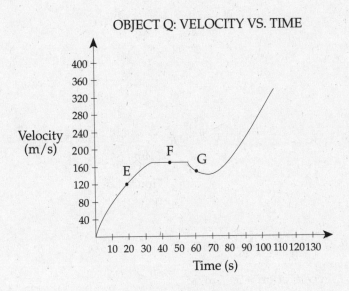

Figure 4.5

Examine the graph. The segment containing point E shows the object Q's velocity increasing with time; it has positive acceleration. The portion containing point F shows the velocity remaining constant at 160 m/s for 30 seconds. The section containing point G shows the object's velocity decreasing; the object is experiencing negative acceleration (which is followed by positive acceleration).

The graph of velocity vs. time demonstrates that acceleration at any point is equal to the *slope* at that point.

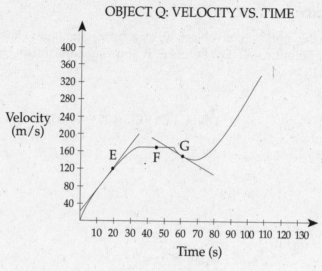

Figure 4.6

At point E, slope = $\dfrac{200-30}{30} = \dfrac{170}{30} = 5.67$

Hence, at point E, acceleration = 5.67 m/s²

At point F, slope = 0, and acceleration = 0 m/s²

At point G, slope = $\dfrac{120-200}{80-40} = \dfrac{-80}{40} = -2$

Hence, at point G, acceleration = –2 m/s²

Remember, object Q is in motion at point F. Because the y-axis represents velocity and not displacement, a slope of zero does not describe an object without velocity. It describes an object for which velocity does not change.

Please solve this problem:

- The motion of an object is depicted on a cartesian plane where the y-axis represents velocity and the x-axis represents time. At the portion of the graph between time = 9 seconds and time = 13 seconds, the graph is linear with a slope of –2. Which of the following represents a proper conclusion regarding the body's motion at time = 11 seconds?

  A. The body is stationary.
  B. The body is experiencing positive acceleration.
  C. The body is experiencing negative acceleration.
  D. The body's acceleration is decreasing.

Problem solved:

C is the correct answer. The question requires that you understand the relationship between velocity and acceleration as shown on a cartesian plane. At any point on a graph, the slope $\left(\dfrac{\Delta Y}{\Delta X}\right)$ represents the rate at which values on the *y*-axis change in relation to those on the *x*-axis; in this example, velocity vs. time. If, for any body, velocity changes over the course of time then during that period of time, then the body experiences acceleration—positive if the velocity increases, and negative if the velocity decreases.

We are told that between time = 9 seconds and time = 13 seconds the graph is linear with a slope of –2. Velocity is decreasing over this entire period at a constant rate of –2. We are not told that the cartesian plane describes the body's motion in SI units (m/s^2), so we cannot know what units have been used to express length and time.

A decrease in velocity over time represents a negative acceleration, which is why choice C is correct. Choice D is *not* correct because it refers to a *change in acceleration*. For a graph that plots *velocity vs. time*, the slope does not depict change in acceleration, but change in velocity. If, on the other hand, a graph plots *acceleration vs. time*, its slope represents change in acceleration. In such a case, a slope of zero does not mean that the body has constant velocity. Rather, it means that the body has constant acceleration—it accelerates at a uniform rate. You should make sure that this subtle difference is clear to you.

4.1.4.2.2 ACCELERATION VS. TIME

If acceleration is plotted as a function of time, the slope at any point on the resulting curve corresponds to **change in acceleration**. Some MCAT questions will require that you understand the difference between a change in velocity and a change in acceleration.

Figure 4.7 depicts the motion of object T on a cartesian plane with acceleration expressed as a function of time. The *x*-axis represents time and the *y*-axis represents acceleration. The points H, I, J, and K were arbitrarily chosen.

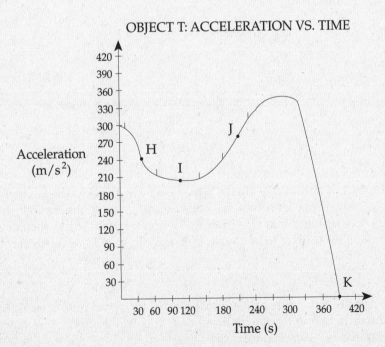

Figure 4.7

The segment containing point H shows object T's acceleration decreasing over time. This *decreasing* acceleration *does not* signify *negative* acceleration; it does not imply reduced *velocity*. During the time between 0 s to 90 s object T's *acceleration* decreases from 300 m/s² to 210 m/s². Yet, at second 90, the object does experience positive acceleration; its velocity is increasing at a rate of 210 m/s².

The segment containing point I shows that object T's acceleration remains constant at 210 m/s² for approximately 60 seconds (90 s to 150 s). During that period, its velocity continues to increase by 210 m/s every second. The segment that contains point J shows that acceleration begins to increase once again, from 240 m/s² to 300 m/s² over a period of 60 seconds (180 s to 240 s).

At point K object T's acceleration falls to zero. That does not mean, however, that *motion* stops. Acceleration of zero means only that *velocity* does not change. At point K, object T experiences constant velocity.

4.1.5 UNIFORMLY ACCELERATED MOTION ALONG A STRAIGHT LINE

If an object moves with constant acceleration, it is said to be in *uniformly accelerated motion*. If such an object moves continuously *in a straight line*, it is said to be in *uniformly accelerated motion along a straight line*.

Examine Figure 4.8, the graph of object Q, plotting *velocity vs. time*.

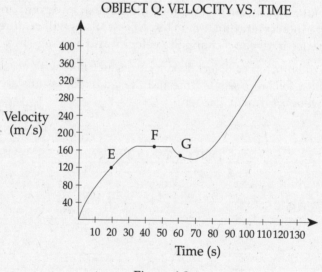

Figure 4.8

At 80 seconds, the curve becomes linear, moving upward and to the right. The straight line means that object Q's velocity increases at a constant rate, which means that the magnitude of its acceleration is constant and that Q is in uniform acceleration. If the object's *direction* is known (from some other source) to be linear, then the object is in uniform acceleration along a straight line.

Therefore:

For any object depicted on a cartesian plane that plots velocity vs. time, a straight line segment indicates uniform acceleration. If the object's direction is known to be linear, then the object is in uniform acceleration *along a straight line*.

Examine Figure 4.9, the graph of object T, plotting acceleration vs. time.

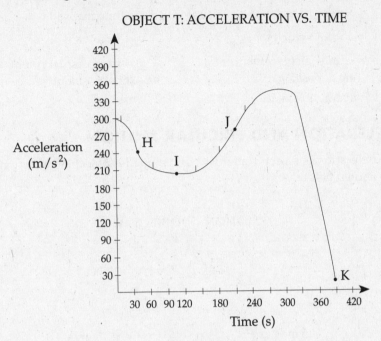

OBJECT T: ACCELERATION VS. TIME

Figure 4.9

At 90 seconds, the curve becomes *horizontal*. The horizontal line means that the magnitude of object T's acceleration is constant. Again, if the object's *direction* is known to be linear, then the object is in uniform acceleration along a straight line.

Therefore:

For any object depicted on a cartesian plane that plots acceleration vs. time, *a horizontal line segment *indicates* uniform acceleration. If the object's direction is known to be linear, it indicates uniform acceleration along a straight line.*

4.1.5.1 Uniformly Accelerated Motion along a Straight Line: Equations

For any object moving in uniform accelerated motion along a straight line, the following equations apply:

$$v_f = v_o + at$$

$$d_f = d_o + v_o t + \frac{1}{2}at^2$$

$$v_f^2 = v_o^2 + 2a(d_f - d_o)$$

$$v = \frac{v_f + v_o}{2}$$

Where:

a = acceleration

v_o = initial velocity

d_o = initial displacement
(initial position)

v = average velocity

t = time elapsed

v_f = final velocity

d_f = final displacement
(final position)

4.1.6 ACCELERATION AND CIRCULAR MOTION

Recall that acceleration is a vector quantity, and consider object W, which moves in a circular path as shown below.

MOTION OF OBJECT W

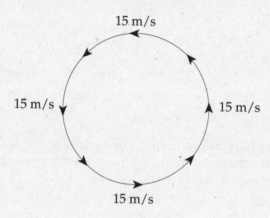

Figure 4.10

An object that travels at a constant velocity in a straight line experiences no acceleration. Object W moves circularly at a constant rate of 15 m/s. The velocity's magnitude is constant, but its direction is not. At every instant, direction is subjected to a change that produces the circular motion. If a body's velocity undergoes change in magnitude, direction, or both it experiences acceleration. Therefore, *the continuous change in W's direction signifies acceleration.*

The maintenance of circular motion requires an acceleration with constant magnitude directed toward the center of the circle. Such acceleration is termed **centripetal acceleration**. The circular motion that results is shown in Figure 4.11.

MOTION OF OBJECT W

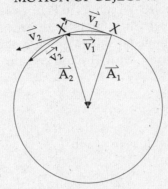

Figure 4.11

On Figure 4.11, imagine point X' moving closer to point X: The secant $\overline{XX'}$ becomes smaller. If we continue this process around the entire circle, the number of sides of the inscribed polygon will tend towards ∞ and a circular path will result.

If, at points X or X', centripetal acceleration were suddenly to cease, object W would move off in a straight line tangent to its original circular path.

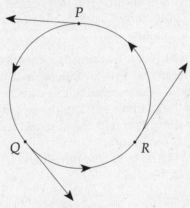

Figure 4.12

The magnitude of centripetal acceleration $= \dfrac{v^2}{r}$ where $v =$ the magnitude of velocity and $r =$ radius of the circle. For circular motion at constant speed, therefore, the following phenomena apply:

- At all moments, the object's velocity vector is tangent to the circular path

- Centripetal acceleration $(a_c) = \dfrac{v^2}{r}$

- $v = \dfrac{d}{t} = \dfrac{2\pi r}{T}$; $T = \dfrac{2\pi r}{v}$

Where:

$v =$ magnitude of velocity

$T =$ period = time required for one complete revolution

Please solve this problem:

- Assume that object W, shown in Figures 4.10, 4.11, and 4.12, travels in a circle with radius of 40 meters. Determine (a) the magnitude of centripetal acceleration, and (b) the period of W's motion.

Problem solved:

You are asked to determine the values of a_c and T. As shown above:

$$a_c = \frac{v^2}{r} = \frac{225 \text{ m}^2\text{s}^2}{40 \text{ m}} = 5.625 \text{ m/s}^2$$

$$T = \frac{2\pi r}{v} = \frac{2(3.14)40 \text{ m}}{15 \text{ m/s}} = 16.75 \text{ s}$$

Please answer this question:

- If a planet revolves about a sun in a perfect circle, which of the following describes the direction of the planet's acceleration?

  A. A tangential vector running in a direction parallel to the planet's instantaneous path.
  B. A tangential vector running in a direction opposite to the planet's instantaneous path.
  C. A vector with its tail at the sun and its head pointing at the planet.
  D. A vector with its tail at the planet and its head pointing at the sun.

Question answered:

D is the correct answer. The question requires that you understand centripetal acceleration. As a body moves in a circular path it experiences an acceleration *toward the center of the circle*; this acceleration is called centripetal acceleration. In the case of a planet moving in a circular path about a sun, the planet's centripetal acceleration is described by a vector running *from* the planet *toward* the sun.

Choice A is not correct, but the vector that is tangent and parallel to the planet's path does have significance: If a body in circular motion is *deprived* of the centripetal acceleration that maintains its motion (if, for example, a planet's sun should disappear), the body will move off at constant velocity in a direction tangential to its path at that instant.

Please answer this question:

- If a satellite's orbit around a planet has a diameter of 800 kilometers and a circular velocity of 900 m/s, what is the approximate value in *meters per second squared* of the centripetal acceleration that maintains the satellite's orbit?

  A. 1.0 m/s²
  B. 2.0 m/s²
  C. 3.0 m/s²
  D. 4.0 m/s²

Question answered:

B is the correct answer. Begin by recognizing that you will need the equation that expresses centripetal acceleration in terms of velocity and radius: $(a_c) = v^2/r$. The diameter of the satellite's orbit is 800 km; its radius is 400km. Apply the equation:

$$(a_c) = \frac{V^2}{r}$$

$$(a_c) = \frac{(900 \text{ m/s})^2}{400,000 \text{ m}} = \frac{810,000 \text{ m}^2/\text{s}^2}{400,000 \text{ m}} = 2.025 \text{ m/s}^2$$

4.1.7 FREE FALL MOTION

Free fall motion describes an object falling from some height, h, to the ground. It is a form of uniformly accelerated motion along a straight line. The acceleration results from the Earth's gravitational field. This acceleration is a constant for all objects near the surface of the Earth: $g = 9.81$ m/s² (often approximated as 10 m/s²). When MCAT questions address free fall motion they will usually instruct you to disregard rotation of the earth, air resistance, and differences in the magnitude of gravity exerted at different heights from the earth.

The acceleration due to gravity is positive (+) or negative (–) depending on perspective. One direction should be chosen as positive and the other negative for all vectors, and that convention should be maintained throughout the problem.

Please solve this problem:

- If an object is dropped from a height of 80 m above the earth, (a) how long does it take to reach the earth, and (b) what is the object's velocity at the instant prior to impact with the earth?

Problem solved:

Examine section **4.1.5.1** and select an equation that allows us to express the unknown values in terms of the known values. Time and final velocity are unknown. Final distance (80 m), initial velocity (zero), and acceleration (approx 10 m/s²) are known.

Part (a) calls for equation 2:

$$d_f = d_o + v_o t + \frac{1}{2}at^2$$

Substituting 80 m for d_f, 0 for d_o, 0 for v_o, and 10 m/s² for a:

$$80 \ m = 0 + 0(t) + \left(\frac{1}{2}\right)\left(10 \ m/s^2\right)\left(t^2\right)$$

$$80 \ m = \left(5 \ m/s^2\right)t^2 \qquad t^2 = \frac{80 \ m}{5 \ m/s^2}$$

$$t^2 = \left(\frac{80 \ m}{1}\right)\frac{s^2}{5 \ m} \qquad t^2 = \frac{80 \ ms^2}{5 \ m}$$

$$t^2 = 16 \ s^2 \qquad t = 4 \ s$$

Part (b) calls for equation 1:

$$v_f = v_o + at$$

Substitute 0 for V_o, 10 m/s² for a, and 4 s for t:

$$v_f = v_o + at$$

$$v_f = 0 + 0 + (10 \ m/s^2)(4s) \qquad v_f = \left(\frac{10m}{s^2}\right)\frac{4s}{1}$$

$$v_f = \frac{40 \ ms}{s^2} \qquad v_f = 40 \ m/s$$

Please solve this problem:

- If an object is launched directly upward from the earth with an initial velocity of 120 m/s, (a) how long will it take to come to rest in mid-air, (b) at what height will it do so, (c) how many seconds after coming to rest in mid-air will it reach the earth again, and (d) with what velocity will it strike the earth?

Problem solved:

The upward trip involves an initial velocity of 120 m/s, a negative acceleration of 10 m/s^2, and a final velocity of 0 m/s.

Part (a) calls for equation 1:

$$v_f = v_o + at$$

Substituting 0 m/s for v_f, 120 m/s for v_0, and –10 m/s^2 for a:

$$0 \text{ m/s} = 120 \text{ m/s} + [(-)10 \text{ m/s}^2 (t)] \qquad -120 \text{ m/s} = (-)10 \text{ m/s}^2 (t)$$

$$t = \frac{120 \text{ m/s}}{10 \text{ m/s}^2} \qquad t = (120 \text{ m/s})\frac{s^2}{10 \text{ m}}$$

$$t = \frac{120 \text{ ms}^2}{10 \text{ ms}} \qquad t = 12 \text{ s}$$

Part (b) calls for equation 2:

$$d_f = d_o + v_o t + \frac{1}{2}at^2$$

Substituting 0 for d_o, 120 m/s for v_o, –10 m/s^2 for a, and 12s for t:

$$d_f = 0 + 120 \text{ m/s}(12 \text{ s}) + \frac{1}{2}(-10 \text{ m/s}^2)(144 \text{ s}^2)$$

$$d_f = 1{,}440 \text{ ms/s} - (5 \text{ m/s}^2)(144 \text{ s}^2)$$

$$d_f = 1{,}440 \text{ ms/s} - (720 \text{ ms}^2/\text{s}^2)$$

$$d_f = 1{,}440 \text{ m} - 720 \text{ m} \qquad d_f = 720 \text{ m}$$

Parts (c) and (d) resemble the *previous* problem. In essence they concern an object that falls freely from a height of 720 m.

Part (c) calls for equation 2:

$$d_f = d_o + v_o t + \frac{1}{2}at^2$$

Substituting –720 m for d_f, 0 for d_o, 0 for v_o, and –10 m/s^2 for a:

$$-720 \text{ m} = 0 + 0(t) + \left(\frac{1}{2}\right)(-10 \text{ m/s}^2)(t)^2$$

$$-720 \text{ m} = (-5 \text{ m/s}^2)t^2 \qquad t^2 = \frac{-720 \text{ m}}{-5 \text{ m/s}^2}$$

$$t^2 = \frac{720 \text{ ms}^2}{5 \text{ m}}$$

$$t^2 = 144 \text{ s}^2 \qquad t = \sqrt{144} \text{ s} = 12 \text{ s}$$

Part (d) calls for equation 1:

Substituting 0 for v_o, -10 m/s^2 for a, and 12 s for t:

$$v_f = v_o + at$$

$$v_f = 0 + (-10 \text{ m/s}^2)(12 \text{ s}) \qquad v_f = (-10 \text{ m/s}^2)\left(\frac{12}{1}\right)$$

$$v_f = -120 \text{ ms/s}^2 \qquad v_f = -120 \text{ m/s}$$

Please solve this problem:

- A body falls freely from a stationary position above the earth. Assume that g = acceleration due to gravity, t = elapsed time, h = height, and m = mass. Which of the following expressions describes the body's velocity the moment before it strikes the earth?

  A. $(g)(t)$

  B. $\frac{1}{2}(gt^2)$

  C. $(h)(t)$

  D. $\frac{1}{2}(mt^2) + mt$

Problem solved:

A is the correct answer. The question requires that you understand free fall motion in relation to the parameters of time, distance, and acceleration. Free fall is a special case of uniformly accelerated motion along a straight line. The acceleration derives from gravity and is approximately 10 m/s^2. (*All* bodies near the surface of the earth are accelerated downward at the same rate: 9.8 m/s^2; mass is irrelevant to the calculation.) For any body in any uniform accelerated motion along a straight line:

final velocity = initial velocity + (acceleration)(time)

$$v_f = v_o + at$$

Since the body started at rest, $v_o = 0$ and $v_f = at$. Acceleration in this case is equal to g and final velocity = gt.

4.1.8 MASTERING PROJECTILE MOTION

4.1.8.1 The Concepts

Projectile motion generally refers to an object launched from the earth with a velocity that has both horizontal and vertical components. The resultant velocity then takes a path like that of a kicked football (which serves as the classic illustration of the projectile):

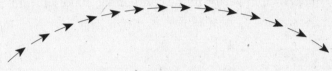

Figure 4.13

MCAT questions usually address idealized projectile motion and will instruct you to ignore the effects of friction and air resistance. You should learn to analyze projectile motion in idealized terms:

1. Initial velocities:

A projectile is launched with an **initial velocity**, which is represented by a vector, with **horizontal and vertical components**. Simple vector analysis allows us to solve problems concerning the status of a projectile at the time it is launched. If we are provided with (a) the angle at which it is launched and (b) the magnitude of its initial horizontal *or* vertical velocity—we do not need both—we can calculate its true observed velocity. If we *are* provided with the initial magnitudes of both the vertical and horizontal velocities, then we can calculate true, observed initial velocity without knowing the angle of launch.

Please solve this problem:

- A projectile is launched at an angle of 35° from the horizontal. The vertical component of initial velocity has a magnitude of 4 meters per second. What is the initial magnitude of the projectile's true observed velocity? (*Note*: cos 55° = approx. 0.57)

Problem solved:

The problem addresses only velocities that apply at the moment of launch. We are told that the vertical velocity is 4 m/s and that the angle to the horizontal is 35°. The angle to the vertical must be 55°, and the problem can be solved through simple vector analysis. Treat the true observed velocity (which in this case is unknown) as a principal vector; draw it in relation to its vertical component (which is known). Visualize a right triangle in which a line segment drawn from the principal vector to the component makes a right angle with the component.

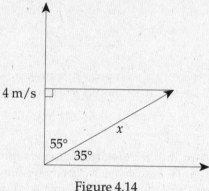

Figure 4.14

It now becomes clear that:

$$\cos 55° = \frac{4 \text{ m/s}}{x} \text{ and that } 4 \text{ m/s} = x(\cos 55°) \text{ m/s}$$

$$x = \frac{4 \text{ m/s}}{\cos 55°} = \frac{4 \text{ m/s}}{0.57} = \text{approx. } 7.0 \text{ m/s}$$

When faced with problems like this, which concern projectiles and their *initial* velocities or angles of orientation, think in terms of vectors and their components.

2. **The Ascent**:

Vertical movement: As a projectile ascends, it experiences the negative (downward) acceleration due to gravity. From the moment an object is launched, therefore, the magnitude of the projectile's *vertical* velocity decreases by approximately 10 m/s² (the approximate acceleration due to gravity as exerted on objects near the surface of the earth). Ultimately, vertical velocity falls to zero, and for that instant the projectile has neither upward nor downward movement.

Horizontal movement: As the projectile ascends, experiencing a constant negative acceleration in the *vertical* direction, it experiences *no acceleration* in the horizontal direction (because the MCAT will assume zero air resistance; in reality, air resistance does impart a negative acceleration). If, therefore, the projectile is launched with an initial horizontal velocity of 30 m/s, the horizontal component of its velocity continues at 30 m/s, throughout the flight. Even as the velocity's vertical component falls to zero, its horizontal component continues undisturbed at 30 m/s. *Horizontal velocity does not change.*

3. **The Descent:**

Vertical movement: When the vertical component of the projectile's velocity becomes zero, gravity continues to exert itself and vertical velocity immediately begins to increase in the downward direction at 10 m/s². In terms of vertical movement, the falling projectile should be conceived as an object in free fall. The time at which it strikes the earth can be determined according to the equations set forth at section **4.1.5.1** solely by calculation of the time of ascent and descent, without regard for horizontal motion.

Note also: For an object in ideal projectile motion, the *time* that elapses during ascent is equal to the time that elapses during descent. If we are told (or we calculate) that an object in projectile motion ascends for 25 seconds, then we know, without further inquiry, that it also descends for 25 seconds.

Horizontal movement: Again, because the projectile experiences no acceleration in the horizontal direction, the magnitude of horizontal velocity continues unchanged from the time of launch. That is, the ideal projectile (experiencing zero air resistance) continues throughout flight with a horizontal velocity equal to that of its initial horizontal velocity—only the vertical velocity changes as we discussed—due to the acceleration of gravity.

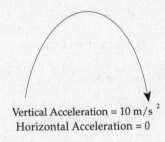

Vertical Acceleration = 10 m/s²
Horizontal Acceleration = 0

Figure 4.16

Please answer this question:

- A bullet is fired from a gun at an angle of 20° to the earth. The magnitude of its horizontal velocity is initially 3.2 x 10⁶ m/s. Ignoring air resistance, the magnitude of its horizontal velocity the moment before it strikes the ground is:

A. 3.2 x 10⁵ m/s
B. 1.6 x 10⁶ m/s
C. 3.2 x 10⁶ m/s
D. Not determinable from the information given.

Question answered:

C is the correct answer. The question requires that you remember this: In ideal projectile motion (projectile motion without air resistance) the moving body experiences no acceleration in the horizontal direction—neither positive nor negative. The magnitude of its horizontal velocity is constant throughout the course of flight. At the moment the projectile—a bullet, in this case—strikes the ground, its *horizontal* velocity remains at 3.2 × 10⁶ m/s.

4.1.8.2 The Equations

Equations pertaining directly to projectile motion are only specialized applications of those that pertain generally to uniform accelerated motion and free fall motion. We provide them for completeness, but you do not need to memorize them.

For all ideal projectiles—

in relation to *horizontal* motion:

$$v_{xo} = v_o(\cos\theta)$$

$$v_x = v_{xo}$$

$$d_x = v_{xo}t$$

Where:

θ = initial angle to the horizontal (earth)

v_{xo} = initial horizontal velocity

v_o = projectile's true observed velocity

v_x = horizontal velocity at any given time

d_x = displacement in horizontal direction

t = elapsed time

in relation to *vertical* motion:

$$v_{yo} = v_o(\sin\theta)$$

$$v_y = v_{yo} - gt$$

$$d_y = v_{yo}t - \frac{1}{2}gt^2$$

Where:

θ = initial angle to the horizontal (earth)

V_{yo} = initial vertical velocity

V_y = vertical velocity at any given time

d_y = displacement in vertical direction

g = acceleration due to gravity = approx. 10 m/s^2

t = time elapsed

Please solve this problem:

- An object with a mass of 10 kg is fired from a cannon. It moves with a true initial velocity of 100 m/s at an angle of 30° to the horizontal. After traveling a projectile path, the object returns to the horizontal, slides another 100 m horizontally and then falls over the edge of a precipice. The height of the precipice is 1,000 m. Neither air resistance nor friction need be accounted for and assume that $g = 10$ m/s². (*Note*: cos 60° = 0.5.)

  The initial magnitude of the object's vertical velocity is:

  A.   0 m/s
  B.   50 m/s
  C.   100 m/s
  D.   200 m/s

Problem solved:

B is the correct answer. You are given the object's true initial velocity with both the magnitude and the direction. Think of the velocity as a vector, and then try to find the vertical component of that vector. Draw a right triangle that includes a leg running from the known vector to the unknown vector, making a right angle at the unknown:

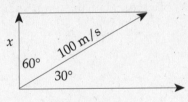

Figure 4.17

$$\cos 60° = \frac{x}{100} \, ; x = 100 \cos 60°$$

$$x = 100 \, (0.5) \text{ m/s} = 50 \text{ m/s}$$

Please solve this problem:

- How long does the object remain in flight before it returns to the horizontal surface from which it was launched?

  A.   2 seconds
  B.   5 seconds
  C. 10 seconds
  D. 20 seconds

Problem solved:

C is the correct answer. The question draws on sections **4.1.5** and **4.1.8.1**. The object has an initial vertical velocity of 50 m/s. It experiences a uniform (negative) vertical acceleration of -10 m/s². Total flight time is equal to the time of ascent plus the time of descent. The ascent ends when the object's vertical velocity has a magnitude of zero:

$$v_f = v_o + (a)(t)$$

$$0 = 50 \text{ m/s} + (-10 \text{ m/s}^2)(t)$$

$$0 - 50 \text{ m/s} = (-10 \text{ m/s}^2)(t)$$

$$\frac{-50 \text{ m/s}}{-10 \text{ m/s}^2} = (t)$$

$$\frac{50 \text{ m/s}}{10 \text{ m/s}^2} = (t) = 5 \text{ s} = \textit{time of ascent}$$

The ascent takes 5 seconds, and the descent, therefore, takes another 5 seconds. The total flight time is 10 seconds.

Please solve this problem:

- In relation to the horizontal from which it is launched, the object reaches a maximum height of:

A. 62.5 m
B. 100 m
C. 125 m
D. 250 m

Problem solved:

C is the correct answer. The question draws on sections **4.1.5** and **4.1.8.1**. Because the projectile takes 5 seconds to reach its maximum height, we apply this equation:

$$d_f = d_o + v_o t + \frac{1}{2}at^2$$

$$d_f = 50 \text{ m/s}(5 \text{ s}) + (\frac{1}{2})(-10 \text{ m/s}^2)(25 \text{ s}^2)$$

$$250 \text{ m} - 125 \text{ m} = 125 \text{ m}$$

4.2 MASTERY APPLIED: SAMPLE PASSAGE AND QUESTIONS

Passage

According to our present-day understanding of aeroballistics and associated aerodynamic force systems, the axis of a moving projectile is not expected to point always along the path of motion of its center of gravity. Rather, the axis is inclined at an angle, the *angle of yaw*—to the direction of motion. Consequently, a force, F, acts at a point P. The force acts in a direction that is inclined to the projectile's axis and its direction of motion.

As shown in Figure 1, F may be resolved into two forces and one torque, each acting at the center of gravity (G). One force resists the projectile's forward motion and acts therefore in the direction opposite to its motion (R). The other force, lift (L), acts in the direction perpendicular to the projectile's motion. The torque (not shown) imposes a turning effect around the projectile's center of gravity G; this gives rise to the *yawing moment*.

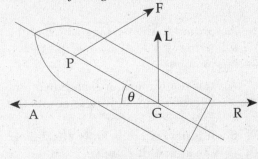

Figure 1

Every aeroballistic projectile has an associated nondimensional drag coefficient, f_R, which depends largely on its Mach number, M, which in turn is equal to $\frac{\text{velocity}}{\text{angle of yaw}}$. The drag coefficient also depends on the shape of the projectile and in particular on the degree to which the projectile's head is blunt or pointed. Figure 2 demonstrates, generally, the relationship of drag coefficient f_R to Mach number (M) (ignoring the effects of the Reynolds number Re, the effects of which are significant only for very long projectiles with large surface areas).

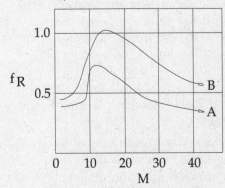

A: Projectile with slender pointed head.
B: Projectile with blunt head.

Figure 2

The drag coefficient tends also to increase with increasing angles of yaw according, approximately, to the formula

$$f_R = F_{Ro} \left(1 + \frac{\theta^2}{200}\right)$$ where F_{Ro} is the zero yaw

drag coefficient and θ is the angle of yaw.

Two other coefficients, the lift and yawing moment coefficients, show a variation with the Mach number similar to that seen in the case of the drag coefficient.

1. An ascending aeroballistic projectile is launched at an initial angle of θ, with an applied initial force F, and no continuing applied force. The vertical component of its initial velocity is 9,000 m/s. Assuming the acceleration due to gravity is 10 m/s², and ignoring the effects of air resistance, what magnitude will be associated with the vertical component of the projectile's velocity at time = t?

   A. 9,000 m/s
   B. 9,000 + (t^2) m/s
   C. 9,000 + 10(t) m/s
   D. 9,000 − 10(t) m/s

2.   Accounting for air resistance, which of the following is true of an aeroballistic projectile when it reaches the highest point in its path, if it is launched from the earth at angle θ with an initial force F, and no continuing applied force?

A. It has vertical acceleration of 0.
B. It has vertical velocity of 0.
C. It has horizontal acceleration of 0.
D. It has horizontal velocity of 0.

3. In Figure 1, the item labeled F represents:

A. a scalar quantity equal to the distance from point G.
B. a scalar quantity equal to the speed away from point G.
C. a vector quantity equal to a component of vector L.
D. a vector equal to the sum of vectors R and L.

4. The angle of yaw tends to impose forces acting in which of the following directions?

A. Upward and backward
B. Upward and forward
C. Downward and backward
D. Downward and forward

5. Two aeroballistic projectiles A and B differ in their angles of yaw, projectile A having one half that of projectile B. According to the passage which of the following will be true of projectile A?

A. Its mass will be equal to (mass of projectile B)^2.
B. It will experience acceleration due to gravity of 0.5 m/s^2.
C. At equal velocities projectile A's Mach number will be twice that of B's.
D. Its velocity will be equal to (Mach number for Projectile B) × 0.5.

6. According to Figure 2, for Mach numbers below 10, increased Mach numbers produce:

A. increased coefficients of drag.
B. increased angles of yaw.
C. decreased coefficients of drag.
D. decreased angles of yaw.

7. By extrapolation, the curves set forth on Figure 2 tend to indicate which one of the following trends?

A. When the Mach number is less than 20, it has a negligible effect on the coefficient of drag.
B. When the Mach number is greater than 20, it has a negligible effect on the coefficient of drag.
C. When the Mach number exceeds 40, further increases tend to have relatively greater effects on the coefficient of drag.
D. When the Mach number exceeds 40, further increases tend to have relatively smaller effects on the coefficient of drag.

8. According to the passage which of the following is true of a projectile's yawing moment?

A. It is nondimensional and therefore exerts little significance on the projectile's motion.
B. It is never significantly affected by the Reynolds number.
C. It tends to produce a turning motion that pivots on the projectile's center of gravity.
D. It is unrelated to Mach number but depends heavily on the value of the lift coefficient.

4.3 MASTERY VERIFIED: ANSWERS AND EXPLANATIONS

1. *D is correct.* The problem bears little relation to the passage *per se*; it concerns projectile motion in general and, in particular, the formula $v_f = v_o + at$. We are told that the projectile is launched with an initial velocity whose vertical component is 9,000 m/s. The only acceleration to which the projectile is subjected in the vertical direction is that of gravity $(g) = 10$ m/s^2. Gravity is exerting a downward acceleration and therefore, in relation to the object's motion, the downward acceleration is negative (–).

$$v_f = v_o + at$$

$$v_f = 9,000 \text{ m/s} + (-)(10 \text{ m/s}^2)(t) = 9,000 \text{ m/s} - 10t \text{ m/s}$$

2. *B is correct.* Again, the question bears little relation to the passage *per se*. Rather it requires that you understand certain fundamental dynamics of projectile motion on the earth. A projectile launched with an initial applied force takes on a vertical and horizontal velocity. With or without air resistance, the projectile experiences a downward acceleration due to gravity (10 m/s^2) and ultimately slows to a halt. At that point where vertical motion stops, the projectile has a velocity of zero (and then begins to descend with acceleration of negative (–) 10 m/s^2). Because the reader is advised to account for air resistance, which does impart a negative acceleration in the horizontal direction, choice C is not correct. In the absence of air resistance, C would also be correct.

3. *D is correct.* The item draws on (a) information in the passage, (b) information in Figure 1, and (c) a knowledge of vectors. The passage indicates that the force F, imposed at point P can be resolved into two forces L and R. R tends to oppose the projectile's forward motion and L tends to lift the projectile. To state that F can be resolved into L and R is to say, reciprocally, that the sum of L and R is F. Moreover, a visual inspection of the vectors F, R, and L indicates that if the head of R were positioned at the tail of L, or the tail of R positioned at the head of L, the resultant would have the magnitude and direction of F.

4. *A is correct.* The question draws on the passage and your understanding of vectors. The second sentence in the passage indicates that the angle of yaw, which represents the angle at which an aeroballistic projectile is inclined relative to the path of its motion, creates a force represented in Figure 1 as F. Visualization of the vector F that results from the angle of yaw indicates that it is directed upward and backward. The passage indicates that the vector resolves into two components: one that tends to draw the projectile backward and the other that tends to impart lift.

5. *C is correct.* This question draws only on your ability to (a) use the formula provided in the passage and (b) understand the simple proportionality it establishes. You don't need to know anything about Mach number, just its *proportionality* to the angle of yaw.

$$\text{Mach number, M} = \frac{\text{velocity}}{\text{angle of yaw}}$$

Instead of succumbing to intimidation by these foreign terms, notice that Mach number (M) is directly proportional to velocity and *inversely proportional to angle of yaw*. This means that when angle of yaw is halved, Mach number is doubled.

6. *A is correct.* You must avoid being intimidated by Figure 2. Look at the curves on Figure 2. Each first slopes upward (positive slope), reaches a peak, and then slopes downward (negative slope). Note that for *Y* value (Mach number) = 10, each curve is to the left of its peak. Now, observe each curve to the left of its peak: Rightward movement (increase) along the *x* axis (Mach number) corresponds to upward movement (increase) in the *y* axis (coefficient of drag).

7. *D is correct.* Observe each curve where *y* axis (Mach number) = 40. Each shows a pronounced tendency to flatten. Extrapolation (reading beyond the values actually shown) indicates that the slope will tend to progress further toward a flat configuration and that additional positive movement along the *x* axis (Mach number) will bring about progressively smaller changes on the *y* axis (coefficient of drag).

8. *C is correct.* The question tests your ability to read relatively complex scientific matter while taking note of relatively simple statements. The passage refers to the drag coefficient as "nondimensional," but this question concerns the yawing moment. The conclusion of the passage's second paragraph states: "Component forces *R* and *L* impose a turning effect around the projectile's center of gravity *G*, this giving rise to the *yawing moment*." Choice C represents a paraphrase of this statement.

4.3.1 STRATEGIC ANALYSIS OF PASSAGE AND QUESTIONS

Notice that the subject of the passage is largely arcane. Most candidates find the MCAT passages similarly strange and foreign in the topics they address. Yet your ability to answer the questions depends only on (a) your knowledge of concepts that you do understand (if you have reviewed Chapter 4) and (b) your ability to avoid the intimidation and confusion that usually arise from unfamiliar subjects, equations, and phenomena.

Neither the first nor second questions drew on the passage at all; instead they called on your understanding of vectors and projectiles. The last question drew on the passage, but not on science; it required only that you read and understand, *as ordinary English*, the last sentence of the second paragraph. The third and fourth questions required you to apply Figure 1 to your understanding of simple vector phenomena (as explained in this chapter). The fifth question drew only on your ability to understand the proportionality inherent in a mathematical equation, not to understand the equation in detail. The sixth and seventh questions pertained to the interpretation of a curve set forth on a Cartesian plane, not on an understanding of the significance of its parameters.

This degree of seeming difficulty is typical of MCAT passages. Some questions require a knowledge of science (the knowledge imparted in this book), some require skillful reading, some require logical reasoning, and a great many require only that you not be intimidated by complex-looking graphs, figures, and pictures.

Notice, finally, that the passage did not test *all* that you have learned in Chapter 4. No single form or administration of the MCAT will test everything you study in this book. Although predicting exactly what any given test form will test is impossible, if you master all that is set forth in this book, the MCAT will offer few surprises.

CHAPTER 5

FORCES

5.1 MASTERY ACHIEVED

5.1.1 THE PHENOMENON OF FORCE AND NEWTON'S FIRST LAW

The definition of **force** as it pertains to the MCAT is simply a "push" or "pull." The MCAT will not require a more sophisticated definition than this. Force is a *vector* quantity: it has both direction and magnitude.

A body—in motion or at rest—retains its velocity indefinitely, unless it is acted on by some force. This principle underlies **Newton's first law**:

> *An object initially at rest or in motion at a constant velocity will remain in its initial state unless acted upon by a non-zero net external force.*

Because change in velocity is equivalent to acceleration (chapter 4), Newton's first law might also be stated thus:

> *If a net positive force acts on a body, the body will experience acceleration.*

As a consequence of Newton's law, objects have a natural tendency *not* to accelerate. That tendency is termed **inertia**, and Newton's first law is sometimes called **the law of inertia**.

5.1.2 NEWTON'S SECOND LAW

Newton's second law provides a quantitative relationship between a force and the **acceleration** it produces. The force is directly proportional to the object's **mass**, and the relationship may be expressed as:

$$\text{applied force} = (\text{object's mass})(\text{acceleration produced})$$

This is equivalent to:

$$\text{force} = (\text{mass})(\text{acceleration})$$

$$F = ma$$

Through algebraic manipulation, any one of the three variables—force, mass, or acceleration—may be determined if the other two are given:

$$F = ma \qquad a = \frac{F}{m} \qquad m = \frac{F}{a}$$

Mass is expressed in the SI unit **kilogram (kg)**, and acceleration is in **m/s²**. It follows that force, which represents mass × acceleration, is expressed in the unit: **kg•m/s²**. For convenience, 1 kg•m/s² is named 1 **newton (N)**. The magnitude of a force is usually expressed in newtons (N).

The MCAT candidate should observe not only the equalities established by Newton's second law, but also the corresponding *proportionalities*. Note that for any body subjected to a force, acceleration is (a) proportional to force and (b) inversely proportional to mass $\left(a = \dfrac{F}{m}\right)$.

Please solve this problem:

- A force of magnitude F is applied to an object of mass m, and produces an acceleration a. If the same force is applied to an object with mass of $0.7m$, what will be the magnitude of the resulting acceleration?

Problem solved:

According to Newton's second law, mass is inversely proportional to acceleration. Since the problem describes a constant force, if mass is multiplied by a factor of 0.7, acceleration must be divided by a factor of 0.7. The resulting acceleration will be:

$$\frac{a}{0.7} = \frac{10a}{7} = 1.428a$$

5.1.3 DISTINGUISHING BETWEEN MASS AND WEIGHT; WEIGHT AS FORCE

Mass represents a quantity of matter. It is a scalar quantity, measured in the SI unit kg. An object's mass is independent of gravity, and so must be distinguished from its weight. For any object, **weight** is the force acting on a mass due to gravitational acceleration of the planet or heavenly body on which the object is situated. On Earth, an object's weight is the force produced by the product of:

(mass of object)(acceleration due to Earth's gravity)

(mass of object)(10 m/s²)

Please solve this problem:

- An object on Earth has a weight of 50 N. What is its mass?

Problem solved:

Weight is equal to the product:

$$\text{(mass)(acceleration due to Earth's gravity)}$$

$$\text{mass} = \frac{\text{weight}}{\text{acceleration due to gravity}}$$

$$m = \frac{50 \text{ N}}{10 \text{ m/s}^2}$$

$$m = \frac{50 \text{ kg} \bullet \text{m/s}}{10 \text{ m/s}^2}$$

$$m = 5 \text{ kg}$$

Please solve this problem:

- An object situated on Planet X has mass of 80 kg and weight of 320 newtons on Planet X. The object is dropped from 18 meters above the surface of Planet X. Find the time before the object strikes the surface of the planet, and find the object's velocity at the instant before impact with the planet's surface.

Problem solved:

To solve this problem, the student will need to understand Newton's second law, free fall, and the relationships among velocity, time, and acceleration.

First, determine the object's acceleration:

$$F = ma$$

$$320 \text{ N} = 80 \text{ kg } (a)$$

$$a = 4.0 \text{ m/s}^2$$

Knowing that the body accelerates at 4.0 m/s^2, calculate t:

$$d = v_o t + \frac{1}{2} at^2$$

$$18 \text{ m} = 0 + \frac{1}{2}(4)(t^2)$$

$$18 \text{ m} = 2t^2$$

$$\frac{18}{2} = t^2$$

$$t^2 = 9$$

$$t = 3$$

Knowing that the object travels for 3 seconds with an acceleration of 4.0 m/s², calculate its final velocity:

$$v_f = v_o + at$$

$$v_f = 0 + (4.0 \text{ m/s}^2)(3s)$$

$$v_f = 12 \text{ m/s}$$

5.1.4 NEWTON'S LAW OF UNIVERSAL GRAVITATION

Newton's law of universal gravitation states that any pair of objects will produce a mutually attractive gravitational force according to this equation:

$$F = G\frac{m_1 m_2}{r^2}$$

where:

F = force of gravity

m_1 = mass of object 1 in kg

m_2 = mass of object 2 in kg

r = distance between the centers of the masses of objects 1 and 2

G = universal gravitational constant = 6.67×10^{-11} N•m²/kg²

The MCAT will not require you to know the value of the universal gravitational constant, but some questions will require an understanding of the proportionalities in Newton's law of gravitation. Note that:

• Gravitational force is directly proportional to the mass of each object.

• Gravitational force is inversely proportional to the square of the distance between the centers of mass of the objects.

Please solve this problem:

• Two objects, A and B, with masses of 0.04 kg and 0.05 kg, respectively, have their centers of mass separated by a distance of 1.2 meters. Object A experiences a force of F due to gravity toward object B. Object B is replaced by C, which has a mass of 0.15 kg. The distance between the center of masses of A and C is then reduced from 1.2 to 0.4 meters. Express, in terms of F, the gravitational force on A due to C.

Problem solved:

The problem draws on proportionalities related to the law of gravitation. The mass of one object is increased by a factor of 3:

$$(3)0.05 \text{ kg} = 0.15 \text{ kg}$$

This change increases the gravitational force by a factor of 3. The distance between the two objects is reduced by a factor of 3. By itself, that change increases the gravitational attraction by a factor of $3^2 = 9$. Together, the two changes increase gravitational force by the factor:

$$(3)(9) = 27$$

$$F_1 = (27)(F)$$

5.1.5 NET FORCE

5.1.5.1 Summation of Forces

An object might experience two or more forces simultaneously, and this results in a net force that is equal to the sum of those forces. Since force is a vector, net force is a **vector sum**.

Please solve this problem:

- An object is subjected to a 40 newton force westward and a 15 newton force eastward. What net force does it experience?

Problem solved:

Since the two forces are exactly opposite in direction, the answer is derived easily with a drawing. An eastward force of 15 N added to a westward force of 40 N yields a westward force of 25 N.

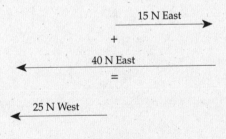

Figure 5.1

Please solve this problem:

- An object is subjected to a 90 newton force to the north and a 35 newton force directed 20° north of east. Draw a vector diagram of the total net force.

Problem solved:

The vector that represents the net force can be depicted by simple vector summation:

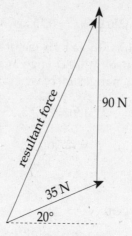

Figure 5.2

5.1.5.2 Newton's Third Law

On the MCAT, net force requires an understanding of **Newton's third law**:

When one body exerts a force on another, the second body will exert an equal and opposite force on the first.

(This law has given rise to that familiar statement: "For every action there is an equal and opposite reaction.")

If an object with weight of 50 newtons rests on a table, it imposes a 50 N downward force on the table, and according to Newton's third law, the table top exerts a 50 N force upward on the object:

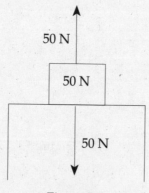

Figure 5.3

Therefore, the object itself experiences *two forces*:

(1) a 50 N downward force (due to gravity)

(2) a 50 N upward force (from the table)

Net force takes into account all contributory forces, including those that are attributable to Newton's third law. Consider the net force imposed on the object that we described immediately above. Account for each contributory force as a vector, with its tail at the object and its head pointed away from the object.

The object experiences a 50 N downward force and a 50 N upward force:

Figure 5.4

Therefore, it experiences a net force of: +50 N upward + (–50 N) downward = 0.

5.1.5.3 Tension

MCAT questions use the word **tension** when discussing connectors like threads, strings, wires, ropes, or cables. A full understanding of tension requires integral calculus, but don't worry, calculus will not be tested on the MCAT.

The two principles of tension that the MCAT will test are:

(1) If equal forces are applied at two ends of any connector, then (a) tension is equal to the force applied at each end (*not the sum of the forces*) and (b) no acceleration results.

(2) If unequal forces are applied at two ends of any connector, then acceleration occurs according to the net force exerted (greater force minus the lesser force).

For each rule, the converse also applies:

(1) If two forces are applied at either end of a connector and no acceleration results, then the forces at each end are equal.

(2) If two forces are applied at either end of any flexible connector, and acceleration does result, then the forces at the two ends are unequal. The rate of acceleration is dependent on the net force.

Consider an object that weighs 100 N and is suspended from the ceiling by a rope. At its lower end, the rope experiences a force of 100 N imposed by the object's weight. (According to Newton's third law, the object experiences a 100 N force upward, imposed by the rope.) The rope conveys that force to the ceiling, and the ceiling therefore experiences a downward force of 100 N. According to Newton's third law, the ceiling then imposes an upward force of 100 N on the rope.

The rope experiences:

(a) at its lower end, a 100 N downward force, imposed by the object's weight

(b) at its upper end, a 100 N upward force, imposed by the ceiling

The forces at each end are equal. Tension in the rope is 100 N, and there is no acceleration.

100 N Imposed
by Ceiling

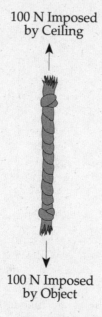

100 N Imposed
by Object

Figure 5.5

Next, consider a rope that is (a) attached to a 100 N object at its lower end and (b) subjected to a lifting force of 120 N at its upper end:

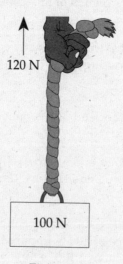

120 N

100 N

Figure 5.6

The forces at the two ends are unequal. Tension in the rope is 120 N, and the object accelerates according to the net force it experiences. That net force is equal to:

100 N downward + 120 N upward = 20 N upward

The object accelerates upward. The magnitude of acceleration is calculated with Newton's second law; first you calculate the object's mass, and then calculate the acceleration that it undergoes.

Calculate the object's mass:

$$F = ma$$

$$100 \text{ N} = (m)(10 \text{ m/s}^2)$$

$$m = 10 \text{ kg}$$

Knowing that a 10 kg object experiences a 20 N upward force, calculate the associated acceleration:

$$F = ma$$

$$20 \text{ N} = (10 \text{ kg})(a)$$

$$a = 2 \text{ m/s}^2$$

Please solve this problem:

- A 1,200 kg object is lowered by cable so that it accelerates downward at 2.8 m/s². What is the tension in the cable?

Problem solved:

The object accelerates downward; therefore, (a) the force at the cable's upper end is less than the force at its lower end.

Using Newton's second law, ascertain the net force exerted on the object. Since the object accelerates downward at 2.8 m/s², it experiences a net downward force of

$$F = mg - T = ma$$

$$F = (1{,}200 \text{ kg})(10 \text{ m/s}^2) - T = (1200 \text{kg})(2.8 \text{m/s}^2)$$

$$F = 12{,}000 \text{ N} - T = 3{,}360 \text{ N}$$

Tension, therefore, equals:

$$T = 12{,}000 \text{ N} - 3{,}360 \text{ N} = 8{,}640 \text{ N}$$

5.1.5.4 Vertical and Horizontal Forces

A single object may be subjected to forces on a horizontal plane, a vertical plane, or both. To determine the net force for an object, assess the net horizontal force and net vertical force.

A human hand applies a 35 N rightward force to an object that weighs 10 N and is situated on a frictionless surface:

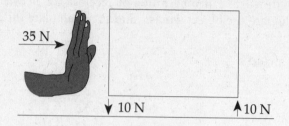

Figure 5.7

The object experiences:

• a downward force of 10 N, imposed by its weight

• an upward force of 10 N, imposed by the table according to Newton's third law

• a rightward force of 35 N imposed by the hand

The object experiences a net vertical force of 0 and a net horizontal force of 35 N rightward.

Please solve this problem:

• A 6 kg object is subjected to an upward force of 100 N. Simultaneously, it is pushed to the right with a 110 N force against a wind blowing to the left with a force of 70 N. Assuming that $g = 10$ m/s², what is the net force on the object?

Problem solved:

Consider vertical and horizontal forces separately.

Vertically, the object experiences:

(1) a downward force equal to its own weight = (6 kg)(10 m/s²) = 60 N

(2) an upward force of 100 N

Therefore, a net force of (100 N – 60 N) = 40 N upward.

Horizontally, the object experiences:

(1) a 110 N force to the right

(2) a 70 N force to the left

Therefore, a net force of (110 N – 70 N) = 40 N to the right.

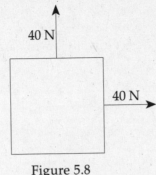

Figure 5.8

Net force is equal to the sum of the net horizontal and net vertical forces:

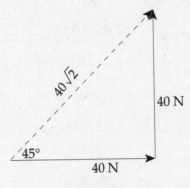

Figure 5.9

The vector diagram produces a right triangle. The hypotenuse represents the resultant. The two legs have length of 40 N each. The 1:1 leg ratio presents a right triangle conforming to the ratio $1:1:\sqrt{2}$, each side being multiplied by a factor of 40. The length of the hypotenuse is therefore $40\sqrt{2}$.

In a $1:1:\sqrt{2}$ right triangle, the angles are 45°, 45°, and 90°. The object therefore experiences a net force of $40\sqrt{2}$ in a direction 45° above the horizontal.

5.1.5.5 Motion on an Inclined Plane

With respect to an object on an inclined plane, you should be familiar with the following relationships:

$$w_g = mg$$

$$N = mg(\cos\theta)$$

$$F_i = mg(\sin\theta)$$

$$a = \frac{F_i}{m}$$

Where:

m = the mass of the object

w = the force imposed on the object directly downward as a result of gravity:

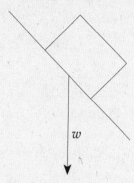

Figure 5.10

N = the normal force or the force exerted on the block by the plane:

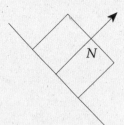

Figure 5.11

θ = the angle of incline:

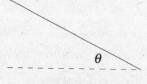

Figure 5.12

F_i = the resultant force experienced by the object down the inclined plane due to w and N:

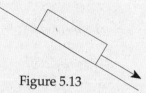

Figure 5.13

These formulas are specialized applications of principles already discussed in this chapter and in chapter 3. If you have an understanding of these principals, you should not need to memorize the formulas.

Consider an 80 kg object on a frictionless plane inclined 30° above the horizontal (note: sin 30° = 0.5; cos 30° = 0.867):

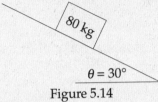

$\theta = 30°$

Figure 5.14

Note that when you know m and θ, you can calculate w, N, F_i, as well as acceleration down the plane, by ordinary vector analysis.

(1) $w = (80 \text{ kg}) \times (10 \text{ m/s}^2) = 800 \text{ N}$

(2) $N = w \cdot \cos 30° = (800 \text{ N})(0.867) = \text{approx. } 694 \text{ N}$

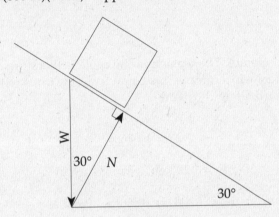

Figure 5.15

(3) $F_i = w \cdot \sin 30° = 800 \text{ N} (.5) = 400 \text{ N}$

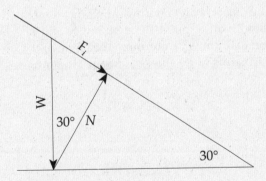

Figure 5.16

(4) $a = \dfrac{F_i}{m} = \dfrac{[(800)(\sin 30°)]\text{N}}{80 \text{ kg}} = \dfrac{400 \text{ N}}{80 \text{ kg}} = 5 \text{ m/s}^2$

Furthermore, the object's velocity at any moment in time, or the distance it travels after any period of time, can be calculated with these formulas:

$$V_f = V_o + at$$

$$d = v_o t + (\frac{1}{2})at^2$$

Please solve this problem:

- A 120 kg object on a frictionless plane inclined at 60° to the horizontal, is pulled by cable upward along the plane at a constant velocity of 0.25 m/s. What is the tension in the cable? (*Note:* sin 60° = approx. 0.866.)

Problem solved:

The object does not accelerate. The tension in the cable is therefore equal to the force that's exerted at either of its ends, which means it is equal to F_i (the force with which gravity tends to pull the object downward along the plane).

Calculate F_i:

$$F_i = w (\sin \theta)$$

$$F_i = (120 \text{ kg})(10 \text{ m/s}^2)(\sin 60°)$$

$$F_i = (1,200 \text{ N})(0.866) = 1,039.2 \text{ N}$$

Note that the answer is unaffected by the object's velocity; any constant velocity signifies zero acceleration. When acceleration = 0, then F (the net force) = $(m)(0)$ = 0.

Please solve this problem:

- A 50 kg object is moved upward along an inclined plane with an applied force of 360 N and acceleration of 0.5 m/s². Determine the angle of the incline in terms of its sine, cosine, or tangent.

Problem solved:

$$F_i = w (\sin \theta)$$

$$\sin \theta = \frac{F_i}{w}$$

$$\theta = \arcsin \frac{F_i}{w}$$

Calculate the values of w and F_i:

$$w = (50 \text{ kg})(10 \text{ m/s}^2) = 500 \text{ N}$$

Because the object accelerates up the plane at 0.5 m/s², it must experience a net force in that direction of:

$$F = ma$$

$$F = (50 \text{ kg})(0.5 \text{ m/s}^2) = 25 \text{ N}$$

The applied force of 360 N upward along the plane must exceed F_i by 25 N, which means that:

$$F_i = 360 \text{ N} - 25 \text{ N} = 335 \text{ N, and}$$

$$\theta = \arcsin 335/500 = \arcsin 0.67$$

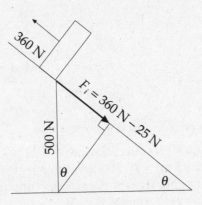

Figure 5.17

5.1.5.6 Rotational Motion and Torque

Torque is force that is associated with rotational motion, the dynamics of which involve an axis, a **lever arm**, l_1 (also called a **moment arm**), and an applied force F_1, as shown in Figure 5.18:

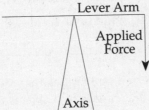

Figure 5.18

You should think of torque as a force exerted around an axis of rotation. Torque has either a clockwise or counterclockwise direction and a magnitude equal to:

(lever arm)(applied force perpendicular to lever arm)

$T = F_1 \times l_1$, where lever arm is the distance from the point of rotation to the perpendicularly applied force.

Since torque is the product of (force) × (length), its unit of measure is N•m.

In any system involving rotational motion, **net torque** around an axis is calculated by taking the difference between the clockwise torque (if any) and the counterclockwise torque (if any).

Although a rotational system might feature a true physical axis, it also features an infinite number of **hypothetical** axes. In the system shown in Figure 5.19, a physical axis is located at the center of a 10 m length of wood. Downward forces of 18 N and 7 N are applied at right and left ends, respectively. An upward force equal to the weight of the apparatus is applied at the fulcrum.

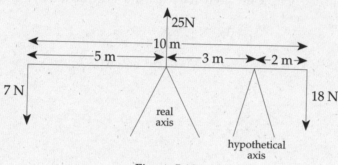

Figure 5.19

The torque around the axis can be calculated as follows:

Clockwise torque = (18 N)(5 m) = 90 N•m clockwise
Counterclockwise torque = (7 N)(5 m) = 35 N•m counterclockwise
The force applied by the fulcrum goes right through the point of rotation and thus has no lever arm. Therefore it results in zero torque.
Net torque = 90 N•m clockwise - 35 N•m counterclockwise = 55 N•m clockwise.

Notice that the torque around a hypothetical point 2 meters from the right end of the wood results in the same torque.

Clockwise torque = (18 N)(2m) + (25 N)(3m) = 111 N•m clockwise
Counterclockwise torque = (7N)(8m) = 56 N•m counterclockwise
Net torque = 111 N•m clockwise – 56 N•m counterclockwise = 55 N•m clockwise.

Torque calculated about any axis will be the same for any system.

5.1.5.7 Friction

Friction is a force that occurs between two bodies that are in contact with each other. You should think of friction as the force that causes two objects to resist moving or sliding "against" one another.

The classic illustration for friction is that of an object on a table. Any attempt to move the object across the table top requires an initial application of force, and any effort to maintain the object in motion across the table top requires a persistant application of force. The necessity for such forces arises from the force of friction, which must be overcome if motion is to be initiated and maintained.

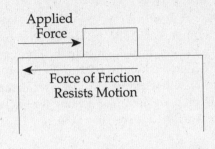

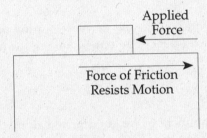

Figure 5.20

Like any force, friction is a vector quantity. Its direction is *opposite* to that of the intended motion, and its magnitude is equal to:

$$F_\mu = \text{(coefficient of friction) (normal force)}$$

$$F_\mu = \mu N$$

Normal force, N, is the force exerted on an object by the surface upon which it rests. The normal force is always perpendicular to that surface. If the object to be moved is situated on a level surface, then the normal force, N, is equal to the magnitude of the object's weight and opposite in direction. If the object is situated on an inclined plane, then the normal force is opposite in direction and equal in magnitude to the component of the object's weight that exerts itself perpendicular to the surface of the plane (mg cos (θ) near the surface of the Earth).

You should recognize that, for any two substances, there are *two* associated coefficients of friction:

(1) the coefficienct of *static* friction, μ_s

(2) the coefficient of *kinetic* friction, μ_k

In terms of the equation $F_\mu = \mu N$, the coefficient of static friction, μ_s, concerns the initiation of motion, and the coefficient of dynamic friction μ_k concerns the maintenance of motion.

Suppose that object A weighs 60 N and rests on a flat surface B. The coefficients of friction are μ_s (the coefficient of static friction) = 0.2 and μ_k (the coefficient of kinetic friction) = 0.12.

The force required to initiate movement of object A along surface B is:

$$F_\mu = \mu_s N$$

$$F_\mu = \mu_s N = (60 \text{ N})(0.2) = 12 \text{ N}$$

The force required to maintain movement of object A along surface B, once it has been initiated, is:

$$F_\mu = \mu_k N = (60 \text{ N})(0.12) = 7.2 \text{ N}$$

Please solve this problem:

- An object with mass of 130 kg slides down a plane inclined at an angle of 30 degrees to the horizontal. If the coefficient of kinetic friction between the surfaces is 0.2, with what magnitude of acceleration does the object move downward along the incline?
  (Note: $\sin 30^0 = 0.5$; $\cos 30^0 = 0.867$.)

Problem solved:

According to Newton's second law, the object's acceleration downward along the incline will be equal to the *net force* it experiences downward along the incline, divided by the object's mass:

$$F = ma \qquad\qquad a = \frac{F}{m}$$

The net force equals the component of weight directed along the incline *minus* the associated force of friction between the object and the plane.

Calculate the component of the object's weight F_i directed downward along the incline:

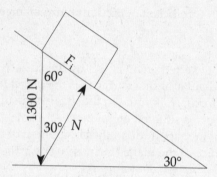

Figure 5.21

$$F_i = w\,(\sin 30°)$$
$$F_i = 1300\ N\,(\sin 30°) = 650\ N$$

Calculate the force of friction (F_μ) that resists the motion of the object down the incline. Start by calculating the normal force, N. Then substitute N into the equation $F_\mu = \mu N$, where μ is the coefficient of friction:

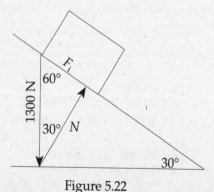

Figure 5.22

$$N = (1300\ \text{N})(\cos 30°) = 1300\ \text{N}\ (0.870) = \text{approx. } 1131\ \text{N}$$

$$F_\mu = \mu_k N = 1131\ \text{N}\ (0.2) = \text{approx. } 226\ \text{N}$$

Net force downward along the incline = 650 N – 226 N = 424 N

Calculate acceleration:

$$a = \frac{F}{m} = \frac{424\ \text{N}}{130\ \text{kg}} = \text{approx. } 3.26\ \text{m} / \text{s}^2$$

You should be aware of the *proportionalities* associated with friction. Since $F_\mu = \mu N$, the force of friction between any two objects is proportional to the normal force between them. In the case of an object resting on a flat surface, the force of friction is pro-portional to weight. Furthermore, since weight is proportional to mass, friction is proportional to mass, as well.

5.1.5.8 Center of Mass

Every object (whether it is regularly or irregularly shaped), has a **center of mass** (sometimes called the center of gravity). MCAT questions do not draw on the mathematical or geometric definition of the center of mass but rather on its practical significance.

The MCAT candidate should think of the center of gravity as the point at which all of an object's mass is concentrated. In day-to-day application it is conceived as the object's "balancing point."

For any object, mass may or may not be uniformly distributed. Consider a solid rectangular steel bar. If such a bar were suspended by a rope that was attached to the bar's mid-point, it would hang in balance:

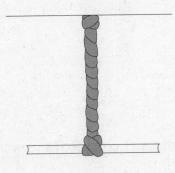

Figure 5.23

For any object whose mass is *uniformly distributed*, the center of mass is at the *geometric center*.

Consider a regularly shaped rectangular bar composed of lead on its left half and aluminum on its right half. If it were suspended by a rope that was attached to its geometric center (as shown in Figure 5.24), it would tilt to the left:

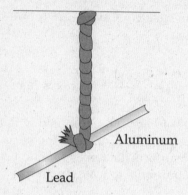

Aluminum

Lead

Figure 5.24

For the object pictured in Figure 5.24, the center of mass is located somewhere to the left side of its center. It would be suspended *in balance* by a rope attached (approximately) at the point pictured in Figure 5.25:

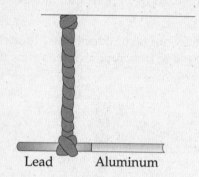

Lead   Aluminum

Figure 5.25

5.1.5.9 Statics: Translational and Rotational Equilibrium

You must be familiar with the concepts of:

- translational equilibrium

- rotational equilibrium

A body (or system of bodies) is in translational equilibrium if it experiences no net force in any direction. A body (or system of bodies) is in rotational equilibrium if it experiences no net torque.

Please solve this problem:

- Ropes 1, 2, and 3 are knotted together, as shown in Figure 5.26. Rope 2 is fastened to a vertical wall, and rope 3 is fastened to a horizontal ceiling. A mass with a weight of 50 N hangs on rope 1. The angle between rope 3 and the ceiling is 60°. Find T_1, T_2, and T_3, the tension in each of the ropes. (Assume that the weight of the ropes is negligible.)

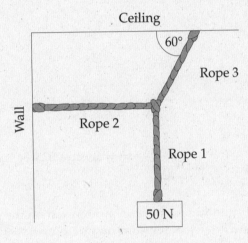

Figure 5.26

Problem solved:

Find T_1:

Because the system is in equilibrium:

upward force on rope 1 = downward force on rope 1 = 50 N

$$T_1 = 50 \text{ N}$$

Find T_3:

Note that the knot, like all components of this system, is in equilibrium. It experiences a downward force of 50 N and must also experience an upward force of 50 N. Rope 2 is attached horizontally; its tension has no vertical component. The entire 50 N upward force imparted to the knot must arise from the vertical component of rope 3. The *vertical component* of the tension in rope 3, therefore, is 50 N. Rope 3 represents a vector whose vertical component is 50 N, which allows for the calculation of T_3.

Remember that we do not seek to evaluate the component of the hypothetical vertical tension that lies 30° to the right of rope 3. *We are looking for the tension whose component 30° to the left is 50 N.* The vector diagram we draw will make a right angle with the vertical—the vertical represents the component, and T_3, the principal vector:

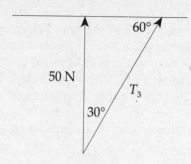

Figure 5.27

$$\cos 30° = \frac{50\ \text{N}}{T_3}$$

$$T_3(\cos 30°) = 50\ \text{N}$$

$$T_3 = \frac{50\ \text{N}}{\cos 30°} = \frac{50\ \text{N}}{0.866} = \text{approx. } 57.7\ \text{N}$$

Find T_2:

T_2 is directed horizontally and imposes a leftward tension on the knot. Because the knot is in equilibrium, it must experience equal tensions on its right and left sides. The only source of rightward tension on the knot is the horizontal component of T_3. Therefore:

$$T_2 = \text{horizontal component of } T_3$$

Knowing that $T_3 = 57.7$ N, calculate its horizontal component:

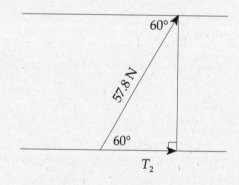

Figure 5.28

$$\cos 60° = \frac{T_2}{57.7\ \text{N}}$$

$$57.7\ \text{N}\ (\cos 60°) = T_2$$

$$T_2 = 57.7\ \text{N}\ (0.5) = 28.9\ \text{N}$$

5.2 MASTERY APPLIED: SAMPLE PASSAGE AND QUESTIONS

Passage

Commercial internal combustion engines vary in form, but all depend on these four features:

- compression of a gaseous mixture containing O_2 (usually air) mixed with fuel

- increase in temperature of the mixture due to compression

- expansion to the initial pressure and volume by combustion

- elimination of exhaust (the product of combustion)

Fuels vary, and engines relying on alcohol, diesel, and coal have been produced. The fuel for the modern internal combustion engine is gasoline.

The classic Otto "four-stroke cycle" combustion engine is based on a piston encased within an otherwise hollow cylinder. Attached to the piston's lower end is a rotary crank shaft (as shown in Figure 1). The rotation of the crank shaft permits the piston to move upward and downward within the cylinder.

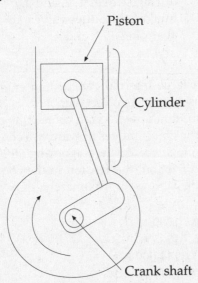

Figure 1

The first, or intake, stroke involves the downward motion of the piston and the intake of air and gas fuel through open inlet valves. The second, or compression stroke, involves upward movement of the piston. Intake and outlet valves are closed and compression of the gaseous mixture occurs. During the third stroke (with all the valves remaining closed), the mixture is ignited by a spark (generally generated by electricity). This is the power stroke: the combustion of the gaseous mixture expands the gases and imposes a downward force on the piston.

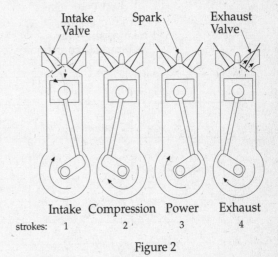

Figure 2

During the fourth, or exhaust, stroke the piston moves upward forcing the products of cumbustion (exhaust) out of the cylinder's open outlet valve. The cylinder is emptied of exhaust, the piston is ready for another intake stroke, and the cycle continues.

The events associated with the four strokes bear a relationship to pressures within the cylinder, roughly equivalent to those shown in Figure 3 (on rectangular coordinates) and Figure 4 (on logarithmic coordinates). In each case, pressure is a measure of force per unit area.

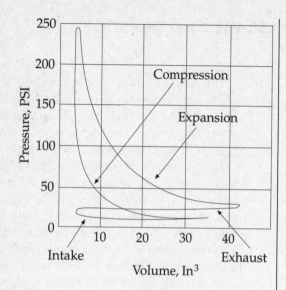

Figure 3

Stroke-pressure relationships on rectangular coordinates

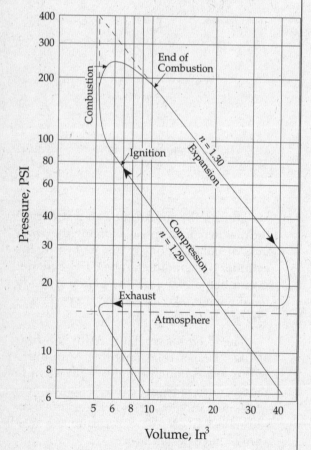

Figure 4

Stroke-pressure relationships on logarithmic coordinates

In order to put the engine to practical use, the crank shaft is usually connected to a device, such as an aircraft propeller, an automobile wheel, a ship's propeller, or a variety of non-locomotive mechanisms.

Thermodynamic theory defines the thermal efficiency of an Otto combustion cycle as:

$$T_e = 1 - \frac{1}{r^{n-1}}$$

The variable r represents the compression ratio. Ordinarily, n is equal to 1.4 (when the engine is operating under earth's atmospheric conditions). The actual efficiency of the engine turns out to be far less than that predicted by the equation.

1. An experimenter examines, in detail, the dynamics of an Otto internal combustion engine. She finds that during strokes 1, 2, and 4, the piston decelerates. Which of the following choices best furnishes a partial explanation for the observation?

   A. The piston has mass and so cannot sustain a constant velocity.
   B. The piston experiences friction with the walls of the cylinder.
   C. The piston experiences no forces during strokes 1, 2, and 4.
   D. Intake and outlet valves are open at strokes 1, 2, and 4.

2. A large internal combustion engine is used to lift an object with mass of 120 kg straight upward via a connecting cable. The object moves upward at a constant velocity of 2.5 m/s. Ignoring all forces of friction, the tension in the connecting cable is approximately:

   A. 0 N
   B. 1200 N
   C. 1225 N
   D. 144,000 N

3. According to Figure 3, which of the following choices is true of the pressure within the cylinder of an Otto internal combustion engine?

   A. The pressure increases significantly with one, but not both, of the downward strokes.
   B. The pressure increases significantly with both downward strokes.
   C. The pressure increases significantly with one but not both of the upward strokes.
   D. The pressure increases significantly with both upward strokes.

4. With reference to Figure 3 and Figure 4, which of the following choices most likely explains the relative constancy of pressure during two of the four strokes?

   A. One of the strokes involves the combustion of gas.
   B. The piston moves in two directions.
   C. Valves are closed during two of the four strokes.
   D. Valves are open during two of the four strokes.

5. If the value of n for an Otto internal combustion engine were changed from 1.4 to 1.8, the thermal efficiency (T_e) would: (assume r > 1)

   A. be positive and increase.
   B. be negative and increase.
   C. be positive and decrease.
   D. be negative and decrease.

6. As described in the passage, which of the following does NOT apply to the crank shaft during the operation of an internal combustion engine?

   A. It is in rotational equilibrium.
   B. It experiences no net translational force.
   C. It experiences a net torque.
   D. It is dependent on the power stroke for its continued motion.

7. Assume that an internal combustion engine is fitted with a small aircraft propeller and attached to a sled. The engine-propeller combination propels the sled forward with a horizantal force of 10,000 N causing the sled to move at a constant velocity of 25m/s. Ignoring air resistance, which of the following alterations would require the engine to apply a 20,000 N force in order to keep the sled moving at 25 m/s?

   A. Reducing, by half, the net force on the piston during the power stroke.
   B. Reducing, by half, the length of the sled.
   C. Doubling the mass of the sled, engine, and propeller.
   D. Doubling the weight of the engine and propeller without altering the weight of the sled.

8. On which of the following substances does the operation of an internal combustion engine depend?

   A. Nitrogen
   B. Oxygen
   C. Coal
   D. Electricity

5.3 MASTERY VERIFIED: ANSWERS AND EXPLANATIONS

1. *B is correct.* According to Newton's first law, a body that is set in motion by a force will remain in motion at constant velocity unless acted upon by some other force. The fact that a body has mass has no bearing on the matter, since all bodies have mass. If, as is suggested in choice C, the piston experienced no forces during strokes 1, 2, and 4, it would not experience any change in velocity. The most obvious force at issue in this instance is that of friction between the piston and the cylinder walls.

2. *B is correct.* Here you should apply Newton's first law and its corollaries that relate to tension. You should understand that to state that an object moves at constant velocity is to state that it does not experience acceleration. If an object, whether stationary or in motion, is suspended by a flexible connector (such as a cable), and the object does not experience acceleration, it can be concluded that the forces exerted at each end of the connector are equal. The object attached to the lower end of the cable has a *weight* of 120 kg $\times 10$ m/s², or 1200 N. Since the object experiences no acceleration, the force exerted by the engine at the top of the cable is equal to 1200 N, and the tension in the cable is also equal to 1200 N. Choice A would be correct if you were asked to calculate the *net force* on the object.

3. *C is correct.* Here you need to examine Figure 3 in connection with the passage's text. The two upward strokes are compression and exhaust. Examination of Figure 3 shows that during the exhaust phase there is little movement along the y-axis (pressure). During the compression phase, however, there is steep movement upward along the y-axis. During the downward strokes—intake and power—pressure is relatively constant in the first and decreases in the second.

4. *D is correct.* Here you are told that, with reference to Figures 3 and 4, pressure is a "measure of force per unit area." (This is the standard definition.) The forces at issue are those first generated by the combustion of fuel. When the intake and outlet valves are closed, the area over which the force has to act is limited to the inside of the cylinder. When the valves are open, the available area expands, as it does when the piston moves. If the available area changes, F/a must change as well. The opening of the valves during the intake and exhaust strokes explains the relative constancy of pressure during those phases of the cycle.

   You should have little reason to examine Figure 4, even though the question leads you to it. The figure would be unfamiliar and intimidating to most MCAT candidates, and scrupulous examination of it would not, in this case, be likely to affect the selection of a correct answer. Indeed, like many figures set forth in MCAT passages, Figure 4 is unnecessary.

5. *A is correct.* The question draws on the student's ability to transcend the apparent complexity of the passage's subject matter and appreciate the dynamics of a mathematical equation quite apart from its context. The entire value for thermal efficiency (T_e) is equal to 1 *minus* a fractional number:

$$1 - \frac{1}{r^{n-1}}$$

Since r is greater than 1, T_e will always be positive.

The larger the fractional number, the smaller is T_e, since it is subtracted from 1. The size of the fractional number depends on the relative values of its numerator and denominator. Its numerator is fixed at 1. Its denominator, however, is subject to two variables, r and n. The problem is an increase in n, which describes an increase in the value of the exponent of r.

Since r is greater than 1, the increased size of the exponent will increase the value of the denominator, decrease the size of the fraction, and *increase* the overall value of

$$1 - \frac{1}{r^{n-1}}.$$

Therefore, if n is increased, it will bring about an increase in thermal efficiency.

6. *A is correct*. The crank shaft (shown in cross section in Figure 1) rotates so that the piston is able to maintain its upward and downward motion. The fact that the acceleration of the piston is not uniform means that the crankshaft is not in rotational equilibrium and that it does experience a net torque. This eliminates choice C, and the student is directed toward choice A. Choice B is a true statement. The crankshaft does not accelerate translationally and thus experiences no net translational force. All motion within the engine is dependent upon the power stroke. D therefore is a true statement.

7. *C is correct*. The net forward force provided by the propeller must be equal to the net backward force imposed by friction for the engine to maintain the sled at a constant velocity. Friction is equal to the product of the normal force and the coefficient of friction. The normal force is proportional to mass, so doubling the mass will double the force of friction. To keep the sled moving forward at constant velocity, the engine and propeller would have to double their forward force from 10,000 N to 20,000 N.

8. *B is correct*. In the passage's first paragraph, you are told that the internal combustion engine depends on a "gaseous mixture containing O_2." Oxygen is a necessity; the fuel may vary. Combustion, you are told, is often attributable to a spark which, in turn, is often generated by electricity. But you are not told that the spark *must* be generated by electricity. Diesel engines do not require an electric spark.

CHAPTER 6

ENERGY, WORK, POWER, AND MOMENTUM

6.1 MASTERY ACHIEVED

6.1.1 WORK

With respect to any body:

work = (force applied in the direction of displacement)(displacement)

$$W = F \cdot d$$

Because work is the product of force and displacement, it is expressed in the SI unit N•m, which is also called the **joule** (J). **Torque** is also expressed in N•m, but is not expressed in joules. This is because torque is a vector quantity. Work is scalar, and the joule is a scalar unit:

$$N \cdot m = 1 \, J$$

Please solve this problem:

- If a 50 kg object is pushed to the right with a 30 N force in the same direction for a distance of 1 kilometer along a frictionless surface, how much work is performed on the object?

Problem solved:

The mass of the object is irrelevant, because the applied force is provided:

$$W = Fd = (30 \text{ N})(1{,}000 \text{ m}) = 30{,}000 \text{ N} \bullet \text{m} = 30{,}000 \text{ J}$$

Attend carefully to the fact that a component of work is **displacement**, which refers to **net movement (4.1.2)**. This fact gives rise to a counterintuitive phenomenon of which the MCAT candidate must be aware. *If a body is subjected to conservative forces that ultimately return the body to its initial position and state of motion, the total work performed on that body is zero.* For example, if an object weighing 10 newtons is lifted from the ground a distance of 5 meters and then lowered again to the ground, displacement is zero, and thus work is zero, as well.

Please solve this problem:

A 10 N force is applied as shown to a 10 kg object. If the object is displaced by 10 meters to the right then how much work has been done? (Assume friction to be negligible.)

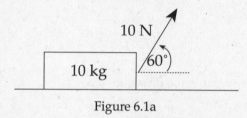

Figure 6.1a

Problem solved:

The work equals only the force applied in the direction of displacement which is 10 N times the cosine of 60 degrees. Thus:

$$W = Fd \cos \theta = (10)(10)(.5) = 50 \text{ J}$$

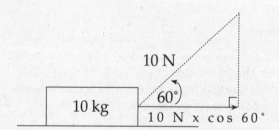

6.1.2 ENERGY

Energy is frequently described as the capacity to do work and is also measured in the SI unit joule (J). Energy may take a variety of forms, including kinetic energy, mechanical potential energy, chemical potential energy, heat energy, and light energy. You should clearly comprehend the relationship between kinetic energy and mechanical potential energy.

6.1.2.1 Kinetic Energy

Kinetic energy (KE) refers to the energy inherent in the movement of an object and can be determined by the formula:

$$KE = \frac{1}{2}mv^2$$

Observe the consistency of units associated with all forms of energy. The value mv² represents the multiplication:

$$(kg)[(m/s)(m/s)] = \frac{kg \bullet m^2}{s^2} = \frac{kg \bullet m}{s^2} \bullet \frac{m}{1} = N \bullet m = J$$

Please solve this problem:

- A 35 kg object falls from a height. When its velocity reaches 18 m/s, what kinetic energy does the object possess?

Problem solved:

Apply the formula:

$$KE = \frac{1}{2}mv^2 = 0.5(35 \text{ kg})(18 \text{ m/s})^2 = 5,670 \text{ J}$$

Please solve this problem:

- What is the kinetic energy of an object that weighs 1,200 newtons travelling at a velocity 90 m/s?

Problem solved:

The object's weight has been supplied but its mass has not. Determine its mass:

$$w = mg = 1,200 \text{ N} = (m)(10 \text{ m/s}^2)$$

$$m = \frac{1,200 \text{ N}}{10 \text{ m/s}^2} = 120 \text{ kg}$$

Apply the formula:

$$KE = \frac{1}{2}mv^2 = 0.5(120 \text{ kg})(90 \text{ m/s})^2 = 486,000 \text{ J}$$

6.1.2.2 Mechanical Potential Energy

The term **mechanical potential energy** describes the energy inherent in the status or position of an object or system. A classic example is a stretched or compressed spring; the spring has the potential to perform work.

Particularly significant to the MCAT candidate is the mechanical potential energy inherent in an object positioned above the earth. This form of mechanical potential energy is called **gravitational potential energy (GPE)**. An object has the capacity to perform work via the force of gravity. For an object situated above the earth, gravitational potential energy =

$$(object's\ mass)(acceleration\ due\ to\ gravity)(object's\ height)$$

$$GPE = mgh$$

Please solve this problem:

- A body with a mass of 75 kg is situated at a height of 30 m above the ground. What is its gravitational potential energy?

Problem solved:

Apply the formula for gravitational potential energy:
$$GPE = mgh = (75\ kg)(10\ m/s^2)(30\ m) = 22,500\ J$$

6.1.2.3 Work as a Function of Kinetic Energy and Gravitational Potential Energy

The quantity of work performed on a body is calcuated with the equation $W = Fd$. When a moving object experiences a change in either its kinetic energy, its potential energy, or both, and there is no change in other forms of energy, work can *also* be described as:

$$(change\ in\ kinetic\ energy) + (change\ in\ potential\ energy)$$

$$W = KE + PE$$

You should be prepared to apply this concept to an object moving upward or downward within the earth's gravitational field when friction and air resistance are negligible. During such an object's travel, it exhibits kinetic energy, and either loses or gains gravitational potential energy, depending on whether it falls or rises, respectively. For such an object, adaption of the equation set forth above yields:

$$W = KE + mgh$$

An object with a mass of 78 kg is initially at rest 40 m above the ground. At Time 1, it is subjected to a force that causes it to move upward at an angle of 20° to the horizontal. At Time 2, the object's height is 65 m and its velocity is 25 m/s (ignore air resistance).

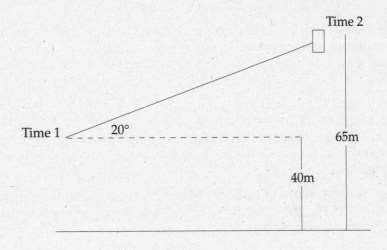

Figure 6.2

The work that has been done on the object between Times 1 and 2 can be determined through the formula $W = \Delta KE + \Delta mgh$. (The 20° angle to the horizontal is irrelevant to this calculation; the MCAT candidate should be aware of this.)

1. Calculate ΔKE:

At Time 1, the object has kinetic energy of zero, and at Time 2 it has kinetic energy =

$$\frac{1}{2}mv^2 = 0.5(78 \text{ kg})(25 \text{ m/s})^2 = 24{,}375 \text{ J}$$

The *change* in kinetic energy = $\Delta KE = 24{,}375 \text{ J} - 0 \text{ J} = 24{,}375 \text{ J}$

2. Calculate ΔGPE:

At Time 1, the object has gravitational potential energy of:

$$GPE = mgh = (78 \text{ kg})(10 \text{ m/s}^2)(40 \text{ m}) = 31{,}200 \text{ J}$$

At Time 2, the object has gravitational potential energy of:

$$GPE = mgh = (78 \text{ kg})(10 \text{ m/s}^2)(65 \text{ m}) = 50{,}700 \text{ J}$$

Change in $GPE = \Delta GPE = 50{,}700 \text{ J} - 31{,}200 \text{ J} = 19{,}500 \text{ J}$

3. Calculate work, according to the formula $W = \Delta KE + \Delta GPE$

$$W = \Delta KE + \Delta GPE = 24{,}375 \text{ J} + 19{,}500 \text{ J} = 43{,}875 \text{ J}$$

6.1.2.4 Conservation of Energy

The law of conservation of energy states:

The energy of an isolated system is constant.

This means that the energy in the universe may change form, but it cannot be destroyed or created. MCAT questions will sometimes draw on the candidate's ability to apply this principle to situations and systems involving the conversion of energy from one form to another.

An object that weighs 12 newtons and is positioned 125 meters above the earth's surface is allowed to fall. Suppose that all of the object's initial gravitational potential energy is converted to kinetic energy; none is converted to heat or any other form of energy. Through conservation of energy, we may calculate, for example, the velocity of the object the moment before it strikes the earth.

Because energy is conserved, and because the object has no gravitational potential energy when it reaches the earth (height = 0: mgh = 0), its kinetic energy at impact must be equal to its initial gravitational potential energy:

$$\frac{1}{2}mv^2 = mgh$$

Knowing that $m = 12$ N, $g = 10$ m/s^2, and $h = 125$ m, we know:

$$\frac{1}{2}(12)\,(v^2) = (12)(10)(125)$$

$$6v^2 = 15{,}000 \text{ J}$$

$$v^2 = 2{,}500 \text{ m}^2/\text{s}^2$$

$$v = 50 \text{ m/s}$$

In practice, an object that falls through the air experiences friction, and so a small portion of gravitational potential energy is converted to heat.

6.1.3 MECHANICAL ADVANTAGE

Recall, once again, that $W = Fd$. Therefore, keeping work constant, applied force is inversely proportional to distance.

Various simple machines afford **mechanical advantage** by reducing the force required, and consequently increasing the distance required by a corresponding factor. Common machines tested on the MCAT are the pulley, the lever, and the inclined plane.

For example, if an 80 newton object is to be lifted a distance of 12 meters, the work required is equal to (80 N)(12 m) = 960 J. If the object were to be lifted directly upward without machinery, the applied force would be 80 N, and the displacement 12 m. If, however, a simple machine is used, *the necessary force is reduced, while the displacement is increased by a corresponding factor.*

On the MCAT, questions concerning mechanical advantage and simple machines draw on the candidate's understanding that using a machine does not reduce the work to be done, it reduces the *force* (and increases the necessary displacement) and the application of inverse proportionality.

These phenomena are most easily illustrated with an inclined plane. Suppose the 80 N object of the previous example was pushed upward along a frictionless plane inclined 20° to the horizontal to a vertical displacement of 12 meters, as shown in Figure 6.3 (sin 20° = 0.342):

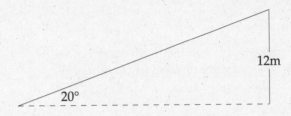

Figure 6.3

Simple trigonometry (**1.1.3**) provides the length of the inclined plane (d):

$$\sin 20° = 12 \, m/d$$

$$(d)(\sin 20°) = 12 \text{ m}$$

$$(d)(0.342) = 12 \text{ m}$$

$$d = 35 \text{ m}$$

Knowing that work of 960 J will be done by moving an 80 N object 35 m up an inclined plane, calculate the force associated with the work thus performed:

$$W = Fd$$

$$960 \text{ J} = F(35 \text{ m})$$

$$F = \frac{960}{35} = \text{approx. } 27.4 \text{ N}$$

To lift an 80 N object 12 m from the ground along a plane inclined at 20° requires the application of approximately 27.4 N. To lift this object without machinery would require the application of 80 N of force.

You should think of mechanical advantage as *a reduction in force and an increase in displacement*.

6.1.4 POWER

Power refers to the quantity of work performed over time.

$$P = W/t$$

It is expressed in joules/second. In the SI system 1 joule per second is renamed the **watt (W)**.

$$1\,J/s = 1\,W$$

Please solve this problem:

- How much power is needed to lift an object with a mass of 75 kg straight upward to a height of 16 m in 22 seconds?

Problem solved:

The object's mass is 75 kg, and its weight is:

$$W = 75\,kg(10\,m/s^2) = 750\,N$$

The lift will involve work of:

$$W = Fd = (750\,N)(16\,m) = 12{,}000\,J$$

If 12,000 joules of work are to be performed in 22 seconds, the associated power =

$$12{,}000\,J/22\,s = 545.45\,W$$

You should follow this analysis of the units associated with power:

(1) "watt" is equivalent to J/s

(2) "joule" is equivalent to N•m, and the watt is therefore equivalent to N•m/s which also represents the product: (force)(velocity).

Note that power is equivalent to (force)(velocity) and that *the quantity of power necessary to maintain any object at constant velocity is equal to the product:*

$$(\text{net force on the object})(\text{velocity})$$

$$P = Fv$$

Please solve this problem:

- An engine that delivers power of 24,750 watts lifts an object straight upward against the force of earth's gravity with a constant velocity of 330 m/s. Determine the mass of the object (and assume friction to be negligible).

Problem solved:

For any object maintained in motion at constant velocity:

$$P = Fv$$

In this instance, power = 24,750 W and velocity = 330 m/s

$$24,750 \text{ W} = F(330 \text{ m/s})$$

$$F = \frac{24,750}{330}$$
$$F = 75 \text{ N}$$

The force applied by the engine to keep the object moving upward at constant velocity = 75 N, which, if we assume no air resistance, means the object's weight = 75 N. This means its mass is:

$$\frac{75 \text{ N}}{10 \text{ m/s}^2} = 7.5 \text{ kg}$$

6.1.5 LINEAR MOMENTUM

For any object, linear momentum equals (mass of body)(velocity):

$$P = mv$$

In terms of SI units the product represents:

$$(\text{kg})(\text{m/s})$$

and momentum is therefore expressed in the SI unit kg•m/s.

Please solve this problem:

- If an object with mass of 110 kg moves to the west with a velocity of 18 m/s, what is its momentum?

Problem solved:

The problem draws on the formula:
$$P = mv$$

$$(110 \text{ kg})(18 \text{ m/s}) = 1,980 \text{ kg•m/s}$$

Because momentum has direction, it is a vector quantity. The MCAT draws on the concept of linear momentum in terms of conservation of momentum when objects collide or separate.

6.1.5.1 Conservation of Linear Momentum

On the MCAT, collisions between two objects are elastic or inelastic. An elastic collision results in the two colliding bodies rebounding with no loss of total kinetic energy. An inelastic collision results in the transformation of at least some of the kinetic energy to heat energy when the two bodies collide.

When two moving bodies collide, they both experience a change in velocity (magnitude, direction, or both). The nature of the change depends on surrounding factors.

For the MCAT, the law of conservation of linear momentum provides that when bodies A and B collide, the total momentum of the two bodies is unchanged by the collision. Therefore:

(momentum of body A *before* collision) + (momentum of body B *before* collision)

=

(momentum of body A *after* collision) + (momentum of body B *after* collision)

Please solve this problem:

- Body A has a mass of 18 kg and travels through space to the left at 14 m/s. Body B has a mass of 27 kg and travels through space to the right (it travels in a direction exactly opposite to that of body A)—at 12 m/s. The two bodies undergo a perfectly inelastic collision and join to become a single body. What is the magnitude and direction (right or left) of the velocity at which the newly formed body moves?

Problem solved:

The problem concerns conservation of linear momentum. The two velocities are of opposite sign. If we decide that the velocity of body A is (+) and that of body B is (−), then:

$$m_1 v_1 + m_2 v_2 \text{ after collision} = (m_1 + m_2)v_f$$

$$(18 \text{ kg})(14 \text{ m/s}) + (27 \text{ kg})(-12 \text{ m/s}) = (18 + 27)(v) = 45v$$

$$45v = (18 \text{ kg})(14 \text{ m/s}) + (27 \text{ kg})(-12 \text{ m/s})$$

$$v = -\frac{72}{45}$$

$$v = -1.6 \text{ m/s} = 1.6 \text{ m/s to the right}$$

6.1.5.1.1 Conservation of Kinetic Energy in Collisions

Momentum is conserved for all collisions, elastic and inelastic. You should know that kinetic energy is conserved in perfectly elastic collisions, but not in inelastic collisions. With respect to two bodies, A and B, undergoing a perfectly elastic collision,

$$\frac{1}{2}mv^2 \text{ (body A)} + \frac{1}{2}mv^2 \text{ (body B)} \qquad \textit{before} \text{ the collision}$$

$$=$$

$$\frac{1}{2}mv^2 \text{ (body A)} + \frac{1}{2}mv^2 \text{ (body B)} \qquad \textit{after} \text{ the collision}$$

In an inelastic collsion, kinetic energy is not conserved; some is converted to heat. Total energy, however, is conserved.

Please solve this problem:

- Body A has a mass of 86 kg and travels through space with a velocity of magnitude 20 m/s. Body B has a mass of 40 kg and travels through space with a velocity of magnitude 12 m/s. The bodies undergo a perfectly inelastic collision at such an angle as to move off together as a single body with velocity of magnitude 15 m/s. In this inelastic collision, how much energy is converted from kinetic energy to heat?

Problem solved:

The problem relies on the concept that all kinetic energy lost in an inelastic collision is converted to heat. Solve by first calculating the total kinetic energy of both bodies before the collision:

$$\frac{1}{2}mv^2 \text{ (body 1)} + \frac{1}{2}mv^2 \text{ (body 2)} =$$

$$0.5(86 \text{ kg})(20 \text{ m/s})^2 + 0.5 (40 \text{ kg})(12 \text{ m/s})^2 =$$

$$17{,}200 \text{ J} + 2{,}880 \text{ J} = 20{,}080 \text{ J}$$

Calculate the kinetic energy of the new body after the collision:

$$\frac{1}{2}mv^2 = 0.5(86 \text{ kg} + 40 \text{ kg})(15 \text{ m/s})^2 = 14{,}175 \text{ J}$$

A total of (20,080 – 14,175 J) = 5,905 J of kinetic energy is lost in the inelastic collision. This means the collision generates 5,905 J of heat.

6.2 MASTERY APPLIED: SAMPLE PASSAGE AND QUESTIONS

Passage

The modern bicycle reflects several centuries of progress in engineering and design. In the early 1880s, a bicycle nicknamed the "ordinary" became popular. It featured an extraordinarily large front wheel and pedals situated relatively close to that wheel's axis of rotation, as shown in Figure 1.

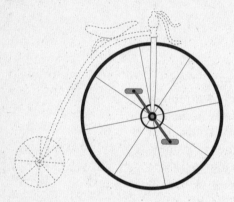

Figure 1

The construction of the "ordinary" meant that each revolution of the rider's legs produced one revolution of the wheel, although the circumference of the rider's revolution was much less than that of the front wheel itself. Variations on the ordinary were undertaken in order to afford the rider more mechanical advantage. One variation extended the lengths of the shafts on which the pedals were held so that the rider's legs would travel a circumference more nearly equal that of the wheel, as shown in Figure 2.

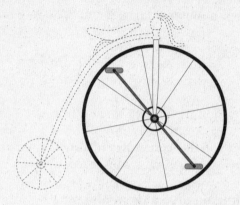

Figure 2

Advances in mechanical engineering led to a bicycle on which the pedals drove a toothed sprocket connected by a flexible chain to a toothed sprocket on the rear wheel. Lateral mobility of the chain at the rear aspect, within the control of the rider, provided the possibility of positioning the rear portion of the chain on relatively larger or smaller sprockets to adjust the mechanical advantage. The relatively larger sprockets on the rear afforded the rider a greater degree of mechanical advantage than did the relatively smaller ones.

More recent models provide multiple gears at the pedaling axis so that the mechanical advantage may be changed. On these vehicles, a rider will have difficulty propelling himself uphill with the chain revolving about the largest front gear since that requires a greater force. Moreover, the design of these multi-geared machines prevents movement of the chain unless the bicycle is in motion.

Increased efficiency was also achieved by the advent of the pneumatic tire and by the subsequent narrowing of its gauge.

1. A bicycle rider with a mass of m_r rides a bicycle with a mass of m_b. He pedals d meters directly up a hill, inclined at an angle of $\theta°$ to the horizontal. On reaching the top of the hill, he has achieved a true vertical *height* of h meters from the point at which he started. Where g = acceleration due to gravity, which of the following expression describes the work the rider has performed in riding up the hill? (Assume friction to be negligible.)

   A. $(g)(h)(m_r + m_b)$
   B. $(m_r^2 + m_b^2)(\cos \theta)$
   C. $(d)\cos \theta (h^2)$
   D. $m_b gd$

2. If the rider described in question 1 above turns around and coasts downward along the incline, what will be the normal force exerted on his bicycle?

   A. dgh
   B. $(\theta)^2 (g)^2 (m_r + gm_b)$
   C. $(\sin \theta) (gm_r + m_b)$
   D. $(\cos \theta) (gm_r + gm_b)$

3. Two riders, A and B, of equal mass, ride (separate) bicycles, also of equal mass. The bicycles are fitted with derailleurs that allow for adjustment of the mechanical advantage by lateral movement of the chain among several gears located on the rear axle. Rider A positions the chain on a smaller rear sprocket than does Rider B, and both riders travel the exact same path covering a displacement over the road of d. (Assume friction to be negligible.) Which of the following is true?

   A. Rider A performs less work on the pedals than does Rider B.
   B. Rider A performs more work on the pedals than does Rider B.
   C. Riders A and B perform equal quantities of work on the pedals.
   D. Neither Rider A nor Rider B performs any work on the pedals.

4. The engineer who designed the modified "ordinary," as shown in Figure 2 most probably attempted to achieve which objective?

   A. Reduce the amount of work performed by the rider
   B. Reduce the amount of force applied by the rider
   C. Increase the velocity attained by the rider for any given quantity of work performed
   D. Increase the acceleration attained by the rider for any given quantity of work performed

5. Rider A rides an old-fashioned "ordinary" (shown in Figure 1) and Rider B rides a modified ordinary (shown in Figure 2). The bicycles are of equal mass. Rider A attains a westward velocity of v_1 and Rider B attains a westward velocity of v_2, which is equal to $2(v_1)$. Assuming that Riders A and B are of equal mass, which of the following is true?

   A. Rider B achieves a momentum equal to one half that of Rider A.
   B. Rider B achieves a momentum twice that of Rider A.
   C. Rider B achieves a momentum equal to that of Rider A.
   D. The sum: (momentum achieved by Rider A + momentum achieved by Rider B) remains constant, even if each rider changes her velocity.

6. An investigator wishes to know which of two innovations afforded the greater advance in efficiency: the introduction of narrow gauge tires or the availability of multiple sprockets. She conducts an experiment in which Subject 1 rides a bicycle with *wide* gauge tires and *no* multiple sprockets; Subject 2 rides a bicycle with *wide* gauge tires *and* multiple sprockets; and Subject 3 rides a bicycle with *narrow* gauge tires and *no* multiple sprockets. In relation to her experiment, which rider constitutes the control?

   A. Subject 1
   B. Subject 2
   C. Subject 3
   D. Subjects 1 and 2 together

7. In terms of mechanical advantage, the use on a modern bicycle of a relatively small sprocket on the axle attached to the pedals is roughly analogous to:

   A. the introduction of pneumatic tires.
   B. the use on a modern bicycle of a relatively small sprocket on the rear axle.
   C. creating a large wheel on the original "ordinary."
   D. increasing the size of the pedal shafts on the modifed "ordinary."

6.3 MASTERY VERIFIED: ANSWERS AND EXPLANATIONS

1. *A is correct.* The work he has performed is equal to Fd, but you are not provided with any variable representing F. He is, however, provided with the variables associated with the gravitational potential energy the rider has garnered in climbing the hill. The gravitational energy, mgh, must be equal to the work the rider has performed. Therefore, the answer is one that reflects the formula mgh.

    In this instance, m is equal to the combined mass of rider and bicycle, $m_r + m_b$. The height $= h$ and $g =$ acceleration due to gravity. Therefore, the answer is

    $$(g) \times (h) \times (m_r + m_b)$$

    You should note that the answer is a formula with which you are familiar: GPE = mgh. It has only been presented in an unfamiliar form. *You should become accustomed to questions that require you to work with abstract variables instead of numerical values.*

2. *D is correct.* The normal force (N) is the force exerted by the plane onto the bicycle. The normal force is equal to the weight of the object times the cosine of the angle of the plane from the horizontal. The combined weight of the bicycle and rider $= (g)(m_r + m_b)$, which, through the distributive property of multiplication, is equal to $(gm_r + gm_b)$. Simple trigonometry reveals that $N = (\cos \theta)(\text{combined weight}) = (\cos \theta)(gm_r + gm_b)$.

3. *C is correct.* Recall that mechanical advantage reduces force, but not work. This concept alone yields the answer to the question.

4. *B is correct.* Like question 3 above, this question can be answered by understanding that mechanical advantage affects force, but not work. The passage states that the extension of the pedal shafts was undertaken in order to afford mechanical advantage. Again, you have to look within the passage and questions for the principles and phenomena that you're familiar with.

5. *B is correct.* The bicycles do not collide, and there is no occasion here to consider conservation of momentum. The fact that the two bicycles differ in design is similarly irrelevant to the problem. Rather, you need only apply the formula:

    $$\text{momentum} = (m)(v)$$

    Remember that momentum is directly proportional to velocity. Since Rider B attains a velocity that has a magnitude twice that of Rider A on equivalent masses, she achieves also a momentum that is twice that of Rider A.

6. *A is correct.* The experimenter is testing the effects of two innovations: narrow gauge tires and multiple sprockets. In order to compare their effects as innovations she must have, as a control, a device that offers *neither feature.* Subject 1 rides a bicycle that lacks both innovations.

7. *D is correct.* The question calls for careful reading. The passage indicates that the modified "ordinary" was designed in order to afford the rider greater mechanical advantage. It also indicates, with reference to the modern bicycle, that "a rider will have difficulty propelling himself uphill with the chain revolving about the largest of sprockets at the front aspect since that tends to require a greater force from him." The reference to greater force means that the large sprocket offers relatively smaller degree of mechanical advantage. The small sprocket, therefore, must offer a greater degree of mechanical advantage and so is analogous to the lengthening of the shafts on the modified "ordinary."

CHAPTER 7

FLUIDS AND SOLIDS

7.1 MASTERY ACHIEVED

7.1.1 SOLIDS

Solids are distinct from fluids in that they do not flow.

7.1.1.1 Density and Specific Gravity

For any solid, density is a measure of mass per volume and is expressed in the SI unit kilogram per cubic meter:

$$\frac{kg}{m^3}$$

The statement that "lead is heavier than cotton" lacks scientific meaning. Rather, lead is *more dense* than cotton: any given volume of lead has greater mass (and hence weight) than the same volume of cotton. For any sample of solid, volume may be obtained, among other methods, by immersing the solid in liquid and observing the volume of liquid that is displaced.

Density can be treated as a *unit conversion ratio*, where mass is calculated on the basis of volume, or volume on the basis of mass.

Please solve this problem:

- If a substance has density of 9.3×10^4 kg/m³, what volume is occupied by 88 kg of the substance?

Problem solved:

$$\text{density} = \frac{\text{mass}}{\text{volume}}$$

$$\text{volume} = \frac{\text{mass}}{\text{density}} = \frac{88 \text{ kg}}{9.3 \times 10^4 \text{ kg}/\text{m}^3} = 9.5 \times 10^{-4} \text{m}^3$$

The density of water is 1,000 kg/m³. For any solid, the value known as **specific gravity** represents the ratio of density of the solid to density of water. A solid whose density is 2,000 kg/m³—twice that of water—has a specific gravity of 2. The same holds for fluids: a fluid whose density is 600 kg/m³—0.60 times that of water—has a specific gravity of 0.60.

Because specific gravity reflects the division:

$$\frac{\left[\text{density}\left(\dfrac{\text{kg}}{\text{m}^3}\right)\right] \text{Solid}}{\left[\text{density}\left(\dfrac{\text{kg}}{\text{m}^3}\right)\right] \text{H}_2\text{O}}$$

the result is expressed without units. Specific gravity is a dimensionless quantity.

Please solve this problem:

- A container with total capacity of 1.0×10^{-3} m³ is half-filled with water so that the fluid level reaches the mark, 0.5×10^{-3} m³. A solid object with mass of 0.2 kg is completely submerged in the water. The presence of the object causes the fluid level in the container to rise to 0.75×10^{-3} m³. What is the density of the object? What is the specific gravity of the object?

Problem solved:

Density = mass/volume. The object's mass is 0.2 kg. Its volume is equal to the volume of liquid it displaces:

$$(0.75 \times 10^{-3} \text{ m}^3) - (0.50 \times 10^{-3} \text{ m}^3) = 0.25 \times 10^{-3} \text{ m}^3$$

Its density is calculated by:

$$\frac{0.2 \text{ kg}}{0.25 \times 10^{-3} \text{ m}^3} = \frac{\left(0.2 \times 10^0\right) \text{kg}}{0.25 \times 10^{-3} \text{ m}^3} = 0.8 \times 10^3 \ \frac{\text{kg}}{\text{m}^3} = 800 \text{ kg/m}^3$$

Thus its specific gravity can be determined:

$$800/1{,}000 = 0.8$$

7.1.1.2 Tensile Stress, Tensile Strain, and Young's Modulus

The subjects of stress, strain and the associated quantity Young's modulus pertain to the application of stretching and compressive forces to elongated solids. You should understand these phenomena inasmuch as they pertain to substances that obey Hooke's law; the MCAT does not address them in contexts beside that.

7.1.1.2.1 Tensile Stress

Tensile stress (T_{ss}) refers to a force that (a) is applied equally at both ends of a solid object, and (b) tends to stretch *or* compress it. Consider stress as it relates to forces applied at either end of an elongated object such as a bar, rod or pole:

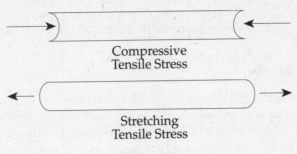

Figure 7.1

Tensile stress is measured in terms of applied force per cross-sectional area of solid. In the SI unit system, it represents the quantity, N/m^2. For convenience, $1 \, N/m^2$ is termed the **pascal (Pa)**:

$$1 \, N/m^2 = 1 \, Pa$$

Tensile stress (T_{ss}) is normally expressed in the unit Pa.

Consider a cylindrical rod with radius of 3 cm (0.03 m). The rod's cross-sectional area is calculated by:

$$\pi r^2 = (3.14)(0.03)^2 = 2.83 \times 10^{-3} \, m^2$$

If the rod is subjected to a 90 newton stretching force at each end, the stress it experiences is found by:

$$\frac{force}{cross\text{-}sectional \; area} = \frac{90 \, N}{2.83 \times 10^{-3} m^2} = \frac{90 \times 10^0 \, N}{2.83 \times 10^{-3} m^2} = 31.80 \times 10^3 \, Pa$$

The same computation applies to both stretching and compressing forces applied to an object:

$$T_{ss} = F/A_{cs}$$

Please solve this problem:

- A rectangular steel bar, the ends of which have two edges measuring 3 cm and 4 cm, respectively, is subjected at each end to a compressive force of 40 N. What tensile stress does the bar experience?

Problem solved:

Use the formula: $T_{ss} = F/A_{cs}$.

Calculate the bar's cross-sectional area (A_{cs}):

$$(0.04 \, m)(0.03 \, m) = 0.0012 \, m^2 = 1.2 \times 10^{-3} \, m^2$$

Since applied force is 40 N, T_{ss}, the tensile stress is:

$$\frac{force}{cross\text{-}sectional \; area} = \frac{40 \, N}{1.2 \times 10^{-3} m^2} = \frac{40 \times 10^0 \, N}{1.2 \times 10^{-3} m^2} = 33.33 \times 10^3 \, Pa$$

In the foregoing illustrations, tensile stress was calculated without regard to the solid object's length. Note that calculation of tensile stress takes into account cross-sectional area (A_{cs}), but not length. Length *is* relevant to the calculation of tensile strain, however, as you will see below.

7.1.1.2.2 TENSILE STRAIN

Tensile strain (T_{sn}) refers to the degree to which tensile *stress* causes a solid object to undergo a change in length. It is measured as a function of change in length relative to the original length. If a solid object of length 2 meters undergoes tensile stress that stretches it, and as a result actually lengthens so that its new length is 2.01 meters, the object experiences tensile strain (T_{sn}) of:

$$\Delta L / L_o = \frac{2.01 \text{ m} - 2.0 \text{ m}}{2.0 \text{ m}} = \frac{.01 \text{ m}}{2.0 \text{ m}} = .005$$

Note that the result shows no units. Strain is a dimensionless quantity; it is expressed without units.

Compressive tensile stress is calculated in the same way.

Please solve this problem:

- A rectangular bar of length 34 meters is subjected to a compressive force at either end, and its length is reduced to 33.97 meters. What tensile strain has the object experienced?

Problem solved:

The object experiences tensile strain (T_{sn}) of:

$$\Delta L / L_o = \frac{34 \text{ m} - 33.97 \text{ m}}{34 \text{ m}} = \frac{0.03 \text{ m}}{34 \text{ m}} = .00088 = 8.8 \times 10^{-4}$$

Note that both cross-sectional area and the magnitude of applied force are irrelevant to the calculation of tensile strain. Observe that:

- The calculation of *stress* draws on applied force and cross-sectional area (A_{cs}).

- The calculation of *strain* draws on change in length and original length.

Tensile stress and tensile strain are related by Young's modulus.

7.1.1.2.3 YOUNG'S MODULUS

For any solid that obeys Hooke's law, **Young's modulus** represents the ratio:

$$\frac{\text{tensile stress}}{\text{tensile strain}}$$

Every substance that obeys Hooke's law is associated with its own Young's modulus—a value which, *for that particular substance*, expresses the degree of strain that will be imposed by a given degree of stress. Because Young's modulus represents:

$$\frac{\text{stress (in Pa)}}{\text{strain (no units)}}$$

it gives rise to the fraction $\frac{Pa}{1}$ = Pa. Therefore, Young's modulus is expressed in pascals.

For any substance, knowledge of Young's modulus permits algebraic calculation of stress, when strain is known, and of strain, when stress is known.

Consider an object composed of substance X, for which Young's modulus is 7.5×10^5 Pa. If it is subjected to a tensile stress of 50 Pa, it will undergo a degree of strain as calculated below:

$$\frac{50 \text{ Pa}}{\text{tensile strain}} = 7.5 \times 10^5 \text{ Pa}$$

$$(\text{tensile strain})(7.5 \times 10^5 \text{ Pa}) = 50 \text{ Pa}$$

$$(\text{tensile strain}) = \frac{50 \text{ Pa}}{7.5 \times 10^5 \text{ Pa}} = 6.67 \times 10^{-5}$$

(The problem does not specify whether the imposed stress was stretching or compressive; the math is the same in either case.)

Please solve this problem :

- A cylindrical rod measures 5 m in length and 1.5 cm in radius. It obeys Hooke's law and has a Young's modulus of 5.2×10^6 Pa. What compressive force is necessary to reduce its length to 4.9981 meters?

Problem solved:

Note that you are asked to identify *force*, not stress. Since stress represents F/A_{cs} force is ascertained by: (1) the calculation of cross-sectional area by reference to the data; and (2) the calculation of strain, by reference to original and modified lengths; which allows for (3) the calculation of stress via Young's modulus; which allows for (4) the calculation of force via the formula $T_{ss} = F/A_{cs}$.

Calculate cross-sectional area (A_{cs}):

$$A_{cs} = \pi r^2 = 3.14 \,(.015)^2 = .00071 \text{ m}^2 = 7.1 \times 10^{-4} \text{ m}^2$$

Calculate strain:

$$\text{strain} = \Delta L/L_o = \frac{5 \text{ m} - 4.9981 \text{ m}}{5 \text{ m}} = \frac{.0019 \text{ m}}{5 \text{ m}} = .00038 = 3.8 \times 10^{-4}$$

Calculate stress:

$$\frac{\text{Stress}}{\text{Strain}} = 5.2 \times 10^6 \text{ Pa}$$

$$\frac{\text{Stress}}{3.8 \times 10^{-4}} = 5.2 \times 10^6 \text{ Pa}$$

$$\text{stress} = (5.2 \times 10^6 \text{ Pa}) \times (3.8 \times 10^{-4}) = 1.98 \times 10^3 \text{ Pa}$$

Calculate force by rearranging $T_{ss} = F/A_{cs}$:

$$F = (T_{ss})(A_{cs}) = (1.98 \times 10^3 \text{ Pa})(7.1 \times 10^{-4} \text{ m}^2)$$

$$F = 1.4 \text{ N}$$

Checking for dimensional consistency in the last calculation, note that:

$$\text{Pa} = \text{N/m}^2$$

and:

$$(\text{Pa})(\text{m}^2) = (\text{N/m}^2) \times (\text{m}^2) = \text{N}$$

7.1.2 FLUIDS

7.1.2.1 Density and Specific Gravity

Any substance that, when poured into a container, takes on the shape of that container can be considered a fluid.

Every fluid, like every solid, is associated with a specific gravity, which is represented by the ratio of the density of fluid to the density of water (which, as noted above, is $\frac{1,000 \text{ kg}}{\text{m}^3}$). A fluid whose density is three times that of water has specific gravity of 3. A fluid whose density is 0.25 times that of water has a specific gravity of 0.25.

For any ordinary liquid (as for any ordinary solid), density is relatively constant under varying conditions of temperature and pressure. For gases, however, density is subject to change. The density of a gas must be described in terms of a given temperature and pressure.

7.1.2.2 Fluid Pressure

Pressure is a measure of force per unit area and is expressed in the SI unit N/m^2, which, as was discussed earlier, is called the pascal (Pa). Pressure, like stress, is expressed in pascals, and you should note that stress and pressure are related.

Fluid pressure refers to the pressure exerted by a fluid on a real or hypothetical body. Fluid exerts a pressure of P on an object submerged in it at depth d. Whether or not an object is in fact situated at depth d, the fluid pressure still exists at d; it represents the pressure that *would* be exerted on an object situated within the fluid at the given depth.

For any resting fluid that is not experiencing any external pressure, the fluid pressure at a specified depth is given by the formula:

P = (density)(acceleration due to gravity)(depth below the surface of the fluid)

Depth is often conceived of as the height (h) of the fluid column above the point in question, and the formula just described is often expressed:

$$P = \rho(g)(h)$$

where:

ρ = fluid density

g = acceleration due to gravity

h = height of the fluid above the point in question

The above pressure is referred to as gauge pressure. In real situations the fluid within which pressure is to be measured will often be exposed to atmospheric pressure at its surface. When measuring the pressure at a depth 'h' below the surface of such a fluid, atmospheric pressure is added directly as follows: $P = (\rho)(g)(h)$ + atmospheric pressure.

This new sum is called **absolute pressure**. It is the actual pressure to which a submerged object is exposed.

Pascal's principle says that *pressure applied to an enclosed fluid is transmitted undiminished to every portion of the fluid and the walls of the containing vessel.*

Accordingly, the following statement is also true:

Fluid pressure at any given depth in a resting fluid is unrelated to the shape of the container in which the fluid is situated.

Observe the proportion in the formula for fluid pressure. Pressure is directly proportional to fluid density and to depth.

Please solve this problem:

- Fluid F has density d. At a given depth x, within a sample of fluid F, fluid pressure is 3000 Pa. What is the fluid pressure at depth $2x$ in a sample of fluid E, whose density is $0.4d$?

Problem solved:

Because fluid pressure is directly proportional to fluid density and depth, the pressure at depth $2x$ in fluid E is calculated from:

$$P = 3{,}000 \text{ Pa} \times (0.4)d \times 2x = 0.8(3{,}000 \text{ Pa}) = 2{,}400 \text{ Pa}$$

7.1.2.3 Buoyancy

Buoyancy refers to a fluid's tendency to propel submerged or partially submerged substances toward the surface of that fluid. The buoyancy force then is an upward force exerted by a fluid on another body or fluid.

For any body immersed in fluid, the magnitude of buoyancy is calculated using **Archimedes' principle**:

Buoyancy $(F_b) = $

(volume of fluid displaced)(density of displaced fluid)(acceleration due to gravity)

$$F_b = (V)(\rho)(g)$$

Observe that the quantity just set forth is in fact equal to the *weight* of the fluid displaced, which is verified by examination for dimensional consistency:

$$(m^3)(kg/m^3)(m/s^2) = (m^4 \cdot kg/m^3 \cdot s^2) = (kg \cdot m/s^2) = \text{newton (N)}.$$

Archimides' principle may thus be restated:

Buoyancy (F_b) = weight of fluid displaced

Therefore, for any body immersed in a fluid, buoyancy represents a force with upward direction and a magnitude equal to the weight of the fluid displaced. In this connection one should recall that a fully submerged body will displace a volume of fluid equal to its own volume.

An object immersed in a fluid experiences a downward force equal to its own weight, and an upward force equal to the force of buoyancy (F_b), as just described. Whether the object accelerates downward (sinks) or upward depends on the relative magnitudes of the downward and upward forces.

Please solve this problem:

- An object with density of 11.3×10^3 kg/m^3 and mass of 57 kg is immersed in water and is subjected to no horizontal or rotational forces.

    (1) What (approximately) is the net force experienced by the object?
    (2) Will it accelerate? If so, with what magnitude?

Problem solved:

(1) The only forces to which the object is subject are those of its own weight, and the upward force of buoyancy.

Calculate the object's weight:

$$wt = 57 \text{ kg} \times 10 \text{ m/s}^2 = 570 \text{ N}$$

We wish next to calculate the magnitude of buoyancy (F_b), but that calculation requires that we figure out the volume of water that was displaced. Recalling that the volume of water displaced is equal to the volume of the solid itself, and noting that the solid has a density of 11.3×10^3 kg/m^3 and a mass of 57 kg, we calculate the volume of the solid (and therefore, the volume of the fluid the solid displaces):

$$\text{volume} = \frac{\text{mass}}{\text{density}}$$

$$\text{volume} = \frac{57 \text{ kg}}{11.3 \times 10^3 \text{kg/m}^3}$$

$$\text{volume} = 5.0 \times 10^{-3} \text{ m}^3$$

Knowing now that the solid object displaces 5.0×10^{-3} m^3 of water, and recalling that the density of water is 1,000 kg/m^3, we calculate F_b with Archimedes' principle:

$$F_b = (\text{volume})(\text{density of fluid})(g)$$

$$F_b = (5.0 \times 10^{-3} \text{ m}^3) \times (1 \times 10^3 \text{ kg/m}^3) \times (10 \times 10^0 \text{ m/s}^2) = 50 \text{ N}$$

The object experiences a downward force of 570 N and an upward force of 50 N. It experiences, therefore, a net force of 520 N downward.

(2)   The object will accelerate downward. Since its downward net force has a magnitude of 520 N, we apply the formula:

$$f = ma$$
$$a = \frac{f}{m}$$
$$a = \frac{520 \text{ N}}{57 \text{ kg}} = \text{approx. } 9.1 \text{ m/s}^2$$

7.1.2.4 Flow and Ideal Flow

Flow (Q) refers to the quantity of fluid that passes a given point in a given period of time. It is expressed therefore in units of $\frac{\text{volume}}{\text{time}}$, and in the SI system, the unit of flow is:

$$\frac{m^3}{s} \quad \text{or sometimes} \quad \frac{m^3}{\min}$$

Simple unit analysis discloses that the fraction $\frac{\text{volume}}{\text{time}}$ results from the computation:

$$(\text{area})(\text{velocity}) = (m^2)(m/s) = \frac{m^3}{s}$$

and you should remember that for any fluid flowing through a vessel (pipe or tube):
Flow = (area of pipe or tube)(velocity of fluid)

The MCAT candidate should comprehend several phenomena associated with *ideal flow*.

Ideal flow:

- flow is constant at all points
- no viscosity
- no turbulence
- no drag (fluid friction)
- flow = (velocity)(area)

7.1.2.4.1 THE BERNOULLI EQUATION AND POISEUILLE'S LAW

Laminar flow refers to flow in which whirlpools and eddies are absent; turbulent flow is flow in which such phenomena do occur.

The Bernoulli equation and Poiseuille equation are given below, but you will not be expected to have them memorized.

The **Bernoulli equation** describes a relationship among flow, pressure, velocity, and vessel height. For any fluid undergoing ideal flow,

$$P + \rho(g)(h) + \frac{1}{2}\rho v^2 = \text{constant}$$

where:

P = pressure of fluid

ρ = density of fluid

h = height of vessel's center above a reference point

v = velocity of fluid

Poiseuille's law describes the relationship among flow, radius of the vessel, P, viscosity, and vessel length:

$$Q = \frac{\pi r^4 (P_1 - P_2)}{8(n)(L)}$$

where:

Q = flow

r = vessel radius

n = coefficient of viscosity

L = vessel length

7.1.2.4.2 CALIBER (WIDTH) OF THE VESSEL:

For an ideal fluid flowing through a vessel or system of vessels in which caliber varies, as shown below:

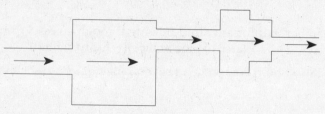

Figure 7.2

areas of smaller caliber represent areas of greater velocity and reduced pressure. When a fluid flows through a system resembling that shown above, the *velocity* of the fluid is greatest in areas of smallest caliber and least in areas of greatest caliber. In contrast, the *pressure* experienced by the fluid is greatest in areas of widest caliber and least in areas of least caliber.

The fact that velocity is less with greater diameter of the vessel is consistent with the idea, as already discussed, that flow = (area) × (velocity).

For fluid flowing within a vessel system of variable caliber, velocity is inversely proportional to cross-sectional area.

Such a proportionality does not hold for pressure and vessel caliber. The relationship between those two parameters can be derived using Q = Av and the Bernoulli equation (see 7.1.2.4.1). In relating pressure and caliber, one must remember that an increase in one corresponds to an increase in the other, but that the relationship is *not proportional*.

Please solve this problem:

- Fluid flows through a system of vessels of various calibers, as shown in Figure 7.3:

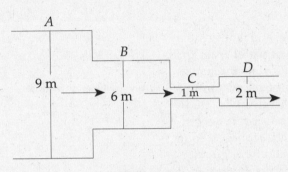

Figure 7.3

(1) In which section of the system is the fluid under the greatest pressure?
(2) Through which section of the system does the fluid travel at the greatest velocity?
(3) If the fluid's velocity is 0.5 m/s through section B, (a) what is its velocity through section D? (b) what is its flow at section D? and (c) what is the flow through section A?

Problem solved:

(1) Where caliber is greatest, pressure is greatest; thus pressure is greatest at section A.

(2) Where caliber is least, velocity is greatest; thus velocity is greatest at section C.

(3)(a) Area and velocity are inversely proportional. Ascertain the ratio:

area of section B : area of section D

Noting that the formula for the area of a circle is πr^2, recognize that area of a circle is proportional to the square of the radius. The *radius* of section B is 3 m, and the radius of section D is 1 m. The two radii bear the ratio 3:1, which means that the ratio of their areas is:

$$3^2 : 1^2 = 9 : 1$$

Since velocity is inversely proportional to area, and the velocity in section B is 0.5 m/s, the velocity in section D:

$$(0.5 \text{ m/s}) \times 9 = 4.5 \text{ m/s}$$

(3)(b) Since flow equals the product of area and velocity, flow in section D equals:

$$(\pi r^2) \times (4.5 \text{ m/s}) = (3.14)(1 \text{ m}^2) \times 4.5 \text{ m/s} = 14.3 \text{ m}^3/\text{s}$$

(3)(c) Flow is equal at all points. Having calculated flow in section D at 14.3 m³/s, we know that flow in all sections including section A is also 14.3 m³/s.

7.2 MASTERY APPLIED: SAMPLE PASSAGE AND QUESTIONS

Passage 1

Tropical fish tanks require regular maintenance. The removal and replacement of a significant amount of water from the fish tank is one aspect of this maintenance. Considering the weight of the water, this can be quite a chore for large tanks. Traditionally, the removal has been accomplished with a siphon. The siphon, a long hose with an equal diameter throughout, is filled with water either by submerging it in the fish tank or by sucking water in from one end like a large straw. Once it is filled with water, one end is left in the fish tank and the water is allowed to drain through the siphon as shown in Figure 1.

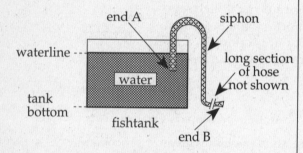

Figure 1 Traditional siphon

Because some fish enthusiasts find starting a siphon to be unpleasant, a commercial device (similar to Figure 2) has been proposed to simplify the process. This device is designed to attach to a faucet. The dotted lines represent the interior of the device. The large arrows represent the flow of water. When the faucet is turned on, in position 1, water flows through the device, draining the tank. The stop valve can then be closed and the tank refilled as shown by position 2. (Assume ideal behavior for all fluids unless otherwise stated.)

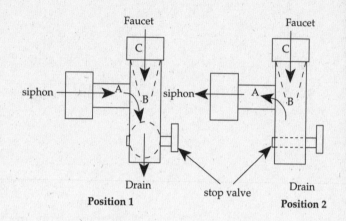

Figure 2 Commercial device

1. In order for the traditional siphon to remove water from the tank in Figure 1, end B must be positioned:

   A. anywhere below the level of the waterline.
   B. only below the level of end A.
   C. anywhere out of the water.
   D. only below the level of the tank bottom.

2. If the fish tank in Figure 1 were filled with a fluid having a higher density than water, then the velocity at end B of the heavier fluid would be:

   A. less than the velocity of water, because a greater force would be required to accelerate the greater mass.
   B. equal to the velocity of water.
   C. greater than the velocity of water, because greater pressure is created by the higher density fluid.
   D. greater than the velocity of water, because the fluid with the greater mass has more potential energy to convert to kinetic energy.

3. If a narrower siphon were used in Figure 1, which of the following would be true about the water at any given point in the narrower siphon, compared to the water at the same point in the larger siphon?

   A. The velocity would be increased and the pressure would be decreased.
   B. Both the velocity and the pressure would be decreased.
   C. Both the velocity and the pressure would be increased.
   D. Both the velocity and the pressure would be the same.

4. Even when positioned above the fish tank, the commercial device in position 1 draws water from the fish tank because:

   A. low pressure is created at B.
   B. low pressure is created at C.
   C. high pressure is created at A.
   D. high pressure is created at B.

5. Which of the following choices is likely to have the greatest pressure?

   A. A in position 1.
   B. A in position 2.
   C. B in position 1.
   D. C in position 2.

6. Why does the commercial device narrow just before point B?

   A. to decrease pressure at point B.
   B. to increase pressure at point B.
   C. to increase flow rate at point B.
   D. to decrease velocity at point B.

7. Aluminum has a Young's modulus of 70 GN/m². If a solid block of aluminum were completely submerged in the fish tank, as the siphon drained the tank, the strain on the block would:

   A. decrease due to an increase in stress.
   B. decrease due to a decrease in stress.
   C. increase due to an increase in stress.
   D. remain unchanged.

8. The pressure at the bottom of a 300 gallon tank that is 2.5 feet tall, compared to that of a 100 gallon tank that is 2.5 feet tall is:

   A. one third as great.
   B. the same.
   C. three times as great.
   D. nine times as great.

7.3 MASTERY VERIFIED: ANSWERS AND EXPLANATIONS

1. *A is correct*. In order for the siphon to work, the pressure at end B must be greater than atmospheric pressure. If we pretend, for a moment, that end B is closed, then we just have an irregularly shaped container. Since we know that the pressure is unrelated to the shape of the container, we can find the pressure at any point by the equation (7.1.2.2):

$$P = \rho\, gh + \text{atmospheric pressure}$$

Where h is the distance below the surface. Now, when end B is opened, only atmospheric pressure opposes the movement of water out of the siphon. Thus the siphon will work if, before the siphon is opened, the pressure, P, at end B is greater than atmospheric pressure. P will be greater than atmospheric pressure if h is not negative; h is positive below the waterline and negative above the waterline. End B must be held below the waterline.

2. *B is correct*. The velocity of an ideal fluid flowing from a container is:

$$v = \sqrt{2gh}$$

Notice that the velocity is unrelated to the mass or density. When considered together, the reasons given in A, C, and D actually offset each other. Greater force is required to accelerate greater mass. However, just like with any falling object, the force accelerating the fluid is proportional to the mass and thus results in the same acceleration for any density of fluid. This is true for energy as well; both potential and kinetic energy are proportional to mass and thus the greater potential energy of a heavier fluid is required to achieve a greater kinetic energy and the same velocity.

3. *D is correct*. Flow rate = (cross-sectional area) x (fluid velocity) (**7.1.2.4**). Since the cross-sectional area of a siphon is the same throughout, the velocity of the water in a siphon is the same throughout. As shown in the explanation for question #3, the velocity is not related to the siphon diameter. However, velocity is related to pressure and, since the velocity does not change, the pressure does not change.

When relating diameter of pipe to velocity and pressure [(i.e. when comparing Bernoulli's equation (**7.1.2.4.1**) and the volume flow equation above (**7.1.2.4.**)], be sure that the comparison is between two points in the same pipe and not the same point in two different pipes. This is because these equations depend on a constant flow rate and, for an ideal fluid, flow rate can change for two different pipes (as in this problem) or for the same pipe under two different circumstances. Flow rate cannot change for two points in the same pipe at the same time. If the same siphon had a different diameter at two points, then the velocities and pressures would be different at those two points.

4. *A is correct*. Of the choices, only low pressure at B could draw water from the fish tank. High pressure at C creates high velocity at B. The high velocity creates low pressure, allowing water to come through the siphon even at some heights above the waterline.

    If we relate Figure 2 to Figure 1, we see that the commercial device attaches to end B of Figure 1. Remember from the explanation to question 1 that end B must be greater than atmospheric pressure for water to leave the siphon. The commercial device simply lowers the pressure that the water at end B must overcome. Thus, for the siphon to work above the waterline, point B must be lower than atmospheric pressure.

    Notice that question 4 suggests that answer choice C to question 1 is incorrect. If you chose C for question 1, you should have gone back and changed your answer after reading question 4. You can and should use information in some questions to answer others on the MCAT.

5. *D is correct*. Position 2 is simply ideal fluid flow represented by $Q = Av$. C has the largest cross-sectional area of all the choices and thus the lowest velocity. From Bernoulli's equation, $K = P + \frac{1}{2} ev^2 + egh$, we see that the lowest velocity corresponds to the largest pressure. A and B at position 1 are both low pressure areas, as explained in the explanation to question 4.

6. *A is correct*. Again, as explained above, the device works by lowering pressure at point B. Pressure is lowered by increasing velocity. Flow rate remains unchanged unless we consider the flow rate before the tank water arrives compared to after it arrives. Answer choice A is the best answer.

    You should be aware that, on the MCAT, two apparently correct answers may arise, as they did in question 6. When faced with this dilemma, you should choose the simplest answer. In this case of question 6, choice C would be a trick answer; it refers to an exceptional situation, the seeming violation of the rule of constant flow in an ideal fluid. Since there is a straightforward answer that relies on a fundamental principle of physics; Bernoulli's equation, the straightforward answer is the better choice.

7. *B is correct*. The original stress on the block was created by the pressure of the water. As the tank drains, the pressure created by the water is removed. A decrease in stress coincides with a decrease in strain, as is shown in the equation for Young's modulus (**7.1.1.2.3.**).

Young's modulus = stress/strain

8. *B is correct*. Pressure in a standing fluid is proportional to height. $P = \rho gh$. Both tanks are the same height and thus have the same pressure.

CHAPTER 8

ELECTROSTATICS

8.1 MASTERY ACHIEVED

8.1.1 ELECTRON MOBILITY: CONDUCTION AND INSULATION

The term **electron mobility** refers to the movement of electrons between and among the atoms or molecules within some sample of a given substance.

Substances (elements and compounds) vary in their degree of electron mobility. Among the elements, metals are characterized by relatively high electron mobility, and nonmetals are characterized by relatively low electron mobility.

Movement of electrical charge is attributable to the movement of electrons. Substances whose electrons are mobile tend, therefore, to conduct the movement of electrical charge and are termed **electrical conductors**. Substances whose electrons are *extremely* immobile tend to resist the conductance of electrical charge and are termed **insulators**.

Electron mobility is a matter of degree. Every substance has some degree of electrical mobility, and so every substance is, in a sense, a conductor. We identify some substances as conductors and others as insulators based on the degree to which they manifest electron mobility. Metals, for example, tend to show a high degree of electron mobility and are considered conductors. Rubber and glass, on the other hand, show an extremely low degree of electron mobility and are insulators.

8.1.2 CONTACT CHARGE AND INDUCTION

8.1.2.1 Contact Charge

Consider a body that acquires an electrical charge—meaning that through some process its supply of electrons comes to be less than or greater than its total supply of protons. The phrase **contact charge** refers to the phenomenon in which such a charged body comes in contact with another body and imparts some or all of its charge to that second body. The first body is said to produce contact charge; it imparts its charge *to* the second body. The second body is said to experience contact charge; it acquires charge *from* the first body. As explained below, the phenomenon arises from this fundamental proposition: bodies of like charge tend to repel one another, and bodies of opposite charge tend to attract one another. *Contact charge proceeds rapidly*—almost instantaneously: the moment one charged conductor comes in contact with another, the second conductor undergoes an immediate alteration in its own charge.

Because contact charge arises from electron mobility, only relatively good conductors will produce and experience it. Consider a negatively charged metal. Its supply of electrons exceeds its supply of protons:

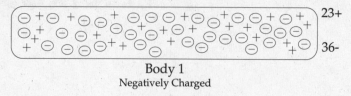

Body 1
Negatively Charged

Figure 8.1

If this metal is placed in contact with another uncharged conductor (another metal, for example), the tendency of its excess electrons to repel one another will cause movement of electrons from it into the second metal:

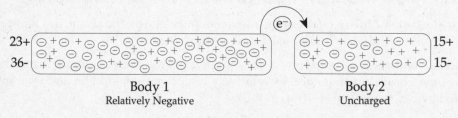

Body 1   Body 2
Relatively Negative   Uncharged

Figure 8.2

Now consider a body that is *positively* charged; its supply of electrons is less than its supply of protons:

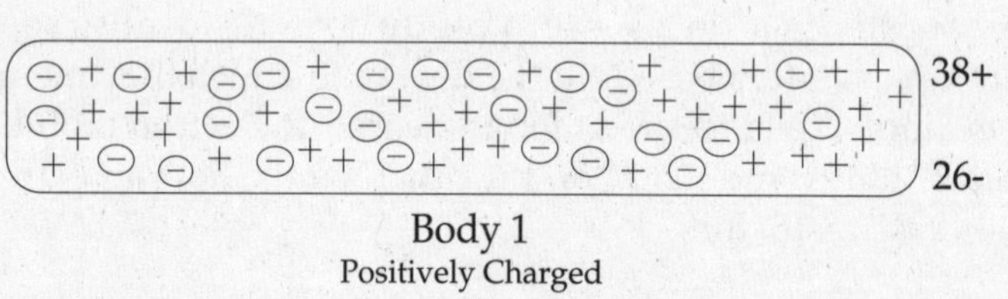

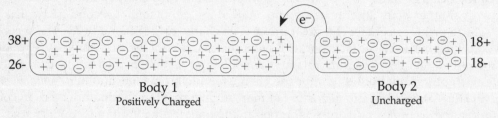

Body 1
Positively Charged

Figure 8.3

If, as before, the body is placed in contact with an uncharged conductor, the overall positive charge of the first body and its attraction for negative charge will cause electrons to move from the second body to the first body:

Body 1   Body 2
Positively Charged   Uncharged

Figure 8.4

The movement of electrons from the second body to the first leaves the second body with a positive charge and the first body with less of a positive charge than it had initially.

If either of the second bodies had not been a good conductor, neither movement of charge nor contact charge would have occurred. That is, because the entire process requires mobility of electrons within both bodies, and because a poor conductor has relatively poor electron mobility, *a poor conductor will neither produce nor experience contact charge.*

Please solve this problem:

- A positively charged body is placed in contact with an uncharged body. Which of the following choices is (are) true?

    I.   If either of the bodies is a poor conductor, each body will tend to maintain its initial charge status.
    II. If, and only if, both bodies are poor conductors each body will tend to maintain its initial charge status.
    III. If both bodies are good conductors, protons will move from the un-charged body to the negatively charged body.

    A. I only
    B. II only
    C. I and III only
    D. I, II, and III

Problem solved:

A is correct. Contact charge between a charged and uncharged body involves the movement of electrons (not protons) from one body to the other and proceeds only if both bodies experience relatively good electron mobility; in other words, both bodies must be good conductors.

The phenomenon of contact charge arises not only between charged and uncharged bodies but between *two charged* bodies if their magnitudes of charge differ. Consider two negatively charged bodies, A and B:

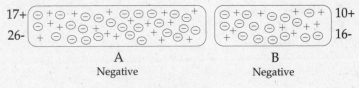

A
Negative

B
Negative

Figure 8.5

Since each body carries an excess of negative charge, both bodies have a tendency to repel electrons. But this tendency is greater for body A than for body B, because body A carries the greater excess of electrons. Electrons will move from body A to body B; body B will undergo contact charge, and the magnitude of its negative charge will increase. Because both bodies began as charged entities, and because each will undergo alteration in its charge, each body produces and experiences contact charge.

In principle, a charged body that is placed in contact with a neutral body also experiences contact charge, since its charge is altered by emission or absorption of electrons. By convention, however, a charged body contacting a neutral body is said to **produce** contact charge, and the neutral body is said to **experience** it:

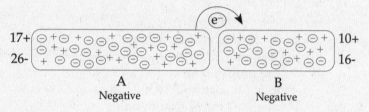

17+
26-

10+
16-

A
Negative

B
Negative

Figure 8.6

The same reasoning applies to (a) two positively charged bodies, if the magnitudes of their charges differ, and to (b) two bodies of opposite charge.

Please solve this problem:

- A negatively charged body, X, and a positively charged body, Y, come into contact. Each body is composed of a metallic substance that features a high degree of electron mobility. Which of the following choices is (are) true?

    I. Body Y will undergo contact charge.
    II. Body X will undergo contact charge.
    III. Electrons will move from body X to body Y.

  A. I only
  B. II only
  C. I and II only
  D. I, II, and III

Problem solved:

D is correct. The question concerns contact charge as applied to a negatively and a positively charged body. Both bodies are good conductors. Body X will impart electrons to body Y, which makes choice III correct. The negative charge on body X will be reduced in magnitude, as will the positive charge in body Y. Choices I and II are also accurate.

8.1.2.2 Induction

Charge induction refers ideally to the phenomenon in which a charged body is brought into proximity with a neutral conductor, whereupon the charged body *induces* uneven distribution of electrons within the conductor, making one end negatively charged relative to the other; one end of the conductor is then apposed to another conductor, thereby imparting or absorbing electrons according to the relative charge at that end. The second conductor is then removed, leaving a net charge on the first.

For example, suppose that a positively charged rod is placed near one end of a conductor as in Figure 8.7. The electrons in the conductor will move toward the positively charged body but be unable to leave the conductor, due to the space between the two bodies.

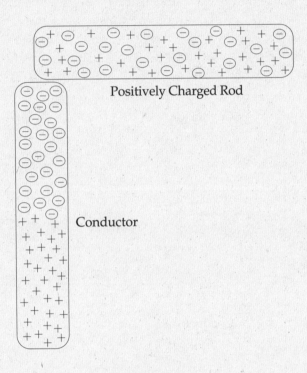

Positively Charged Rod

Conductor

Figure 8.7

Consequently, the conductor, although neutral as an entire entity, is negatively charged at the end nearest the rod and positively charged at its other end. If the charged rod is removed from the vicinity of the conductor, the conductor will return to its normal state, with electrons evenly distributed.

If, while the positively charged rod remains near the conductor (now labeled A), another conductor (labeled B) is touched to the opposite end of conductor A, electrons will be induced to move from conductor B to conductor A.

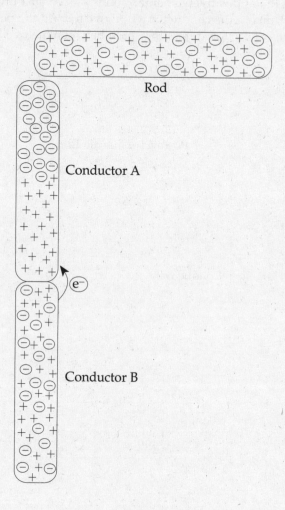

Figure 8.9

In absolute terms, then, conductor A will have an excess of electrons and conductor B will have an electron deficit: A will be negatively charged, and B will be positively charged. If all elements are then separated, the charged rod will remain charged, as it was before the process was initiated, but the two conductors, which are *initially neutral*, will now be *charged*: Conductor A will be *negatively* charged and conductor B will be *positively* charged.

Note that induction does not require that the two conductive elements be neutral at the outset; it requires that their charge *differ* from that of the rod.

Please solve this problem:

- A negatively charged object, A, is brought near the end of a conductive metal object B, which has no charge. At its opposite end, object B is connected directly to another metal object, C. Object C is removed first and then object A is removed. Which of the following statements is true at the end of this experiment?

    I. Object A is negatively charged.
    II. Object A has no charge.
    III. Object B is negatively charged.

  A. I only
  B. II only
  C. I and III only
  D. I, II, and III

Problem solved:

A is correct. The question concerns charge by induction. Object A neither gains nor loses electrons throughout the process and so maintains its original negative charge. Some of the electrons in object B are repelled by the negative charge of object A and passed to object C. When object C is removed, Object B is left positively charged.

8.1.3 CHARGE AND COULOMB'S LAW

Charge is expressed in the SI unit **coulomb (C)**. As already noted, like charges repel, and unlike charges attract; these attractive and repulsive forces are called **Coulomb's forces**. Coulomb's law provides that the force with which two charged particles repel or attract each other is equal to:

$$F = \left(\frac{1}{4\pi\varepsilon_0}\right)\left(\frac{q_1 q_2}{r^2}\right)$$

where:

ε_0 = permittivity constant
q_1 = charge on object 1
q_2 = charge on object 2
and r = distance between the centers of charge.

The value of the permittivity constant is *entirely unimportant* on the MCAT but we'll provide it just to satisfy your curiosity:

$$\varepsilon_0 = 8.85 \times 10^{-12} \text{ C}^2/\text{N} \bullet \text{m}^2$$

You should think of Coulomb's law as a law of *proportionality*, and, for all intents and purposes, ignore the fraction:

$$\left(\frac{1}{4\pi\varepsilon_0} \right)$$

since it operates only as a constant and hence contains no variables that you might need for problem solving. Thought of this way, Coulomb's law provides that for any two point charges:

$$F = K \frac{q_1 q_2}{r^2} \text{ where } K \text{ equals } \left(\frac{1}{4\pi\varepsilon_0} \right)$$

Observe that the force on each is directly proportional to the charge on each of the bodies, and inversely proportional to the square of the distance between them. (Note also that in its mathematical operation, Coulomb's law is closely analogous to Newton's universal law of gravitation, which provides that for any two bodies, the attractive force is directly proportional to the mass of each body and inversely proportional to the square of the distance between their centers of mass.)

Please solve this problem:

- A particle with a charge of −4 C lies 3 cm from a particle with a charge of −3 C. The particles affect each other with a repulsive force, F_{r1}. Assume the distance between the particles is decreased to 0.75 cm, thus modifying the repulsive force, so that it acquires a new value, F_{r2}. Write an equation that expresses F_{r2} in terms of F_{r1}.

Problem solved:

The problem draws on the proportionalities associated with Coulomb's law. The repulsive (or attractive) force created by two point charges is inversely proportional to the square of the distance between them. In this instance, the distance has been *reduced* by a factor of $\frac{3}{0.75} = 4$, which means that the repulsive force is increased by a factor of $4^2 = 16$, so that

$$F_{r2} = 16 F_{r1}$$

Please solve this problem:

- Two charged particles, A and B, separated by a distance, D, carry charges of +X coulombs and -Y coulombs, respectively. Another pair of charged particles, G and H, separated by a distance, 0.5 D, carry charges of +3X and +6Y, respectively. Write an equation that expresses the magnitude of the attractive force $F_{a(ab)}$ created by particles A and B in terms of the repulsive force $F_{r(gh)}$ created by particles G and H.

Problem solved:

As noted in the problem, particles A and B experience an attractive force, since their charges are of opposite sign; and particles G and H experience a repulsive force, since their charges are of like sign. The question concerns the relationship between the magnitude of these forces, and the answer lies in the proportionalities associated with Coulomb's law:

$$F = K \frac{q_1 q_2}{r^2}$$

In relation to the first pair of particles, the second pair of particles generates a numerator that is $(3) \times (6) = 18$ times as large. *Of itself*, that difference would create the relationship:

$$F_{a(ab)} = \left(\frac{1}{18}\right)\left(F_{r(gh)}\right)$$

However, the second pair of particles are separated by one half the distance that separates the first pair. Since the applicable force is inversely proportional to the square of the distance between the particles:

$$F_{a(ab)} = \left(\frac{1}{(2)^2}\right)\left(F_{r(gh)}\right) = \left(\frac{1}{4}\right)\left(F_{r(gh)}\right)$$

combine the effects of numerator and denominator:

$$F_{a(ab)} = \left(\frac{1}{4}\right)\left(\frac{1}{18}\right)\left(F_{r(gh)}\right)$$

$$F_{a(ab)} = \left(\frac{F_{r(gh)}}{72}\right)$$

Please solve this problem:

- Two charged particles experience a repulsive force of 33 N. If the charge on one of the particles is tripled, and the distance between the particles is also tripled, what will be the magnitude of the repulsive force experienced by the two particles?

Problem solved:

According to Coulomb's law, tripling the magnitude of charge on one of the particles will triple the repulsive force between the particles. Tripling the distance between the particles reduces the force by a factor of $(3)^2 = 9$. Multiply the new force by $> \frac{3}{9}$ or $\frac{1}{3}$:

$$33\text{N} \cdot \frac{1}{3} = \frac{33}{3} = 11 \text{ N}$$

8.1.4 ELECTROSTATIC FIELDS AND ELECTROSTATIC FIELD STRENGTH

A charged particle situated at any given location establishes an **electrostatic field**—a surrounding area of force that would exist between it and any other charged particle located somewhere in its vicinity, according to Coulomb's law, as previously discussed:

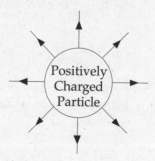

Figure 8.10

With reference to any point at a given distance from such a charged particle, electrostatic field refers, generally, to the hypothetical attractive or repulsive force that the charged body would exert on a particle carrying a (+1) coulomb charge, situated at that point. The phrase **electrostatic field strength** refers specifically to the *magnitude* of that force. It is expressed in **newtons per coulomb (N/C)**.

When calculating electrostatic field strength, you should calculate force in newtons (N), and then, recalling that the force was calculated on the basis of an imagined particle of charge (+1) C, express the electrostatic field strength in newtons per coulomb (N/C).

Consider a particle, X, with a charge of (–3) coulombs, and a point P, 2 cm (.02 m) from it. The electrostatic field strength created by X at P is ascertained by imagining a particle with charge (+1) C at point P and calculating the force that would exist on the hypothetical particle due to X.

The magnitude of the force is given by Coulomb's law:

$$F = \left(\frac{1}{4\pi\varepsilon_0}\right)\left(\frac{(q_1)(q_2)}{r^2}\right)$$

Taking as 3.14 and the permittivity constant as 8.85×10^{-12} $C^2/N \times m^2$, the value of the fraction $\left(\frac{1}{4\pi\varepsilon_0}\right)$ is approximately equal to $9 \times 10^9 \dfrac{N \cdot m^2}{C^2}$

The total force that would act upon the hypothetical particle situated at point P is given as:

$$\left(\frac{(-3)C \times (+1)C}{(.02 \text{ m})^2}\right) = -6.75 \times 10^{13}\, N$$

The magnitude of the force is approximately 6.8×10^{13} N. Since magnitude is at issue, the (–) sign is unimportant.

Verification of dimensional consistency shows that:

$$\left(\frac{1}{C^2/N \bullet m^2}\right)\left(\frac{(C)(C)}{m^2}\right) = \left(\frac{1}{C^2}\right)\left(\frac{N \bullet m^2}{1}\right)\left(\frac{C^2}{m^2}\right) = \frac{N \bullet m^2}{m^2} = N$$

As such, the electrostatic field strength exerted by particle X at point P is 6.8×10^{13} N/C.

The MCAT will probably not require you to compute electrostatic field strength, but it may require you to solve problems on the basis of mathematical relationships and, more particularly, by using the proportionalities inherent in Coulomb's law.

Please solve this problem:

- A particle, A, carries a charge of magnitude x coulombs. At a point P_1, located y meters from particle A, particle A creates an electrostatic field strength of .008 N/C.

  (a) What electrostatic field strength does particle A exert at point P_2, located $6y$ meters from particle A?

  (b) Among the following choices, the equation that properly expresses x in terms of y, , and ε_0 is:

  A. $\quad x = \dfrac{y(0.008)}{(\pi\varepsilon_0)}$

  B. $\quad x = \dfrac{y^2(0.008)}{\left(\pi^2\varepsilon_0{}^2\right)}$

  C. $\quad x = y^2(0.008)(4\pi\varepsilon_0)$

  D. $\quad x = y(0.004)\left(2\pi\varepsilon_0{}^2\right)$

Problem solved:

The problem requires that you use the mathematical relationships inherent in Coulomb's law.

Part (a): The force between two charged particles is inversely proportional to the square of the distance between them. The ratio $6y{:}y$ is equivalent to the ratio 6:1. Since $(6)^2 = 36$, the electrostatic field strength at $P_2 = \dfrac{x}{36}$.

Part (b): *C is correct.* Using Coulomb's law:

$$F = \frac{1}{4\pi\varepsilon_0} \times \frac{(q_1)(q_2)}{r^2}$$

The problem allows for the replacement of F with 0.008 and q_1 with x, the value for which we are to solve. Since the question asks for electrostatic field strength, q_2 is thought of as $(+1)$C. The value for r is given as y. With the variables replaced, Coulomb's law gives us:

$$0.008 \text{ N} = \frac{1}{4\pi\varepsilon_0} \times \frac{(x)(1)}{y^2}$$

Solving for x is a matter of simple algebra:

$$0.008 \div \frac{1}{4\pi\varepsilon_0} = \frac{(x)(1)}{y^2}$$

$$\frac{(0.008)(4\pi\varepsilon_0)}{1} = \frac{(x)}{y^2}$$

$$x = y^2(0.008)(4\ \varepsilon_0)$$

Since electrostatic field strength is expressed in the SI unit N/C, the force experienced by any charged particle located at a position of known electrostatic field strength is:

(electrostatic field strength)(charge on particle), or

$$F_{es} = E_{fs}(q)$$

Please solve this problem:

- A positively charged particle situated at point P establishes an electrostatic field with strength = 6 N/C at point P_1. What is the magnitude of force experienced by a particle with a charge of 0.0022 C located at point P_1?

Problem solved:

The problem can be solved by using the equation:

$$F_{es} = \text{(electrostatic field strength)(charge on particle)}$$

$$F_{es} = E_{fs}\,(q)$$

$$F_{es} = (6\ \text{N/C}) \times (0.0022\ \text{C})$$

$$F_{es} = 0.0132\ \text{N}$$

8.2 MASTERY APPLIED: SAMPLE PASSAGE AND QUESTIONS

Passage

The human heartbeat is produced by a cyclic series of electrical events. An initiating impulse is issued approximately once every 0.83 seconds at the sinoatrial node, located in the right atrium, and conducted around both right and left atrial chambers more or less simultaneously. The impulse is then conducted to the atrioventricular node, to the transitional fibers, and to the "A-V" (atrioventricular) bundle of myocardial fibers.

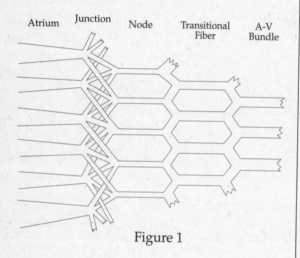

Figure 1

The conduction between atria and the atrioventricular bundle is a frequent site of pathologic difficulty, giving rise to cardiac arrhythmias, some of them life-threatening. A microanatomic depiction of the normal route through which the impulse travels from atria to ventricles is set forth schematically in Figure 1, and a macroscopic view of the associated structures is set forth schematically in Figure 2. The atrioventricular node produces a conduction *delay*, so that the impulse does not travel too quickly from atria to ventricles; too rapid transmission might produce dangerous arrhythmias.

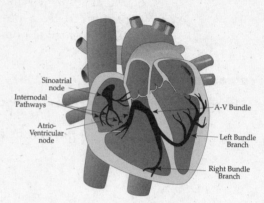

Figure 2

From the atrioventricular node, the impulse is conducted throughout both right and left ventricles. The conduction produces contraction of the two chambers, and this propels blood from the right ventricle into the pulmonary circulation and from the left ventricle into the systemic circulation.

Ideal function of cardiac muscle would require that the impulse originating at the sinoatrial node reach all portions of the ventricle simultaneously. Practically, however, the impulse reaches almost all portions of the ventricle within a very small span of time. The first muscle fiber within the ventricle receives the impulse only 0.06 seconds before the last fiber. The actual time during which the muscle remains contracted is approximately 0.30 seconds, and so the rapid spread of the impulse causes both ventricles to contract almost simultaneously.

This sort of synchronicity is important to the effectiveness of cardiac function. If the impulse were to travel through the ventricles slowly, the heart would lose a great deal of its effectiveness.

1. A researcher constructs an artificial heart in which heart muscle fibers are replaced by finely drawn threads of a conductive metal. She initiates a simulated cardiac cycle by imparting an electrical charge to the region of her model that is anatomically analogous to the sinoatrial node. In view of her model's construction, the impulse will be conducted by means of:

   A. induction produced by the insulating effects of the metal.
   B. contact charge produced by the electron mobility of the metal.
   C. electrostatic field force produced by charge at the simulated sinoatrial node.
   D. Coulomb's forces produced by separation of metal threads.

2. If, when first initiating an impulse, the sinoatrial node were regarded momentarily as a single charged particle, any charged particle in its vicinity would be subject to:

   I. conduction.
   II. Coulomb's forces.
   III. an electrostatic field.

   A. I only
   B. II only
   C. I and II only
   D. II and III only

3. An experimenter notes that conduction through the atrioventricular node is delayed. Among the following choices, the hypothesis best supported by the observation is:

   A. the cardiac impulse does not move through the atrioventricular node via classic contact charge.
   B. the atrioventricular node is positively charged at the time the impulse reaches it.
   C. the muscle fibers of the atrioventricular node permit no electron mobility.
   D. the muscle fibers of the atrioventricular node feature extraordinarily high electron mobility.

4. An investigator measured the electrostatic force on a point charge at various distances from the SA node. Assuming the charge on the SA node was the same for each measurement, which of the following graphs would most accurately reflect the magnitude of the force experienced by these charges as a function of their distance from the SA node?

A.
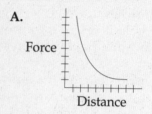

B.
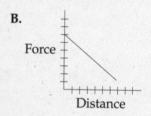

C.
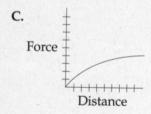

D.
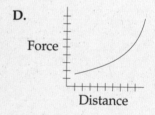

5. An experimenter determines that cardiac muscle is NOT composed of an insulating material. Which of the following conclusions about cardiac muscle most logically follows from his observation?

   A. It will donate or receive protons if exposed to a charged body made of a conductive material.
   B. It will neither donate nor receive electrons if exposed to a charged body made of a conductive material.
   C. If no insulating substance exists between the heart muscle and the SA node, any charge on the SA node will cause a charge to conduct across the heart muscle.
   D. It is metallic in nature.

6. Taken together with Figure 1, the passage indicates which of the following about the normal heart?

   A. It sends an impulse from the A-V bundle to the transitional fibers.
   B. It experiences a delay in conduction between the atria and the A-V bundle.
   C. It cannot conduct an impulse through the atrioventricular node.
   D. Its electrical impulses are directed from the ventricles toward the atria.

7. An investigator works with a laboratory animal suffering from excessively rapid conduction through the atrioventricular junction and abnormally slow conduction through the ventricles proper. The animal suffers from an arrhythmia termed **paroxysmal ventricular tachycardia (PVT)**, and the investigator posits that the condition is due to the abnormality at the atrioventricular junction. Which of the following measures should she take in order to best confirm or deny her hypothesis?

A. Determine the statistical frequency of inborn defects in atrioventricular conduction and ventricular conduction.

B. In an animal of a different species, determine whether PVT can be induced by slowing conduction through the ventricles proper.

C. Examine an animal of a different species afflicted with PVT, and look for additional signs of cardiac abnormality.

D. In a normal animal of the same species, induce rapid conduction through the atrioventricular node without otherwise affecting the animal, and look for PVT.

8. According to the passage, the normal heart beats approximately how many times per minute?

A. 83
B. 72
C. 67
D. 60

8.3 MASTERY VERIFIED: ANSWERS AND EXPLANATIONS

1. *B is correct*. The cardiac cycle depends on the movement of electrical impulses through a network of conductive substance; the movement of electrical charge is a function of contact charge, which is attributable to electron mobility.

2. *D is correct*. The sinoatrial node is hypothesized as the charged particle. Charged particles produce an electrostatic field, so any other charged particle within the field's vicinity will be subject to an attractive or repulsive Coulomb's force. Choice I refers to conduction, which is a process that requires contact between the bodies.

3. *A is correct*. The means of conduction is not classic contact charge, which, as explained in **8.1.2.1**, is virtually immediate.

4. *A is correct*. The attractive or repulsive force between any two charged particles varies inversely with the square of the distance that separates them; such a relationship between variables is depicted in cartesian coordinates.

    Choices C and D are eliminated, because they show force tending to *increase* with distance. Choice B depicts a *linear* relationship, not a proportional one. Only choice A shows force varying inversely with the square of distance.

5. *C is correct*. Any conducting material will conduct a charge as described in **8.1.1**. Choice A is incorrect, because the movement of charge involves movement of electrons, not protons. Choice B is incorrect, because a material that is not an insulator will receive and donate electrons if exposed to a charged conductor. Choice D states that metals are good conductors, but that is not to say that all good conductors are metals.

6. *B is correct*. It is clear that the impulse passes from the atria to the ventricles via the pathway just mentioned. Figure 1 serves only to confirm that which the text sets forth.

7. *D is correct*. The investigator is faced with an animal that shows two observable abnormalities in conduction and an identifiable syndrome (PVT). The investigator hypothesizes that the syndrome arises from one of the abnormalities and not the other. She should (1) obtain an animal otherwise resembling the one at issue (of the *same* species, therefore), (2) induce the abnormality that she suspects as the cause of the syndrome, and (3) examine the animal for the appearance of the syndrome. If the animal manifests the syndrome, the investigator has confirmed her hypothesis. If the animal does not manifest the syndrome, the investigator has disaffirmed it.

8. *B is correct*. The passage states that the normal heartbeat proceeds from a cycle initiated at the sinoatrial node once every 0.83 seconds, which means it occurs 1.20 times per second. Noting that there are 60 seconds per minute, multiply $(1.20)(60) = 72$.

CHAPTER 9

CAPACITORS

9.1 MASTERY ACHIEVED

9.1.1 ELECTROSTATIC FIELD STRENGTH

The topic of **capacitors** refers generally to the electrostatic field and associated considerations of force and energy associated with two charged plates that are equal in area, of equal and opposite charge, and, relative to their own size, close to one another. Two such plates together constitute a capacitor and are represented in the diagram below as **A** (a positively charged plate) and **B** (a negatively charged plate).

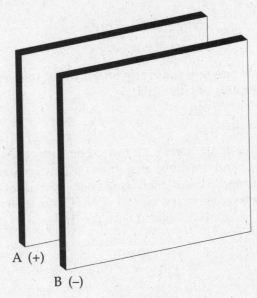

A (+)

B (−)

Figure 9.1

Although capacitors may in fact be structured with non-rectangular plates, *MCAT questions require only an understanding of the dynamics of the capacitor with parallel plates.*

The strength of the electric field produced between such a pair of plates (equal in size and of equal and opposite charge) is equal to the quotient:

$$\text{Electric field strength} = \frac{\text{charge on one plate}}{(\varepsilon_0)(\text{area of plate})}$$

$$E = \frac{Q}{(\varepsilon_0)(A)}$$

where:

Q = the magnitude of charge on either plate
ε_0 = permittivity constant
(A) = area of either plate

Noting that charge is expressed in coulombs, area in m², and the permittivity constant in $\frac{C^2}{N \cdot m^2}$, a verification for dimensional consistency reveals that:

$$\frac{\text{charge}}{(\varepsilon_0)(\text{area})} = \frac{C}{\left(\frac{C^2}{N \cdot m^2}\right)(m^2)} = \left(\left(\frac{C}{m^2}\right) \times \frac{N \cdot m^2}{C^2}\right) = \frac{N}{C}$$

which constitutes a correct expression for electrostatic field strength as discussed in Chapter 8.

Note the proportionalities established by the formula just provided; that for any two closely spaced plates of equal area and equal but opposite charge, the electrostatic field strength between them is proportional to the fraction:

$$\frac{\text{charge on either plate}}{\text{area of one plate}} = \frac{(Q)}{(A)}$$

As such, electrostatic field strength is directly proportional to the charge on either plate and inversely proportional to the area of either plate.

Please solve this problem:

- Two plates, A and B, each measuring 1.5 cm × 2 cm, are closely spaced, one carrying a charge of (+)1 × 10⁻⁵ C, and the other, a charge of (–)1 × 10⁻⁵ C. A separate pair of plates, C and D, each measuring 1.8 cm × 2 cm, are closely spaced, one carrying a charge of +1.2 × 1⁻⁵ C, and the other, a charge of (–) 1.2 × 10⁻⁵ C. Write an expression that describes the electrostatic field strength associated with the first pair of plates (E_1) in terms of that associated with the second (E_2).

Problem solved:

The charge on each plate in the first pair in relation to the charge on each plate in the second pair gives rise to the ratio $1:1.2 = \dfrac{5}{6}$. The area of each plate in the first pair in relation to the area of each plate in the second pair gives rise to the ratio $3.0:3.6 = \dfrac{5}{6}$. This second ratio is the ratio of the areas, which is inversely proportional to the electric field and, thus, should be inverted. The electric field strength associated with the first pair of plates in relation to that associated with the second creates the ratio $\dfrac{5}{6} \times \dfrac{6}{5} = 1$.

The equation for the electrostatic field, E_1, in terms of E_2 is simply $E_1 = E_2$

9.1.2 ELECTROSTATIC POTENTIAL

For any capacitor, **electrostatic potential** is equal to the product, (electrostatic field strength) × (separation of plates), or:

$$V = Ed$$

where:

V = electrostatic potential

E = electrostatic field strength

d = distance between the plates

Electrostatic potential is expressed in the unit joule per coulomb $\left(\dfrac{J}{C}\right)$ and one joule per coulomb is renamed one volt (V):

$$\frac{1J}{C} = 1V$$

With electrostatic field strength expressed in newtons per coulomb, and length expressed in meters, verification for dimensional consistency reveals that:

$$(\text{newton per coulomb}) \times (\text{meter})$$

$$= m \bullet \frac{N}{C} = \frac{\text{joules}}{\text{coulomb}} = \text{volt (V)}$$

In addition, electrostatic potential for a capacitor refers to the potential energy that would be possessed by a massless particle with charge of magnitude 1 C, situated on the plate of like charge.

Consider a capacitor, and imagine a massless charge of (–)1 coulomb situated on the positively charged plate. The hypothetical particle is attracted to the positively charged plate and held there with a force equal to the capacitor's electrostatic field strength. Suppose, as shown below, that the plates of a particular capacitor have such area and charge as to produce an electrostatic field strength of 800 $\frac{N}{C}$. Suppose further that the plates are separated by a distance of 1.5 cm (.015 m), as shown below:

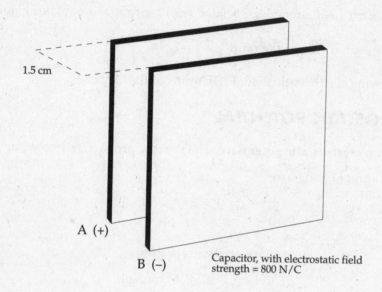

Capacitor, with electrostatic field strength = 800 N/C

Figure 9.2

A massless particle with charge of (–)1C situated on the positively charged plate will be held to the plate with a force of 800 N. To move the (–1)C particle from the positive plate to the negative plate—*thereby opposing the force imposed by the electrostatic field*—one would have to perform work on the particle equal to:

$$800 \text{ N} \times (.015 \text{ m}) = 12 \text{ N} \cdot \text{m} = 12 \text{ J}$$

If the particle was moved across the capacitor and held to the *negatively* charged plate, its *tendency* to move back to the positively charged plate, through the ordinary operation of Coulomb's forces, as shown below, would represent potential energy equal, once again, to:

$$800 \text{ N} \times (.015 \text{ m}) = 12 \text{ N} \cdot \text{m} = 12 \text{ J}$$

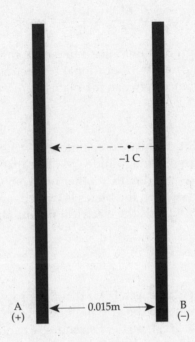

A
(+)   ← 0.015m →   B
(−)

−1 C

Figure 9.3

If, as just explained, we conceive of the capacitor in terms of the potential energy that would be possessed by a hypothetical particle with a (−1)C charge, located on the *negatively* charged plate (the plate of like charge), we describe the capacitor as having electrostatic potential of 12 joules per coulomb $\left(\dfrac{12 \text{ J}}{\text{C}} \right)$.

Coulomb's forces (Chapter 6) dictate that the force with which the hypothetical particle would be repelled from the plate of like charge and attracted to the plate of opposite charge is proportional to the charge on the particle. If, then, the hypothetical particle carried a charge not of (−)1 C but of (−)3 C, the Coulomb's forces would be equal to (800 N) × (3) = 2,400 N. The potential energy possessed by such a particle, if located on the negatively charged plate, would be equal to three times 12 J:

$$2400 \text{ N} \times (.015 \text{ m}) = 36 \text{ J}$$

If the hypothetical particle carried a charge of (–)5.5 coulombs, Coulomb's force would be equal to (800 N) × (5.5) = 4,400 N. The potential energy possessed by such a particle, if located on the negatively charged plate, would be equal to 5.5 times 12 J:

$$4,400 \text{ N} \times (.015 \text{ m}) = 66 \text{ J}$$

For this capacitor, however, the *ratio* of potential energy to charge remains:

$$\frac{6 \text{ J}}{3 \text{ C}} = \frac{66 \text{ J}}{5.5 \text{ C}} = \frac{12 \text{ J}}{\text{C}} = 12 \text{ volts}$$

You should be aware of the proportionalities inherent in the formula: $V = Ed$. For a capacitor, electrical potential is directly proportional to electrostatic field strength and is also directly proportional to the distance between the plates.

Please solve this problem:

- A capacitor is composed of two plates separated by a distance d, each plate having an area A and carrying a charge of magnitude Q_1. The capacitor's electrostatic potential is V_1. If (1) the capacitor is replaced with another for which the area of each plate is doubled, (2) the distance between the plates is tripled, and (3) the charge between the plates is maintained at Q_1, what is the electrical potential, V_2, of the new capacitor, expressed in terms of V_1?

Problem solved:

Recall that (1) electrostatic field strength (E) is directly proportional to the charge on either plate (Q) and inversely proportional to the area of either plate (A), and (2) electrical potential (V) is directly proportional to electrostatic field strength (E) and also directly proportional to the distance between the plates (d). V is directly proportional to the fraction:

$$\frac{(Q)(d)}{A}$$

The doubling of (A) tends to reduce V by a factor of 2, and the tripling of d tends to increase V by a factor of 3. The alterations therefore multiply V by the fraction $\frac{3}{2} = 1.5$, which means that:

$$V_2 = (1.5)(V_1)$$

9.1.3 CAPACITANCE

The term **capacitance** refers qualitatively to the degree to which a capacitor stores electric charge *in relation to its electrostatic potential*. For any capacitor, capacitance (C) is proportional to the quotient:

$$\frac{\text{charge}}{\text{electrostatic potential}} = \frac{Q}{V}$$

As is indicated by the fraction $\frac{Q}{V}$, capacitance is expressed in coulombs per volt $\left(\frac{C}{V}\right)$ and, one coulomb per volt is renamed a **farad**.

Consider the effect on capacitance of plate size:

- The area of the plates is inversely proportional to electric field strength (E).

- The electric field strength is directly proportional to electrostatic potential (V).

- The electrostatic potential is inversely proportional to capacitance (C); *increased size of the capacitor's plates is directly proportional to capacitance*. The relevant algebra is shown below:

C is proportional to $\dfrac{Q}{V}$

V is proportional to $(E)(d)$

E is proportional to $\dfrac{Q}{(\varepsilon_0)(A)}$

C is plainly proportional to:

$$Q \div \frac{(d)(Q)}{(\varepsilon_0)(A)} = \frac{(Q)(\varepsilon_0)(A)}{(d)(Q)} = \frac{(\varepsilon_0)(A)}{d}$$

which is proportional to A.

Dielectric constant refers to the material situated between the capacitor's plates. No capacitor can maintain a charge on its plates unless the material or mixture of materials between them has some tendency to insulate. The dielectric constant (k) represents the degree to which a substance or common mixture of substances tends to reduce the electric field between the plates. Hence, *capacitance is directly proportional to the dielectric constant*, and the true quantitative definition of capacitance is:

$$C = \frac{(K)(\varepsilon_0)(A)}{d}$$

where:

K = dielectric constant of material between plates

ε_0 = permittivity constant

A = equal area of either plate

d = distance between plates

The formula reveals that capacitance is:

- directly proportional to the dielectric constant

- directly proportional to the area of the plates

- *inversely* proportional to the distance between the plates

(Because the dielectric constant of air is close to 1, and because some authors assume the material between the plates to be air, unless otherwise stated, it is sometimes written that:

$$C = \frac{(\varepsilon_0)(A)}{d})$$

9.1.4 CAPACITORS: ENERGY

Electrostatic potential (see **9.1.2**) represents considerations of potential energy, and a capacitor is said to store energy. Do not memorize the equations that quantify the energy of a capacitor (u). If any such equation is relevant to an MCAT question, it will be provided. But understand that capacitors do store energy and that the energy storage is related to the electrical potential difference between the plates.

Three common equations that describe the energy of a capacitor are below :

$$(\text{energy of a capacitor}) = \frac{(\text{charge})(\text{electrostatic potential})}{2}$$

(1) $u = \frac{1}{2}(Q)(V)$

(2) $u = \frac{1}{2}CV^2$

(3) $u = \frac{Q^2}{2C}$

9.1.5 CAPACITORS: DIELECTRIC BREAKING POINT

One should appreciate the significance of a dielectric's **breaking point**. When the electrostatic field is raised to a sufficiently high level, discharge will occur: electrons will move through the dielectric from the negatively charged plate to the positively charged plate. For any dielectric, the breaking point represents the electrostatic field at which discharge occurs.

9.2 MASTERY APPLIED: SAMPLE PASSAGE AND QUESTIONS

Passage

Modern understanding of electrostatics identifies lines of force that arise from two or more charged particles placed in some given position relative to one another. All such lines of force are ultimately traceable to Coulomb's forces.

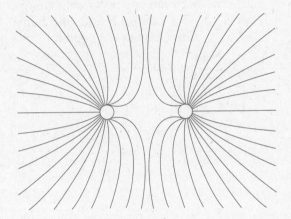

Figure 1

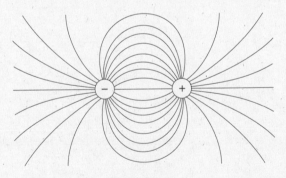

Figure 2

Figure 1 shows the lines associated with a repulsive force between two such particles with charges of equal magnitude. Figure 2 shows the lines associated with an attractive force between two such particles with charges of equal magnitude. Figure 3 shows the lines associated with an attractive force between two such particles with charge magnitudes differing by a factor of 4.

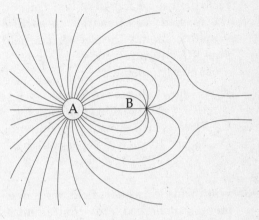

Figure 3

The potential difference between two points within an electric field may be defined to be the work in ergs, joules, or other applicable units that is required to move a charged particle of one coulomb from one point to the other. The work required is identical for all paths between the two points. That proposition is fundamental to the law of conservation of energy; if it were not so, the work *required* to move a particle from one position to the other might differ from the work *produced* by returning the particle to its original position.

1. If a particle with charge of (+) 3×10^{-7} C is first situated on the negative plate of a 100-volt capacitor and then moved to the positive plate, the amount of work performed on it will be:

   A. 3.0×10^{-5} joules.
   B. 9.0×10^{-5} joules.
   C. 1.5×10^{-4} joules.
   D. 1.8×10^{-4} joules.

2. Assuming that the value of the permittivity constant, $\varepsilon_0 = 8.85 \times 10^{-12}\ C^2/N \cdot m^2$, consider two parallel plates of equal area and equal but opposite charges. Each plate measures 10 cm × 9 cm, and the magnitude of charge on each is 9×10^{-4} coulomb. The electrostatic field strength produced by such a pair is most nearly equal to:

A. 0.1 newtons per coulomb.
B. 1.13×10^{10} newtons per coulomb.
C. 71.65×10^5 newtons per coulomb.
D. 88.5×10^{12} newtons per coulomb.

3. Within an electrostatic field, the movement of a charged body from point A to point B requires work of 40 joules. The movement of the charged body back to point A from point B produces 38 joules of work. Which of the following best explains the finding?

A. The sign of the body's charge is positive.
B. The charged body acquired 78 joules of potential energy when it moved from point A to point B.
C. The charged body followed two different pathways in traveling between points A and B.
D. Two joules of energy were lost as heat.

4. Among the following, Figure 1 might depict:

I. the lines of force that arise between one body with charge (+) 1 coulomb and one body with charge (−) 1 coulomb.
II. the lines of force that arise between one body with charge (−) 1 coulomb and one body with charge (−) 1 coulomb.
III. the lines of force that arise between one body with charge (+) 1 coulomb and one body with charge (+) 1 coulomb.

A. I only
B. II only
C. I and II only
D. II and III only

5. Two charged bodies, A and B, are located near one another. Body A has charge of (+) 6×10^{-6} C and body B has charge of (−) 2.4×10^{-5} C. Among the following figures, the associated force lines are best represented by:

A.

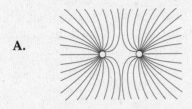

B.

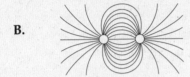

C.

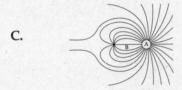

D.

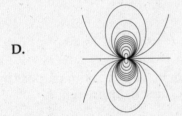

6. An investigator makes appropriate electrical connections between a capacitor and an electrical lifting device so that energy stored within the capacitor may be used to lift a 5 kg object. She hypothesizes that if the capacitor causes the machine to lift the object a total distance of 2 meters upward, it will, in the process, lose more than 100 joules of potential energy. Is the hypothesis plausible?

A. Yes, because the first law of thermodynamics is inapplicable to charged plates so long as they are spaced relatively close together.

B. Yes, because the operation of the machine itself will occasion the performance of work and the generation of heat.

C. No, because the gravitational potential energy of the object would then be greater than the potential energy expended.

D. No, because gravitational potential energy cannot be related mathematically to electrical potential energy.

9.3 MASTERY VERIFIED: ANSWERS AND EXPLANATIONS

1. *A is correct.* The designation "100-volt capacitor" signifies a capacitor in which a hypothetical particle with charge of magnitude 1 coulomb would acquire 100 joules of potential energy when moved from the plate with charge of opposite sign to the plate with charge of like sign.

   The question concerns a hypothetical particle with charge of (−) 3×10^{-7} coulomb. If situated on the positive plate, the repulsive force it experiences is far less than that which would be experienced by a hypothetical particle with charge of 1.0 C. The difference is indeed a function of proportion:

$$100 \text{ V} = \frac{100 \text{ J}}{\text{C}}$$

$$100 \text{ J/C} \times 3 \times 10^{-7} \text{ C} = 300 \times 10^{-7} \text{ J} = 3.0 \times 10^{-5} \text{ J}$$

2. *B is correct.* Knowing that electrostatic field strength is equal to the fraction:

$$\frac{Q}{(\varepsilon_0)(A)}$$

calculate:

$$\frac{9 \times 10^{-4} \text{C}}{\left(8.85 \times \dfrac{10^{-12} \text{C}^2}{\text{N} \bullet \text{m}^2}\right)\left(9 \times 10^{-3} \text{m}^2\right)} = \frac{90 \times 10^{-5} \text{C}}{79.65 \times \dfrac{10^{-15} \text{C}^2}{\text{N}}}$$

$$= 1.13 \times \frac{10^{10} \text{N}}{\text{C}}$$

In this case, all choices are expressed in newtons per coulomb, so there is no purpose in verification for dimensional consistency. Moreover, electrostatic field strength is expressed in $\dfrac{\text{N}}{\text{C}}$. If, however, you had forgotten the unit in which electrostatic field strength is expressed and one of the answer choices provided the correct numerical response but the incorrect unit (for instance, coulombs per farad), you could go through the following computations to determine the correct units:

$$\frac{\text{C}}{\left(\dfrac{\text{C}^2}{\text{N} \bullet \text{m}^2}\right)(\text{m}^2)} = \frac{\text{C}}{\dfrac{\text{C}^2 \text{m}^2}{\text{N} \bullet \text{m}^2}} = \frac{\text{C}}{\dfrac{\text{C}^2}{\text{N}}} = \text{C} \div \frac{\text{C}^2}{\text{N}}$$

$$= \text{C} \times \frac{\text{N}}{\text{C}^2} = \frac{\text{C} \bullet \text{N}}{\text{C}^2} = \frac{\text{N}}{\text{C}}$$

3. *D is correct.* If the movement of a charged body between two points in an electrostatic field requires work, then the body is acquiring potential energy equal to the amount of work required *minus* any energy that's converted to other forms, *such as heat.* In no event can the body acquire potential energy greater than the work performed on it. When the charged body is allowed to move back to its original position, its potential energy might be harnessed to perform work. The maximum amount of work that might be performed is equal to the potential energy which, in turn, is equal, at maximum, to the amount of work originally performed to move the object *from* its original position. If the work done by the object during its "return" trip is less than that done on the object during its initial movement, the explanation might be that the potential energy it acquired has been converted, in part, to heat, and not directed to the production of work.

4. *D is correct.* The lines in Figure 1 represent a *repulsive* force, so the two charged bodies that they relate to must be of like charge: they might both be positive or negative, but the charge of one cannot be negative and that of the other positive. The lines also reflect two bodies whose charges are of equal magnitude.

5. *C is correct.* The question refers to two bodies that exert an attractive force on one another; their charges are of opposite sign. The difference in magnitude is 4, since:

$$\frac{2.4 \times 10^{-5}}{6 \times 10^{-6}} = \frac{24 \times 10^{-6}}{6 \times 10^{-6}} = 4 \times 10^{0} = 4$$

One should search among the answer choices for a figure that closely resembles Figure 3.

6. *B is correct.* The investigator intends to apply the energy stored within a capacitor (the potential energy represented by its electrical potential) toward the performance of work. The lifting of a 5 kg body 2 meters upward imparts gravitational potential energy of:

$$(m)(g)(h) = (5 \text{ kg})(10 \text{ m/s}^2)(2 \text{ m}) = 100 \text{ joules}$$

which corresponds to 100 joules of potential energy. Since the operation of the machine itself will require the performance of work and hence the conversion of potential energy, it is plausible that the actual amount of potential energy lost by the capacitor will be greater than that acquired by the lifted object.

CHAPTER 10

ELECTROMAGNETISM

10.1 MASTERY ACHIEVED

10.1.1 ELECTRIC CIRCUITS

When two entities of different electrical potentials are connected by a conductor, electric current will flow between them. The potential difference just described, which promotes the flow of current, is called **electromotive force (emf)**, or E. You should recognize that electromotive force is not a Newtonian force; electromotive force is measured in volts, and not in Newtons.

If an electrical device is interposed within the connection between potentials, then it will be made to operate. The arrangement of such a device along with an electromotive force and conductors is called an **electric circuit**. The two sources of diverse potential are termed positive and negative **poles**, or positive and negative **terminals**.

In an electrical circuit, electrons flow from the negative terminal, through the circuit, to the positive terminal. The role of the electromotive force (*emf*) is to take the electrons at the positive terminal and move them back to the negative terminal. Without the *emf*, the flow of electrons would stop.

As a matter of convention, the flow of current is defined as the "flow of positive charge." Current flow is *opposite* in direction to electron flow. Although there is no *actual* flow of positive charge, you should be familiar with the concept of current.

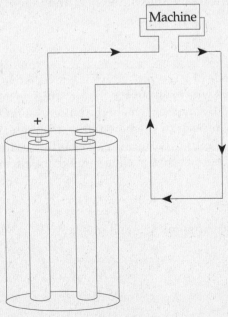

Figure 10.1

A battery may be described in terms of its voltage, which reflects the electrical potential difference between its cathode(+) and anode(–). In a 2-volt battery, for instance, the cathode and anode differ in electrical potential by a magnitude of 2 volts.

You should be familiar with this seemingly paradoxical concept: *every conductor, even as it mediates and facilitates the flow of current, simultaneously resists it*. By analogy, you might imagine a crowded four-lane highway during rush hour, merging onto a one-lane bridge that conducts traffic across a river. The loss of three lanes impairs the traffic flow: the bridge produces a "resistance." Without the bridge, however, traffic could not traverse the river: the bridge "conducts" the traffic, even as it resists it.

10.1.1.1 Current

The flow of current is promoted by the potential difference between positive and negative poles; increased potential difference between positive and negative poles increases current flow. The flow of current is impaired by resistance, and increased resistance decreases current flow. The relationships just described constitute the essence of **Ohm's law**, which provides that when two entities of differing potential are connected by a conductor:

$$I = \frac{V}{R}$$

where:

$I =$ current (amperes—A)

$V =$ voltage (volts—V)

$R =$ resistance (ohms—Ω)

Problem solving on the MCAT often calls for algebraic manipulation of the Ohm's law equation, and you should be familiar with these relations:

$$R = \frac{V}{I} \qquad\qquad V = IR$$

Once again, note the *proportionalities* inherent in these equations. Current is directly proportional to voltage (electrical potential difference) and inversely proportional to resistance.

Please solve this problem:

- The cathode of a 12-volt battery is connected by a conductive wire to an electric motor, which is then connected by another wire to the battery's anode. The total resistance of the circuit—through the wire, motor, and battery—is 2 . What is the magnitude of current traveling through the circuit?

Problem solved:

The problem requires simple application of Ohm's law:

$$\frac{V}{R} = I \qquad\qquad \frac{12V}{2\Omega} = 6A$$

Please solve this problem:

- A piece of equipment requires for its operation a minimum current of 4,800 amperes. It draws electricity from an 1,800-volt source. What is the maximum resistance of the system under which the equipment will remain operational?

Problem solved:

This problem, like the preceding one, draws on Ohm's law:

$$4800 \text{ A} = \frac{1800 \text{ V}}{R} \qquad R(4800 \text{ A}) = 1800 \text{ V} \qquad R = \frac{1800 \text{ V}}{4800 \text{ A}} = 0.375 \ \Omega$$

If the resistance in the circuit exceeds 0.375 ohms, current will fall below 4,800 A, and the equipment will not operate.

Note that the problem may be solved by initially applying the following form of the Ohm's law equation:

$$R = \frac{V}{I}$$

$$R = \frac{1800 \text{ V}}{4800 \text{ A}} = 0.375 \ \Omega$$

Please solve this problem:

- Consider a power source of 50 volts that drives equipment with current of 40 amperes. What is the total resistance in the circuit through which the equipment operates?

Problem solved:

Once again, the problem involves the simple application of Ohm's law:

$$R = \frac{V}{I}$$

$$R = \frac{50 \text{ V}}{40 \text{ A}} = 1.25 \ \Omega$$

Please solve this problem:

- An electrical device is driven by a power source of voltage V. The circuit through which it operates has resistance R and carries current of I. Assuming that the conductor in the circuit is modified so that the total resistance of the circuit is $3R$, and the power source is modified so that its voltage is $\frac{1}{2}V$, write an equation that expresses the resulting modified current, I_1, in terms of the original current I.

Problem solved:

The problem requires an appreciation of the proportionalities of Ohm's law. Current is directly proportional to voltage and inversely proportional to resistance. Since resistance is multiplied by a factor of 3, and voltage by a factor of $\frac{1}{2}$, the new current, I_1, comes from the original current, I, divided by a factor of 3 and multiplied by a factor of $\frac{1}{2}$:

$$I_1 = (I) \times \left(\frac{0.5}{3}\right)$$
$$I_1 = 0.167(I)$$

10.1.1.2 Electrical Circuits and Power

Power represents the quantity of work per unit time, and is expressed in the SI unit **watt** (**W**). One must be able to derive and manipulate **power, P,** using the electrical variables current, voltage, and resistance.

The power of electricity flowing through a circuit is equal to the product of current and voltage:

$$P = IV$$

If we know the resistance of the system, we can derive another expression for electrical power:

$$P = I(IR)$$

and

$$P = I^2R$$

Since Ohm's law can also be expressed as:

$$I = \frac{V}{R}$$

the following substitution can be made, giving a third expression for power:

$$P = \frac{V}{R}(V)$$

$$P = \frac{V^2}{R}$$

Please solve this problem:

- A 200-watt device is operated within a circuit that draws 1.60 amperes. What is the voltage of the power source?

Problem solved:

The problem is solved by simple application of the equation that relates power, current, and voltage:

$$P = IV$$

$$V = \frac{P}{I}$$

$$\frac{200 \text{ W}}{1.60 \text{ A}} = 125 \text{ V}$$

Note that power does *not* represent one concept in the context of electricity and another in the context of force and motion. Power has the same meaning in *both* cases, and can therefore be expressed in both electrical and mechanical terms. If, for example, you are told that an electric motor lifts a 45 kg object a distance of 8 meters over a period of 2 seconds, you can determine the motor's power by:

$$P = \frac{\text{work}}{\text{time}} = \frac{\text{force} \times \text{distance}}{\text{time}} = \frac{(\text{mass} \times \text{acceleration}) \times \text{distance}}{\text{time}}$$

for vertical lifting.

Using $g = 10 \text{ m/s}^2$:

$$P = \frac{(45 \text{ kg} \times 10 \text{ m/s}^2)(8 \text{ m})}{2\text{s}} = 1800 \frac{(\text{kg} \cdot \text{m/s}^2)}{\text{s}} = 1800 \text{ N} \cdot \text{m/s}$$
$$P = 1800 \text{ J/s} = 1800 \text{ W}$$

If the current in the system is known to be 6 amperes, you can also determine the voltage of the circuit:

$$P = IV$$

$$1800 \text{ W} = (6 \text{ A}) \times (V)$$

$$V = \frac{1800 \text{ W}}{6 \text{ A}} = 300 \text{ V}$$

The circuit's resistance may be determined by applying Ohm's law, $R = \frac{V}{I}$, or by applying the formula, $P = I^2R$. Using the first approach:

$$R = \frac{V}{I}$$

$$R = \frac{300 \text{ V}}{6 \text{ A}} = 50 \ \Omega$$

Using the second approach:

$$P = I^2R, \text{ or } R = \frac{P}{I^2}$$

$$R = \frac{1800 \text{ W}}{36 \text{ A}^2} = 50 \text{ }\Omega$$

Please solve this problem:

- An electric lifting device operates from a 3,000-volt power source, and the circuit through which it operates has total resistance of 1,200 ohms. If the lift is attached to a mass of 200,000 kg, during what time period will it raise the mass to a height of 8 meters? (Assume that no energy is lost to heat and that $g = 10$ m/s².)

Problem Solved:

Solving this problem requires that you relate electrical terms and mechanical terms through their respective formulae for power. In mechanical terms, the time required to lift a given mass a specified distance depends upon the power of the lift, as specified by:

$$P = \frac{\text{work}}{t} = \frac{W}{t}$$

which can be rearranged to:

$$t = \frac{W}{P}$$

Power can be readily derived from the information provided in the problem, by using the formula:

$$P = \frac{V^2}{R}$$

$$P = \frac{(3000 \text{ V})^2}{1200 \text{ }\Omega} = 7500 \text{ W}$$

which by definition:

$$= 7500 \text{ J/s}$$

Work can also be derived from the information given, using:

$$W = (\text{force})(\text{distance})$$

$$= [(200,000 \text{ kg})(10 \text{ m/s}^2)] \, [8 \text{ m}]$$

$$= 1.6 \times 10^7 \text{ J}$$

Substituting these results into our previously rearranged formula, we find:

$$t = \frac{1.6 \times 10^7 \text{ J}}{7500 \text{ J/s}}$$

$$= 2133 \text{ s}$$

$$\approx 36 \text{ minutes}$$

10.1.1.3 Resistors

MCAT questions will require that you understand quantitative relationships that arise from the placement of **resistors** within electric circuits.

Resistors are objects that conduct electricity poorly. All conductors inherently *resist* current (electron) flow to some extent. Thus, all conductors are resistors, and all resistors are conductors. Whether an object is considered a "resistor" or a "conductor" is based on a matter of degree. That which conducts well is considered a conductor (even though it also resists) and that which conducts poorly is considered a resistor.

Materials such as wood, rubber, and glass are all very poor conductors of electricity, and are thus termed resistors. As earlier noted, resistance is expressed quantitatively in the SI unit ohm (Ω).

In any electric circuit, one should appreciate the difference between a group of resistors connected **in series** and a group connected in parallel. To state that a group of resistors is connected in series means that they are arranged sequentially, as shown in Figure 10.2:

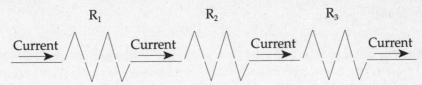

Figure 10.2

To state that a group of resistors is connected in parallel means that one end of each resistor is connected at a common junction and the opposite ends are attached to another common junction, as shown in Figure 10.3:

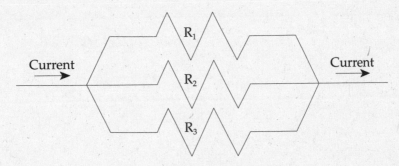

Figure 10.3

When two or more resistors are placed in series, the total resistance they offer is equal to the sum of the resistance of each.

The electric circuit shown in Figure 10.4 features two resistors connected in series, plus a light bulb. The resistors have resistances of 8 Ω and 2 Ω, respectively, and the light bulb has a resistance of an additional 1 Ω. The light bulb (like any device or mechanism driven by electricity) has resistance of its own. The light bulb is connected in series with the two resistors, and the circuit thus features three resistors connected in series:

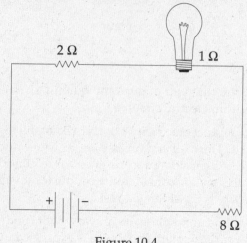

Figure 10.4

To ascertain the total resistance in the circuit (ignoring that of the conducting wire itself and the battery), simply sum the resistances of each of the resistors:

$$R_t = R_1 + R_2 + R_3 + \dots$$

Thus, in this case:

$$8\,\Omega + 2\,\Omega + 1\,\Omega = 11\,\Omega$$

The mathematics are more complicated in cases where resistors connected in parallel. When two or more resistors are connected in parallel, total resistance is equal to the reciprocal of the sum of reciprocals of individual resistances.

The electric circuit depicted in Figure 10.5 features a power source and a set of four parallel resistors. The resistors have resistances of 9 Ω, 7 Ω, 5 Ω, and 2 Ω, respectively:

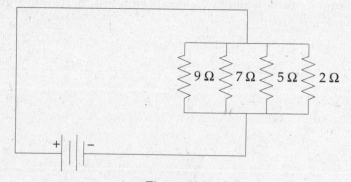

Figure 10.5

Total resistance, R_t, is calculated according to the formula:

$$\frac{1}{R_t} = \frac{1}{R_1} + \frac{1}{R_2} + \frac{1}{R_3} + \dots$$

If one ignores all other resistance in the circuit (such as that of the conducting wire and power source, for example), the total resistance, R_t, is calculated from the individual resistances according to this equation:

$$\frac{1}{R_t} = \frac{1}{9\,\Omega} + \frac{1}{7\,\Omega} + \frac{1}{5\,\Omega} + \frac{1}{2\,\Omega}$$

You calculate the result by (1) taking the sum set forth on the right side of the equation, and then (2) taking the reciprocal of the result. The denominators 9, 7, 5, and 2 have a common denominator of 630. Hence, the sum:

$$\frac{1}{9\,\Omega} + \frac{1}{7\,\Omega} + \frac{1}{5\,\Omega} + \frac{1}{2\,\Omega}$$

is equivalent to:

$$\frac{70}{630\,\Omega} + \frac{90}{630\,\Omega} + \frac{126}{630\,\Omega} + \frac{315}{630\,\Omega} = \frac{601}{630\,\Omega}$$

R_t is found by taking the reciprocal of the sum:

$$R_t = \frac{1}{\dfrac{601}{630\,\Omega}}$$

$$R_t = 1.05\ \Omega$$

Notice that the total resistance is less than the smallest resistor in parallel. This will always be the case. The bridge example in section 10.1.1 explains this nicely. If another bridge is added across the river, then the overall resistance to traffic flow will be decreased.

10.1.1.4 Circuitry

The student should be able to calculate the total resistance of a circuit of complex organization by applying the following principle, which derives from the formulas just described: If, *within a single set of resistors connected in parallel* two or more resistors are connected *in series*, then one first takes the sums of the resistances aligned in series and then uses those sums in calculating the resistances arranged in parallel.

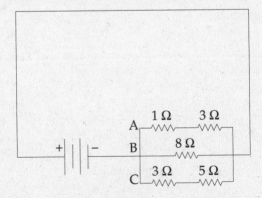

Figure 10.6

Referring to the circuit depicted in Figure 10.6, note that entities A and C each carry two resistors in series. That is, A carries a 1 Ω resistor and a 3 Ω resistor, and its total resistance is 4 Ω. C carries a 3 Ω resistor and a 5 Ω resistor, and its total resistance is 8 Ω. Thus, the set of five resistors can be interpreted more simply as three resistors connected in parallel, the first with resistance of 4 Ω, the second with 8 Ω, and the third with 8 Ω. The total resistance of the set can then be calculated according to the equation for resistances in parallel:

$$\frac{1}{R_t} = \frac{1}{R_1} + \frac{1}{R_2} + \frac{1}{R_3}$$

$$\frac{1}{R_t} = \frac{2}{8\,\Omega} + \frac{1}{8\,\Omega} + \frac{1}{8\,\Omega} = \frac{4}{8}\Omega$$

$$\frac{1}{R_t} = 0.5\,\Omega$$

Thus:

$$R_t = 2\,\Omega$$

Please solve this problem:

- The electric circuit depicted in Figure 10.7 presents a 220-volt power source that operates an article of equipment having 3 ohms of resistance. The circuit further features a 3 Ω resistor, a 2 Ω resistor, and the set of resistors connected in parallel, as shown. *Within* the set of resistors connected in parallel, are resistors connected in series. Ignoring any resistance offered by the conducting wire itself or the power source, please find (a) the total resistance in the circuit, (b) the total current drawn by the device, and (c) the total power associated with the circuit.

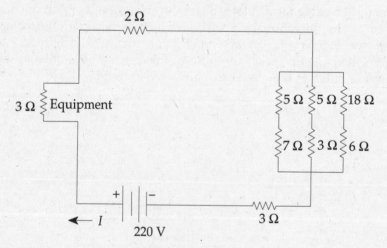

Figure 10.7

Problem solved:

(a) The total resistance within the circuit is the sum of the four resistors connected in series, including, as one resistor, the equipment itself, and as another resistor, the set of resistors connected in parallel. The resistors other than those connected in parallel have a total resistance of:

$$3\,\Omega + 2\,\Omega + 3\,\Omega = 8\,\Omega$$

The set connected in parallel features three resisting entities, each composed of two resistors in series. Find the resistance of each of the parallel resisting entities by summing their respective resistances in series. The series on the right has a resistance of $6\,\Omega + 18\,\Omega = 24\,\Omega$; the middle series, $5\,\Omega + 3\,\Omega = 8\,\Omega$; and the series on the left, $5\,\Omega + 7\,\Omega = 12\,\Omega$. The entire set, therefore, is equivalent to three parallel resistors of $24\,\Omega$, $8\,\Omega$, and $12\,\Omega$, respectively.

To determine the total resistance of the parallel resistors, apply the equation:

$$\frac{1}{R_t} = \frac{1}{R_1} + \frac{1}{R_2} + \frac{1}{R_3}$$

$$\frac{1}{R_t} = \frac{1}{24\,\Omega} + \frac{1}{8\,\Omega} + \frac{1}{12\,\Omega}$$

Since 24 is the common denominator, the equation may be rewritten:

$$\frac{1}{R_t} = \frac{1}{24\,\Omega} + \frac{3}{24\,\Omega} + \frac{2}{24\,\Omega}$$

$$= \frac{6}{24\,\Omega}$$

$$\frac{1}{R_t} = \frac{1}{4\,\Omega}$$

The reciprocal of $\frac{1}{4}$ is 4, and therefore the total resistance of the set is equal to $4\,\Omega$. Adding the $4\,\Omega$ to the $8\,\Omega$ of the circuit's other resistors, you can determine that the total resistance within the circuit is $12\,\Omega$.

(b) Knowing now that the circuit's total resistance is $12\,\Omega$, one can calculate the current of the circuit using Ohm's law:

$$I = \frac{V}{R}$$

$$I = \frac{220\,V}{12\,\Omega}$$

$$I = 18.33\,A$$

(c) Knowing that the circuit's resistance is $12\,\Omega$, and its current 18.33 A, power can now be calculated using either of the equations $P = I^2R$ or $P = IV$.

The first equation gives us:

$$P = I^2R$$

$$P = (18.33 \text{ A})^2 \times (12 \ \Omega)$$

$$P = 4{,}032 \text{ W}$$

The second equation gives us:

$$P = IV$$

$$P = (18.33 \text{ A}) \times (220 \text{ V})$$

$$P = 4{,}032 \text{ W}$$

Please solve this problem:

- The electric circuit depicted in Figure 10.8 presents a 450-volt power source that operates an article of equipment having 7 Ω of resistance. The circuit further features a 3 Ω resistor, and two sets of resistors connected in parallel as shown. Within the second set of parallel resistors are two resistors connected in series. Ignoring any resistance offered by the conducting wire itself or the power source, please find (a) the total resistance in the circuit, (b) the total current drawn by the device, and (c) the total power associated with the circuit.

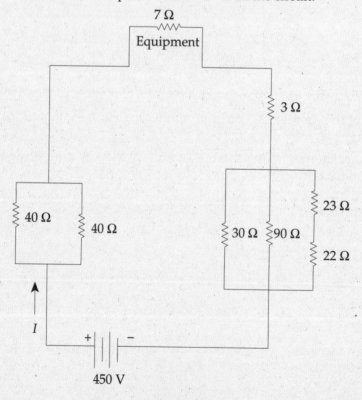

Figure 10.8

Problem solved:

(a) The circuit features two sets of parallel resistors. The total resistance of the circuit is equal to the sum of all resistors connected in series, which means the sum of (1) the first set of parallel resistors, (2) the equipment with resistance of 7 Ω, (3) the 3 Ω resistor, and (4) the second set of parallel resistors. Total resistance of the first set of parallel resistors is:

$$\frac{1}{R_t} = \frac{1}{40\ \Omega} + \frac{1}{40\ \Omega}$$

$$\frac{1}{R_t} = \frac{2}{40\ \Omega}$$

$$R_t = 20\ \Omega$$

Total resistance of the second set of parallel resistors is determined by first summing two resistors connected in series:

$$R = 22\ \Omega + 23\ \Omega$$

$$R = 45\ \Omega$$

The parallel set is thus equivalent to a set consisting of a 45 Ω resistor, a 90 Ω resistor, and a 30 Ω resistor. Total resistance of the set is:

$$\frac{1}{R_t} = \frac{1}{R_1} + \frac{1}{R_2} + \frac{1}{R_3}$$

$$\frac{1}{R_t} = \frac{1}{45\ \Omega} + \frac{1}{90\ \Omega} + \frac{1}{30\ \Omega}$$

The denominators 45, 90, and 30 have 90 as a common denominator; thus, the equation may be rewritten:

$$\frac{1}{R_t} = \frac{2}{90\ \Omega} + \frac{1}{90\ \Omega} + \frac{3}{90\ \Omega}$$

$$\frac{1}{R_t} = \frac{6}{90\ \Omega}$$

The fraction $\frac{6}{90\ \Omega}$ represents $\frac{1}{R_t}$, so the total resistance is equal to its reciprocal,

$$\frac{90}{6}\ \Omega = 15\ \Omega.$$

Total resistance of the circuit is the equal to 20 Ω + 7 Ω + 3 Ω + 15 Ω = 45 Ω.

(b) Knowing that the circuit's total resistance is 45 Ω, its current is calculated by reference to Ohm's law:

$$I = \frac{V}{R}$$

$$I = \frac{450\ V}{45\ \Omega}$$

$$I = 10\ A$$

(c) Knowing that the circuit's current is 10 A, the associated power is calculated according to the equation, $P = I^2R$, or $P = IV$.

The first equation generates the result:

$$P = I^2R$$

$$P = (10 \text{ A})^2 \times (45 \text{ }\Omega)$$

$$P = 4{,}500 \text{ W}$$

The second equation generates the result:

$$P = IV$$

$$P = (10 \text{ A}) \times (450 \text{ V})$$

$$P = 4{,}500 \text{ W}$$

10.1.1.4.1 VOLTAGE DROP

Over the course of an electric circuit, voltage drops progressively. A true evaluation of voltage drop between any two points in the circuit would have to take into account the resistance offered by the conducting wire itself. (MCAT questions, however, will not consider resistance within the conducting wire or power source unless the relevant information is provided to the test-taker.)

As current within a circuit moves across any individual resistor, however, the voltage drops according to Ohm's law:

$$V = IR$$

where:

V represents the voltage drop between any two points in the circuit

I represents the circuit's current (which is constant throughout)

R represents the resistance between the two points under consideration

Consider the circuit described in the previous problem:

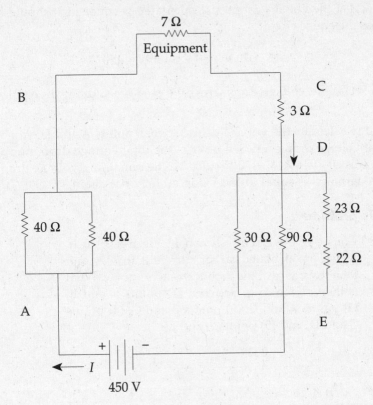

Figure 10.9

As calculated earlier, the current is 10 amperes. The voltage drop between points A and B as shown in figure 10.9 is calculated using Ohm's law equation, $V = IR$. The total resistance between points A and B is equal to the resistance offered by the parallel set of resistors that intervenes, which was calculated to be 20 Ω. Therefore, the voltage drop between points A and B =

$$IR = (10 \text{ A}) \times (20 \text{ Ω}) = 200 \text{ V}$$

Similarly, the voltage drop between points B and C is:

$$V = (10 \text{ A}) \times (7 \text{ Ω}) = 70 \text{ V}$$

The voltage drop between points C and D is equal to:

$$V = (10 \text{ A}) \times (3 \text{ Ω}) = 30 \text{ V}$$

The voltage drop between points D and E is equal to:

$$V = IR$$

$$V = (10 \text{ A}) \times (15 \text{ Ω}) = 150 \text{ V}$$

Note that the total of the voltage drops just calculated is equal, as it should be, to the total voltage drop across the entire circuit:

$$200 \text{ V} + 70 \text{ V} + 30 \text{ V} + 150 \text{ V} = 450 \text{ V}$$

which, as you can see, is the voltage drop across the positive and negative poles of the power source.

If you are asked to calculate the voltage drop between points A and D, you only need to sum the individual voltage drops between points: the total voltage drop interposed between points A and D is thus 200 V + 70 V + 30 V = 300 V. The remaining voltage drop between point D and the negative terminal is equal to 150 V, for a total, once again, of 300 V + 150 V = 450 V.

Please solve this problem :

- Consider the circuit shown in Figure 10.10 in which, as calculated earlier, current is 18.33 A, and total resistance of the parallel resistors is 4 Ω. What is the voltage drop between (1) points A and B, (2) points A and C, (3) points B and C, (4) points C and D, and (5) points A and D?

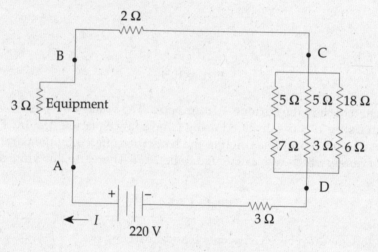

Figure 10.10

Problem solved:

Apply the principle just explained, recalling that voltage drop between any two points is a function of the product IR:

(1) The voltage drop between points A and B is equal to the product:

$$V = (18.33 \text{ A}) \times (3 \text{ }\Omega) = 55 \text{ V}$$

(2) The voltage drop between points A and C is determined in the same way. The total intervening resistance is 3 Ω + 2 Ω = 5 Ω. Therefore:

$$V = (18.33 \text{ A}) \times (5 \text{ }\Omega) = \text{approx. } 92 \text{ V}$$

(3) Since the total intervening resistance is 2 Ω:

$$V = (18.33 \text{ A}) \times (2 \text{ }\Omega) = \text{approximately } 37 \text{ V}$$

(4) Since the total intervening resistance is 4 Ω:

$$V = (18.33 \text{ A}) \times (4 \text{ }\Omega) = \text{approximately } 73 \text{ V}$$

(5) The voltage drop between points A and D is determined by adding the voltage drops A–B, B–C, and C–D, as calculated above:

$$55 \text{ V} + 37 \text{ V} + 73 \text{ V} = 165 \text{ }\Omega$$

Alternatively, the value might have been calculated by noting that the total intervening resistance between points A and D is 3 Ω + 2 Ω + 4 Ω = 9 Ω and applying Ohm's law:

$$V = (18.33 \text{ A}) \times (9 \text{ }\Omega) = 165 \text{ V}$$

Note that if the 165 voltage drop between A and D as just calculated is added to the voltage drop between the negative terminal itself and point D, where a 3 Ω resistor is interposed, the result is:

$$165 \text{ V} + [(18.33 \text{ A}) \times (3 \text{ }\Omega)] = 165 \text{ V} + 55 \text{ V} = 220 \text{ V}$$

which represents the voltage drop associated with the entire circuit.

10.1.2 MAGNETISM, MAGNETIC FIELDS, AND CURRENT

A moving charged particle creates its own magnetic field. Electrons moving through a wire constitute a stream of moving, charged particles in which the magnetic field created will be strongest near the wire and diminish with distance.

Magnetic field strength is given in units called **tesla (T)**, where T = N/A•m. The strength of the magnetic field, B, arising from a current in a wire has direction as well as strength inversely proportional to the distance from the wire.

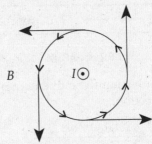

Figure 10.11

It is important to remember that the magnetic field generated by the current in the wire is continuous at all distances from the wire, so that it can be thought of as an infinite series of circles from the wire outward (see Figure 10.12).

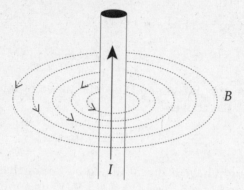

Figure 10.12

The reader should also be aware that there are two possible directions for the magnetic field, as shown in Figure 10.13.

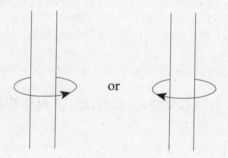

Figure 10.13

Imagine a current—a stream of positive charge—flowing through a conducting wire to the left, as shown in Figure 10.14.

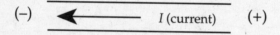

Figure 10.14

Recall, for theoretical purposes only, that the movement of the current *truly* represents the flow of electrons in the opposite direction:

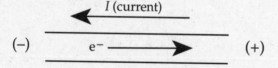

Figure 10.15

To identify the direction of the magnetic field B surrounding the wire, apply what is called the **right hand rule**. This rule is applied by positioning the right hand so that the thumb points in the direction of the current in the wire. If the hand grasps the wire in this way, the bend of the fingers around the wire will indicate the direction of the induced field surrounding the wire.

Application of the right hand rule is demonstrated in Figure 10.16 with respect to a current flowing to the left. The magnetic field occupies a path that corresponds to the circle suggested by the curve of the fingers:

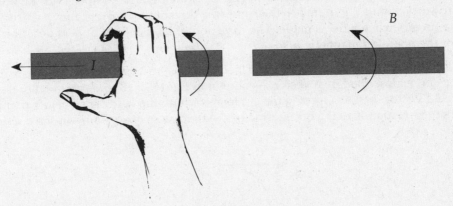

Figure 10.16

Please solve this problem:

- Consider a current moving through the conducting wire shown in Figure 10.17 and determine which of the illustrations that follows it correctly depicts the direction of the resulting magnetic field.

$I \longrightarrow$

Figure 10.17

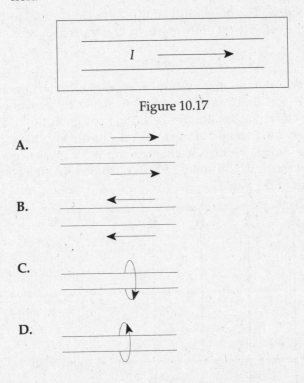

A.

B.

C.

D.

Problem solved:

C is the correct answer. Use the right hand rule. The illustration depicts a current moving through a conducting wire to the reader's right. With the right hand open and the fingers pointing upwards, point the thumb to the right (the direction of current flow). Observe the bend of the fingers when a fist is made. The direction of the bending fingers describes the direction of the resulting magnetic field.

Although the total magnetic field is described by concentric circles, the magnetic field at any given point is described by a vector. As shown in figure 10.18, each arrow represents a magnetic field vector that is *tangent to* the circle describing the field. The vectors point in a direction that corresponds to the orientation of the field at an exact point on the circle:

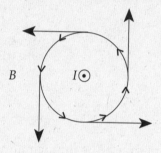

Figure 10.18

You should understand the interaction between a magnetic field and a moving or changing electrical field. When a charged particle moves through a magnetic field, the magnetic field exerts a force upon that particle. The magnitude of this force (F) is equal to the product of the charge of the particle (q), the velocity (v) of the particle, and the magnetic field strength (B).

$$F = qvB$$

The direction of the force is determined by another right hand rule. Orient your right hand so that your fingers point in the direction of the magnetic field vectors and your thumb extends in the direction of current (opposite the direction of electron flow). The direction in which your palm is facing is the direction of the force on a positively charged particle. In the example below, since an electron is negatively charged and will experience a force opposite of that of a positively charged particle, you should have concluded that the electron will be deflected towards you—out of the page.

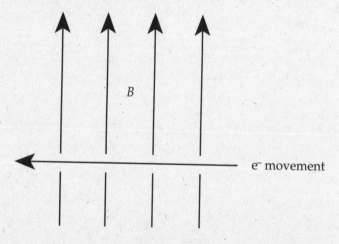

Figure 10.19

Please solve this problem:

- Consider an electron which moves upward, as shown in Figure 10.20. Assume that the particle passes through a magnetic field causing the electron to be deflected away from the reader—into the page. Characterize by illustration the direction of the magnetic field the particle encounters.

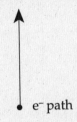

Figure 10.20

Problem solved:

Since you know the direction of deflection, you can place your right hand with your palm facing in this direction. Next, point your thumb in the direction of the current (opposite the direction of electron flow). Your fingers should be pointing to the left. This is the direction of the magnetic field.

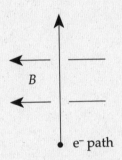

Figure 10.21

10.2 MASTERY APPLIED: SAMPLE PASSAGE AND QUESTIONS

PASSAGE

Electric current is produced by electromotive force (ε). The term "force," in this context, however, does not carry its usual meaning and cannot be measured in newtons; rather, it is measured using the unit joule/coulomb (J/C).

In an ordinary battery, for instance, energy is stored as chemical energy. When the positive and negative terminals of the battery are connected across, some resistance of this chemical energy can be used to do work.

The chemical reaction that takes place inside a battery is often reversible. Any reversible process experiences an equilibrium state in which its course might be reversed through an alteration in the system's environment. A battery, for example, may be charged or discharged. A generator may be operated mechanically to produce electrical energy; alternatively, it can be driven backwards to operate as a motor.

Kirchoff's second rule, also known as the **loop rule**, dictates that the sum of changes in potential associated with the completion of a full loop through an electric circuit equals zero.

All seats of emf have internal resistance, r, which is to be distinguished from external resistance, R, imposed by a conventional resistor. Calculations of real emf must include the internal resistance. Figure 1 depicts an electric circuit, with internal resistance labeled r:

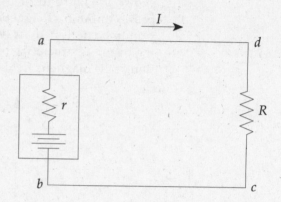

Figure 1

Accounting for r in the loop theorem, and beginning arbitrarily at point b of Figure 2:

$$\varepsilon - Ir - IR = 0$$

In Figure 2, the circuit of Figure 1 is represented as a straight line, with corresponding changes in potential plotted along a vertical line:

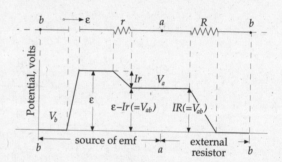

Figure 2

Experiment 1:

An investigator assembles an electrical circuit, attaching to it an electric motor, as shown below in Figure 3:

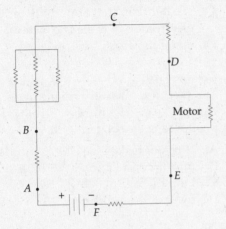

Figure 3

Measuring voltage drop across various sections of the circuits, she obtains the following plot (Figure 4):

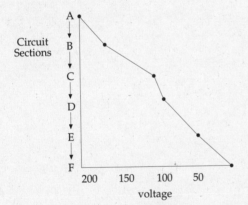

Figure 4

1. With reference to Figure 1, the magnetic field generated by the current between points a and d is oriented:

   A. around the conducting wire directed (a) out of the page above the wire and (b) into the page below the wire.

   B. around the conducting wire directed (a) into the page above the wire and (b) out of the page below the wire.

   C. parallel to the conducting wire and directed to the left.

   D. parallel to the conducting wire and directed to the right.

2. If, at a very small distance r from the conducting wire shown in Figure 1, the associated magnetic field has strength of B tesla, what is the strength of the magnetic field at a distance $2.5r$ from the conducting wire?

   A. $I^2B^2\pi$ tesla
   B. $(2.5\pi)B^2$ tesla
   C. $(2.5)B$ tesla
   D. $(0.4)B$ tesla

3. Which of the following conclusions is justifiable on the basis of the investigator's data as shown in Figure 4 as they relate to Figure 3?

   A. The current between points A and B is greater than the current between points B and C.

   B. The current between points A and B is less than the current between points B and C.

   C. The electric motor offers greater resistance than does the resistor situated between points C and D.

   D. The electric motor offers less resistance than does the resistor situated between points C and D.

4. According to Kirchoff's second rule as described in the passage which of the following would accurately represent the strength of a real electromotive force?

   A. $I (r + R)$
   B. $I/(r + R)$
   C. Eq
   D. $K (qq)/r^2$

5. With reference to Figure 3, which of the following choices best characterizes the set of resistors situated between points B and C?

   A. As a set they are connected in parallel with the electric motor.
   B. As a set they are connected in series with the electric motor.
   C. As a set they are connected in series with one another.
   D. As a set they must necessarily offer less resistance than any other resistive element in the circuit.

6. According to Figure 2, as it relates to Figure 1, the electrical potential at point A is:

   A. greater than that at point B.
   B. less than that at point B.
   C. greater than that at point B, only if electromotive force is constant.
   D. equal to zero.

7. The fact that a battery might undergo charge or discharge illustrates phenomena associated with:

   A. external resistance.
   B. internal resistance.
   C. loop theory.
   D. reversible equilibria.

10.3 MASTERY VERIFIED: ANSWERS AND EXPLANATIONS

1. *A is the correct answer.* The solution requires the right hand rule. Examining the segment of conducting wire between points A and D in Figure 1, the investigator sees that with reference to the page, the current is directed to the right. She should, then, extend her thumb to the right and direct her fingers upward (which means her palm will face her). The natural curve of her fingers will then suggest the circle followed by the magnetic field surrounding the wire. Her fingers point toward her as they go over the wire and away from her (into the page) as they pass under the wire.

2. *D is the correct answer.* The question tests your ability to apply the proportional relationships associated with the equation that describes field strength, B. Strength is *inversely* proportional to r, the distance from the conducting wire. If at distance r, field strength equals B, then at a distance of 2.5 r, the field strength will equal $\frac{1}{2.5}B$ or $(0.4)B$.

3. *C is the correct answer.* Figure 4 describes the voltage drop between various sectors of the circuit. Voltage drop is determined by Ohm's law: $V = IR$. Since current (I) is identical between any two labelled points in the circuit, the greater the drop between any two points in the circuit, the greater the resistance between those points. The electric motor is positioned between points D and E, and the voltage drop between D and E as shown in Figure 4 is approximately 50 volts (100 V – 50 V). The voltage drop between points C and D, on the other hand, is clearly less than that amount, as indicated by the markedly greater slope of the line segment corresponding to points C and D.

4. *A is the correct answer.* Examine the equation associated with Kirchoff's second rule (as supplied in the passage) and rearrange it through simple algebra:

$$E - Ir - IR = 0$$

$$E = Ir + IR$$

$$E = I(r + R)$$

5. *B is the correct answer.* The question tests knowledge of the distinction between resistors connected in parallel and those connected in series. Although the set of resistors between points B and C is one of parallel resistors (with one segment consisting of two resistors connected in series), *the entire set as a unit* is connected in series with all other resisting elements of the circuit.

6. *A is the correct answer.* Figure 2 relates electrical potential to various points within the circuit shown in Figure 1. Electrical potential is described by the vertical axis. Notice that the position associated with point A is higher than that associated with point B.

7. *D is the correct answer.* The chemical reactions that take place within a battery are often reversible, and thus often susceptible to an equilibrium state, and the direction of a reaction may be altered by a change in environment. As an example, the author refers to the charge and discharge of a battery. The question, then, calls only for reading comprehension in a scientific context.

CHAPTER 11

WAVES, OSCILLATIONS, AND SIMPLE HARMONIC MOTION

11.1 MASTERY ACHIEVED

11.1.1 DYNAMICS OF THE WAVE

You should understand the characteristics of **transverse waves** and **longitudinal waves**. The accepted model for a transverse wave conforms to the traditional wave-like appearance that you are familiar with. It can be represented schematically as in Figure 11.1.

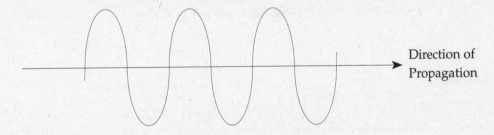

Figure 11.1

The arrow indicates that the wave is moving to the right. The medium through which the wave moves (whether it be a rope, string, or wire) does *not* move in the direction associated with the wave's movement. Rather, it **oscillates** cyclically, corresponding to the wave's movement.

If, for example, with respect to the diagram presented above, one imagines that the wave is propagated through a rope, the rope itself does *not* move rightward. Rather, it moves cyclically in vertical orientation, repeatedly creating crests and troughs, whose *locations within the medium move* rightward, without any rightward movement of the medium itself.

A transverse wave is said to have a **cycle**; its cycle is most easily understood in terms of the movement of its medium, as just described. The fact that the medium exhibits a rightward-moving series of peaks and troughs represents a repetition of events, and each such repetition describes a cycle. One such cycle is associated with the generation of one crest and one trough.

The transverse wave's cycle is expressed in terms of its **period**. The wave's period represents the time associated with one cycle, or the time in which a point in the medium experiences the cycle of crest-trough-crest. In other words, the time that intervenes between one crest and the next represents the wave's period.

Period expresses the ratio time per cycle (time/cycle) although, by convention, the reference to the cycle is taken for granted and so is omitted from the expression. Period is measured simply in units of time. The SI unit for period is the **second (s)**, and to state that a wave has a period of 4 seconds is to state that it undergoes one cycle in 4 seconds (4 seconds per cycle).

Frequency is the reciprocal of period. It expresses the number of cycles the wave undergoes in one second. If, for example, a wave undergoes 1 cycle in 4 seconds, then it undergoes 0.25 cycles in one second, and its frequency is 0.25 cycles per second. The phrase "cycles per second" is renamed **hertz (Hz)**, and the frequency of such a wave would most commonly be described as 0.25 Hz.

Please solve this problem:

- A transverse wave travels through a visible medium. An observer directs her attention to one point on the medium, and with the appearance of a given crest which she numbers as the first, she marks the time as zero. Including the first crest, she notes that a total of 5 crests pass her view in a period of 8 seconds Find the wave's (a) period and (b) frequency.

Problem solved:

Part (a): The appearance of 5 crests in a period of 8 seconds indicates that the wave has undergone 4 (not 5) cycles in 8 seconds. The first crest does not represent a cycle. Rather, the appearance of 2 crests represents a cycle, and the appearance of 5 crests represents 4 cycles, as shown below:

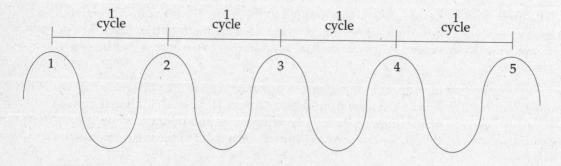

Figure 11.2

The wave undergoes 4 cycles in 8 seconds. The fraction $\frac{8 \text{ seconds}}{4 \text{ cycles}}$ is equivalent to the fraction $\frac{2 \text{ seconds}}{1 \text{ cycle}}$, and the period of the wave is 2 seconds.

Part (b): If you know that the wave's period is 2 seconds, you know that it undergoes 1 cycle in 2 seconds. To ask a wave's frequency is to ask how many cycles it undergoes in 1 second, which is to ask for the reciprocal of the period. The reciprocal of $\frac{2 \text{ seconds}}{1 \text{ cycle}}$ is $\frac{1 \text{ cycle}}{2 \text{ seconds}}$ = 0.5 cycles/second. The wave's frequency, therefore, is 0.5 Hz.

Please solve this problem:

- A transverse wave travels through a visible medium. An observer directs her attention to one point on the medium, and with the appearance of a given trough, which she numbers as the first trough, she marks the time as zero. Including the first trough, she notes that a total of 13 troughs pass her view in a period of 60 seconds. Find the wave's (a) period and (b) frequency.

Problem solved:

The second of the 13 troughs that pass the observer's view represents the completion of 1 cycle, and the 13 troughs in total represent the completion of 12 cycles. The wave, therefore, undergoes 12 cycles in 60 seconds.

Part (a): The wave's period is derived from the fraction $\frac{60 \text{ seconds}}{12 \text{ cycles}}$ = 5 seconds/cycle, which is conventionally expressed as 5 seconds.

Part (b): The wave's frequency is the reciprocal of its period. The reciprocal of $\frac{5}{1}$ is $\frac{1}{5}$ = 0.2, and the frequency, therefore, is 0.2 Hz.

It follows that when a wave's period is less than 1 second, its frequency is greater than 1. If a given wave undergoes 1 cycle in 0.7 seconds, its frequency is approximately $\frac{1}{0.7}$ Hz = 1.43 Hz.

For any wave, **wavelength** represents the distance from one crest to the next (or from one trough to the next) and, generally, from one position within a single wave unit to the corresponding position of the next.

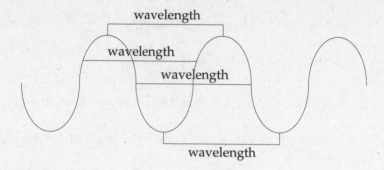

Figure 11.3

Wavelength is symbolized by the Greek letter **lambda** (λ) and is measured in meters. (More precisely, wavelength is a measure of meters per cycle; but by convention the reference to cycles is understood and omitted from the expression.)

With respect to any wave, **speed** refers to the rapidity (measured in units of distance per time) with which the wave moves through its medium. Since wavelength represents the distance from crest to crest, and frequency represents the time during which two crests (representing one cycle) pass a given point within the medium, the speed of any transverse wave is equivalent to the product:

$$v = (\text{frequency})(\text{wavelength})$$

For any transverse wave $v = f\,\lambda$

Verification for dimensional consistency shows us that:

$$v = (\text{frequency})(\text{wavelength}) = \text{speed}$$

$$\left(\frac{\text{cycles}}{\text{second}}\right)\left(\frac{\text{meters}}{\text{cycle}}\right) = \frac{\text{meters}}{\text{second}}$$

Please solve this problem:

- A given transverse wave has a period of 4×10^{-5} seconds and a speed of 680 m/s. Find (a) its frequency and (b) its wavelength.

Problem solved:

Part (a): The wave's period is 4×10^{-5} seconds, and its frequency is the reciprocal:

$$\frac{1}{4 \times 10^{-5}} = \frac{1 \times 10^{0}}{4 \times 10^{-5}}$$

$$= 0.25 \times 10^{5}$$

$$= 2.5 \times 10^{4}\,\text{Hz}$$

which means that it undergoes 25,000 cycles per second.

Part (b): Knowing that the wave's frequency is 25,000 Hz, and that its speed is 680 m/s, calculate its wavelength by reference to the equation:

$$speed = (frequency)(wavelength)$$

$$wavelength = \frac{speed}{frequency} = \frac{680 \text{ m/s}}{25,000 \text{ Hz}}$$

$$\frac{680 \times 10^{0}}{2.5 \times 10^{4}} = 2.72 \times 10^{-2} \text{m}$$

With respect to any transverse wave, **amplitude** represents the wave height: the distance from the central portion of one wave unit to the crest or the distance between the central portion of the wave unit and the trough.

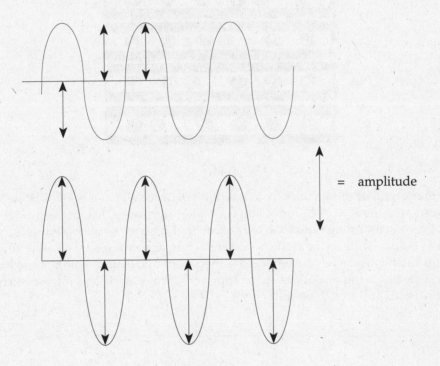

= amplitude

Figure 11.4

11.1.1.1 Longitudinal Compression Waves

A **longitudinal compression wave** is a wave that travels parallel to the plane in which its own medium oscillates, and gives rise cyclically to areas of increased and decreased density. The phenomenon is best visualized by reference to a cylindrical steel bar that is fixed at one end and free at the other. If the bar is struck at the free end, then at the point of impact it will momentarily compress—its density will increase. The compression will travel longitudinally through the bar, so that along its length, the bar experiences a moving area of increased density.

Since the overall mass of the bar does not change, each region of increased density must leave behind it an area of reduced density (just as the peak of a transverse wave leaves a trough immediately behind it). The area of reduced density is called an area of **rarefaction**, and for a longitudinal compression wave, the analogs to crest and trough are compression and rarefaction, respectively.

Figure 11.5 depicts a steel bar, with the six circles inside representing the molecules that comprise it. The six drawings show the bar in its initial state (1), a moment after it is struck at the left end (2), and successive moments thereafter (3)–(6).

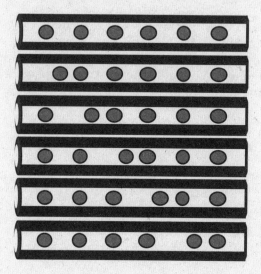

Figure 11.5

Observe the second of the six bars. The first two "molecules" have been compressed. The third bar shows that the area of compression is moving rightward, leaving behind it an area of rarefaction. The fourth through the sixth bars show that the area of increased density—the compression—is advancing to the right, with rarefaction appearing immediately to its left, and that areas still further to the left are recovering their normal density. Think of the longitudinal compression wave as being analogous to the transverse wave, and showing a cyclic pattern of crests (compression) and troughs (rarefaction).

Figure 11.6 schematically depicts the analogy.

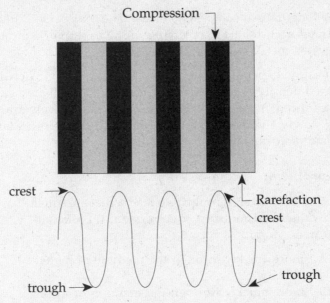

Figure 11.6

The longitudinal compression wave has the five essential features of a transverse wave: period, frequency, wavelength, speed, and amplitude. Do not invest effort in acquiring a true conceptual appreciation of those phenomena as they relate to longitudinal compression waves. Instead, in all contexts concerning period, frequency, wavelength, speed, and amplitude, visualize it as a transverse wave.

Please solve this problem:

- If a particular sound wave has a period of approximately 0.0286 seconds and speed of 1190 meters per second, find (a) its frequency and (b) its wavelength.

Problem solved:

Part (a): Knowing that the wave has a period of 0.0286 seconds (meaning that it undergoes one cycle in 0.0286 seconds), identify its frequency by taking the reciprocal of that number:

$$\frac{1}{0.0286} = \text{approx. } 3.5 \times 10^1 \, \text{Hz}$$

approx. $3.5 \times 10^1 \, \text{Hz} = 35 \, \text{Hz}$

Part (b): Knowing that the wave's frequency is 35 Hz (meaning that it undergoes 35 cycles in one second) and that its speed is 1190 meters per second, its wavelength (which is in reality meters/cycle) is calculated by the equation:

$$(\text{speed}) = (\text{frequency}) \times (\text{wavelength})$$

$$\text{wavelength} = \frac{\text{speed}}{\text{frequency}} = \frac{1190 \ \text{m/s}}{35 \ \text{Hz}} = 34 \, \text{m}$$

11.1.2 SOUND WAVES

Sound travels as a longitudinal compression wave and may do so through a variety of media. Humans are most accustomed to receiving sound as it travels through air, but it may also travel through water, metals, wood, and other media.

The speed of sound depends on two features of its medium: **density** and **resistance to compression**. Increased density of the medium decreases speed. Increased resistance to compression increases speed. In general, then, a medium of relatively greater density tends to conduct sound more slowly, and a medium that is relatively more resistant to compression tends to conduct sound more quickly.

Please solve this problem:

- If sound travels through two media that are equal in their resistance to compression, then it will travel:

  A. more quickly through the medium of higher density.
  B. more quickly through the medium of lower density.
  C. at equal speed through the two media.
  D. more quickly or less quickly through the medium of higher density, depending on the mass of each medium.

Problem solved:

The correct answer is B. Since the two media are equally resistant to compression, density is the only factor affecting speed. The higher the density of the medium, the slower the conduction.

Please solve this problem:

- If sound travels through two media, one more resistant to compression than the other, then it will travel:

  A. more quickly through the medium that is more resistant to compression.
  B. more quickly through the medium that is less resistant to compression.
  C. at equal speed through the two media.
  D. more quickly or less quickly through the medium that is more resistant to compression, depending on the densities of the two media.

Problem solved:

The correct answer is D. The speed of sound is dependent not only on the medium's resistance to compression, but on its density as well.

11.1.2.1 Loudness and Intensity

Sound has both **loudness** and **intensity**. Loudness [β] is measured in the unit **decibel (dB)**, and intensity [I], in the unit **watts per square meter (W/m²)**.

At the threshold of human hearing, sound intensity is approximately 10^{-12} W/m²; and for any level of intensity, loudness is equal to the product:

$$10 \times \log \left[\frac{\text{Intensity}}{10^{-12} \text{W/m}^2} \right]$$

As noted, the value 10^{-12} W/m² represents the threshold of human hearing and is assigned the symbol I_o. Therefore, the conventional equation relating loudness to intensity is:

$$\beta = 10 \log \frac{I}{I_o}$$

where:

β = loudness (in decibels)

I = intensity in watts/square meter

I_o = threshold of human hearing = 10^{-12} W/m²

One should understand that according to the above equation:

If any given intensity, I_1, corresponds to a particular loudness, β_1, then for any x >1, a new intensity I_2, which is equal to $(I_1)(10^x)$, corresponds to a new loudness, β_2, which is equal to $(B_1 + 10x)$.

With respect to the paragraph above, consider the variable x. Suppose, for example, one is told that a sound wave of intensity Z W/m² corresponds to a loudness of Y dB. The relationship between loudness and intensity is such that:

intensity		loudness	
100(Z) W/m²	corresponds to	Y + 20 dB	(x = 2)
1,000 (Z) W/m²	corresponds to	Y + 30 dB	(x = 3)
10,000(Z) W/m²	corresponds to	Y + 40 dB	(x = 4)

Study the pattern just presented; it represents the context in which the equation

$\beta = 10 \log \frac{I}{I_o}$ will most likely be tested on the MCAT.

Please solve this problem:

- A whistle has loudness of 88 decibels. If its loudness is increased to 108 decibels, its intensity will be:

  A. multiplied by a factor of 200.
  B. multiplied by a factor of 100.
  C. increased by 200.
  D. increased by 100.

Problem solved:

The correct answer is B. Again, for any $x > 1$, a new intensity I_2, which is equal to $(I_1)(10^x)$ corresponds to a new loudness, β_2, which is equal to $\beta_1 + 10x$. In this instance, loudness has been increased by 20, which is equal to $10(2)$. The x value, therefore, is 2. Intensity, therefore, is multiplied by 10^x, which, in this instance, is $10^2 = 100$.

Please solve this problem:

- An engine's sound has intensity of 8×10^{-12} W/m². If the intensity is increased to 8×10^{-9} W/m², the associated loudness, in decibels, will be:

  A. multiplied by a factor of 300.
  B. divided by a factor of 3,000.
  C. increased by 30.
  D. increased by 3,000.

Problem solved:

The correct answer is C. The x value as used in this context is 3. When intensity is multiplied by 1,000, loudness is increased by $10x$, or 30.

11.1.2.2 Pitch and the Doppler Effect

Sound has **pitch**, which in common terms refers to how high or low it sounds. For any given sound wave, pitch corresponds to frequency; with respect to sound, the two words are virtually synonymous. Pitch, therefore, is described in the unit hertz (Hz), as is frequency. The higher the frequency, the higher the pitch; the lower the frequency, the lower the pitch. The range of human hearing is approximately 10 to 20,000 hertz. Because sound was historically conceived as a phenomenon significant to human beings, a frequency below 10 Hz (the lower limit of human hearing) is called **infrasonic**, and a frequency above 20,000 Hz (the upper limit of human hearing) is called **ultrasonic**.

The **Doppler effect** arises when a source of sound moves in relation to an observer (listener). From the observer's perspective, as a source of sound approaches, the wavelength shortens, and the frequency increases. The apparent increased frequency causes the observer to hear an elevated pitch. From the observer's perspective, as the sound source recedes, the wavelength increases, the apparent frequency decreases, and the observer experiences a declining pitch.

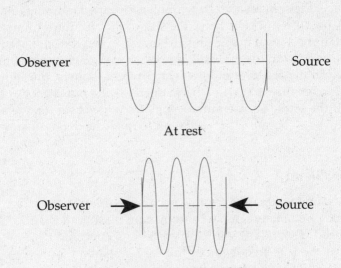

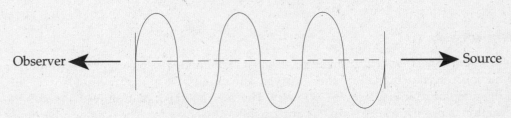

Figure 11.7

The Doppler effect is expressed as:

$$f_o = f_s \left(\frac{v \pm v_o}{v \pm v_s} \right)$$

where:

f_o is the frequency perceived by the observer

f_s is the frequency as actually emitted

v is the speed of the wave in the given medium (usually air)

v_o is the velocity at which the observer moves, which is (+) if the observer moves toward the source, and (–) if the observer moves away from it

v_s is the velocity at which the source moves, which is (–) if the source moves toward the observer, and (+) if it moves away from the observer

The (+) and (–) signs are assigned on the basis of the following. Any motion that tends to draw the source and the observer closer should make the fraction larger. If the observer moves toward the sound source, the sign associated with his movement—the sign between v and v_o—should be positive (+), because it will increase the size of the fraction's numerator and hence the size of the fraction. If the source moves toward the observer, the sign between v and v_s should be negative (–), and it will decrease the size of the denominator, raising the value of the fraction. Conversely, if the observer moves away from the source, the sign between v and v_o should be negative (–), because that will tend to decrease the numerator and reduce the value of the fraction. If the sound source moves away from the observer, the sign between v and v_s should be positive (+), because that will tend to raise the denominator and reduce the value of the fraction.

Please solve this problem:

- A sound source moves toward an observer at a rate of 80 meters per second. Assuming that the speed of sound in air is 340 meters per second and that the true frequency of the source's sound is 400 hertz, what frequency would the observer perceive?

Problem solved:

The problem concerns the Doppler effect as just explained. The observer is stationary and the sound source is moving *toward* the observer. The numerator of the fraction is v = (340 m/s), and the denominator is (340 m/s – 80 m/s). The subtraction of 80 from 340 *increases* the size of the fraction, since the sound source is approaching the observer. The equation becomes:

$$f_o = (400 \ \text{Hz}) \times \frac{340 \ \text{m/s}}{340 \ \text{m/s} - 80 \ \text{m/s}}$$

$$f_o = (400 \ \text{Hz}) \frac{340 \ \text{m/s}}{260 \ \text{m/s}}$$

$$f_o = 400 \ \text{Hz} \ (1.3) = \text{approx. } 520 \ \text{Hz}$$

Please solve this problem:

- A sound source emits a sound with frequency of 280 hertz. It moves away from a listener at a rate of 30 meters per second, but the listener moves toward the source at a rate of 70 meters per second. Assuming that the speed of sound in air is 340 meters per second, what frequency would the observer perceive?

Problem solved:

Both sound source and observer are in motion. The sound source moves away from the observer, which means the sign within the numerator will be positive (+), reducing the size of the fraction. The observer moves toward the sound source, which means the sign in the numerator will also be positive (+), increasing the size of the fraction:

$$f_o = (280 \text{ Hz}) \times \frac{340 \text{ m/s} + 70 \text{ m/s}}{340 \text{ m/s} + 30 \text{ m/s}}$$

$$f_o = (280 \text{ Hz}) \frac{410 \text{ m/s}}{370 \text{ m/s}}$$

$$f_o = 280 \text{ Hz} (1.1) = \text{approx. } 310 \text{ Hz}$$

11.1.3 OSCILLATIONS AND SIMPLE HARMONIC MOTION

The phrase **simple harmonic motion** refers to a certain form of oscillatory motion classically illustrated by a swinging pendulum. Were it not for relevant forces of friction, the pendulum would oscillate endlessly. When the pendulum is at the rightmost position of its path, it is momentarily stationary, but the force of gravity draws it down to the bottommost position of its path, where velocity reaches a maximum. It continues, swinging leftward and upward, and reaches the uppermost position on the left side of its path, where velocity is again momentarily zero. The force of gravity, however, sends it downward once again, its velocity now increasing, until it reaches the bottommost position of its path, where velocity is again at a maximum. The pendulum then moves upward, and to the right, and the oscillatory motion continues without end (ignoring, once again, applicable forces of friction).

Simple harmonic motion is by no means limited to the operation of a pendulum. One might envision an object affixed to the end of a spring that moves in a horizontal path rightward and leftward in response to the cyclic stretching, relaxation, and compression of the spring. Again, if forces of friction are ignored, the oscillatory motion continues without end. When the spring is fully compressed, the object is momentarily stationary. The force associated with the spring's compression causes the spring to move toward its relaxation point, the object being propelled with it.

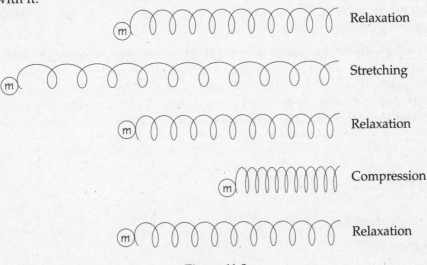

Figure 11.8

The mass attains a maximum velocity at the relaxation point (which is analogous to the bottommost point of a pendulum's path). As motion continues in the same direction, the spring begins to stretch, during which period the velocity decreases until the spring's motion ceases momentarily. The force associated with the stretching of the spring, however, causes the spring to move backward—again toward its relaxation point (just as gravity causes the pendulum to move downward from the uppermost position of its path). The attached object follows, and its velocity increases. The spring again reaches its relaxation point, at which time velocity is maximum. Motion continues, the spring compresses, and velocity decreases, until the spring reaches maximum compression.

11.1.3.1 Simple Harmonic Motion as a Wave

The oscillation of an object in simple harmonic motion has features analogous to those of a wave. An object in simple harmonic motion is said to have a period, frequency, and amplitude. The period represents the time taken to complete one full cycle. In the case of a pendulum, it might be measured as the time taken for the pendulum to complete its travel from rightward end to rightward end (which involves two passages through its bottommost position) or, alternatively, from its leftward end to its leftward end. If the time associated with one full cycle of the pendulum's travel is 2 seconds, its period is 2 seconds.

The same principle applies to the object attached to the end of a spring. The period of the associated simple harmonic motion is the time taken for the spring to complete one full cycle, which might be measured as the time associated with its travel from its point of maximum compression to its point of maximum compression. Alternatively, it might be expressed as the time taken for the spring to travel from its point of maximum stretch to its point of maximum stretch.

As in the case of a wave, the frequency associated with simple harmonic motion is the reciprocal of the period representing the number of oscillations (cycles) that occur in one second. If an object in simple harmonic motion has a period of 5 seconds (meaning, in fact, $\frac{5 \text{ seconds}}{1 \text{ cycle}}$), then its frequency is $\frac{1}{5} = 0.2$ cycles per second.

11.1.3.2 Simple Harmonic Motion: Force and Energy

Simple harmonic motion is associated with force. In the case of a pendulum, the associated force is the pendulum's weight. In the case of the object affixed to a spring, the associated force is the tension within the spring.

The force associated with any point in the oscillation of simple harmonic motion is a function of **displacement**, which refers to the distance from the point of maximum velocity, and the **spring constant**, which, while initially named in relation to a spring, applies whether or not the simple harmonic motion involves a true spring. The spring constant is expressed in the SI unit **newtons/meter (N/m)**. The equation from which force is derived is **Hooke's law**:

$$F = -k(x)$$

where:

F = force

k = spring constant

x = displacement

For any instance of simple harmonic motion, you will be supplied with the spring constant, because it will differ depending on the entity in motion. In the case of a pendulum, the spring constant is approximately equal to the fraction, $\dfrac{\text{weight of pendulum}}{\text{length of pendulum}}$.

Hooke's law may only be applied to a spring or other object if the spring or other such object obeys Hooke's law. When a spring is the instrument of motion and it conforms to Hooke's law, it is actually called a **Hooke's law spring**. (MCAT problems will not ask you to solve problems in which Hooke's law is not obeyed, unless the relevant information is supplied.)

Please solve this problem:

- A Hooke's law spring has a spring constant of 2500 newtons/meter. It is stretched to a position located 0.06 meters from its relaxation point. What is the force that acts to restore the spring to its relaxation point?

Problem solved:

The problem calls for the application of Hooke's law:

$F = -(k)(x)$. The spring constant is given as 2.5×10^3 N/m, and the displacement as 0.06 m. The solution then requires simple algebra:

$$F = (-2500 \text{ N/m})(0.06 \text{ m}) = -150 \text{ N}$$

(The (−) sign in the Hooke's law formula indicates that force is opposite the direction of displacement. The force at issue is **restorative**; it tends to restore the moving object to the point at which it has no potential energy. The force of a swinging pendulum is downward as the pendulum moves upward. The force of a spring is toward the relaxation point as the spring moves away from it.)

Envision a pendulum at the rightward end of its path. It is raised, and relative to the bottommost position of its path, has a gravitational potential energy equal to the product of:

$$(\text{mass})(g)(\text{height}) = mgh$$

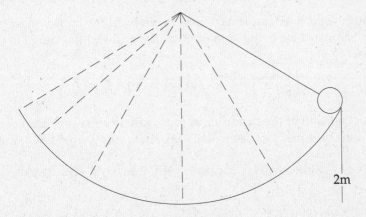

2m

Figure 11.9

Imagine that the pendulum has a mass of 25 kilograms and that its height at the upward end of its motion is 2 meters, as shown. Its gravitational potential energy (relative to the bottommost position of its path) = (25 kg)(10 m/s²)(2 m) = 500 joules (J). The pendulum has the same gravitational potential energy, 500 joules, when it swings fully leftward and occupies a position at the left end of its path.

When the pendulum reaches the bottommost position of its path, all of its potential energy has been converted to kinetic energy; potential energy is zero, and kinetic energy is at a maximum. The mathematical corollary is that $(m)(g)(h)$ at the point of maximum potential energy is equal to $\frac{1}{2}mv^2$ at the point of maximum kinetic energy. Moreover, since the total sum (kinetic energy) + (potential energy) is unchanged at all points in the path, *the sum of $(m)(g)(h)$ and $\frac{1}{2}mv^2$ is constant throughout the path of simple harmonic motion.*

For simple harmonic motion depending on some instrument other than a pendulum, the same principle applies; but the potential energy at issue will not necessarily be *gravitational* potential energy. Whatever the source and form of the simple harmonic motion, however, you must be aware that: (1) there is a perpetual conversion between potential and kinetic energy; (2) at the point of maximum velocity, kinetic energy is at a maximum, and potential energy is at a minimum; (3) at the point of minimum velocity, potential energy is at a maximum, and kinetic energy is at a minimum, and; (4) throughout the motion, the sum of potential energy and kinetic energy is constant.

Please solve this problem:

- A pendulum swings in simple harmonic motion and has a mass of 240 kg. Each time it passes the bottommost point in its path, it has speed of 8 m/s. Ignoring all forces of friction, determine the maximum height it reaches on each side of its path.

Problem solved:

In the case of a swinging pendulum, the potential energy to be considered is gravitational potential energy = $(m)(g)(h)$. Kinetic energy, as always, = $\frac{1}{2}mv^2$. The sum: $(m)(g)(h) + \frac{1}{2}mv^2$ is constant throughout the path of simple harmonic motion. At the bottommost position, potential energy is zero, and the entire sum of potential and kinetic energy is attributable to kinetic energy alone:

$$\left(\frac{1}{2}mv^2\right) = \frac{1}{2} \times (240 \text{ kg}) \times (8^2) = 7{,}680 \text{ J}$$

At the uppermost portion of the pendulum's path, kinetic energy is zero and potential energy, therefore, must be equal to 7,680 J. Knowing that $(m)(g)(h) = 7{,}680$ J, the student may solve for h:

$$(m)(g)(h) = 7{,}680 \text{ J} \qquad (240 \text{ kg}) \times (10 \text{ m/s}^2) \times (h) = 7{,}680$$

$$2{,}400 \, (h) = 7680 \qquad h = \frac{7{,}680}{2{,}400} = 3.2 \qquad h = 3.2 \text{ meters}$$

11.2 MASTERY APPLIED: SAMPLE PASSAGE AND QUESTIONS

Passage

The superposition phenomenon involves the coincident use of one space by more than one wave. That is, more than one wave may travel and occupy the same space at the same time, each independent of the other.

Illustrations of the superposition principle are numerous, radio waves and sound waves furnishing good examples. Large numbers of radio broadcasting facilities commonly operate at the same time, and the "tuning" of a radio to one such station involves adjusting the receiver, so that it receives only *one* of the many frequencies traveling through the surrounding space. Similarly, the perceived sound that emerges from an orchestra involves the contemporaneous travel through the air of a large number of longitudinal waves which the human ear is capable of perceiving as a cacophony, but which it may also resolve into the individual sounds of orchestral instruments.

The medium through which independent waves move is displaced according to the sum of the displacements that would be associated with each one of them independently. Indeed, the term "superposition" refers to the vector summation that accompanies the summed displacement. This superposition principle, however, does not always hold. It applies to waves in deformable media only when a relation of proportionality exists between the deformation and the restorative force. The relationship would then be manifest mathematically in a linear equation of the form $y = mx + b$. Hooke's law represents a linear equation, and it fails to operate when wave disturbance is sufficiently large as to distort the normal linear laws of mechanical action. Superposition applies to electromagnetic waves, for example, because the relations between electric and magnetic fields are linear.

1. One musical instrument sounds a frequency of 440 cycles per second and another simultaneously sounds a frequency of 600 cycles per second. Both instruments are located on a vehicle that travels toward a listener at a rate of 90 meters per second. Assuming the speed of sound through air is approximately 340 meters per second, which of the following numbers best approximates the factor by which each frequency is multiplied in order to yield the apparent frequency perceived by the listener?

   A. 0.2
   B. 0.8
   C. 9.0
   D. 1.36

2. An investigator discovers a particular wave that does not conform to the superposition principle. Which of the following choices would LEAST likely be true of such a wave?

   A. Amplitude and restorative force would bear a proportional relationship.
   B. Speed and wavelength would bear a directly proportional relationship.
   C. Frequency and period would bear an inversely proportional relationship.
   D. The wave would not obey Hooke's law.

3. Two longitudinal compression waves, 1 and 2, travel through the same space simultaneously. Wave 1 has a period of P_1, and a speed of S_1 Wave 2 has a period of P_2 and a speed of S_2. If the wavelengths of Waves 1 and 2 are represented by WL_1 and WL_2 respectively, which of the following represents the ratio $WL_2 : WL_1$?

A. $S_1 S_2 : P_1 P_2$

B. $S_2 P_2 : S_1 P_1$

C. $\dfrac{S_2}{P_1} : (P_2 P_2)$

D. $\dfrac{P_2}{P_1} : (S_1 P_1)$

4. An experimenter designs a pendulum according to a carefully devised set of specifications. In a variety of experimental trials, she demonstrates that when the pendulum swings and is raised above the lowest position of its path, the force tending to draw it downward is NOT proportional to its displacement. The investigator concludes that the pendulum she has designed does not conform to Hooke's law. Is her conclusion justified?

A. No, because Hooke's law applies to simple harmonic motion involving a spring.

B. No, because the conclusion cannot be drawn unless the investigator has calculated the pendulum's spring constant.

C. Yes, because according to Hooke's law, restorative force and displacement are proportional.

D. Yes, because the absence of the proportionality indicates the absence of a spring constant.

5. A laboratory worker experiments with a spring and mass that exhibit classic simple harmonic motion. For several positions relating to the path of motion, he records the tension in the spring and the corresponding displacement from the spring's relaxation point. On a Cartesian plane, he then plots his results, with force recorded on the y-axis and displacement on the x-axis. Which of the following descriptions would most likely characterize the resulting graph?

A. The graph would be linear, with a slope of 1.

B. The graph would be linear, with a slope of magnitude equal to the spring constant.

C. The graph would be linear, with an x intercept equal to the spring constant.

D. The graph would be nonlinear.

6. Which of the following choices best explains the fact that waves of electromagnetic radiation conform to the superposition principle?

A. For waves of electromagnetic radiation, period and frequency are inversely proportional.

B. Electromagnetic waves move at the speed of light.

C. Magnetic and electric fields may occupy the same space simultaneously.

D. Magnetic and electric fields bear a linear relationship.

11.3 MASTERY VERIFIED: ANSWERS AND EXPLANATIONS

1. *D is correct.* Although the question concerns two sound waves traveling simultaneously, the passage indicates that for most practical purposes such waves may be treated separately. Each sound source moves toward the observer at a rate of 90 m/s. The perceived frequencies will be greater than the true frequencies emitted by the instruments. The factor by which each frequency is multiplied to yield the apparent frequency is equal to the fractional component of the Doppler formula: $f_o = f_s \left(\dfrac{v \pm v_o}{v \pm v_s} \right)$.

    Since the observer does not move, the sum $(v + v_o)$ is equal to $v = 340$ m/s. Since the sound source is moving toward the observer, frequency will increase, and the denominator must be reduced to reflect an increase in the overall size of the fraction. The sign employed in the denominator, therefore, must be $(-)$, and the fraction becomes:

    $$\frac{340}{340-90} = \frac{340}{250} = 1.36$$

2. *A is correct.* The superposition principle applies only when there is a proportional relationship between deformation and restorative force. Choice A states that amplitude and restorative force are proportional. Such is said not to be the case of waves for which the superposition principle does not operate. Choices B and C are truths that apply to all waves with which one is expected to be familiar; but in relation to this question (which essentially asks for false statements), they are incorrect answers. Choice D might be true, since Hooke's law does manifest a relationship of proportion and is specifically cited by the author in that regard.

3. *B is correct.* The question tests only your mastery of (a) algebraic manipulation, and (b) the relationships among period, speed, frequency, and wavelength.

    Recalling that period is the reciprocal of frequency, and that

    $$(\text{speed}) = (\text{wavelength})(\text{frequency})$$

    then,

    $$(\text{speed}) = (\text{wavelength})\,\frac{1}{\text{period}}$$

    Solve for wavelength in terms of speed and period by multiplying each side of the equation by period.

    $$(\text{speed})(\text{period}) = (\text{wavelength})$$

    Wavelength is directly proportional to speed and directly proportional to frequency, so the ratio of WL_1 to WL_2 is simply $S_2 P_2 : S_1 P_1$.

4. *C is correct.* For any oscillatory motion that conforms to Hooke's law, restorative force and displacement are proportional. The question describes a swinging pendulum for which restorative force and displacement are *not* proportional. It is a simple logical deduction, therefore, that the pendulum does not conform to Hooke's law—for the reason as stated in choice C that "according to Hooke's law, restorative force and displacement are proportional."

5. *B is correct.* The passage characterizes a linear equation as one that takes the form $y = mx + b$. It further states that Hooke's law represents a linear equation. Since Hooke's law, $F = -(k)(x)$, represents such an equation, where:

$$m = -k$$

and x = displacement

the graph drawn by the laboratory worker will be linear.

For any linear equation, the slope has magnitude equal to m, which, in connection with Hooke's law, is $-k$, the spring constant. The graph drawn by this laboratory worker will be linear and will have a slope equal to the magnitude of the spring constant.

6. *D is correct.* In this case, the last sentence provides the answer in rather a straightforward fashion: "Superposition applies to electromagnetic waves, for example, because the relations between electric and magnetic fields are linear."

CHAPTER 12

LIGHT AND OPTICS

12.1 MASTERY ACHIEVED

12.1.1 GENERAL CHARACTERISTICS OF LIGHT

12.1.1.1 Wavelength and Speed

Visible light is a form of electromagnetic radiation that is normally conceived of as a wave. Electromagnetic radiation has the essential features associated with waves: period, frequency, wavelength, and speed. Electromagnetic radiation whose wavelength falls between 390×10^{-9} meters and 700×10^{-9} meters is visible light.

White light represents a mixture of all wavelengths within the spectrum of visible light. Within the spectrum of visible light, variable wavelength corresponds to diversity of color. Wavelength of 390 nm corresponds roughly to the color violet, 500 nm to the color green, 600 nm to orange, and 700 nm to red. The term **infrared** light refers to electromagnetic radiation with wavelength somewhat above 700 nm, and the term **ultraviolet** light refers to electromagnetic radiation, falling somewhat below 390 nm.

When moving through space, electromagnetic radiation has a speed of approximately 3×10^8 meters/second, which is known as the **speed of light** and is assigned the symbol c. For any given wavelength of electromagnetic radiation or light, frequency is determined by the formula that relates speed and wavelength for waves in general:

$$\text{frequency} = \frac{\text{speed}}{\text{wavelength}}$$

For light:

$$\text{frequency} = \frac{3 \times 10^8 \, \text{m/s}}{\text{wavelength}}$$

The spectrum of visible light is depicted in Figure 12.1 in terms of wavelength and corresponding frequency.

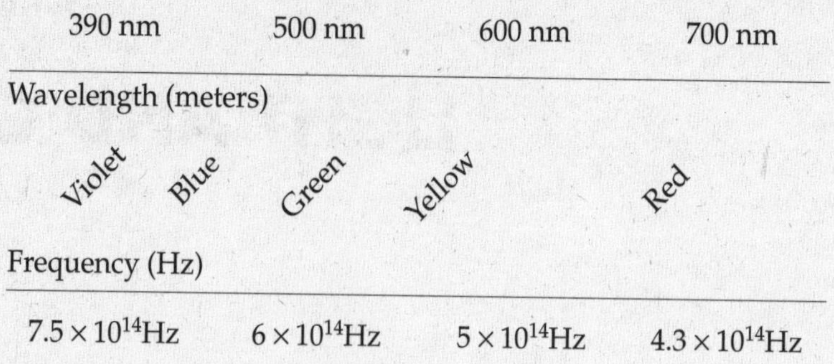

390 nm	500 nm	600 nm	700 nm

Wavelength (meters)

Violet   Blue   Green   Yellow   Red

Frequency (Hz)

$7.5 \times 10^{14} Hz$	$6 \times 10^{14} Hz$	$5 \times 10^{14} Hz$	$4.3 \times 10^{14} Hz$

Figure 12.1

12.1.1.2 The Index of Refraction

As noted previously, the speed of light through a vacuum is 3×10^8 m/s. Its speed through some physical medium is reduced according to the medium's **refractive index**. The index of refraction is defined in terms of the degree to which it slows the travel of light. For any medium, it is equal to the fraction:

$$\frac{\text{speed of light in vacuum}}{\text{speed of light in medium}}$$

$$n = \frac{c}{v}$$

where:

n = refractive index of medium

c = speed of light in vacuum (3×10^8 m/s)

v = speed of light in medium

Index of refraction is dimensionless (without units), as is evidenced by the fraction $\frac{c}{v}$, in which the units in the numerator and denominator both are (m/s), and thus cancel out.

For any medium, the index of refraction varies slightly with the frequency of light that traverses it.

Please solve this problem:

- The speed of light through water is approximately 2.26×10^8 meters per second. Find the refractive index of water.

Problem solved:

The question requires algebraic manipulation of the equation just presented:

$$n = \frac{c}{v} = \frac{3 \times 10^8 \, m/s}{2.26 \times 10^8 \, m/s} = \frac{3}{2.26} = \text{approx. } 1.33$$

Please solve this problem:

- The refractive index of fused quartz is approximately 1.46. At what speed does light travel through the substance?

Problem solved:

The problem once again relies on the equation that defines refractive index and in this instance provides refractive index, requiring one to calculate speed:

$$n = \frac{c}{v}$$

$$1.46 = \frac{3 \times 10^8 \, \text{m/s}}{v}$$

$$v = \frac{3 \times 10^8 \, \text{m/s}}{1.46 \times 10^0 \, \text{m/s}} = \text{approx. } 2.05 \times 10^8 \, \text{m/s}$$

In most contexts light is conceived of as a wave, but within the field of optics, it is best depicted as a **ray**. The sections and subsections that follow deal with optics, so light will be referred to as a ray.

12.1.1.3 Refraction and Reflection

Refraction refers to the phenomenon in which a light ray, on passing from one medium to another, bends as shown in Figure 12.2.

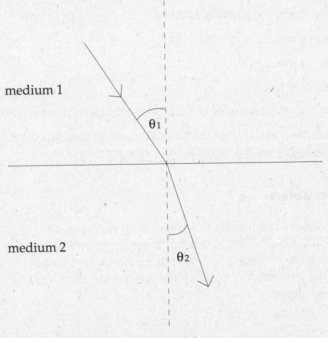

Figure 12.2

In Figure 12.2, the angles θ_1 and θ_2 represent the **angles of incidence** and **angles of refraction**, respectively.

Reflection refers to the phenomenon in which a light ray, while traveling through one medium encounters another, and bounces, as shown below:

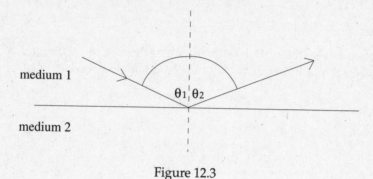

medium 1

$\theta_1 \, \theta_2$

medium 2

Figure 12.3

In Figure 12.3, θ_1 and θ_2 represent the angle of incidence and angle of reflection, respectively.

With respect to refraction, the angles of incidence and refraction are related by **Snell's law** which provides that for each such angle, there is equality between the product:

$$\sin\theta \times \text{index of refraction}$$

Thus,

$$n_1\sin\theta_1 = n_2\sin\theta_2$$

where:

n_1 is the index of refraction for medium 1

n_2 is the index of refraction for medium 2

θ_1 is the angle of incidence

θ_2 is the angle of refraction

With respect to reflection, the angles of incidence and reflection are equal.

The angles of incidence, refraction, and reflection are all measured by reference to an imaginary line oriented perpendicular to the medium interface.

Please solve this problem:

- A light ray travels through a first medium and, on encountering a second, is reflected so that it makes an angle of 75° with the interface between the two media. What is the associated angle of incidence?

Problem solved:

The 75° angle to which the problem refers is made between the reflected ray and the interface between the two media. It is not the angle of reflection. Rather the angle of reflection falls between the reflected ray and a line that runs perpendicular to the interface. The angle of reflection is complementary to the 75° angle mentioned in the problem:

$$90° - 75° = \text{angle of reflection} = 15°$$

Please solve this problem:

- A light ray traveling through a medium encounters a second medium, forming an angle of 60° with the interface between the two media. If the first medium has a refractive index of R_1 and the second, a refractive index of R_2, which of the following expressions best characterizes θ_2, the angle of refraction (sin 30° = 0.5; sin 60° = 0.867)?

A. $\arccos (0.867) \times \dfrac{R_1}{R_2}$

B. $\arccos (R_1)(R_2) (0.867)$

C. $\arcsin (90 - 60) (R_2)$

D. $\arcsin \dfrac{R_1}{2R_2}$

Problem solved:

D is the correct answer. The 60° angle to which the problem refers does not constitute the angle of incidence, as it is formed by the media interface and the incident light ray. The angle of incidence is equal to the difference between that angle and 90°, as shown in Figure 12.4:

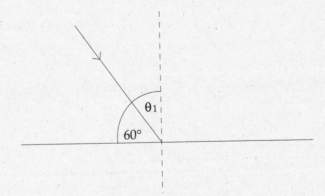

Figure 12.4

The angle of incidence, then, is 90° – 60° = 30°. The sin of 30° is 0.5. Using Snell's Law:

$$n_1 \sin\theta_1 = n_2 \sin\theta_2 \quad R_1(0.5) = R_2 \sin\theta_2 \quad \frac{(0.5)(R_1)}{R_2} = \sin\theta_2$$

$$\left(\frac{1}{2}\right) \times \left[\frac{(R_1)}{R_2}\right] = \sin\theta_2 \quad \frac{(R_1)}{2(R_2)} = \sin\theta_2$$

$$\theta_2 = \arcsin \frac{(R_1)}{2(R_2)}$$

12.1.1.3.1 Total Internal Reflection and the Critical Angle

Total internal reflection refers to a ray of light that travels through a medium and encounters a second medium with a lower index of refraction than the first. If the angle between the incident ray and the line perpendicular to the interface exceeds the **critical angle** (θ_{cr}), all of the incident light will be reflected back into the first medium.

Total internal reflection is depicted qualitatively in Figure 12.5, which shows three light rays, 1, 2, and 3, emanating from a source located within medium A, each approaching an interface with medium B. Ray 1 reaches the interface and is refracted. (If the angle of incidence were known, the angle of refraction could be calculated, as already demonstrated, through application of Snell's law.) Ray 2 strikes the interface, and forms with the perpendicular an angle that is equal to the critical angle (θ_{cr}) for these two media. The consequent refraction causes the ray to run parallel to the interface and hence make a 90° angle with the perpendicular as shown. Ray 3 strikes the interface at an angle that exceeds the critical angle, and the consequence is total internal reflection, as shown:

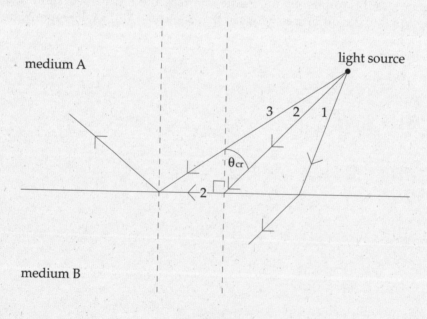

Figure 12.5

The quantitative aspects of total internal reflection pertain to the evaluation of the critical angle for any two interfaces, and are calculated with a modification of Snell's law, with the angle of refraction equal to 90° (its sin is set to 1):

$$\sin \theta_{cr} = \frac{n_b}{n_a}$$

where:

θ_{cr} is the critical angle that applies to the two media in question

n_b is the index of refraction for the second medium

n_a is the index of refraction for the first medium

12.1.2 MIRRORS: CONVEX AND CONCAVE

In the area of **optics**, a variety of fundamental tenets are associated with mirrors. Recall that mirrors may be **flat** or **spherical** and that spherical mirrors in turn may be **convex** or **concave**. A convex mirror is one whose exposed surface curves outward, and a concave mirror is one whose exposed surface curves inward, as shown in Figure 12.6:

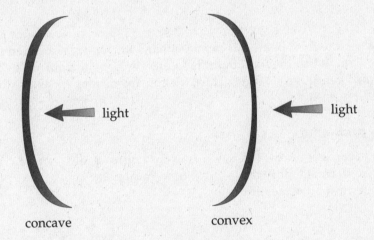

concave   convex

Figure 12.6

12.1.2.1 Focal Length of a Mirror

All spherical mirrors feature a **focal length,** at the end of which sits a **focal point**. The focal length is equal to one half the mirror's radius of curvature:

$$f = \frac{1}{2} R_c$$

where:

f = focal length

R_c = mirror's radius of curvature

For a convex mirror, the focal length extends into the mirror, and the focal point is said to be located behind it. For a concave mirror, the focal length is directed away from the mirror, and the focal point is said to be located in front of it. That is, with respect to an observer who faces the surface of a convex mirror, the side on which he stands is opposite to that on which the focal point is located. With respect to an observer who faces the surface of a concave mirror, the side on which he stands is the same as that on which the focal point is located.

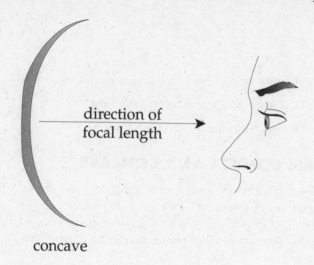

direction of focal length

concave

Figure 12.7

By convention, when the focal point is located behind a mirror, its associated focal length is given a negative (–) sign. When the focal point is located in front of a mirror, its associated focal length is assigned a positive (+) sign. Thus, for convex mirrors, focal length is negative; for concave mirrors, it is positive.

Please solve this problem:

- A concave mirror has a radius of curvature equal to 40 cm. Identify the location of its focal point in terms of distance and sign.

Problem solved:

The mirror is concave, and its focal point is located in front of the mirror, which gives it a positive sign. Absolute value of focal length is easily calculated with the above equation:

$$f = \frac{1}{2} R_c = \frac{40 \text{ cm}}{2} = 20 \text{ cm}$$

The focal length is +20 cm.

Please solve this problem:

- A convex mirror has a radius of curvature equal to 162 cm. Identify the location of its focal point in terms of distance and sign.

Problem solved:

The problem is analogous to the previous one, but involves a convex mirror. The focal length is directed into the mirror, and the focal point therefore carries a (–) sign. The absolute value of the focal length is equal to:

$$f = \frac{1}{2}R_c = \frac{162 \text{ cm}}{2} = 81 \text{ cm}$$

The focal point is located –81 cm from the mirror.

12.1.2.2 Conformation, Orientation, Location, and Magnification of Mirror Images

The location of a mirror's focal point is not neccessarily the location of the image the mirror produces. Rather, the position of a mirror image produced by some object is determined by the **thin lens equation**, which, despite its name, applies to mirrors (as well as to lenses, which will be discussed in subsequent subsections):

$$\frac{1}{f} = \frac{1}{o} + \frac{1}{i}$$

where:

f is the mirror's focal length

o is the distance of the object from the mirror

i is the distance of the image from the mirror

Although a concave mirror has its focal point located in front of the mirror, it may produce images behind the mirror.

One should be familiar with the distinction between **real** and **virtual** images. A mirror image that is located behind a mirror—which means, that it is visible in the mirror—is termed virtual. A mirror image that is located in front of the mirror—(which means that it cannot be seen in the mirror but rather on a screen held in front of the mirror—is termed real. In addition, the signs (+) and (–) are assigned to the location of mirror images as they are assigned to the location of focal points: an image located behind a mirror carries a negative (–) sign, and an image located in front of a mirror carries a positive (+) sign.

Any virtual mirror image is **upright** and any real image is **inverted**. The association of "real" with "inverted" and "virtual" with "upright" is somewhat counterintuitive, as one might expect that a real image should more accurately reproduce an object. For this reason, take special care not to be confused by terminology. Make these associations:

mirror image location	real/virtual	orientation	sign
behind mirror	virtual	upright	(–)
in front of mirror	real	inverted	(+)

Table 12.1

Please solve this problem:

- A convex mirror has a radius of curvature equal to 80 cm, and an object is situated 20 cm in front of it. Identify the location of the resulting image in terms of distance and sign.

Problem solved:

First, determine the absolute value of the focal length according to the simple equation $f = \frac{1}{2}(R_c)$. The absolute value is 40 cm. The mirror is convex, and its focal point is located behind it. The focal length carries a negative (–) sign. Focal length = –40 cm. Next, apply the thin lens equation set forth above to locate the mirror image:

$$\frac{1}{f} = \frac{1}{o} + \frac{1}{i}$$

$$\frac{1}{-40 \text{ cm}} = \frac{1}{20 \text{ cm}} + \frac{1}{i}$$

$$\frac{-1}{40 \text{ cm}} - \frac{1}{20 \text{ cm}} = \frac{1}{i}$$

$$\frac{1}{i} = \frac{-1}{40 \text{ cm}} - \frac{2}{40 \text{ cm}}$$

$$\frac{1}{i} = \frac{-3}{40 \text{ cm}}$$

$$i = \frac{-40 \text{ cm}}{3} = \text{approx. } -13.33 \text{ cm}$$

The negative sign indicates that the image is behind the mirror and thus virtual and upright.

Spherical mirrors may produce **magnification** and the size of an image may therefore vary from the size of the object that generates it. Magnification is a dimensionless quantity, and for any object and mirror, it is equal to the fraction:

$$- \frac{\text{distance of image from mirror}}{\text{distance of object from mirror}}$$

The distance is taken in terms of its absolute value, so the sign is ignored:

$$m = \frac{-i}{o}$$

where:

i = distance of image from mirror

o = distance of object from mirror

Please solve this problem:

- A convex mirror has a radius of curvature equal to 60 cm, and a 20 cm object is positioned 15 cm in front of it. Determine the size of the image that results.

Problem solved:

First, calculate i, the distance of the image from the mirror. You make that calculation, as before, by first ascertaining the relevant focal length. Its absolute value is equal to

$\frac{1}{2}(R_c) = \frac{60}{2} = 30$ cm. The mirror is convex, and the focal length carries a negative (–) sign; focal length = –30 cm. The value for i is then calculated by the thin lens equation:

$$\frac{1}{f} = \frac{1}{o} + \frac{1}{i}$$

$$\frac{1}{-30 \text{ cm}} = \frac{1}{15 \text{ cm}} + \frac{1}{i}$$

$$\frac{-1}{30 \text{ cm}} - \frac{1}{15 \text{ cm}} = \frac{1}{i}$$

$$\frac{-1}{30 \text{ cm}} - \frac{2}{30 \text{ cm}} = \frac{1}{i}$$

$$\frac{1}{i} = \frac{-3}{30 \text{ cm}}$$

$$i = \frac{-30 \text{ cm}}{3} = -10 \text{ cm}$$

The magnification is calculated by the equation:

$$m = \frac{-i}{o}$$

$$= \frac{10 \text{ cm}}{15 \text{ cm}} = 0.67$$

Since the object's true size is 20 cm, the mirror image will have size equal to:

$$(0.67)(20) = 13.4 \text{ cm}$$

A negative magnification would indicate an inverted image.

12.1.3 LENSES

12.1.3.1 Converging and Diverging Lenses

A **lens** is a structure with two refracting surfaces. **Thin lenses** are lenses for which the two refractory surfaces are so closely spaced as to render the intervening space optically negligible. All matters discussed in sections and subsections to follow concern thin lenses.

Lenses may be **converging** or **diverging;** each term refers to the effect of the given lens on light rays that pass through it. Converging lenses produce the convergence of rays toward the lens's central axis. Diverging lenses produce the divergence of rays away from the central axis. As shown in Figure 12.8, convergence corresponds to convexity, and divergence, to concavity. Lens A is convex and converging. Lens B is concave and diverging.

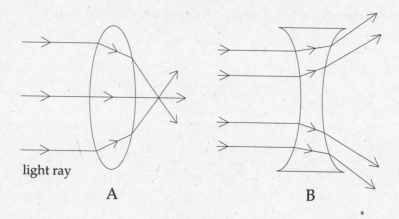

Figure 12.8

Like mirrors, every lens, converging or diverging, is associated with a **focal length**, the terminus of which represents the **focal point**. For a converging lens, the focal point is that point at which parallel rays traversing the lens will come together through refraction. For a diverging lens, the focal point represents that point at which parallel rays that have traversed the lens, and so have been subjected to divergence, will meet by hypothetical linear extension in the reverse direction.

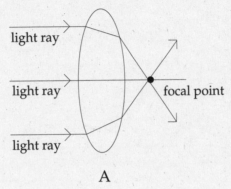

A

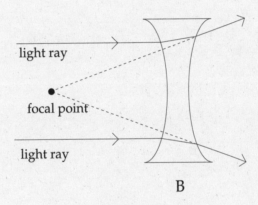

B

Figure 12.9

Light rays emanating from a common source diverge in all directions. If a lens is very close to the source, light rays will remain markedly divergent at the time they reach it. The closer the lens is to the source, the greater the divergence at the time the rays reach the lens. If a lens is removed some distance from a source, many of the rays that reach it will miss the path in which it stands. Moreover, those rays that do reach it will show a markedly reduced degree of divergence.

Figure 12.10 illustrates the point.

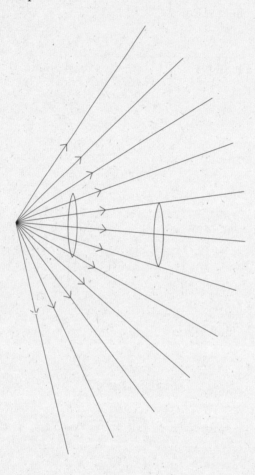

Figure 12.10

A source of light is shown at the left, emitting widely divergent rays. If a lens is positioned some small distance away from the source, many widely divergent light rays reach it. (The lens's tendency to refract the rays is not illustrated, so that the status of the rays in the absence of the lens might be understood at a more distant position, where a second lens is positioned.) If a lens is placed at a considerable distance from the light source, most of the emitted rays miss its path. Those rays that do reach the lens show relatively small divergence and are considered parallel (although some divergence is evident).

The side from which light approaches a lens is considered the **front**. If an object is subjected to light, then the object itself constitutes a source of light. Consequently, when an object is viewed through a lens, the object serves as source of light and is said to be at the front of the lens. Divergent lenses have their focal points located at the front, and convergent lenses, at the back.

Through the **lensmaker's equation**, the focal length of a lens is determined through (a) the refractive index that applies to the material of which the lens is made and (b) the radius of curvature associated with each side of the lens. For each side of a lens, radius of curvature represents the radius of a circle that would be completed if the curve were extended to suggest the circle of which it is a part, as shown in Figure 12.11.

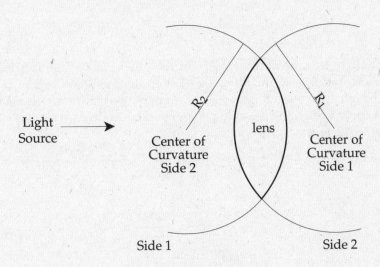

Figure 12.11

The designation "side 1" is assigned to the first of the lens surfaces to be struck by incident light (the "incoming side"), and the designation "side 2" is assigned to the second surface (the outgoing side). In the foregoing illustration, the light source is positioned to the left, which means that the left surface of the lens is side 1, and the right surface is side 2. Had the light source been positioned to the right, the right surface would be side 1, and the left surface, side 2. The lensmaker's equation provides that:

$$\frac{1}{f} = (n-1)\left(\frac{1}{R_1} - \frac{1}{R_2}\right)$$

where:

f is focal length

n is refractive index of the lens material

R_1 is the radius of curvature for side 1

R_2 is the radius of curvature for side 2

Each radius of curvature R_1 and R_2 is associated with a sign, positive (+) or negative (–), in accordance with this rule: *with reference to the movement of light, the curved surface whose center of curvature is on the outgoing side has a positive (+) sign, and the side whose center of curvature is on the incoming side has a negative (–) sign.*

If, as shown in Figure 12.11, light travels from left to right through a convex lens, the left side is side 1, and side 1 has its center of curvature on the outgoing side—the right side. R_1, therefore, is positive (+). Side 2 has its center of curvature on the incoming side, and so R_2 is negative (–).

Please solve this problem:

- The left side of a convergent glass lens has a 20 cm radius of curvature, and the right side has a 5 cm radius of curvature. Assuming that the refractive index of glass is 1.5, find the focal length of the lens.

Problem solved:

If we imagine that light is incident from the right side, then side 1 is on the right, and $R_1 = 5$ cm. Side 2 is on the left, and $R_2 = 20$ cm. Since side 1 is on the right (and is convex), its center of curvature is on the left—the outgoing side—and it takes a positive sign, $R_1 = +5$ cm. R_2, then, with center of curvature on the incoming side, takes a negative (–) sign, and is equal to –20 cm. Application of the lensmaker's equation yields:

$$\frac{1}{f} = (n-1)\left(\frac{1}{R_1} - \frac{1}{R_2}\right)$$

$$\frac{1}{f} = (1.5-1)\left(\frac{1}{5} - \frac{1}{-20}\right)$$

$$\frac{1}{f} = (0.5)\left(\frac{-4}{-20} - \frac{1}{-20}\right)$$

$$\frac{1}{f} = (0.5)\left(\frac{-5}{-20}\right)$$

$$\frac{1}{f} = (0.5)\frac{1}{4} \qquad \frac{1}{f} = \frac{1}{8}$$

$$f = 8.0 \text{ cm}$$

12.1.3.2 Conformation and Orientation of Images

Again lenses are unlike mirrors, because an image formed behind a lens is real and inverted. An image formed in front of a lens is virtual and upright.

You should memorize Table 12.2 so you are not confused about sign, focal point, and image orientation as they apply to mirrors, on the one hand, and lenses on the other:

	Type	Image	Focal Point
For Mirrors	concave	* in front: real, inverted	in front (+)
	convex	behind: virtual, upright	behind (-)

	Type	Image	Focal Point
For Lenses	diverging	in front: virtual, upright	in front (-)
	converging	* behind: real, inverted	behind (+)

Table 12.2

*For concave mirrors and converging lenses, objects placed within the focal distance will create a virtual, upright image.

It should be apparent that for mirrors and lenses alike, all real images are inverted and all virtual images are upright.

The location and magnification of an image produced by a lens are determined by the equations discussed in connection with mirrors. Keeping in mind the differences between lenses and mirrors as just discussed, therefore, you could locate a lens image by using the thin lens equation, $\frac{1}{f} = \frac{1}{o} + \frac{1}{i}$, and identify the magnification of an image by using the equation, $m = \frac{-i}{o}$.

Please solve this problem:

- A divergent glass lens has a focal length of 80 cm. A 40 cm object is held in front of it at a distance of 20 cm. Ascertain the location and size of the image, and determine whether it will be real, virtual, upright, or inverted.

Problem solved:

The absolute value of the lens's focal length is 80 cm; because the lens is divergent, the sign is negative (–). The focal length, therefore, is –80 cm. To locate the image, apply the equation:

$$\frac{1}{f} = \frac{1}{o} + \frac{1}{i}$$

$$\frac{-1}{80 \text{ cm}} = \frac{1}{20 \text{ cm}} + \frac{1}{i}$$

$$\frac{-1}{80 \text{ cm}} - \frac{1}{20 \text{ cm}} = \frac{1}{i}$$

$$\frac{-1}{80 \text{ cm}} - \frac{4}{80 \text{ cm}} = \frac{1}{i}$$

$$\frac{-5}{80 \text{ cm}} = \frac{1}{i}$$

$$i = \frac{-80}{5 \text{ cm}} = -16 \text{ cm}$$

The image is located at a position of –16 cm from the lens, which means it is 16 cm in front of the lens. Any image located in front of a lens is virtual and upright.

The size of the image is obtained by taking the product:

object size × magnification

Magnification is determined by the equation:

$$m = \frac{-i}{o} = \frac{-(-16) \text{ cm}}{20 \text{ cm}} = 0.8$$

$$(0.8) \times (40 \text{ cm}) = 32 \text{ cm}$$

12.1.3.3 Focal Power

Focal power, P, expresses the degree to which a lens imposes a convergence or divergence on the light rays that traverse it. The converging lens of relatively greater power produces greater convergence than does one of relatively lesser power; the diverging lens of relatively greater power produces greater divergence than does one of relatively lesser power.

Focal power is expressed in the unit **diopter**, and it is equal to the reciprocal of the focal length:

$$P = \frac{1}{f}$$

where:

P = focal power

f = focal length (expressed in meters)

Since the focal length associated with a diverging lens is negative (–), so is its power. Since the focal length associated with a converging lens is positive (+), so is its power.

- **Power of converging lens carries positive (+) sign**

- **Power of diverging lens carries negative (–) sign**

Please solve this problem:

- A lens brings parallel light rays to a focus, as shown below. Determine its focal power.

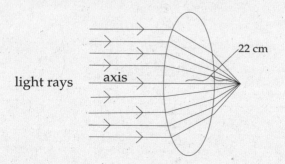

Figure 12.12

Problem solved:

The illustration reveals a convergent lens with a focal length of +22 cm. Expressed in meters, the focal length is +0.22 m, and the focal power is:

$$\frac{1}{0.22}\ \text{diopters}$$

$$= \text{approx. } 4.5 \text{ diopters}$$

12.2 MASTERY APPLIED: SAMPLE PASSAGE AND QUESTIONS

Passage

The human eye mediates the sense of vision by focusing incoming light rays reflected from objects within the environment onto the retina. As indicated below, the necessary refractive power is attributable to several interfaces: between the air and the anterior surface of the cornea; between the posterior surface of the cornea and the aqueous humor; between the aqueous humor and the anterior surface of the lens; and between the posterior surface of the lens and the vitreous humor which, in turn, contacts the retina.

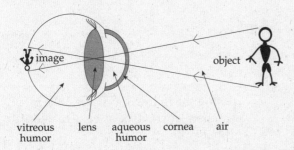

vitreous humor   lens   aqueous humor   cornea   air

For optic analysis, all refractive components of the eye are summed algebraically to form a hypothetical construct called the **reduced eye**, in which the eye's refractory power is imagined to arise from a single lens located approximately 17 mm anterior to the retina and to have positive focal power of approximately 59 diopters in the absence of any effort to increase it by muscular activity. Of those 59 diopters, the eye's own lens proper provides only 15 diopters; the majority of refractory power arises from the anterior surface of the cornea.

The eye's lens proper is convex, and its principal importance lies in the adjustability of its focal power. Through muscular mechanisms, the individual may increase its convexity through a process known as *accommodation*. During childhood, for example, the individual may increase the lens's focal power from 15 diopters to 49 diopters. In middle and older age, the

power of accommodation tends to diminish, and the average 55 year–old can perhaps accommodate to the extent of 2 diopters. A very aged individual will frequently lose his power of accommodation entirely, a condition called *presbyopia*.

The lens is susceptible, also, to other deficiencies, among them a phenomenon termed *chromatic aberration*, illustrated below.

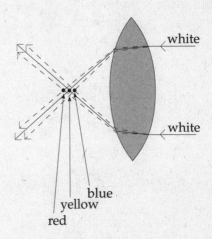

white

white

blue
yellow
red

The condition arises from the fact that the lens's focal power varies slightly depending on the color of the light passing through it.

Early investigators were at a loss to explain the fact that the individual with two eyes focused on an object sees a single image just as he does with one eye closed. The phenomenon of *fusion*, in which the individual sees one image with two eyes open, is mediated by centers within the brain.

1. Each choice in the figure below schematically represents light rays moving from an object toward a human eye. For which set of light rays would the human eye tend to accommodate most?

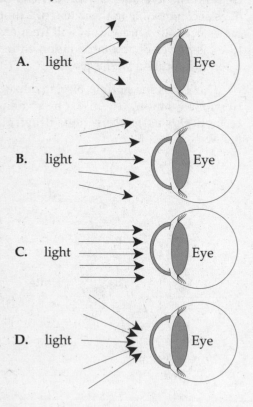

A. light   Eye

B. light   Eye

C. light   Eye

D. light   Eye

2. The image formed on the retina is most likely:

   A. virtual and inverted.
   B. virtual and upright.
   C. real and inverted.
   D. real and upright.

3. The condition of hypermetropia arises when the eye's refractory components have a focal point that falls behind the retina, as shown schematically below:

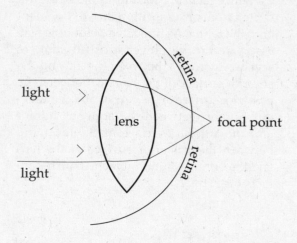

light

light

lens

retina

retina

focal point

Among the following choices, the most effective corrective measure would probably be:

   A. surgical adjustment of the retina's location, so that it is moved forward.
   B. obliteration of the eye's lens with laser technology.
   C. a corrective lens with negative focal power.
   D. a corrective lens with positive focal power.

4. A patient complains of blurred vision when viewing objects located in the distance, but reports visual clarity when viewing objects located close to his eye. A physician hypothesizes that the difficulty is attributable to a condition in which the right retina is located at an abnormally large distance from the anterior surface of the right eye. Which of the following findings would best confirm her hypothesis?

   A. The patient reports improvement when a convex lens is placed in front of his right eye.
   B. The patient reports improvement when a concave lens is placed in front of his right eye.
   C. The patient reports improvement when he opens his eyes more widely.
   D. The patient reports that he does not experience the symptom when either eye is closed and the other remains open.

5. Which of the following most probably explains the phenomenon of chromatic aberration?

   A. The model of the "reduced eye" does not account for the fact of separate refractory components.
   B. The eye cannot diffract white light into its component wavelengths.
   C. The eye's refractory apparatus offers different focal power for different light wavelengths.
   D. Different portions of the eye's retina vary in their degree of sensitivity to color.

6. Which of the following would most likely be useful in focusing the image of a remote object onto the retina?

   I. Structures anterior to the lens with a refractive index different from that of air
   II. The lens's capacity for accommodation
   III. The retina's capacity to create an image

   A. I only
   B. I and II only
   C. I and III only
   D. I, II, and III

7. Which of the following choices best characterizes the deficiency associated with presbyopia?

   A. Inability to diverge converging rays
   B. Inability to increase focal power
   C. Positive focal length
   D. Focal length that does not coincide with focal point

12.3 MASTERY VERIFIED: ANSWERS AND EXPLANATIONS

1. *A is the correct answer.* When the individual accommodates, he increases the convexity of his lens and so increases the degree to which his eye will produce convergence. The greater the divergence among incoming rays, the greater the eye's need to produce convergence in order that the rays be focused. The correct figure is the one that depicts the greatest degree of divergence among the incoming light rays.

2. *C is the correct answer.* The image formed on the retina is a product of light traversing that which amounts to a converging lens. Any image formed behind a lens is real and inverted. (An image formed behind a mirror, on the other hand, is virtual and upright.) Moreover, all real images are inverted and all virtual images are upright. Choices A and D are clearly erroneous, for they refer to images that are virtual and inverted, and real and upright, respectively.

   If one chooses B, one may be working from some intuitive belief that the image formed on the retina should be upright, since human beings are not accustomed to seeing their surroundings in inverted terms. The fact that human beings do not perceive inverted images is a function of processing that occurs at the level of the brain—subsequent to the retina's receipt of an inverted image. As the passage indicates, the same is so for the phenomenon of fusion.

3. *D is the correct answer.* As described and depicted in the question, hypermetropia indicates that the eye's refractory components give rise to a focal length that is too long to allow for focus on the retina. The theoretical solutions are to relocate the retina so that it is further back (not further forward as mentioned in choice A) or to decrease the combined focal length of the eye's refractory components. The latter solution would involve increasing the focal power of the sight system by (a) increasing the convexity of the eye's internal system or (b) supplementing the system with an artificial lens that is convex. Convex lenses have positive focal power.

4. *B is the correct answer.* The patient is unable to focus objects in the distance, suggesting that as parallel light rays traverse the refractive components of his eye, they experience such convergence as produces a focal point anterior to the retina. Either one or both of his eyes has excessive focal power or his retina is located too far back.

   That the patient clearly sees objects located near to him tends to confirm the physician's hypothesis, since, as an object comes closer to a lens, the rays that emanate from it show increased divergence in relation to one another. For such rays, the focal point would be moved backward and might focus *on* the retina as they should.

   If the physician's hypothesis is correct—that in relation to the retina's location, parallel rays of light are focused too far forward—some improvement should accompany the placement of a concave lens in front of the eye. The lens would diverge the incoming light rays before they reached the eye, and would present the eye with rays that, in their divergence, resemble rays that come from objects situated close to it. If the placement of a concave lens brings improvement, the hypothesis is supported.

5. *C is the correct answer.* The passage describes and illustrates chromatic aberration as a condition in which light may be focused at different points, depending on its color. Specifically, the passage states that, "The condition arises from the fact that the lens's focal power varies slightly depending on the color of the light passing through it." Variation of color is a function of variation of wavelength. As such, the statement in the passage becomes equivalent to: The condition arises from the fact that the lens's focal power varies slightly, depending on the wavelength of the light passing through it.

6. *A is the correct answer.* Choice I reflects an accurate statement. Taken together with Figure 1, the passage states that much of the eye's refractory power is attributable to structures anterior to the lens itself. Indeed, in a later paragraph, one learns that, of the 59 diopters inherent in the eye's apparati of focus, the majority is attributable to the anterior surface of the cornea, which is far anterior to the lens.

Choice II refers to the lens's capacity for accommodation. Accommodation represents the process by which the eye adjusts the focal power of its own lens proper, but no such adjustment is necessary when viewing a remote object.

Choice III refers to the retina's capacity to create an image. The retina's capacity to form an image is not relevant to the eye's ability to focus light. It is fair to conclude that the purpose of focusing light is to form a focused image on the retina, but the retina itself does not contribute to the focus.

7. *B is the correct answer.* Presbyopia is the inability to increase convexity of the lens. To increase convexity is to increase focal power, and so choice B is correct.

CHAPTER 13

ATOMS, ELEMENTS, AND THE PERIODIC TABLE

13.1 MASTERY ACHIEVED

13.1.1 ATOMIC MASS, ATOMIC WEIGHT, ISOTOPES, AND IONS

13.1.1.1 Atoms and Subatomic Particles

Chemistry is the study of matter. **Atoms** are the building blocks of all matter. Atoms, in turn, are made up of **electrons**, **neutrons**, and **protons**. The center of an atom, called the atomic **nucleus**, contains protons and neutrons. The nucleus is surrounded by a cloud of electrons. Some important properties of these three subatomic particles are summarized in Table 13.1.

PARTICLE	LOCATION	CHARGE	MASS	MCAT MASS
electron	outside nucleus	–1	$\frac{1}{1840}$ amu	zero
neutron	in nucleus	zero	$\frac{1856}{1840}$ amu	1 amu
proton	in nucleus	+1	$\frac{1853}{1840}$ amu	1 amu

Table 13.1

Amu stands for atomic mass unit. By convention, the most abundant isotope of carbon (carbon-12) is assigned a mass of exactly 12 amu and the masses of all other atoms or subatomic particles are determined from this standard. 1 amu = 1.66×10^{-27} kg.

When representing an element by its one- or two-letter symbol, we can also include information about its numbers of electrons, neutrons, and protons:

$$_{P}^{N+P}X^{P-E}$$

where N = number of neutrons,

P = number of protons,

and, E = number of electrons.

The number of protons is given in the subscript. This number is also known as the **atomic number (AN)** because the number of protons in an atom distinguishes one element from another. The number of protons plus the number of neutrons is given in the left superscript. Since the protons and neutrons are the major constituents of atomic mass (the electrons can be considered massless), this number is also known as the **mass number (MN)**. Unlike atomic number, the mass number of the atoms of a particular element is not always the same. When two atoms of the same element differ in mass number (therefore, in their number of neutrons) these atoms are said to be **isotopes** of one another. $^{12}_{6}C$ and $^{13}_{6}C$ are two isotopes of carbon; the former contains six neutrons and the latter contains seven neutrons. Both contain six protons.

The right superscript of a chemical symbol is reserved for the number of protons minus the number of electrons. Since protons are positively charged and electrons are negatively charged, this difference tells us the net **charge (C)** on an atom. When the number of protons is equal to the number of electrons, the atom is neutral. All atoms in their elemental form are neutral. When the number of protons exceeds the number of electrons, the charge is positive and we refer to the atom as being **electron deficient**. When the number of electrons exceeds the number of protons, the charge is negative and we refer to the atom as **electron rich**. An electron deficient atom has a positive charge and is referred to as a **cation**. An electron rich atom has a negative charge and is referred to as an **anion**.

Please solve this problem:

- What is the charge on an aluminum atom that contains 10 total electrons?

Problem solved:

The charge on an aluminum atom that contains 10 total electrons is +3. We can determine this by referring to the periodic table (**13.1.2**). The atomic number of aluminum is 13; therefore aluminum atoms contain 13 protons. This makes an aluminum atom with 10 electrons a cation, or electron deficient species. Its charge is 13 − 10 = +3.

Considering atomic number, mass number, and charge, we can also interpret an atomic symbol as:

$$^{MN}_{AN}X^{C}$$

It is important to note that mass number is not equal to atomic weight. The **atomic weight** of an element is a weighted average of the mass numbers of all naturally occurring isotopes for that element. There are two isotopes that contribute to the atomic weight of chlorine: $^{35}_{17}Cl$ and $^{37}_{17}Cl$. In a sample of pure chlorine, approximately three-quarters of the atoms are the isotope with a mass number of 35, the remainder are the chlorine–37 isotope. By taking the weighted average, we can compute the atomic weight of chlorine as 35.453 amu.

Please solve this problem:

- A scientist is attempting to determine the accurate atomic mass of a sample of naturally occurring chlorine. Which of the following would introduce the most error into her measurements?

  A. Neglecting the mass of the electrons.
  B. Neglecting the mass of the neutrons.
  C. Neglecting the mass of the protons.
  D. Neglecting the mass of the chlorine–36 isotope.

Problem solved:

B is the correct answer. We see from Table 13.1 that neutrons are slightly heavier than protons, which are substantially heavier than electrons. Neglecting the mass of the chlorine–36 isotope is an MCAT "trap" answer. While it appears to address the question at hand, it is factually incorrect, as the chlorine–36 isotope is not naturally occurring. You must be wary of such traps. If an MCAT answer sounds too complicated relative to the other three answer choices, or unrelated to the other three answer choices, it is probably wrong. In this case, you should recognize that choices A, B, and C all deal with subatomic particles while choice D does not.

13.1.2 THE PERIODIC TABLE

13.1.2.1 Mendeleev's Periodic Table

The first version of the periodic table of the elements was proposed in 1869 by the Russian scientist Dmitri Mendeleev. Since that time, the periodic table has become a permanent fixture in the science classrooms of the world. A periodic table is presented below. (Note: as of early 1995 elements 108–112 have been made in a laboratory. These new elements are not included in the table reproduced here because they will not be important on the MCAT.)

PERIODIC CHART OF THE ELEMENTS

1 H 1.0																	2 He 4.0
3 Li 6.9	4 Be 9.0											5 B 10.8	6 C 12.0	7 N 14.0	8 O 16.0	9 F 19.0	10 Ne 20.2
11 Na 23.0	12 Mg 24.3											13 Al 27.0	14 Si 28.1	15 P 31.0	16 S 32.1	17 Cl 35.5	18 Ar 39.9
19 K 39.1	20 Ca 40.1	21 Sc 45.0	22 Ti 47.9	23 V 50.9	24 Cr 52.0	25 Mn 54.9	26 Fe 55.8	27 Co 58.9	28 Ni 58.7	29 Cu 63.5	30 Zn 65.4	31 Ga 69.7	32 Ge 72.6	33 As 74.9	34 Se 79.0	35 Br 79.9	36 Kr 83.8
37 Rb 85.5	38 Sr 87.6	39 Y 88.9	40 Zr 91.2	41 Nb 92.9	42 Mo 95.9	43 Tc (98)	44 Ru 101.1	45 Rh 102.9	46 Pd 106.4	47 Ag 107.9	48 Cd 112.4	49 In 114.8	50 Sn 118.7	51 Sb 121.8	52 Te 127.6	53 I 126.9	54 Xe 131.3
55 Cs 132.9	56 Ba 137.3	57 La 138.9	72 Hf 178.5	73 Ta 180.9	74 W 183.9	75 Re 186.2	76 Os 190.2	77 Ir 192.2	78 Pt 195.1	79 Au 197.0	80 Hg 200.6	81 Tl 204.4	82 Pb 207.2	83 Bi 209.0	84 Po 209.0	85 At 210.0	86 Rn 222.0
87 Fr 223.0	88 Ra 226.0	89 Ac 227.0															

Lanthanum Series

58 Ce 140.1	59 Pr 140.9	60 Nd 144.2	61 Pm 145.0	62 Sm 150.4	63 Eu 152.0	64 Gd 157.3	65 Tb 158.9	66 Dy 162.5	67 Ho 164.9	68 Er 167.3	69 Tm 168.9	70 Yb 173.0	71 Lu 175.0

Actinium Series

90 Th 232.0	91 Pa 231.0	92 U 238.0	93 Np 237.0	94 Pu (244)	95 Am (243)	96 Cm (247)	97 Bk (247)	98 Cf (251)	99 Es (252)	100 Fm (258)	101 Md (258)	102 No (259)	103 Lr (260)

Table 13.2

Each element is represented by its one- or two-letter chemical symbol. Above each chemical symbol is the atomic number (number of protons) for that element. Below each chemical symbol is that element's atomic weight. There is no need for you to memorize the periodic table for the MCAT, because both the Biological Sciences section and the Physical Sciences section of the exam will include a periodic table inside the front cover for your use. However, it may serve you well to be familiar with the location of more popular elements: H, Li, C, N, O, F, Na, Mg, P, S, Cl, K, Ca, Fe, Cu, Br, Ag, and I.

13.1.2.2 Periods and Groups

Each horizontal row in the periodic table is called a **period**. The outermost electrons of every atom in a period have the same principal quantum number, or shell number (**13.1.3.1**). Each vertical column in the periodic table is called a **group**. Every member of a group has the same number of valence electrons (**13.1.3.1**) and may be expected to have similar chemical properties to other members of the group (**13.1.3.9**). In addition to the designation of groups, we can designate blocks of the periodic table. The blocks are designated by the letter that corresponds to the subshell presently being filled (**13.1.3.2**). The two rows furthest to the left (and He) are designated the *s* block, the next ten rows the *d* block, the six rows furthest to the right are designated the *p* block and the actinides and lanthanides are designated the *f* block.

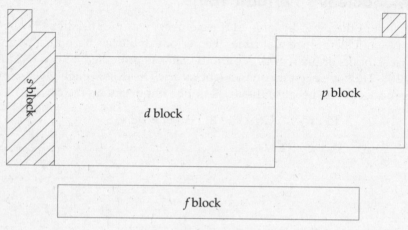

Figure 13.1

13.1.3 QUANTUM NUMBERS AND THE AUFBAU PRINCIPLE

Quantum numbers are used to designate the "address" of each electron within an individual atom. The first, or principal, quantum number refers to the **shell**. The second, or azimuthal, quantum number refers to the **subshell**. The third, or magnetic, quantum number refers to the **orbital**. And, the fourth, or spin, quantum number refers to the **electron spin**. Each of these four concepts is explored in detail below.

13.1.3.1 The Principal Quantum Number (Shell)

In the broadest sense, the address of an electron is given by the **shell** in which it resides. A shell is equivalent to a row in the periodic table. The principal quantum number is designated n and can take the value of any positive integer. The currently known elements require the use of $n = 1$ through $n = 7$. A low principal quantum number indicates electrons that are close to the nucleus. As n increases, the size of the shell also increases. Shells which are entirely filled with electrons are not usually of chemical interest. These shells are termed **core shells** and the electrons in them are **core electrons**. Shells that are only partially full are called **valence shells**. The electrons in these shells are called **valence electrons**. The valence electrons are the focus of most chemists; these electrons impart most of the atom's chemical properties.

13.1.3.2 The Azimuthal Quantum Number (Subshell)

Subordinate to n, the principal quantum number, is the second quantum number, ℓ, which designates a **subshell** within a particular shell and can take any integral value from zero to $n - 1$. So if $n = 2$, then $\ell = 0$ or $\ell = 1$. Each value of ℓ corresponds to a particular subshell, so there are two subshells ($\ell = 1$ and $\ell = 0$) in the second ($n = 2$) shell. (There are n subshells in the nth shell.) At present, all known elements are accommodated by $\ell = 0, 1, 2,$ or 3. Subshells are so important in the study of chemistry that they are also labeled by a lettering system:

$$
\begin{array}{ccccc}
\ell & 0 & 1 & 2 & 3 \\
letter & s & p & d & f
\end{array}
$$

These letter designations also correspond to the blocks in the periodic table (**13.1.2.2**).

13.1.3.3 The Magnetic Quantum Number (Orbital)

Subordinate to the azimuthal quantum number is the magnetic quantum number, m_ℓ, which designates an **orbital** within a particular subshell. An orbital is the region surrounding an atom's nucleus where an electron is most likely to be. The possible values of m_ℓ are any integral value from $-\ell$ to $+\ell$, including zero. Therefore, there are $2\ell + 1$ orbitals in the ℓth subshell.

For example, when $\ell = 1$, the values of m_ℓ are $-1, 0,$ and 1. Each value of m_ℓ corresponds to an orbital. From this, we can see that, per shell, there is only one orbital in the s ($\ell = 0$) subshell:

One orbital in the s ($\ell = 0$) subshell

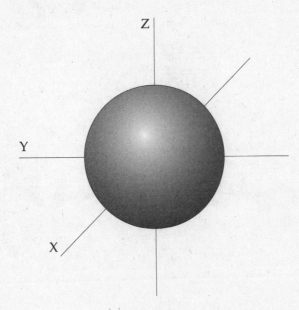

Figure 13.2

Three p ($\ell = 1$) orbitals:

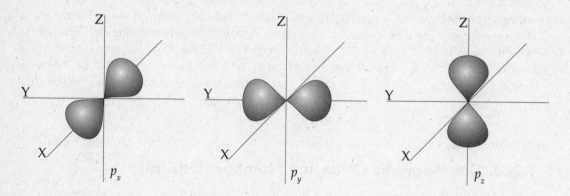

Figure 13.3

Five d ($\ell = 2$) orbitals:

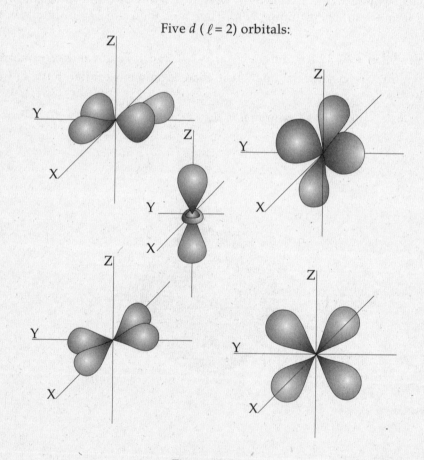

Figure 13.4

There are seven f ($\ell = 3$) orbitals, the shapes of which are similar to the shapes of the d orbitals. The f orbital shapes will not be important on the MCAT.

13.1.3.4 The Spin Quantum Number (Electron Spin State)

The first three quantum numbers are derived from theory. The fourth quantum number, m_s, is experimentally derived and designates the **spin** state of a particular electron within a particular orbital. There are two possible values of m_s: $+\frac{1}{2}$ and $-\frac{1}{2}$.

13.1.3.5 Tabular Summary of Quantum Numbers

Symbol and Name	Possible Values	Related Quantities
n shell	{positive integers}	
ℓ subshell	$\{0, 1, 2, ..., n-1\}$	n subshells per shell
m_ℓ orbital	$\{-\ell, ..., 0, ..., +\ell\}$	$2\ell+1$ orbitals per subshell, n^2 orbitals per shell
m_s electron spin	$\{^{+}_{-}\frac{1}{2}\}$	2 electrons per orbital $4\ell+2$ electrons per subshell, $2n^2$ electrons per shell

Table 13.3

13.1.3.6 The Pauli Exclusion Principle and Hund's Rule

According to the **Pauli exclusion principle**, no electron in any one atom may have all four quantum numbers identical to a second electron in the same atom. Electrons will always be added to the lowest available energy level (as defined by the four quantum numbers). While it is possible to have two electrons with the same n, ℓ, and m_ℓ, these two electrons must differ in m_s. Two electrons that differ only in spin quantum number are said to be spin paired. Spin paired electrons share an orbital within a subshell of a particular shell in the same atom. **Hund's rule** states that no two electrons will become spin paired unless there are no empty orbitals at the energy level of the orbitals that are presently being filled. To illustrate this, consider the three 2p orbitals of carbon. Each of these orbitals has the same energy as the other two orbitals. When orbitals have identical energies, they are called **degenerate orbitals**. Applying Hund's rule, you should recognize that when filling the 2p subshell, one electron goes first into each of the three p orbitals; it is not until a fourth electron is placed into a p orbital that spin pairing would occur in the 2p subshell of carbon.

When an atom contains only electrons that are spin paired, that atom is **diamagnetic**. When an atom contains one or more electrons that are not spin paired, that atom is **paramagnetic**. You should recognize that an atom that contains an odd number of electrons is, by necessity, paramagnetic; however, an atom that contains an even number of electrons may be either diamagnetic or paramagnetic.

13.1.3.7 The Aufbau Principle and Electron Configuration

In order to determine the electron configuration of a particular atom, you need to understand the **aufbau principle**, or "building-up" principle. Electrons are placed into orbitals from lowest energy orbital to highest energy orbital. The aufbau principle is summarized by:

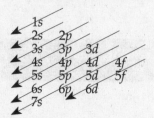

Figure 13.5

Orbitals are filled in the order 1s, 2s, 2p, 3s, 3p, 4s, 3d, 4p, 5s, 4d, 5p, 6s, 4f, 5d, 6p, 7s, 5f, 6d as indicated by the arrows in the figure. In order to determine the lowest possible electron configuration for an atom, you should determine the number of electrons to be put into orbitals (equal to the atomic number for neutral atoms), and use Figure 13.6:

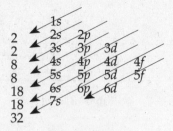

Figure 13.6

Consider vanadium (AN = 23). Its electron configuration must end somewhere in the fifth arrow (2 + 2 + 8 + 8 = 20 and 2 + 2 + 8 + 8 + 18 = 38). The electron configuration is therefore: $1s^22s^22p^63s^23p^64s^23d^3$ (and notice that the sum of the superscripts gives the electron total of the atom). You should be aware that the electron configuration just determined for vanadium is the **ground state** configuration. Any other configuration that contains 23 electrons and does not violate the filling rules (e.g., by putting more than 6 electrons in a p subshell) is an **excited state** electron configuration for vanadium. It is often an excited state configuration that is asked for when electron configuration questions are given on the MCAT.

Please solve this problem:

- Which of the following represents a possible electron configuration of a neutral magnesium atom?

    A. $1s^22s^22p^8$
    B. $1s^22s^22p^6$
    C. $2s^22p^63d^4$
    D. $1s^22s^12p^6$

Problem solved:

The correct answer is C. First, any configurations that do not contain twelve electrons should be eliminated, since the atomic number of magnesium is twelve. This eliminates B and D. Next, configurations that violate filling rules should be eliminated. A is an invalid configuration since the *p* subshell can only contain six electrons. This leaves only answer C. While answer C is not the ground state electron configuration of magnesium, it is still a *possible* electron configuration for magnesium. A is invalid. B is the ground state electron configuration of neon or an **isoelectronic** ion to neon (that is, one which contains the same number of electrons as neon). For example, Mg^{+2}, Na^{+1}, F^{-1}, O^{-2}, and N^{-3} would all be isoelectronic to neon and each other. Choice D is a non-ground state electron configuration (excited state) of fluorine or an ion isoelectronic to fluorine.

13.1.3.8 Periodic Trends

There are five periodic trends that are governed by electron configuration: **electronegativity**, **atomic radius**, **ionization energy**, **metallic character**, and **electron affinity**. Here is a mnemonic device that should help you. Those trends that contain a word beginning with the letter "e" increase from left to right across the periodic table and from bottom to top, those trends that do not contain a word beginning with the letter "e" do the opposite, they increase from right to left and from top to bottom. This is illustrated in Figure 13.7.

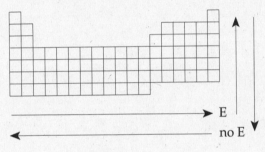

Figure 13.7

Electronegativity can be thought of as the affinity of a particular atom for electrons when that atom is engaged in a chemical bond. Electronegativity is not a directly measurable quantity. The most electronegative atom, fluorine, is assigned an electronegativity of 4.0. The most electropositive (therefore, least electronegative) atom, francium, is assigned an electronegativity of 0.7. Since the noble gases rarely form chemical bonds, they are not included in electronegativity tables. Any two atoms with an electronegativity difference equal to or *greater than 1.7* are said to **bond ionically**. Any two bound atoms with an electronegativity difference *less than 1.7*, but not equal to 0, are said to be involved in a **polar covalent bond**. A **nonpolar covalent bond** can only occur between atoms of **identical electronegativity**—that is, this case can only occur when the two bound atoms are atoms of the same element. In an ionic, or polar covalent bond, the electrons forming the bond spend more time close to the atom with the greater electronegativity (**14.1.1.2**).

Atomic radius decreases from left to right within a period. While this may seem counterintuitive, because the number of electrons within a shell increases from left to right within a period, it is due to the fact that there is an increasing number of protons in the nucleus while the amount of shielding exerted by the core shells remains constant. Therefore, the valence electrons are more strongly attracted to the nucleus and spend more time closer to it. As more shells are added, the electron cloud does get larger; therefore, atomic radius increases from the top of the periodic table to the bottom.

Ionization energy is that energy necessary to release the outermost electron from an atom. Ionization energy generally increases from left to right across a period. As atoms decrease in size (remember that shells *contract* as protons more strongly attract the valence electrons), the valence electrons become more strongly attracted to the nucleus, and more energy is required to liberate an electron.

Metallic character refers to the ease with which an atom loses valence electrons. Atoms with low ionization energies are strongly metallic. Conversely, as ionization energy increases, metallic character decreases.

Electron affinity is the tendency of an atom to gain an additional electron. An atom that would move closer to the electron configuration of a noble gas by gaining an electron is more likely to do so than an atom that would move away from the nearest noble gas electron configuration by picking up an electron.

13.1.3.9 Group Names

Certain columns within the periodic table are assigned group names, and there are two systems of naming the groups. The current system, used by contemporary chemists, is fairly straightforward; the older system, which is still at times used by MCAT writers, is slightly less straightforward. In the newer system, groups are numbered sequentially from 1 to 18 from left to right:

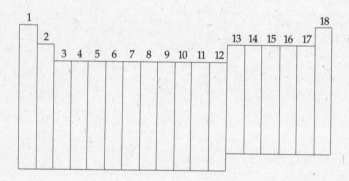

Figure 13.8

In the older system, the groups are numbered I through VIII and denoted as either "A" or "B." All "A" groups are in the *s* and *p* blocks, all "B" groups are in the *d* block:

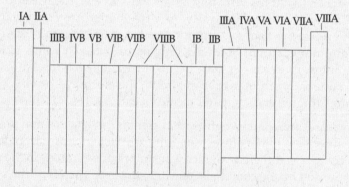

Figure 13.9

In addition to these systematic group names, certain groups have common names. Group 1 is the **alkali metals**. Group 2 is the **alkaline earth metals**. Group 17 is the **halogens**. Group 18 is the **noble gases**. Groups 1, 2, and 13–18 are the **representative elements**, or main block elements. Groups 3–12 are the **transition metals**. The actinides with atomic numbers greater than 92 are called **transuranium elements**. Elements in the same group can be expected to have chemical properties similar to one another.

13.1.4 THE ATOM IN MODERN PERSPECTIVE

With the advent of **quantum mechanics**, our understanding of the atom has changed dramatically. An important precursor to the field of quantum mechanics was the atomic theory of Max Planck. According to Planck, electrons are able to exist only at discrete energy levels. In fact, energy itself can occur only in discrete units. These discrete units of energy are called **quanta**. Planck theorized that electrons are able to move from one energy level to the next only when they are given enough energy to jump to that level; an electron cannot absorb an excess of energy that is not sufficient for a transition to a higher energy level. This is summarized by the equation:

$$\Delta E = hf$$

where ΔE is the difference in energy between two allowed energy levels for an electron, h is Planck's constant, and f is the frequency of the electromagnetic radiation used to increase the energy of the electron. Each allowable energy level is therefore separated by a quanta of energy, hf. Since (wavelength)(frequency) = velocity, and electromagnetic radiation travels at the speed of light (c) we can arrive at the equation

$c = \lambda f$, where λ is the wavelength of the electromagnetic radiation.

Substituting for f, the quantum equation becomes:

$$\Delta E = h\frac{c}{\lambda}$$

13.1.4.1 The Bohr Theory of the Atom and the Uncertainty Principle

Using the work of Planck, Niels Bohr theorized that if electrons are confined to discrete energy levels, then electrons must travel in spherical orbits around the nucleus at distances corresponding to these energy levels. This is known as the **Bohr theory of the atom**. While it has since been supplanted, it remains a convenient method for visualizing the atom.

Utilizing the Schrödinger wave equation, Werner Heisenberg determined that it is impossible to simultaneously determine both the position and the momentum of an electron. This is known as the **Heisenberg uncertainty principle**, and is mathematically stated:

$$\partial p \partial x \geq \frac{h}{4\pi}$$

where ∂p is the uncertainty in momentum, and ∂x is the uncertainty in displacement (position). Heisenberg showed that an electron's location in space at any given time may be determined with certainty only at the expense of the determination of its momentum at that instant. Since it is theoretically impossible to determine both of these variables simultaneously, we cannot assume that electrons travel in spherical orbits. (Using simple geometry, both the position and momentum are absolutely determinable at all times for an electron traveling in a spherical orbit.) Application of the Heisenberg uncertainty principle and the Schrödinger wave equation gives rise to **probability density orbitals** (pictured in

Figure 13.2). These orbitals are usually pictured at the 90 percent confidence level, which is to say that "I am 90 percent sure that the electron is somewhere inside this volume at any moment in time." The darker the shading of the volume, the higher the probability that the electron is within that section of volume.

13.1.4.2 The de Broglie Hypothesis

In 1924, Louis de Broglie posited that any particle traveling with a momentum p, should have a wavelength:

$$\lambda = \frac{h}{p}$$

Since $p = mv$, we may also write this equation as:

$$\lambda = \frac{h}{mv}$$

The significance of the de Broglie hypothesis is that not only do wave phenomena, like light, have particle characteristics but that the converse is true as well: moving particles exhibit wave characteristics.

13.1.4.3 Nuclear Chemistry and Radioactivity

Atoms seek to have a balance between protons and neutrons in their nuclei. For relatively light nuclei, a neutron to proton ratio of one to one will tend to be stable. For heavier nuclei, a neutron to proton ratio of greater than one to one about 1.5 to 1, is needed for ideal stablity. If an isotope has too many neutrons relative to protons, it may seek either to shed some of those neutrons or to convert some of those neutrons to protons. Likewise, if an isotope has too many protons, it may seek either to shed a proton or convert a proton to a neutron. These and related processes are collectively known as **radioactive decay**.

13.1.4.3.1 THE IMPORTANT RADIOACTIVE DECAY PROCESSES

If an isotope is unstable simply because of its nuclear size, it will often seek to shed both neutrons and protons in the process of **alpha decay**. An alpha particle is a helium ion, $_2^4\alpha$ or $_2^4\text{He}^{2+}$. An example of alpha decay is:

$$_{84}^{210}\text{Po} \rightarrow {}_2^4\alpha + {}_{82}^{206}\text{Pb}$$

If an isotope has too many neutrons, it may seek to convert a neutron to a proton via **beta decay**. A beta particle is an electron and can be represented as $_{-1}^0\beta$ or as $_{-1}^0e$. An example of beta decay is:

$$_{82}^{210}\text{Po} \rightarrow {}_{-1}^0\beta + {}_{83}^{210}\text{Bi}$$

Notice that the resulting bismuth −210 isotope has the same mass as the lead −210, but the bismuth isotope has a higher atomic number: a neutron has been converted to a proton. If a relatively light isotope has too many protons, it may seek to convert a proton to a neutron via **positron emission**. A positron is an antimatter electron. It has the same mass as an electron, but a +1 charge. It can be represented as $_{+1}^0\beta$ or as $_1^0e$. An example of positron emission is:

$$_{20}^{39}\text{Ca} \rightarrow {}_{+1}^0\beta + {}_{19}^{39}\text{K}$$

Another method to eliminate an excess of protons (particularly for heavier nuclei) is **electron capture**. An example of electron capture is:

$$^{55}_{26}\text{Fe} + {}^{0}_{-1}\text{e} \rightarrow {}^{55}_{25}\text{Mn}$$

Associated with each of the above processes is the concomitant release of a photon, or **gamma particle**. A gamma particle is effectively massless and therefore does not affect the chemical symbol:

$$^{55}_{26}\text{Fe} + {}^{0}_{-1}\text{e} \rightarrow {}^{55}_{25}\text{Mn} + {}^{0}_{0}\gamma$$

13.1.4.3.2 TABULAR SUMMARY OF RADIOACTIVE DECAY PROCESSES

Decay Type	Symbol	Change in Mass Number	Change in Atomic Number
alpha emission	$-\left({}^{4}_{2}\alpha\right)$	-4	-2
beta emission	$-\left({}^{0}_{-1}\beta\right)$	0	$+1$
positron emission	$-\left({}^{0}_{+1}\beta\right)$	0	-1
electron capture	$+\left({}^{0}_{-1}\text{e}\right)$	0	-1
gamma emission	$-\left({}^{0}_{0}\gamma\right)$	0	0

Table 13.4

It should also be noted that, of the particles involved in radioactive decay, gamma particles have the least mass and the highest energy; alpha particles have the greatest mass and the lowest energy.

13.1.4.3.3 NUCLEAR BINDING ENERGY, MASS DEFECT, AND EINSTEIN'S EQUATION

We have all heard the famous equation:

$$E = mc^2$$

The only times that you will use this equation on the MCAT are in cases involving the computation of **nuclear binding energies** or cases of **mass defect**. It takes energy to break up a nucleus into its constituent protons and neutrons: This energy is the nuclear binding energy, E. It has also been observed that the mass of an atomic nucleus is less than the sum of the masses of the individual protons and neutrons of which it is constituted: This difference in mass is the mass defect, m. Einstein showed that these two quantities, energy and mass, are related by the square of the speed of light.

13.2 MASTERY APPLIED: SAMPLE PASSAGE AND QUESTIONS

Passage

Groups 3–12 in the periodic table are the transition elements. These elements are characterized by a partially filled outermost shell and a partially filled (or completely filled, in the case of group 12) next-to-outermost d subshell. All of these elements exhibit metallic properties.

The first ionization energy of an atom is that energy input required to remove a valence electron from a neutral atom. The second ionization energy is the energy input necessary to remove a second electron from the valence shell. Figure 1 depicts the first ionization energy of the fourth period transition elements.

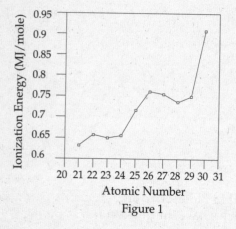

Ionization Energy (MJ/mole) vs. Atomic Number

Figure 1

In general, transition elements react:

$$1s^2 2s^2 2p^6 3s^2 3p^6 3d^n 4s^2 \rightarrow 1s^2 2s^2 2p^6 3s^2 3p^6 3d^n$$

This is true not only of the first transition series, but also of the later transition series. The aufbau principle suggests that the $4s$ energy level is lower than the $3d$ energy level, so why would the $4s$ electrons be lost before the $3d$ electrons? An often-posited explanation for this is that the $3d$ energy level decreases in energy as it fills, such that at AN = 29 the energy levels invert. While this explains why copper and

zinc would lose their $4s$ electrons before losing their $3d$ electrons, it fails to address the other eight first transition series elements.

A more satisfactory explanation of this phenomenon is that what is important is not the relative energies of the $4s$ and the $3d$ levels taken individually as electrons are put in, but rather the relative energies of these levels as electrons are taken out to form cations. When this scenario is considered, it becomes clear that the $4s$ level is higher in energy than the $3d$ level relative to cation formation and that the $3d$ level is higher than the $4s$ level relative to anion formation.

1. Every element in the first period of transition elements except scandium (AN = 21) forms a +2 cation. Scandium most likely does not form this cation because:

   A. the two electrons removed are $4s$ electrons.
   B. removing two electrons from scandium would make it isoelectronic with potassium.
   C. the first ionization energy of scandium is low, the second ionization energy of scandium is high.
   D. the third ionization energy of scandium is low.

2. From the information in Figure 1, which of the following is NOT true?

   A. Iron forms a +1 cation more easily than does cobalt.
   B. Zinc is the least likely of the fourth period transition elements to form a +1 cation.
   C. Nickel forms a +1 cation more easily than does iron.
   D. Cr^{+1} is favored by a d^5 valence shell configuration.

3. Ionization energy is expected to increase from left to right across a period. The most likely explanation for the discrepancies observed in Figure 1 is:

   A. electrons will fill empty orbitals before pairing.
   B. the $4s$ orbital is higher in energy than the $3d$ orbital for all the fourth period transition elements.
   C. the $4s$ orbital is higher in energy than the $3d$ orbital for the fourth period transition elements as they form ions.
   D. electrons will move from a paired orbital into an empty orbital even if the empty orbital is higher in energy.

4. The first ionization energy of potassium (K) is 0.4189 MJ/mol. The first ionization energy of barium (Ba) is 0.5029 MJ/mol. Therefore:

   A. barium is more metallic than potassium.
   B. potassium is more metallic than barium.
   C. barium has a greater electron affinity than potassium.
   D. potassium has a greater electron affinity than barium.

5. Would methane or ethane be expected to have the higher ionization energy?

   A. Methane, because a methyl cation is more stable than a primary cation.
   B. Methane, because a methyl anion is more stable than a primary anion.
   C. Ethane, because a primary cation is more stable than a methyl cation.
   D. Ethane, because a primary anion is more stable than a methyl anion.

6. The most common ions of iron are Fe^{2+} and Fe^{3+}. Are these ions diamagnetic or paramagnetic?

   A. Fe^{2+} is diamagnetic, Fe^{3+} is paramagnetic.
   B. Fe^{3+} is diamagnetic, Fe^{2+} is paramagnetic.
   C. Both ions are diamagnetic.
   D. Both ions are paramagnetic.

7. As seen in Figure 1, zinc (AN = 30) has a high first ionization energy. This is most likely caused by:

   A. the formation of a paramagnetic ion from a diamagnetic atom.
   B. the formation of a paramagnetic ion from a paramagnetic atom.
   C. the formation of a diamagnetic ion from a paramagnetic atom.
   D. the formation of a diamagnetic ion from a diamagnetic atom.

8. Electronegativity is expected to have which relationship to ionization energy?

   A. Inverse
   B. Direct
   C. Inverse squared
   D. Squared

13.3 MASTERY VERIFIED: ANSWERS AND EXPLANATIONS

1. *D is the correct answer.* Choice A represents a true statement. However, this statement does not answer the question. Choice B is also true, but also does not answer the question. Choice C is true, since the second ionization energy of any atom is higher than the first ionization energy. However, it fails to address why a +2 cation is not formed, since it would imply that a +1 cation is the most common ion for scandium. Choice D is the correct answer since the most common cation formed from scandium is the +3 ion. Therefore, the +2 ion is not formed, because if it was formed it would be immediately transformed into the +3 ion, which corresponds to a noble gas configuration for scandium. The noble gas configuration is the most favored electron configuration for any atom that can assume it.

2. *A is the correct answer.* According to Figure 1, iron (AN = 26) has a higher first ionization energy than cobalt (AN = 27), therefore, cobalt will form a +1 cation more easily than iron. Therefore choice A is *false*. According to Figure 1, zinc has the highest first ionization energy. Therefore, zinc (AN = 30) is the least likely of the fourth period transition elements to form a +1 cation. Therefore, choice B is *true*. Nickel (AN = 28) has a lower first ionization energy than iron, thus it will more easily form a +1 cation. Therefore, choice C is *true*. Chromium (AN = 24) has a ground state elemental electron configuration of $1s^22s^22p^63s^23p^63d^54s^1$. When a single electron is removed from this atom to make the +1 cation, the electron configuration for the ion is $1s^22s^22p^63s^23p^63d^5$. Therefore choice D is also *true*.

3. *C is the correct answer.* Choice A is true, however, it does not directly address the question. According to the passage, choice B is false—the $3d$ level drops below the 4s level for copper (AN = 29) and zinc (AN = 30). According to the passage, choice C is true—the energy levels that must be considered when taking an electron out of an atom are not necessarily equal in energy to the energy levels seen when that electron was being put into the atom via the aufbau principle. Choice D is false. Although it costs energy to pair electrons, electrons will not avoid pairing by inserting into higher energy levels—if they did, electrons would never pair!

4. *B is the correct answer.* Metallic character has to do with the tendency of an atom to give up electrons. A low first ionization energy indicates a valence electron that can be easily lost. Electron affinity is the willingness of an atom to gain an electron. While it may seem straightforward to assume that an atom that is less willing to give up an electron must be more willing to take an electron, it is not quite so clear. By knowing the first ionization energy of an atom we can say nothing about the electron affinity of that atom.

    Considering these facts, it is clear that neither C nor D can be the correct answer, because we cannot determine electron affinity from an ionization energy measurement. It should also be clear that an atom with a lower ionization energy is more metallic. For this reason, choice B is a better answer than choice A.

5. *C is the correct answer.* This question requires that you integrate your organic chemistry knowledge with your inorganic chemistry knowledge. The MCAT will frequently require you to do this.

    First, to eliminate choices B and D, we need only consider the fact that we are removing electrons, thus making cations, not anions.

From organic chemistry, we remember that a tertiary cation is more stable than a secondary cation, a secondary cation is more stable than a primary cation, and a primary cation is more stable than a methyl cation. Therefore, in deciding between choices A and C, it is clear that choice A is false, while choice C is true.

6. *D is the correct answer.* Iron has an atomic number of 26. Therefore, Fe^{2+} has 24 electrons and Fe^{3+} has 23 electrons. An atom, or ion, with an odd number of electrons cannot be diamagnetic (all electrons paired). For this reason, choices B and C are thrown out, leaving choices A and D. Since we know that Fe^{3+} must be paramagnetic, the question reduces to: Is Fe^{2+} diamagnetic or paramagnetic?

   Since iron is filling a *d* subshell, it has five orbitals to fill before it will electron pair. Fe^{2+} has six electrons past the nearest noble gas configuration. Whether two of these electrons are paired in the $4s$ orbital, or one electron is in the $4s$ orbital, or no electrons are in the $4s$ orbital, is irrelevant. In any case, the remaining 4, 5, or 6 electrons, respectively, will not all pair in the $3d$ orbitals. Therefore, Fe^{2+} is paramagnetic and the answer must be D.

7. *A is the correct answer.* Using similar reasoning to question 6, we can answer this question. Elemental zinc has an electron configuration of $1s^22s^22p^63s^23p^63d^{10}4s^2$—in other words, since all of its valence electrons shells that are partially filled are entirely filled, it is a diamagnetic atom. This eliminates choices B and C. The loss of a single electron from a diamagnetic species *must* lead to a paramagnetic species. Therefore, the answer *must* be A.

   As proof, remember that all diamagnetic species must have an even number of electrons. While it is not sufficient that a species have an even number of electrons for diamagneticity, it is necessary. Recall, also, that a paramagnetic species may have either an odd number of electrons or an even number of electrons. Recall, also, that an odd number of electrons is sufficient for a species to be paramagnetic. If you remove one electron from any diamagnetic species, you get, of necessity, a paramagnetic species.

8. *B is the correct answer.* Recall the periodic trends presented in the chapter. Those properties that contain words which begin with the letter "e" are expected to exhibit the same trend: increasing from left to right and from bottom to top. Therefore, since both electronegativity and ionization energy contain words that begin with the letter "e," the relationship between these two periodic trends is direct. An inverse relationship exists between those trends that contain a word beginning with the letter "e" and those trends that do not contain a word beginning with the letter "e."

BONDING AND MOLECULAR FORMATION

14.1 MASTERY ACHIEVED

14.1.1 ATOMIC AND MOLECULAR INTERACTIONS: BONDING

Elements that form chemical bonds do so through an alteration of their electron configurations. This alteration occurs only if it leads to a more stable arrangement of electrons. As we saw in Chapter 13, noble gases represent the most stable electron configurations available to the main block (s and p block) elements. For this reason, the most stable ions, or other electron configurations, are isoelectronic with the noble gases.

14.1.1.1 Lewis Dot Structures and the Octet Rule

Lewis dot structures are often useful when considering the bonding requirements of individual atoms. However, you should be aware that Lewis structures begin to break down for atoms that violate the octet rule.

The **rule of eight**, or the **octet rule**, states that each atom would like to have a valence, or outer, shell configuration that matches that of the noble gases. For elements that are in the p block (**13.1.2.2**), this corresponds to a filled valence shell of eight electrons. G. N. Lewis devised a clever way of denoting the number of electrons in the valence shell of an atom by placing dots (one for each electron) around the chemical symbol for that atom. Thus, the Lewis dot structures for the second period elements are:

$$\text{Li}\cdot \quad \text{Be}: \quad \cdot\dot{\text{B}}\cdot \quad \cdot\dot{\underset{\cdot}{\text{C}}}\cdot \quad \cdot\dot{\text{N}}: \quad :\dot{\ddot{\text{O}}}: \quad :\ddot{\text{F}}\cdot \quad :\ddot{\text{Ne}}:$$

Notice that it does not matter where we place the dots around the element, as long as those electrons that do not appear in the same subshell are not paired in the dot structure. The Lewis dot structure for beryllium (Be) shows the electrons paired, because both of these electrons are in the s subshell. The Lewis dot structures for boron (B) and carbon (C) do not show paired electrons, since once the p subshell is made available, by the first electron entering it, the electrons have a tendency to "spread out" via a process known as **hybridization**. Hybridization will be discussed in greater detail in Chapter 33.

An octet may be achieved in the three ways outlined below:

1. A metal may lose electrons to form a cation that is isoelectronic with the previous noble gas. An example of this is the Mg^{2+} cation, which is isoelectronic with neon (Ne). The formation of this ion is given by the equation:

$$Mg\!:\ \longrightarrow\ Mg^{2+} + 2e^-$$

2. A nonmetal may gain electrons to form an anion that is isoelectronic to the next noble gas. An example of this is the F^{1-} anion, which is isoeletronic with neon. The formation of this ion is given by the equation:

$$:\!\ddot{F}\!\cdot\ + e^- \longrightarrow\ :\!\ddot{F}\!:^-$$

3. Atoms (typically two nonmetals) may share electrons with one another such that each atom effectively becomes isoelectronic with the next noble gas. Two examples of this are given below in the HF and NH_3 molecules.

Using the octet rule, we can see that fluorine would like to gain a single electron, while nitrogen would like to gain three electrons. As a result, the following dot structures can be constructed of these elements bonding with hydrogen:

$$H\overset{x}{:}\ddot{F}\!:\qquad H\overset{\cdot}{:}\overset{\cdot\cdot}{N}\overset{\cdot}{\underset{x\,\cdot}{:}}H$$
$$H$$

where the dots came originally from the fluorine or the nitrogen, and the x's came originally from the hydrogens.

Please solve this problem:

- An atom has the electron configuration $1s^2 2s^2 2p^6 3s^2 3p^6 4s^2$. This configuration could represent any of the following species EXCEPT:

  A. Ca$:$
  B. Ti$:^{2+}$
  C. Mn$:^{5+}$
  D. K$:^-$

Problem solved:

D is the correct answer. The electron configuration given is the ground state electron configuration for a calcium atom. This electron configuration also represents possible electron configurations for the dipositive titanium ion and the pentapositive manganese ion. While this would also be the correct electron configuration for the potassium ion depicted in choice D, you should recognize that potassium forms a cation, not an anion.

14.1.1.2 Intramolecular Bonds: Ionic and Covalent

It is convenient to think of the interactions between atoms that allow them to form molecules as bonds. In the broadest sense there are eight types of bonds, the most familiar of which are **covalent** and **ionic bonds**.

In an ionic bond, one atom receives an electron from another atom; the former atom becomes negatively charged, and the latter atom becomes positively charged. This is an ion-ion bond. An example of an ionic bond is the bond between Na and Cl to form sodium chloride:

$$Na\bullet \; + \; :\!\overset{\bullet\bullet}{\underset{\bullet\bullet}{Cl}}\!\bullet \; \longrightarrow \; Na^+ \; + \; :\!\overset{\bullet\bullet}{\underset{\bullet\bullet}{Cl}}\!:^-$$

In a covalent bond, an electron pair is shared between two atoms. The diagrams above of HF and NH_3 are examples of covalent bonding.

What determines whether a bond will be ionic or covalent is electronegativity. If two atoms with identical electronegativities come together to form a bond, this bond will be a true covalent bond. If two atoms with a large difference in electronegativities come together to form a bond, this bond will be an ionic bond. For any two atoms with an electronegativity difference in excess of 1.7, the bond between these atoms is considered an ionic bond. In the case of a true covalent bond, the two electrons constituting the bond each spend an equal amount of time associated with each of the two atomic nuclei.

However, when the two atoms forming a covalent bond differ in electronegativity, the two electrons forming the bond will spend a larger amount of time associated with the more strongly electronegative atom than with the more electropositive atom. This is termed a **polar** covalent bond. When a polar covalent bond is formed, a **dipole** is also formed. The symbol for a dipole is an arrow with a perpendicular line through its tail. The head of the arrow is pointed in the direction of the more electronegative atom.

Consider the possibility of a polar covalent bond between hydrogen and chlorine. This bond could be written:

$$H \longmapsto\!\!\!\!\rightarrow Cl$$

This may also be represented in one of two ways:

$$\overset{\delta^+}{H} \qquad \overset{\delta^-}{Cl}$$

$$(H \qquad Cl)$$

In the upper representation, δ^+ is used to show a partial positive charge on the hydrogen atom, and δ^- is used to denote a partial negative charge on the chlorine atom. In the lower representation, the outline represents the shape of the electron cloud that is formed by the electrons in the bond.

Note that a dipole may be either **permanent** or **induced**. Consider the following set of diagrams:

$$F^- \qquad H-H$$

$$F^- \; \overset{\delta^+}{H}-\overset{\delta^-}{H}$$

Initially, the H_2 molecule has no net dipole—it is a purely covalent molecule. As a fluoride ion is brought closer to the hydrogen on the left, the electrons in the H_2 molecule are repelled by this negatively charged ion. The net result is an induced dipole in the H_2 molecule.

Please solve this problem:

- Which of the following molecules is expected to have the largest individual bond dipole moment?

    A. N_2
    B. CH_4
    C. NaH
    D. H_2O

Problem solved:

C is the correct answer. The nitrogen molecule will not have an overall dipole moment, nor will it have a bond dipole moment. The two nitrogens are equivalent, and they share a pure covalent bond. Methane (CH_4) will not have an overall dipole moment, due to the symmetry of the molecule; however, it will have an individual bond dipole in each of the C-H bonds. These dipoles result from the difference in electronegativity of carbon and hydrogen. It is important that you recognize that carbon is slightly more electronegative than hydrogen, so each dipole points in the direction of the carbon atom.

Sodium has an electronegativity of 0.93 on the Pauling scale (relative to fluorine, which has an electronegativity of 4.0). The electronegativity of hydrogen is 2.20. The difference in electronegativity between these two atoms is therefore 1.27. Recalling that we want an electronegativity difference of greater than 1.7 for an ionic bond, we can state that this is a highly polar covalent bond.

The electronegativity difference between hydrogen and oxygen is 1.24. This is close to the difference between sodium and hydrogen, but not quite as large. You will not be expected to know values of electronegativity for the MCAT, but you must recognize that electronegativity is a periodic trend that increases from bottom to top and from left to right (**13.1.3.8**). Also, be aware that when considering the electronegativity of hydrogen, you should imagine hydrogen as falling between boron and carbon in the periodic table. Using this scenario, without resorting to electronegativity values, we can see that Na—H is the most polar bond in the above question since these elements (with hydrogen imagined between boron and carbon) are the farthest apart in the periodic table.

14.1.1.3 Intermolecular Bonds

Ions, dipoles, and induced dipoles can interact in six ways: **ion-ion**, **ion-dipole**, **ion-induced dipole**, **dipole-dipole**, **dipole-induced dipole**, and **induced dipole-induced dipole**. We have already discussed the strongest of these six interactions: the intramolecular ion-ion. The other five types of interaction are between separate molecules or are intermolecular. Each of these six interactions is summarized in Table 14.1. The interactions are organized from strongest to weakest.

Type of interaction	Example
ion-ion	Na^+/Cl^-
ion-dipole	Na^+/H_2O
dipole-dipole	H_2O/H_2O
ion-induced dipole	Na^+/CCl_4
dipole-induced dipole	CH_3OH/CCl_4
induced dipole-induced dipole	CCl_4/CCl_4

Table 14.1

As can be seen from Table 14.1, even molecules that do not possess a permanent dipole have interatomic or intermolecular forces that are created by induced dipole-induced dipole interactions. These forces are also known as **London dispersion forces**. These are the weakest intermolecular forces.

Please solve this problem:

- The sodium cation, Na^+, is more soluble in water than the silver cation, Ag^{2+}. The best explanation for this fact is:

   A. sodium has a greater electronegativity than silver.
   B. silver has a greater electronegativity than sodium.
   C. the sodium cation experiences ion-dipole interactions with the water.
   D. the silver cation is larger than the sodium cation.

Problem solved:

B is the correct answer. Because silver is more electronegative than sodium, we expect sodium to maintain itself as a "naked" cation (not accepting electron density from the water). This leads to a large ion-dipole interaction between the sodium and the water. Choice C is true; however, it does not provide the complete explanation of the problem at hand, since the silver cation also experiences ion-dipole interactions with water.

Water is a polar molecule; as such, it will solvate polar entities (the more polar, the better). The extremely low electronegativity of sodium makes the sodium cation a better "positive charge" than the silver cation.

In terms of choice D, we must remember that our periodic trend (**13.1.3.8**) was in terms of atomic radius, *not* ionic radius.

14.1.1.4 Hydrogen Bonding

So far, we have discussed seven types of bonding. The eighth, and final, type is **hydrogen bonding**.

A hydrogen bond consists of two components: a hydrogen atom attached to an electronegative atom X and a second electronegative atom Y that contains a lone electron pair. Since the hydrogen that is attached to X is participating in a net dipole with X, the hydrogen possesses a net partial positive charge. The electrons that form the bond between the hydrogen and the electronegative atom spend a majority of time associated with the electronegative atom:

$$\overset{\delta^+}{H}-\overset{\delta^-}{X}$$

When the electron-rich Y comes into the vicinity of this electron-poor hydrogen, it is willing to donate a portion of its lone electron pair to the hydrogen. The hydrogen accepts the electron density from Y, because the hydrogen is electron-deficient. Atom Y is willing to donate a portion of its electron density to the hydrogen, because it can, in effect, give up only a small portion of this electron density while gaining the stability of an additional bond:

$$Y{:}\longrightarrow \overset{\delta^+}{H}-\overset{\delta^-}{X} \Longrightarrow Y\cdots H-X$$

Hydrogen bonds vary in strength, from nearly the strength of a covalent or ionic bond to the strength of only a very weak bond (approximately the strength of dipole-induced dipole bonds). The high strength of hydrogen bonds in water accounts for the peculiar chemical properties of water.

Please solve this problem:

- The boiling point of water is 373 K. The boiling point of ethanol (C_2H_5OH) is 351.5 K. The difference in boiling points observed is most likely accounted for by the fact that:

  A. water is involved in hydrogen bonding, ethanol is not.
  B. both are involved in hydrogen bonding, but the hydrogen bonds in water are stronger.
  C. ethanol has a higher molecular weight than water and therefore is expected to have a lower boiling point.
  D. ethanol has a higher molecular weight than water and therefore is expected to have a higher boiling point.

Problem solved:

B is the correct answer. Both molecules can form hydrogen bonds with themselves, since they both contain a hydrogen attached to an electronegative oxygen atom, and they both contain an electronegative oxygen with lone pairs to donate to the hydrogen. The hydrogen bonds in water are much stronger than the hydrogen bonds in ethanol, which makes the boiling point of water higher than the boiling point of ethanol. Choice D is a true statement, but it does not solve the problem that has been presented.

14.1.2 MULTIPLE BONDS, RESONANCE, AND POLYATOMIC IONS

14.1.2.1 Multiple Bonds

When an atom is in need of more than one electron, it may form multiple covalent bonds with another atom. When two atoms share a single pair of electrons, as was discussed above, this is a **single bond**. When two atoms share two pairs of electrons, this is a **double bond**. The sharing of three pairs of electrons is a **triple bond**.

Examples of double and triple bonds are:

$$N \equiv N$$

$$\begin{array}{ccc} H & & H \\ & C = C & \\ H & & H \end{array}$$

It is important that you understand the relationship between single, double, and triple bonds in terms of bond length and bond strength. Triple bonds are the shortest bonds, single bonds are the longest bonds. As a result, triple bonds are stronger than double bonds, which are stronger than single bonds.

Please solve this problem:

- Which of the following gases is expected to have the strongest intramolecular bonds?

  A. H_2
  B. N_2
  C. O_2
  D. F_2

Problem solved:

B is the correct answer. If we consider the Lewis dot structures of each of these molecules, we see:

$$H - H \qquad \ddot{N} \equiv \ddot{N} \qquad \ddot{O} = \ddot{O} \qquad \ddot{F} - \ddot{F}$$

Both hydrogen gas and fluorine gas have single bonds. Oxygen gas has a double bond. Nitrogen gas has a triple bond.

14.1.2.2 Polyatomic Ions

Just as an atom may bond with more than one other atom in order to form a neutral molecule, an atom may also bond with more than one other atom to form an ion. Consider the molecule $NaNO_3$. The Lewis structure may at first be thought of as:

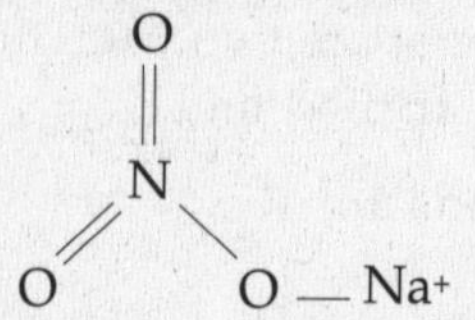

$$
\begin{array}{c}
O \\
\parallel \\
N \\
O \quad \diagdown \quad O - Na^+
\end{array}
$$

However, considering the criterion for the formation of an ionic bond (an electronegativity difference of 1.7 or larger), we can see that sodium is expected to form an ionic bond, not a covalent bond, with oxygen. Therefore, the corrected Lewis structure is:

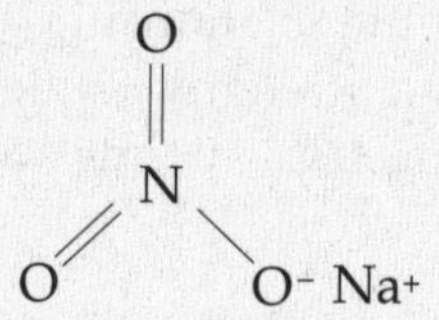

$$
\begin{array}{c}
O \\
\parallel \\
N \\
O \quad \diagdown \quad O^- \; Na^+
\end{array}
$$

where a negative charge is left on one of the oxygen atoms. The resultant structure, neglecting the sodium cation, is the polyatomic nitrate anion, NO_3^{1-}.

The names and formulas of some of the more important polyatomic ions are given in Table 14.2.

Name	Formula
ammonium	NH_4^{1+}
nitrate	NO_3^{1-}
carbonate	CO_3^{2-}
sulfate	SO_4^{2-}
phosphate	PO_4^{3-}

Table 14.2

14.1.2.3 Resonance

We can see in the above depiction of the nitrate ion that there are three possible locations for the "remaining" negative charge; that is, the charge may be located on any one of the three oxygens. This delocalization of charge density is referred to as **resonance**. The three possible resonance structures of the nitrate ion are:

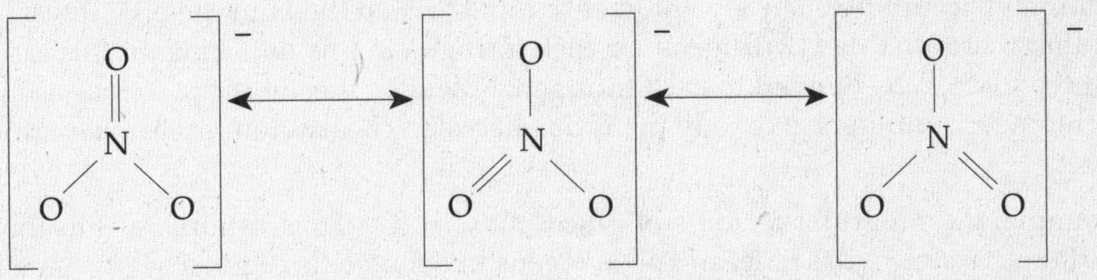

The double-headed arrow is used to indicate that these structures are resonance structures of one another.

We may also represent the three resonance structures of the nitrate ion in a single structure:

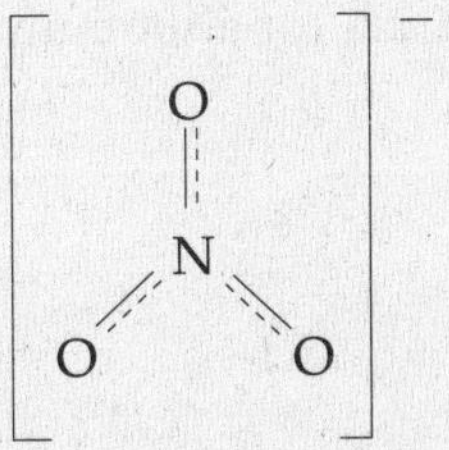

Resonance affects in the chemical properties of materials by imparting **stability** to molecules, making them less susceptible to chemical reaction. This stabilizing influence is referred to as **resonance stabilization.**

Please solve this problem:

- How many resonance structures exist for the phosphate ion (PO_4^{3-})?

    A. 1
    B. 2
    C. 3
    D. 4

Problem solved:

D is the correct answer. We can envision a structure with a central phosphorus atom and four attached oxygen atoms. Since the phosphate ion has a net charge of negative three, only one of these oxygens will have a double bond to phosphorus in any resonance structure, and each of the other three oxygens will form a single bond with phosphorus. Since there are four different oxygen atoms that could form the double bond, we have four resonance structures.

14.1.3 THE FORMATION OF MOLECULES

14.1.3.1 Stoichiometry Within Molecules

As we saw while discussing Lewis dot structures (**14.1.1.1**), nitrogen will form one bond with each of three or four hydrogens, while fluorine will form only one bond with only one hydrogen. The resulting molecular formulas are NH_3 and HF. The subscript number is known as a **stoichiometric number**. The stoichiometric number 3 on the H in the NH_3 molecule indicates that there are three hydrogens for each nitrogen in this molecule. In this case, there are also three hydrogens **bonded** to each nitrogen; however, the subscript 3 does not tell us this: stoichiometric numbers give only the **ratios** between constituent atoms, *not* information on bonding.

For example, the molecular formula of glucose is $C_6H_{12}O_6$. This formula tells us that there are six carbons, twelve hydrogens, and six oxygens in a molecule of glucose; it also tells us that there are two hydrogen atoms and one oxygen atom for every carbon atom in a molecule of glucose. But this formula tells us nothing about how these elements are arranged to form glucose.

Please solve this problem:

- The chemical formula for aluminum sulfate is:

  A. Al_3SO_4
  B. $Al_2(SO_4)_3$
  C. $Al_3(SO_4)_2$
  D. $AlSO_4$

Problem solved:

B is the correct answer. Since aluminum is a group 13 element, it has a valence state of 3^+. From Table 14.2, we know that the complex ion, sulfate, has a charge of 2^-. From this, we can see that we need two aluminum ions ($3^+ \times 2 = 6^+$) for every three sulfate ions ($2^- \times 3 = 6^-$).

14.1.3.2 Molecular Geometry and the VSEPR Model

After we have drawn a Lewis dot structure for a molecule, we can determine the geometry of the molecule based on the valence properties of the central atom. A central atom can possess from one to six electron pairs. In turn, each of these electron pairs will be either a bonding pair (involved in a bond between two atoms) or a nonbonding pair (or lone pair). Once the total number of pairs is known, and the state (bonding or nonbonding) of each pair has been determined, we employ **Valence Shell Electron Pair Repulsion (VSEPR)** to determine the geometry of the molecule. VSEPR allows geometry to be determined by considering the repulsive forces between electron pairs in the central atom of a molecule. These repulsive forces cause the attached atoms, or ligands, to fill a three-dimensional space in which they are as far away from one another as possible. Accounting for both lone pairs and bonding pairs of electrons, we can see that there are three separate repulsive forces: **lone pair-lone pair**, **lone pair-bonding pair**, and **bonding pair-bonding pair**. Since a portion of the electron energy in a bonding pair is used to perpetuate the bond, and none of the electron density in a lone pair is being used for bonding purposes, lone pair-lone pair repulsions are the strongest repulsive forces, while bonding pair-bonding pair repulsions are the weakest repulsive forces. The geometries possible for molecules with a single central atom are summarized in Table 14.3.

Total Pairs	Bonding Pairs	Lone Pairs	Shape	Example
1	1	0	linear	H_2
2	2	0	linear	CaH_2
2	1	1	linear	no molecular example
3	3	0	trigonal planar	BH_3
3	2	1	bent	no molecular example
3	1	2	linear	no molecular example
4	4	0	tetrahedral	CH_4
4	3	1	trigonal pyramidal	NH_3
4	2	2	bent	H_2O
4	1	3	linear	HF
5	5	0	trigonal bipyramidal	SbF_5
5	4	1	see-saw	SeF_4
5	3	2	T-shaped	IF_3
5	2	3	linear	XeF_2
5	1	4	linear	RhI
6	6	0	octahedral	SF_6
6	5	1	square pyramidal	BrF_5
6	4	2	square planar	XeF_4
6	3	3	T-shaped	CoF_3

Table 14.3

Each of the representative molecules in Table 14.3 is graphically depicted in Figure 14.1:

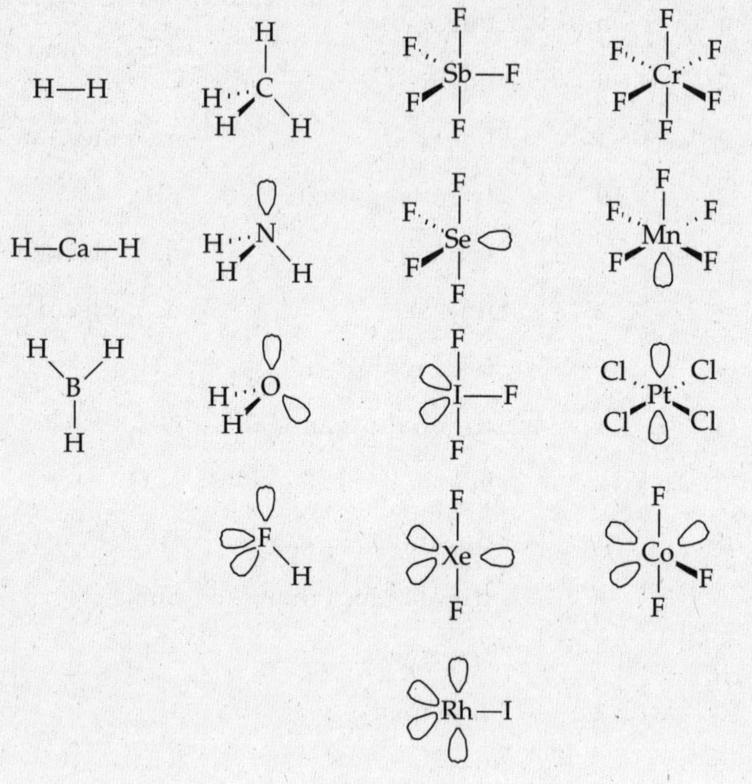

Figure 14.1

$\bigcirc$ = lone pair of electrons

$'''\cdots$ = bond extending into the page

$\diagup$ = bond extending out of the page

——— = bond in the plane of the page

Please solve this problem:

- The predicted molecular geometry of MnBr$_3$ is:

    A. trigonal planar.
    B. trigonal pyramidal.
    C. seesaw.
    D. T-shaped.

Problem solved:

D is the correct answer. From the periodic table, we see that manganese has seven valence electrons. Since three of these electrons will be spent in bonding to the three bromines, we have three bonding pairs and four nonbonding electrons, or two lone pairs. This gives us a total of five electron pairs: three bonding pairs and two lone pairs. From Table 14.3, we see that this coincides with a T-shaped geometry.

14.2 MASTERY APPLIED: SAMPLE PASSAGE AND QUESTIONS

Passage

For years, the newspaper business has been plagued by the problem of ink that smudges. Millions of dollars have been spent to develop a high-speed ink that will not smudge. Recent advances in this area have come from the arena of bonding phenomena. The Dayton Tinker Corporation has invented an ink that does not smudge. In this new process, a positively charged dye is chemically bound to a negatively charged paper.

Traditional newspaper inks never dried to the paper. These inks consisted of an oil mixed with carbon black (soot). While the oil would eventually be absorbed by the paper, the soot remained unattached to the paper.

Paper is mostly composed of cellulose, a sugar. Sugars contain many alcohol groups and are susceptible to hydrogen bonding. The negatively charged paper used in conjunction with the new smudgeless inks is a simple modification of the normal cellulose paper, where protons are removed from the various alcohol groups, creating a negative charge.

1. The bonding responsible for the smudgeless ink is:
   A. pure covalent.
   B. polar covalent.
   C. ionic.
   D. ion-dipole.

2. Carbon black is the carbon residue that remains after the complete burning of carbon-containing compounds; it is composed entirely of carbon. The bonds between individual carbon atoms in carbon black are MOST likely:
   A. nonpolar covalent.
   B. polar covalent.
   C. ionic.
   D. dipole-dipole.

3. The bonding between carbon black and newsprint is most likely:
   A. ion-dipole.
   B. dipole-dipole.
   C. dipole-induced dipole.
   D. induced dipole-induced dipole.

4. Suppose a new ink is developed that involves a polar covalent bond between the ink and the paper. This ink is expected to:
   A. adhere to the paper more strongly than both the traditional ink and the smudgeless ink.
   B. adhere to the paper more strongly than the traditional ink, but less strongly than the smudgeless ink.
   C. adhere to the paper more strongly than the traditional ink, but it cannot be predicted whether it will be held more or less strongly than the smudgeless ink.
   D. adhere to the paper less strongly than both the traditional ink and the smudgeless ink.

5. The oil used in traditional newspaper inks is a nonpolar substance. The oil is preferred over water as a solvent for the carbon black because:

A. the oil is nonpolar, while carbon black is polar.

B. the oil is nonpolar, while carbon black is nonpolar.

C. the oil is nonpolar, while the paper is polar.

D. the oil is nonpolar, while the paper is nonpolar.

6. Colored smudgeless inks have also been developed. These inks are susceptible to fading after two days of exposure to sunlight. This is most likely due to:

A. a change in the chemical composition of the oil holding the ink to the paper.

B. a change in the bond between the ink and the paper.

C. a change in the chemical bonding within the ink.

D. a change in the chemical bonding within the paper.

14.3 MASTERY VERIFIED: ANSWERS AND EXPLANATIONS

1. *C is the correct answer.* As stated in the passage, a negatively charged ink is bound to a positively charged paper. While this could also result in the formation of a polar covalent bond, we do not have enough information to choose polar covalent in preference to ionic, so ionic is the best answer.

2. *A is the correct answer.* In the question, we are told to consider carbon black as consisting entirely of carbon. A material that is composed of a single element cannot have polar covalent or ionic bonds. Such a material also cannot contain a permanent dipole. Therefore, by process of elimination, choice A is correct.

3. *C is the correct answer.* From question 2, we know that carbon black does not contain ions or dipoles; this eliminates choices A and B. From the passage, we know that the paper has many alcohol groups, which means that it possesses many dipoles. Since a dipole can induce a dipole in another material, we choose choice C and eliminate choice D.

4. *C is the correct answer.* A polar covalent bond is definitely stronger than the dipole-induced dipole bond of the traditional ink. We cannot say for sure whether this polar covalent bond will be weaker or stronger than the ionic bond in smudgeless ink.

5. *B is the correct answer.* This question refers to the common statement "like dissolves like." Since carbon black is nonpolar, it is more likely to dissolve in a substance that is also nonpolar. The paper is polar, but this has little to do with the choice of oils.

6. *C is the correct answer.* When the color of these inks fades, it is due to a change in the chemical bonds within the ink. These bonds impart the color to the ink, therefore it must be these bonds that change to effect a change in color. Choice A is incorrect, since this inking process does not involve an oil. This can be deduced from our knowledge that oils are nonpolar and the smudgeless inks are charged. Therefore, an oil would not be a good solvent for smudgeless ink. Choice B is incorrect, as a change in the bonds between the ink and the paper might cause the ink to smudge, not fade. Choice D is incorrect. A change in the internal structure of the paper may lead to brittleness and cracking, but it will not lead to a change in the color of the ink.

CHAPTER 15

CHEMICAL REACTIONS I: FUNDAMENTAL PHENOMENA

15.1 MASTERY ACHIEVED

15.1.1 REACTION CLASSES

In broad terms, there are five types of chemical reactions.

- Synthesis

- Decomposition (analysis)

- Single replacement

- Double replacement (ion exchange)

- Oxidation-reduction

Oxidation-reduction, or redox reactions, which may take the form of any of the four other classes, are the subject of **15.1.3**; the other types of reactions are discussed below.

15.1.1.1 Synthesis

A **synthesis reaction** is the direct combination of two or more compounds, or elements, to form a new chemical compound. The general form of a synthesis reaction is:

$$A + B \rightarrow AB$$

Examples of synthesis reactions include the reaction between hydrogen and oxygen gases to form water:

$$2H_2(g) + O_2(g) \rightarrow 2H_2O(l)$$

and the reaction between barium oxide and water to form barium hydroxide:

$$BaO(s) + H_2O(l) \rightarrow Ba(OH)_2(aq)$$

Please solve this problem:

- All of the following are examples of synthesis reactions EXCEPT:

  A. $2Na(s) + Cl_2(g) \rightarrow 2NaCl(s)$
  B. $4FeO(s) + O_2(g) \rightarrow 2Fe_2O_3(s)$
  C. $FeCl_3(s) + 3Na(s) \rightarrow Fe(s) + 3NaCl(s)$
  D. $H_2O(l) + O_2(g) \rightarrow H_2O_2(aq)$

Problem solved:

The correct answer is C. The reaction given in choice C is an example of a single replacement reaction (**15.1.1.3**).

15.1.1.2 Decomposition

A **decomposition reaction**, or analysis reaction, is the opposite of a synthesis reaction. In a decomposition, two or more compounds, or elements, are formed from a single chemical compound. The general form of a decomposition reaction is:

$$AB \rightarrow A + B$$

Examples of decomposition reactions include the electrolysis of water to form hydrogen and oxygen gases:

$$2H_2O(l) \rightarrow 2H_2(g) + O_2(g)$$

and the decomposition of aluminum trichloride to form aluminum metal and chlorine gas:

$$2AlCl_3(s) \rightarrow 2Al(s) + 3Cl_2(g)$$

Please solve this problem:

- All of the following are examples of unbalanced decomposition reactions EXCEPT:

  A. $Fe_2O_3(s) \rightarrow FeO(s) + O_2(g)$
  B. $FeO(s) \rightarrow Fe(s) + O_2(g)$
  C. $HIO_3(aq) + O_2(g) \rightarrow HIO_4(aq)$
  D. $HIO_4(aq) \rightarrow HIO_3(aq) + O_2(g)$

Problem solved:

The correct answer is C. The reaction given in choice C is an example of a synthesis reaction (**15.1.1.1**).

15.1.1.3 Single Replacement

In a **single replacement reaction**, an element reacts with a compound to form a new compound and a different element. The general form of a single replacement reaction is:

$$A + BX \rightarrow AX + B$$

Examples of single replacement reactions include the reaction between copper metal and sulfuric acid to form hydrogen gas and copper(II) sulfate:

$$Cu(s) + H_2SO_4(aq) \rightarrow CuSO_4(aq) + H_2(g)$$

and the replacement of bromine by chlorine in sodium bromide:

$$2NaBr(aq) + Cl_2(g) \rightarrow 2NaCl(aq) + Br_2(l)$$

Please solve this problem:

- All of the following are examples of single replacement reactions EXCEPT:

  A. $Na(s) + KCl(s) \rightarrow NaCl(s) + K(s)$
  B. $3NaOH(aq) + FeBr_3(aq) \rightarrow 3NaBr(aq) + Fe(OH)_3(s)$
  C. $2Mn(s) + 10HCl(aq) \rightarrow 2MnCl_5(s) + 5H_2(g)$
  D. $16NaCl(s) + S_8(s) \rightarrow 8Na_2S(aq) + 8Cl_2(g)$

Problem solved:

The correct answer is B. The reaction given in choice B is an example of a double replacement reaction (**15.1.1.4**).

15.1.1.4 Double Replacement

In a **double replacement reaction**, two compounds exchange ions with one another. The result is the formation of two new chemical compounds. The general form of a double replacement reaction is:

$$AX + BY \rightarrow AY + BX$$

Examples of double replacement reactions include the neutralization reaction between sodium hydroxide and hydrochloric acid:

$$NaOH(aq) + HCl(aq) \rightarrow NaCl(aq) + H_2O(l)$$

and the reaction between silver nitrate and sodium chloride to form silver chloride and sodium nitrate:

$$AgNO_3(aq) + NaCl(aq) \rightarrow NaNO_3(aq) + AgCl(s)$$

Please solve this problem:

- All of the following are examples of double replacement reactions EXCEPT:

 A. $KBr(aq) + NaOH(aq) \rightarrow KOH(aq) + NaBr(aq)$
 B. $AlCl_3(s) + 3NaOH(aq) \rightarrow Al(OH)_3(s) + 3NaCl(aq)$
 C. $FeS(s) + 2NaOH(aq) \rightarrow Na_2S(s) + Fe(OH)_2(aq)$
 D. $2AlCl_3(s) + 3FeBr_2(aq) \rightarrow 2AlBr_3(s) + 3FeCl_2(aq)$

Problem solved:

The correct answer is A. Since both reactants and both products are in the aqueous phase, it would be impossible to tell if this reaction had occurred. In a case such as this, there is no reason to believe that any trading of ions has occurred; therefore, this is an invalid double replacement reaction.

15.1.2 BALANCED EQUATIONS AND LIMITING REAGENTS

15.1.2.1 Balancing Equations

The subscript 3 in NH_3 is termed a **stoichiometric number** (see **14.1.2.1**). When we want chemicals to react with one another, stoichiometry must be considered. In this case, we cannot change the stoichiometric numbers that designate atomic ratios within molecules, so we must rely on stoichiometric coefficients. A **stoichiometric coefficient** is a determinant of the molar ratio between two or more separate molecules in a **balanced reaction**.

The mass of the reactants in a chemical equation must equal the mass of the products. We can use stoichiometric coefficients to check this mass balance. Consider the reaction of nitrogen gas (N_2) and hydrogen gas (H_2) that produces ammonia (NH_3). This reaction, when run in an industrial setting, is known as the **Haber process** and the unbalanced reaction is:

$$N_2 + H_2 \rightleftharpoons NH_3$$

We can see that this reaction is unbalanced (does not obey the law of conservation of matter) because there are two atoms of nitrogen on the left, but only one atom of nitrogen on the right. Similarly, there are two hydrogen atoms on the left, but there are three hydrogen atoms on the right. In order to balance this equation, we must ensure that there are equal numbers of nitrogen atoms on each side of the equation and equal numbers of hydrogen atoms on each side of the equation. If we consider the ratio of N_2 to NH_3, there is a ratio of two to one in nitrogen atoms. If we consider the ratio of H_2 to NH_3, there is a ratio of two to three hydrogen atoms. These two ratios indicate that in order for the atoms to balance on each side, we must invert each ratio.

$$N_2 + H_2 \rightleftharpoons NH_3$$
$$1 \qquad\qquad 2$$
$$3 \qquad 2$$

Once we have written these ratios, it is clear that since the stoichiometric coefficient prescribed for ammonia in each case is 2, we are finished balancing the equation:

$$N_2 + 3H_2 \rightleftharpoons 2NH_3$$

We can now say that if one mole of nitrogen gas is allowed to react with three moles of hydrogen gas, the product will be two moles of ammonia. It is important to remember that stoichiometric coefficients are measured in terms of moles or atoms, not grams!

Please solve this problem:

- Iron (III) hydroxide may be formed via a reaction between sodium hydroxide and iron (III) bromide. In the balanced equation, what is the ratio of $Fe(OH)_3$ to NaBr?

   A. 1:1
   B. 1:2
   C. 1:3
   D. 3:1

Problem solved:

The correct answer is C. To solve this problem, we must balance the equation:

$$FeBr_3 + NaOH \rightarrow Fe(OH)_3 + NaBr$$

In the unbalanced reaction, there is one iron on each side—iron is balanced. Next, we can balance bromine. There are three bromines on the left, but only one on the right. To balance Br, we get:

$$FeBr_3 + NaOH \rightarrow Fe(OH)_3 + 3NaBr$$

Next, we can balance sodium:

$$FeBr_3 + 3NaOH \rightarrow Fe(OH)_3 + 3NaBr$$

Checking for a balance of oxygen and hydrogen, we can see that this equation is now balanced. From the balanced equation, we can see that the ratio of $Fe(OH)_3$ to NaBr is 1:3

15.1.2.2 Limiting Reagents

Once we have a chemically balanced reaction, we need to concern ourselves with the amounts of reagents that are available to perform the desired reaction. Often, one will add an excess of one reagent relative to the other reagent(s). The reagent that is present in the smallest quantity (based on equivalents) is termed the **limiting reagent**—it limits the extent of the reaction. Consider again the Haber process. If 28 grams of nitrogen gas are allowed to react with 4 grams of hydrogen gas to produce ammonia, which is the limiting reagent?

First, convert all gram masses into moles:

$$\frac{28 \text{ g } N_2}{28 \text{ g}/\text{mole}} = 1 \text{ mole } N_2$$

$$\frac{4 \text{ g } H_2}{2 \text{ g}/\text{mole}} = 2 \text{ mole } H_2$$

Divide each molar quantity by the appropriate stoichiometric coefficient to arrive at a number of "equivalents." An **equivalent** is the amount of each substance that is needed in the balanced reaction.

$$\frac{1 \text{ mole } N_2}{1 \text{ mole}/\text{equivalent}} = 1 \text{ equivalent } N_2$$

$$\frac{2 \text{ mole } H_2}{3 \text{ mole}/\text{equivalent}} = 0.667 \text{ equivalents } H_2$$

Since there are fewer equivalents of hydrogen gas than equivalents of nitrogen, hydrogen is the limiting reagent—it will be entirely consumed first. There is an excess of 0.333 equivalents of nitrogen gas, so at the end of the reaction (when all of the hydrogen gas has been consumed), 0.333 moles (or 9.333 grams) of nitrogen gas will remain unreacted.

To calculate the amount of ammonia produced, we multiply the number of equivalents of the limiting reagent by the stoichiometric coefficient of ammonia.

$$0.667 \text{ equivalents} \times \frac{2 \text{ mole } NH_3}{\text{equivalent}} = 1.333 \text{ mole } NH_3$$

or

$$1.333 \text{ mole } NH_3 \times \frac{17 \text{ grams}}{\text{mole}} = 22.667 \text{ grams } NH_3$$

We can verify this result by checking for mass balance. We put in 28 grams of nitrogen and 4 grams of hydrogen, therefore our reagents had a mass of 32 grams. We produced 22.667 grams of ammonia and left 9.333 grams of nitrogen unreacted, therefore our post-reaction mass is also 32 grams and we have a mass balance.

Please solve this problem:

- 100 grams of calcium carbonate are allowed to react with 100 grams of sodium hydroxide in 100 grams of water to form calcium hydroxide and sodium carbonate. In this reaction, the limiting reagent is:

A. calcium carbonate.
B. sodium hydroxide.
C. water.
D. sodium.

Problem solved:

The correct answer is A. To solve this problem, first write the balanced equation:

$$CaCO_3 + 2NaOH \rightarrow Ca(OH)_2 + Na_2CO_3$$

Because water does not appear in the balanced equation, we can eliminate choice C.

Determine the number of moles of each reagent that are available for the reaction by dividing the masses in grams by their respective molecular weights:

$CaCO_3$:	100 g ÷ 100 g/mol = 1 mol
NaOH:	100 g ÷ 40 g/mol = 2.5 mol

Next, we must find the number of equivalents of each reactant that are available:

$CaCO_3$:	1 mol ÷ 1 mol/equivalent = 1 equivalent
NaOH:	2.5 mol ÷ 2 mol/equivalent = 1.25 equivalents

Since $CaCO_3$ is available in the least number of equivalents, $CaCO_3$ is the limiting reagent.

15.1.3 OXIDATION-REDUCTION REACTIONS

15.1.3.1 Oxidation Numbers

The **oxidation number** of an atom indicates the number of electrons that this atom would have either gained or lost in the formation of the molecule of which it is a part if the molecule were assumed to be entirely composed of ions. *Positive* oxidation numbers indicate a *loss* of electrons. *Negative* oxidation numbers indicate a *"gain"* of electrons. For a neutral molecule, all oxidation numbers must add up to zero. When the oxidation numbers do not add up to zero, the result is a charged molecule or a complex ion.

Most atoms have more than one possible oxidation number. For the transition metals (*d* block), oxidation numbers are easiest to determine from the oxidation numbers of the other elements to which the transition metal is bound. Fortunately, certain elements have only one oxidation number:

- All group 1 elements have an oxidation number of +1.

- All group 2 elements have an oxidation number of +2.

- All group 3 elements have an oxidation number of +3.

- Fluorine always has an oxidation number of –1.

- Oxygen almost always has an oxidation number of –2 (oxygen has a –1 oxidation state in peroxides, e.g., H_2O_2).

- Hydrogen has an oxidation number of either +1 or –1. Use this rule of thumb: +1 when bonded to non-metals, –1 when bonded to metals.

In a molecule with one of these elements, you can figure out the oxidation numbers of other atoms by summing to get zero (or the overall charge on the molecule).

Consider $K_2Cr_2O_7$. Since we know that oxygen has an oxidation number of –2 and potassium, being a group 1 element, has an oxidation number of +1, we can solve for the oxidation number of chromium:

K	2	+1	+2
O	7	–2	–14
Cr	2	__	+12 (since the sum must be zero)

The oxidation state of chromium in $K_2Cr_2O_7$ is +6.

Please solve this problem:

- What is the oxidation number of iodine in periodic acid (HIO_4)?

  A. –5
  B. –1
  C. +5
  D. +7

Problem solved:

The correct answer is D. Since we know oxygen has an oxidation number of –2 and hydrogen has an oxidation number of +1, we can solve for the oxidation number of iodine:

H	1	+1	+1
O	4	–2	–8
I	1	__	+7 (since the sum must be zero)

The oxidation state of iodine in HIO_4 is +7.

15.1.3.2 Redox Reactions

Sometimes the oxidation state of an atom changes during a reaction. When this occurs, the reaction is termed an **oxidation-reduction reaction**, or a **redox reaction**. If the oxidation number of an atom increases during a reaction, it is said to be **oxidized**. If the oxidation number of an atom decreases during the reaction, it is said to be **reduced**. An increase in oxidation number indicates a loss of electrons. A decrease in oxidation number indicates a gain of electrons. Oxidation always occurs in tandem with reduction—the total number of electrons does not change, rather, the electrons are redistributed among the participating atoms.

An atom that undergoes a loss of electrons is being **oxidized**. Because this atom must also then be causing another atom's reduction, the oxidized atom is called the **reducing agent**, or **reductant**. Conversely, an atom that undergoes a gain of electrons is being **reduced**. Since this atom is also causing another atom to be oxidized, this atom is called the **oxidizing agent**, or **oxidant**.

Consider the following redox reaction:

$$Cu(NO_3)_2(aq) + Zn(s) \rightarrow Zn(NO_3)_2(aq) + Cu(s)$$

In this reaction, we can see that copper undergoes a change in oxidation state from +2 to 0, while zinc undergoes a change in oxidation state from 0 to +2. Therefore, copper is reduced (gains electrons) and zinc is oxidized (loses electrons). For this reaction, we can write two **half reactions**:

The half reaction for the reduction of copper is:

$$Cu^{2+} + 2e^- \rightarrow Cu^0$$

and the half reaction for the oxidation of zinc is:

$$Zn^0 \rightarrow Zn^{2+} + 2e^-$$

In this case, each half reaction is a two electron transfer:

$$Cu^{2+} + Zn^0 + 2e^- \rightarrow Cu^0 + Zn^{2+} + 2e^-$$

or

$$Cu^{2+} + Zn^0 \rightarrow Cu^0 + Zn^{2+}$$

The reaction is balanced as written.

Consider the oxidation-reduction reaction between potassium dichromate and hydrogen iodide:

$$K_2Cr_2O_7 + HI \rightarrow KI + CrI_3 + I_2 + H_2O$$

In order to balance this reaction, we must first determine which atoms have been oxidized and which have been reduced. We do this by assigning oxidation numbers to each atom:

K_2	Cr_2	O_7	+	H	I	$\rightarrow$	K	I	+	Cr	I_3	+	I_2	+	H_2	O
+1	+6	−2		+1	−1		+1	−1		+3	−1		0		+1	−2

We can see that chromium is reduced from a +6 oxidation state to a +3 oxidation state, and that some of the iodine is oxidized from a −1 oxidation state to a 0 oxidation state. Therefore the two half reactions for this equation are:

$$Cr^{6+} + 3e^- \rightarrow Cr^{3+}$$

and

$$2I^{1-} \rightarrow I_2 + 2e^-$$

These two half reactions are not balanced in terms of electrons—balancing the electrons is our first step:

$$2 \times (Cr^{6+} + 3e^- \rightarrow Cr^{3+})$$

$$3 \times (2I^{-1} \rightarrow I_2 + 2e^-)$$

$$\overline{\phantom{2Cr^{6+} + 6I^{1-} + 6e^- \rightarrow 2Cr^{3+} + 3I_2 + 6e^-}}$$

$$2Cr^{6+} + 6I^{1-} + 6e^- \rightarrow 2Cr^{3+} + 3I_2 + 6e^-$$

or

$$2Cr^{6+} + 6I^{1-} \rightarrow 2Cr^{3+} + 3I_2$$

Therefore, the minimum number of chromium atoms on each side of the balanced equation is two and the minimum number of iodine atoms on each side of the balanced equation is six. Using this, we get:

$$K_2Cr_2O_7 + 6HI \rightarrow KI + 2CrI_3 + 3I_2 + H_2O$$

Balancing for potassium, this becomes:

$$K_2Cr_2O_7 + 6HI \rightarrow 2KI + 2CrI_3 + 3I_2 + H_2O$$

Balancing for oxygen, this becomes:

$$K_2Cr_2O_7 + 6HI \rightarrow 2KI + 2CrI_3 + 3I_2 + 7H_2O$$

And, finally, balancing for hydrogen, we get the completely balanced equation:

$$K_2Cr_2O_7 + 14HI \rightarrow 2KI + 2CrI_3 + 3I_2 + 7H_2O$$

Although the MCAT will not directly ask you to balance such equations (given the multiple choice nature of the test), it is definitely to your benefit to be able to balance complex redox equations.

Please solve this problem:

- The ratio of copper to nitric acid (HNO_3) in the redox reaction between these substances to form copper (II) nitrate, water, and nitric oxide:

  A. 1:4
  B. 3:8
  C. 8:3
  D. 4:1

Problem solved:

The correct answer is B. To solve this problem we must balance the reaction:

$$Cu + HNO_3 \rightarrow Cu(NO_3)_2 + H_2O + NO$$

The oxidation half reaction is:

$$Cu \rightarrow Cu^{2+} + 2e^-$$

The reduction half reaction is:

$$N^{5+} + 3e^- \rightarrow N^{2+}$$

Balancing for electrons, we get:

$$3Cu + ?HNO_3 \rightarrow 3Cu(NO_3)_2 + H_2O + 2NO$$

The question mark is inserted to show that since not all of the N^{5+} is reduced, we do not know with certainty what this stoichiometric coefficient is simply from an electron balance. In order to determine this value, we need to balance nitrogen. There are 6 + 2 = 8 nitrogens on the right, so there need to be 8 nitrogens on the left:

$$3Cu + 8HNO_3 \rightarrow 3Cu(NO_3)_2 + H_2O + 2NO$$

At this point, even though we are not finished balancing the equation, we can see that the ratio of copper to nitric acid is 3:8.

To check, we can complete the balancing, using either hydrogen or oxygen:

$$3Cu + 8HNO_3 \rightarrow 3Cu(NO_3)_2 + 4H_2O + 2NO$$

15.1.4 REACTION KINETICS: RATE, RATE LAWS, AND CATALYSIS

15.1.4.1 Kinetics: The Study of Reaction Rates

Kinetics is the study of the rates of chemical reactions. The field of kinetics focuses on both the speed at which a reaction occurs and the mechanism by which it occurs.

The amounts of products formed, or the equilibrium amounts of products and reactants (Chapter 18), are not accounted for by kinetics. The thermodynamics of an overall reaction (Chapter 17) also have no bearing on the rate of reaction. Likewise, the stoichiometry of the balanced equation of the reaction is irrelevant to kinetics.

15.1.4.2 Reaction Mechanisms

A chemical reaction involves the breaking of existing chemical bonds and the formation of new chemical bonds. Breaking a chemical bond requires the input of energy, while the formation of a chemical bond involves the release of energy. Many different factors contribute to the strength of a chemical bond (Chapter 14). The breaking or making of bonds may be accomplished in a variety of ways; this results in many different reaction paths from reactants to products. A **reaction mechanism** is the pathway by which reactants are converted to products. Each reaction has available to it a number of different mechanistic pathways. Each mechanism will have different steps, different rates, and different combinations of possible products. The particular mechanism that prevails, or predominates (since often a reaction will proceed simultaneously along competitive pathways) depends on the conditions of the reactions. The reaction conditions include concentrations, pressure, temperature, and the absence or presence of a catalyst.

Each mechanism is comprised of a series of steps. These steps are called **elementary processes**. Consider the overall reaction:

$$2AB + C \rightleftharpoons A_2C + B_2$$

One possible mechanism for this reaction is:

Step 1:	$AB \rightarrow A + B$
Step 2:	$A + C \rightarrow AC$
Step 3:	$AC + A \rightarrow A_2C$
Step 4:	$B + B \rightarrow B_2$

Another possible mechanism for this reaction is:

Step 1:	$AB + C \rightleftharpoons ABC$
Step 2:	$ABC \rightleftharpoons AC + B$
Step 3:	$AB \rightarrow A + B$
Step 4:	$AC + A \rightarrow A_2C$
Step 5:	$B + B \rightarrow B_2$

Elementary processes are distinguished by the number of reactant molecules involved in that particular step. A step involving only one reactant molecule, such as step 1 in the first mechanism or step 2 or 3 in the second mechanism above, is called a **unimolecular process**. A step involving two reactant molecules, such as step 2, 3, or 4 in the first mechanism or step 1, 4, or 5 in the second mechanism above, is called a **bimolecular process**. Elementary processes involving more than two reactant molecules are rare: therefore, most mechanistic steps are either unimolecular or bimolecular.

For each elementary process, or step, in a mechanism there is an energy barrier that must be overcome in order for that step to proceed. This energy barrier is termed the **activation energy** for that step. The higher the activation energy of a step the less likely that step is to occur and, therefore, the slower that step will be. For any mechanism, the step with the highest activation energy is the slowest step. The slowest step in a series of steps will limit the overall progression from reactants to products, so this step is termed the **rate-determining step**. Because steps are dependent on reaction conditions, the rate-determining step under a given set of reaction conditions may change as reaction conditions change.

Another important feature of elementary processes is **microscopic reversibility**. While an overall chemical reaction may not be considered to be reversible, given the order and combination of mechanistic steps, *all* elementary processes are reversible. The reversibility of elementary processes is termed the principle of microscopic reversibility. This principle states that for every forward process, the reverse process also occurs in *exactly* the reverse manner.

If $AB \rightarrow A + B$

then $A + B \rightarrow AB$ by reversing the path.

During the elementary processes of a mechanism, products may be formed and later consumed. An example of this is product ABC of step 1 of the second mechanism above. Such a substance is termed an **intermediate**. An intermediate is an isolable (or at least detectable) substance that is neither reactant nor product and that is formed and then consumed within a mechanistic pathway. The detection of such intermediates is often crucial in determining the mechanism of a reaction.

An intermediate should not be confused with a **transition state**. The latter is a high-energy species found at the peak of the reaction curve. Intermediates are found in the troughs of reaction curves. This is discussed in greater detail when reaction diagrams are presented in **17.1.2.**

Please solve this problem:

- All the following affect reaction kinetics EXCEPT:

    A. catalysts.
    B. temperature.
    C. microscopic reversibility.
    D. stoichiometry.

Problem solved:

The correct answer is D. Kinetics is *not* concerned with the stoichiometry of the reaction under investigation. Kinetics is affected by catalysts and other reaction conditions such as temperature and pressure. Kinetics is concerned with the mechanism of reactions. Mechanisms of reactions are comprised of steps, or elementary processes. All elementary processes are reversible.

15.1.4.3 Reaction Rates

The rate of a chemical reaction is the answer to the question "How much does this reaction move from reactants to products in a given amount of time?" We can express this quantity either as the amount of product formed in a given amount of time or as the amount of reactant consumed in a given amount of time.

Consider the general reaction:

$$aA + bB \rightarrow cC + dD$$

The rate at which the reaction proceeds can be measured as the rate at which reactant A or reactant B is consumed, or as the rate at which reactant C or reactant D is formed:

$$\text{Rate of Reaction} = \frac{-\Delta[A]}{a\Delta t} = \frac{-\Delta[B]}{b\Delta t} = \frac{\Delta[C]}{c\Delta t} = \frac{\Delta[D]}{d\Delta t}$$

To see this more clearly (especially when stoichiometry applies to the rate expression), consider the following example:

$$N_2O_4(g) \rightarrow 2NO_2(g)$$

The rate of this reaction is given by:

$$\text{Rate of Reaction} = \frac{-\Delta[N_2O_4]}{\Delta t} = \frac{\Delta[NO_2]}{2\Delta t}$$

We can see that for every one mole of N_2O_4 consumed, two moles of NO_2 are produced.

Please solve this problem:

- The rate of the reaction $2NO(g) + O_2(g) \rightarrow 2NO_2(g)$
  is given by:

  A. $\dfrac{\Delta[NO]}{2\Delta t}$

  B. $\dfrac{\Delta[O_2]}{\Delta t}$

  C. $\dfrac{\Delta[NO_2]}{2\Delta t}$

  D. $\dfrac{\Delta[N_2]}{\Delta t}$

Problem solved:

The correct answer is C. The rate of reaction is given by either the rate of disappearance of reactants in a given time, or the rate of formation of products in a given time. Choices A and B would be rate of reaction expressions for the reverse reaction. Choice D is nonsense.

15.1.4.4 The Effect of Concentration: The Rate Law

Concentration has a marked effect on the rate of reaction. In general, a reaction will slow down as time passes because reactants are being consumed. As the concentration of reactants decreases, there are fewer collisions between reactant molecules.

The quantitative implication of reaction rate decreasing as concentration of reactants decreases is that rate is proportional to reactant concentration. Considering the general reaction:

$$aA + bB \rightarrow cC + dD$$

the **rate law** is given by:

$$\text{Rate} = k[A]^x[B]^y$$

where $[A]$ and $[B]$ are the concentrations of A and B respectively. The value of x is the *order of the reaction with respect to A* and the value of y is the *order of the reaction with respect to B*. The **overall order** of this reaction is given by the sum of x and y. The values of x and y must be experimentally determined.

The values of x and y bear *no* relationship to the stoichiometric numbers a and b!

For instance, it has been experimentally determined that the rate law expression for:

$$3NO(g) \rightarrow N_2O(g) + NO_2(g)$$

is given by:

$$\text{Rate} = k[NO]^2$$

The final quantity in the above general rate law expression, k, is the **specific rate constant** (or sometimes just the **rate constant**) for the reaction at a particular temperature. Note that if the temperature of the reaction is changed, a new k must be calculated. The following are the important points to remember about rate constant, k:

- The value of k is unique to each reaction at a given temperature.

- The value of k will change if the temperature is changed.

- The value of k does *not* change with time.

- The value of k is not dependent on the concentrations of either reactants or products.

- The value of k *must* be determined experimentally.

- The units of k depend on the overall order of the reaction.

Since k must be determined experimentally, a common method for doing so is the **method of initial rates**. As stated above, k does not change with time, therefore the value of k found from the initial concentration conditions will hold at any later time during the course of the reaction.

Please solve this problem:

- All of the following factors do not affect the specific rate constant, k, EXCEPT:

    A. temperature.
    B. time.
    C. initial concentration of reactants.
    D. volume of reaction system.

Problem solved:

The correct answer is A. Be careful of the double negative questions on the MCAT. You should rephrase this question: "Which of the following affects k?" Then, the answer is clearly "temperature."

15.1.4.5 The Effect of Temperature: The Arrhenius Equation

A change in the temperature of a reaction will lead to a change in the value of the rate constant, k. The average kinetic energy of the molecules in a reaction system is proportional to the temperature (in Kelvin) of the system (Chapter 20). This is because kinetic energy provides the movement for collisions to occur. It is also necessary to provide sufficient energy during the collision such that the activation energy for the reaction, or reaction step, is available for reaction.

From experimental evidence, Svante Arrhenius was able to develop the mathematical relationship between activation energy, absolute temperature (Kelvin), and the rate constant at that temperature. The result is the **Arrhenius equation**:

$$k = Ae^{-\frac{E_a}{RT}}$$

which, in terms of log, base ten, may be written:

$$\log k = \log A - \frac{E_a}{2.303\,RT}$$

This equation is used to determine the rate constant, k_2, at a temperature, T_2, when the rate constant, k_1, is known at temperature T_1. In this case, the Arrhenius equation becomes:

$$\log \frac{k_2}{k_1} = \frac{E_a}{2.303\,R}\left(\frac{T_2 - T_1}{T_1 T_2}\right)$$

If you are expected to use the Arrhenius equation on the MCAT, it will be provided. The important points to remember here are that the rate constant of a reaction is different for different temperatures, and the magnitude of the change in the rate constant is directly proportional to the activation energy of the reaction—the larger the activation energy, the greater the change in rate constant for the same temperature change.

Please solve this problem:

- As temperature is increased:

  A. k increases for all reactions.
  B. k increases for some reactions.
  C. k decreases for some reactions.
  D. k decreases for all reactions.

Problem solved:

The correct answer is A. Given the Arrhenius equation:

$$\log \frac{k_2}{k_1} = \frac{E_a}{2.303\,R}\left(\frac{T_2 - T_1}{T_1 T_2}\right)$$

because temperature is measured in Kelvin, the temperature term must always be positive when temperature increases ($T_2 > T_1$). By definition, activation energy, E_a, is always positive, as is the gas constant, R. Therefore, for increasing temperature, the right side of the Arrhenius equation is always positive. We can now reduce the Arrhenius equation to:

$$\log K = P$$

where $K = k_2/k_1$, and P is meant to designate the positive value of the right side of the equation. Solving for K:

$$K = 10^P$$

By definition, 10^P is always greater than 1. Therefore, K must always be greater than 1, implying that the numerator (k_2) must always be greater than the denominator (k_1).

15.1.4.6 The Effect of Catalysts

Catalysts are substances that are added to reaction systems either to *increase or decrease* the rate of reaction. While catalysts are usually thought of as speeding a reaction, it *must* be recognized that a catalyst may also *slow* a reaction. A catalyst that's used to slow down a reaction is called an **inhibitory catalyst**, or **inhibitor**. The following discussion will focus on catalysts that speed up reactions. You should be aware that an inhibitor will have the reverse effect on a reaction.

A catalyst that increases the rate of reaction acts by allowing the reaction to occur via an alternative pathway. This alternative pathway serves to lower the overall activation energy of the reaction system. Although a catalyst may react with reactants or intermediates along the path of the reaction, it does not appear in the balanced equation for the reaction. If a catalyst does react with a reactant or intermediate, it is regenerated in subsequent steps. If what might appear at first to be a catalyst is not regenerated, it is not a catalyst, it's a reactant.

- A catalyst is neither consumed nor produced during the course of a reaction.

Catalysts may be classified into two categories: **homogeneous catalysts** and **heterogeneous catalysts**. A homogeneous catalyst exists in the same phase as the reactants. An example of a homogeneous catalyst is an acid or a base added catalytically to an organic reaction. **Enzymes** are proteins that act as homogeneous catalysts for specific biochemical reactions.

A heterogeneous, or **contact catalyst,** exists in a different phase than the reactants. Heterogeneous catalysts are usually solids that operate by supplying a surface upon which the reaction may occur. An example of a contact catalyst is "poisoned palladium" (palladium with added graphite) which is often used as a hydrogenation catalyst in organic chemistry.

The most important thing to remember about catalysts is that they operate by altering the activation energy of a reaction. Catalysts have no effect on the equilibrium concentrations of reactants and products (Chapter 18).

Please solve this problem:

- A catalyst does NOT:

    A. affect the mechanism of a reaction.
    B. affect the activation energy of a reaction.
    C. affect the concentration of products at equilibrium.
    D. affect the elementary processes of a reaction.

Problem solved:

The correct answer is C. Catalysts operate by altering the activation energy of a reaction. This alteration in activation energy is achieved by providing an alternative mechanism—via altered elementary processes. Catalysts do not affect equilibrium.

15.2 MASTERY APPLIED: SAMPLE PASSAGE AND QUESTIONS

Passage

The rate of chemical reactions involving gas phase reactants, gas phase products, or both gas phase reactants and gas phase products is easily measured by a change in pressure as the reaction proceeds.

In a reaction involving gas phase reactants, the partial pressures of the reactant gases were varied while the initial reaction rate was recorded. The results for this reaction at 1099°C are tabulated in Table 1. The stoichiometry of this reaction is:

$$2AB(g) + 2C(g) \rightarrow A_2(g) + 2BC(g)$$

Trial #	P_C (torr)	P_{AB} (torr)	Initial Rate (torr/s)
1	200	400	0.160
2	300	400	0.240
3	400	400	0.320
4	400	200	0.040
5	400	300	0.135

Table 1

1. What is the rate law for this reaction?
   A. Rate = $k[AB]^3[C]$
   B. Rate = $k[AB]^2[C]^2$
   C. Rate = $k[AB]^2[C]$
   D. Rate = $k[AB]^3$

2. What is the rate constant, k, in $s^{-1}torr^{-3}$, for this reaction?
   A. 1.25×10^{11}
   B. 5.00×10^3
   C. 2.32×10^{-4}
   D. 1.25×10^{-11}

3. If the total pressure in the container were increased by reducing the volume, the rate of the reaction would:
   A. increase.
   B. decrease.
   C. remain the same.
   D. not be predictable.

4. If the total pressure in the container were increased by adding a nonreactive gas, the rate of the forward reaction would:
   A. increase.
   B. decrease.
   C. remain the same.
   D. not be predictable.

5. If a sixth trial of the reaction is conducted with $P_{AB} = 500$ torr and $P_C = 100$ torr, the initial rate is expected to be:
   A. 0.006 torr/s
   B. 0.062 torr/s
   C. 0.156 torr/s
   D. 0.625 torr/s

6. If an inhibitory catalyst were added to the reaction system:
   A. the equilibrium concentration of $A_2(g)$ would increase.
   B. the equilibrium concentration of $A_2(g)$ would decrease.
   C. the activation energy would increase.
   D. the activation energy would decrease.

15.3 MASTERY VERIFIED: ANSWERS AND EXPLANATIONS

1. *The correct answer is A.* Comparing trial 1 to trial 3, we can see that when P_C is doubled and P_{AB} is held constant, the rate is doubled. Therefore, we can say,

$$\text{rate} \propto P_C \text{ and } P_C \propto [C], \text{ therefore rate} \propto [C]$$

Comparing trial 4 to trial 3, we can see that when P_{AB} is doubled and P_C is held constant, the rate is increased by a factor of 8 (2^3). Therefore, we can say,

$$\text{rate} \propto P_{AB}^3 \propto [AB]^3$$

The rate law says that:

$$\text{rate} = k[AB]^3[C]$$

2. *The correct answer is D.* To solve this problem, we can use our answer from question 1 and plug in numbers for [AB] and [C] from any of the five trials. Using trial 1:

$$\text{rate} = 0.160 = k[400]^3[200] = k(1.28 \times 10^{10})$$

$$\text{Therefore, } k = 0.160 \div (1.28 \times 10^{10}) = 1.25 \times 10^{-11}$$

3. *The correct answer is A.* If the total pressure of the container is increased by decreasing the volume, the frequency of collisions between reactant molecules will increase. The more often the reactant molecules collide, the more likely they are to collide in the proper orientation for a successful reaction. Therefore, as pressure is increased, the rate of the reaction is also increased.

4. *The correct answer is C.* Adding a nonreactive gas would not change the partial pressures of the reacting gases and would not affect the rate of reaction.

5. *The correct answer is C.* Using the rate law derived from question 1 and the rate constant obtained from question 2:

$$\text{rate} = (1.25 \times 10^{-11})[500]^3[100] = 0.156$$

6. *The correct answer is C.* A catalyst acts by affecting the activation energy of a reaction. An inhibitory catalyst increases the activation energy of a reaction by forcing the reaction to take a mechanistic pathway that is less energetically favorable than the pathway available in the absence of the catalyst. Catalysts do *not* affect equilibrium concentrations of reactants or products.

CHAPTER 16

CHEMICAL REACTIONS II: EQUILIBRIUM DYNAMICS

16.1 MASTERY ACHIEVED

16.1.1 EQUILIBRIUM

When appropriate reactants are placed together, they react to form products. The reactants must collide with each other in the correct orientation and with sufficient energy to break old bonds and to form new bonds. Once products are formed, they too can collide with one another in the correct orientation and with sufficient energy to reform the reactant molecules.

As a reaction progresses, a time is reached at which the rate of formation of products from reactants is equal to the rate of formation of reactants from products. From this time forward, in the absence of outside influence, there is no net change in the concentrations of products relative to the concentrations of reactants. The reaction system is not static: reactants are still forming products, and products are still re-forming reactants. It is the *ratio* of products to reactants that is static. This state is called **chemical equilibrium**.

Depending on the starting conditions of the reaction system or the activities performed upon it prior to equilibrium, the absolute concentrations of reactants and products may vary while the relative concentrations—expressed as the ratio of products to reactants—remain constant.

To summarize the equilibrium condition:

- Equilibrium is a *dynamic condition*—forward and reverse reactions occur simultaneously and at the same rate.

- Equilibrium is *independent of the path taken to reach equilibrium*—the ratio of products to reactants will not change as long as temperature and, in some cases, pressure and volume do not change.

Please solve this problem:

- Equilibrium is:

    A. a static condition in which the concentration of the reactants is equal to the concentration of the products.
    B. a dynamic condition in which the concentration of the reactants is equal to the concentration of the products.
    C. a static condition in which the rate of formation of the reactants is equal to the rate of formation of the products.
    D. a dynamic condition in which the rate of formation of the reactants is equal to the rate of formation of the products.

Problem solved:

The correct answer is D. This is the definition of chemical equilibrium.

16.1.2 EQUILIBRIUM CONSTANTS

16.1.2.1 The Equilibrium Constants (K_{eq}, K_c, K_p)

The equilibrium constant, K_{eq}, is the ratio of product concentrations to reactant concentrations that exists at equilibrium. For the general reaction:

$$aA + bB \rightarrow cC + dD$$

the equilibrium constant is given by:

$$K_{eq} = \frac{[C]^c [D]^d}{[A]^a [B]^b}$$

The concentrations are the equilibrium concentrations (not the initial concentrations), and they are usually measured in molarity (M). Pure liquids and pure solids do not appear in the equilibrium equation; these are assumed to have a concentration of 1 M. If all reactants and products are gases, the partial pressures of the gases can be used in place of molarity. When this is done, however, the value of K_{eq} is different from the value of K_{eq} that would have been calculated using molar concentrations. The relationship between these two quantities is:

$$K_p = K_c (RT)^{\Delta n}$$

where K_p is the equilibrium constant calculated from the partial pressures (in atm), K_c is the equilibrium constant calculated from the molar concentrations, R is the gas constant (0.082 L•atm/mol•K), T is the absolute temperature, and Δn is the change in the total number of moles of gas from the reactants to the products.

All K_{eq}'s on the MCAT are K_c's, unless otherwise noted.

The magnitude of K_{eq} is independent of the amounts of reactants and products, but it is *not independent* of changes in temperature and, in some cases, pressure or volume. A change in one of these factors does not *necessarily* correspond to the change in K_{eq}. For example, some reactions will have a *decrease* in K_{eq} with an *increase* in temperature.

The value of the equilibrium constant tells us the relative amounts of reactants and products. If K_{eq} is much larger than 1, then the ratio of product concentrations to reactant concentrations is high. If K_{eq} is close to 1, the relative concentrations of products and of reactants are similar, and, if K_{eq} is much smaller than 1, then the ratio of product to reactant concentrations is low.

In summary:

- If $K_{eq} \gg 1$, then products are favored over reactants

- If $K_{eq} \approx 1$, then neither reactants nor products is favored

- If $K_{eq} \ll 1$, then reactants are favored over products

Please solve this problem:

- Consider the following unbalanced reaction: $CuSO_4 + Fe_2O_3 \rightleftharpoons CuO + Fe_2(SO_4)_3$. The equilibrium concentrations are: $[CuSO_4] = 1.2\ M$, $[Fe_2O_3] = 0.4\ M$, $[CuO] = 1.5\ M$, and $[Fe_2(SO_4)_3] = 0.5\ M$. The resulting equilibrium:

 A. favors reactants.
 B. favors products.
 C. favors neither reactants nor products.
 D. cannot be determined from the information given.

Problem solved:

The correct answer is B. To solve this problem, we must first balance the equation:

$$3\,CuSO_4 + Fe_2O_3 \rightleftharpoons 3\,CuO + Fe_2(SO_4)_3$$

We then see that the equilibrium constant is given by:

$$K_{eq} = \frac{[CuO]^3[Fe_2(SO_4)_3]^1}{[CuSO_4]^3[Fe_2O_3]^1} = \frac{[1.5]^3[0.5]^1}{[1.2]^3[0.4]^1} = \text{approx. } 2.44$$

Since this value is greater than 1, the equilibrium favors products.

16.1.2.2 The Reaction Quotient

The reaction quotient, Q, is related to the equilibrium constant, K_{eq}. While K_{eq} gives the ratio of products to reactants at equilibrium, the reaction quotient gives the same ratio at all times other than at equilibrium. The reaction quotient at equilibrium is K_{eq}. If the equation for the reaction is:

$$aA + bB \rightleftharpoons cC + dD$$

The equation for the reaction quotient is:

$$Q = \frac{(C)^c (D)^d}{(A)^a (B)^b}$$

Parentheses are used instead of brackets to designate concentrations other than equilibrium concentrations.

The reaction quotient can be calculated for any concentrations of reactants and products. The relationship between Q and K_{eq} is described in Table 16.1:

Relationship	Interpretation	Change as Reaction Approaches Equilibrium
$Q > K_{eq}$	Products in excess	Decrease in products, increase in reactants
$Q = K_{eq}$	At equilibrium	No change
$Q < K_{eq}$	Reactants in excess	Decrease in reactants, increase in products

Table 16.1

Please solve this problem:

- At high temperatures, $K_{eq} = 1 \times 10^{-13}$ for: $2\,HF\,(g) \rightleftharpoons H_2\,(g) + F_2\,(g)$. At a certain time, the following concentrations were detected: $[HF] = 0.5\,M$, $[H_2] = 1 \times 10^{-6}\,M$, $[F_2] = 1 \times 10^{-4}\,M$. In order to reach equilibrium:

  A. HF must react to form more hydrogen and fluorine gases.
  B. hydrogen and fluorine gases must react to produce more HF.
  C. nothing needs to happen—the reaction is at equilibrium.
  D. the temperature of the reaction should be lowered.

Problem solved:

The correct answer is B. To solve this problem, we must first determine Q.

$$Q = \frac{(H_2)(F_2)}{(HF)^2} = \frac{\left(1 \times 10^{-6}\right)^1 \left(1 \times 10^{-4}\right)}{(0.5)^2} = \frac{1 \times 10^{-10}}{0.25} = 4 \times 10^{-10}$$

Since we were told that $K_{eq} = 1 \times 10^{-13}$, we know that $Q > K_{eq}$. When this is the case, the products are in excess. Therefore, to reach equilibrium, H_2 and F_2 need to react to form HF.

16.1.2.3 Modifications in the Equilibrium Constant

The equilibrium constant of a chemical reaction system is affected by changes in the chemical equation.

For the general reaction:

$$aA + bB \rightarrow cC + dD$$

the equilibrium constant is given by:

$$K_{eq} = \frac{[C]^c [D]^d}{[A]^a [B]^b}$$

For the reaction:

$$cC + dD \rightarrow aA + bB$$

$$K_{eq}' = 1/K_{eq}$$

The equilibrium constant of a multistep reaction may be determined from the equilibrium constants of the individual steps. Consider the following two-step reaction:

$$aA + bB \rightarrow cC + dD \qquad K_{eq} = K_1$$

$$cC + dD \rightarrow eE + fF \qquad K_{eq} = K_2$$

The equilibrium constant of the reaction:

$$aA + bB \rightarrow eE + fF$$

is given by:

$$K_{eq}'' = K_1 K_2$$

Please solve this problem:

- The equilibria $H_2SO_4 \rightleftharpoons H^+ + HSO_4^-$ and $HSO_4^- \rightleftharpoons H^+ + SO_4^{-2}$ have equilibrium constants of 2.4×10^2 and 5.0×10^{-5}, respectively. The equilibrium constant for H_2SO_4 is:

  A. 5.0×10^{-5}
  B. 1.2×10^{-2}
  C. 2.4×10^2
  D. 4.8×10^6

Problem solved:

The correct answer is B. The equilibrium constant of a two-step reaction is equal to the product of the equilibrium constants of each step:

$$K_{eq} = K_1 K_2 = (2.4 \times 10^2)(5.0 \times 10^{-5}) = 1.2 \times 10^{-2}$$

16.1.3 LE CHATELIER'S PRINCIPLE

16.1.3.1 Basic Le Châtelier

Once a reaction is at equilibrium, a variety of factors may cause a shift away from equilibrium. Addition or removal of either a reactant or a product will affect the concentration of that substance, but it will not affect the value of K_{eq}. Therefore, when a product or reactant is added or removed, the system will seek ways in which to reestablish the equilibrium condition. The tendency of a system to return to a condition of chemical equilibrium is **Le Châtelier's principle**. A statement of Le Châtelier's principle is:

- When a system at equilibrium is subjected to a stress, the equilibrium will shift in a direction that tends to alleviate the effect of that stress.

Consider the general reaction:

$$A + B \rightleftharpoons C + D$$

which is originally at equilibrium.

The addition of more A to the system will have the effect of producing more C and more D. Therefore, the addition of A will also have the effect of reducing the equilibrium concentration of B, since C and D are made from both A and B:

$$A + [A + B \rightleftharpoons C + D]$$

leads to:

$$\uparrow A + \downarrow B \rightleftharpoons \uparrow C + \uparrow D$$

Likewise, an increase in the concentration of B would have a similar result:

$$\downarrow A + \uparrow B \rightleftharpoons \uparrow C + \uparrow D$$

Addition of more A and more B has the effect of driving the equilibrium to the right:

$$\uparrow A + \uparrow B \rightleftharpoons \uparrow\uparrow C + \uparrow\uparrow D$$

Addition of more C to the system increases production of A and B. Therefore, the addition of C will also have the effect of reducing the equilibrium concentration of D, since A and B are made from both C and D:

$$C + [A + B \rightleftharpoons C + D]$$

leads to:

$$\uparrow A + \uparrow B \rightleftharpoons \uparrow C + \downarrow D$$

Increasing the concentration of D will have a similar result:

$$\uparrow A + \uparrow B \rightleftharpoons \downarrow C + \uparrow D$$

Adding more C and more D has the effect of driving the equilibrium to the left:

$$\uparrow\uparrow A + \uparrow\uparrow B \rightleftharpoons \uparrow C + \uparrow D$$

The above scenarios all consider the addition of a substance to the reaction system. The scenarios work in exactly the opposite fashion when a substance is removed from the system.

Remove A: $\downarrow A + \uparrow B \rightleftharpoons \downarrow C + \downarrow D$

Remove B: $\uparrow A + \downarrow B \rightleftharpoons \downarrow C + \downarrow D$

Remove A and B: $\downarrow A + \downarrow B \rightleftharpoons \downarrow\downarrow C + \downarrow\downarrow D$

Remove C: $\downarrow A + \downarrow B \rightleftharpoons \downarrow C + \uparrow D$

Remove D: $\downarrow A + \downarrow B \rightleftharpoons \uparrow C + \downarrow D$

Remove C and D: $\downarrow\downarrow A + \downarrow\downarrow B \rightleftharpoons \downarrow C + \downarrow D$

Please solve this problem:

- In the aldol cycloaddition reaction of isobutyraldehyde with methyl vinyl ketone to form 4,4-dimethyl-2-cyclohexen-1-one and water, water is removed using a Dean-Stark trap to:

    A. decrease the yield of 4,4-dimethyl-2-cyclohexen-1-one.
    B. increase the yield of 4,4-dimethyl-2-cyclohexen-1-one.
    C. increase the yield of isobutyraldehyde.
    D. increase the yield of methyl vinyl ketone.

Problem solved:

The correct answer is B. In order to answer this problem, one need only understand simple applications of Le Chatelier's principle. It is unimportant to this problem that you understand any of the chemistry involved—although this is not always the case.

16.1.3.2 Recognizing the Effect of a Change in pH

For an aqueous solution, an increase in pH means a lowering of H^+ concentration and a raising of OH^- concentration. A decrease in the pH of an aqueous solution means a higher H^+ concentration and a lower OH^- concentration.

Consider the general acid dissociation reaction:

$$HA \rightleftharpoons H^+ + A^-$$

The effect of increasing the H^+ concentration within this system is to lower the pH:

$$\uparrow HA \rightleftharpoons \uparrow H^+ + \downarrow A^-$$

The effect of decreasing the H^+ concentration within this system is to raise the pH:

$$\downarrow HA \rightleftharpoons \downarrow H^+ + \uparrow A^-$$

Please solve this problem:

- The equilibrium constant of the reaction CH_3CO_2H $\rightleftharpoons H^+ + CH_3CO_2^-$ is 1.76×10^{-5}. NaOH is added until a pH of 10 is achieved. The equilibrium concentration of $CH_3CO_2^-$ has:

    A. increased.
    B. remained unchanged.
    C. decreased.
    D. the effect of the addition of NaOH is impossible to predict from the given information.

Problem solved:

The correct answer is A. A change to pH = 10 is an increase in pH. (This is discussed in detail in Chapter 21.) Regardless of what reactant is added, if the pH of the solution increases, the H^+ concentration decreases. Using Le Châtelier's principle, if $[H^+]$ decreases, $[CH_3CO_2H]$ must also decrease and $[CH_3CO_2^-]$ must increase.

16.1.4 EFFECTS OF PRESSURE, VOLUME, AND TEMPERATURE ON EQUILIBRIUM

16.1.4.1 Effects of Pressure and Volume

For a gaseous mixture at equilibrium, the overall pressure within a container can be changed by either adding more gas to the container or by decreasing the volume of the container.

The effects of adding a gas that is already a reactant or product in the reaction can be predicted by simply following Le Châtelier's principle as described in 16.1.3.1. However, if the gas added to the mixture is a nonreactive gas then the pressure will increase without changing the equilibrium concentrations. Since the equilibrium state can be represented by partial pressures of the products over the reactants, and the addition of a nonreactive gas does not change the partial pressures of either the products or the reactants, the equilibrium is unaffected.

To predict changes in equilibrium resulting from pressure changes due to change in volume, Le Châtelier's principle can be used as follows:

- If volume is decreased then pressure is increased. The reaction will be pushed in the direction resulting in lower moles of gas.

- If volume is increased then pressure is decreased and the reaction will shift in the direction with more moles of gas.

So when using Le Châtelier's principle to predict changes in equilibrium that result from change in pressure due to change in volume, pressure can be thought of as a variable on the side of the balanced reaction equation with the greater number of gaseous molecules.

If both sides contain equal number of gaseous moles, then there is no change in equilibrium when pressure is charged.

Please solve this problem:

- The **Haber process** is the industrial method for the production of ammonia: $3\,H_2(g) + N_2(g) \rightarrow 2\,NH_3(g)$. If the pressure in a vessel containing hydrogen gas and nitrogen gas is increased, how is the Haber process affected?

  A. It is favored.
  B. It is disfavored.
  C. It is unaffected.
  D. It is impossible to tell from the information given.

Problem solved:

The correct answer is A. To solve this problem, we must first determine the total number of moles of gas on both the reactant side and the product side of this reaction. Since the number of moles of gas on the reactant side is 4, and the number of moles of gas on the product side is 2, pressure moves the reaction to the right to compensate.

16.1.4.2 Effects of Temperature

The effects of temperature on the equilibrium of a system are more complicated than the effects of pressure. To determine the effects of temperature, one must first determine whether a reaction is endothermic or exothermic. These terms are discussed in greater detail in Chapter 17. For now, it is sufficient to define an endothermic reaction as a reaction that *consumes* heat and an exothermic reaction as a reaction that *gives off* heat. Stating this in Le Châtelier terms:

- An endothermic reaction requires heat as a reactant.

- An exothermic reaction produces heat as a product.

16.1.4.2.1 EFFECTS OF TEMPERATURE ON AN ENDOTHERMIC REACTION

Consider the following equilibrium, where the forward reaction is endothermic:

$$J + K \rightleftharpoons L + M$$

Because the forward reaction is endothermic, this equilibrium can be rewritten as:

$$J + K + heat \rightleftharpoons L + M$$

If the temperature of this system is raised, products are favored:

$$\downarrow J + \downarrow K + \uparrow heat \rightleftharpoons \uparrow L + \uparrow M$$

Likewise, if the temperature of this system is lowered, reactants are favored:

$$\uparrow J + \uparrow K + \downarrow heat \rightleftharpoons \downarrow L + \downarrow M$$

Please solve this problem:

- The production of hydrogen and oxygen gases from water is an example of an endothermic reaction. As the temperature of this reaction is increased:

  A. more water is formed.
  B. less hydrogen gas is produced.
  C. more hydrogen gas is produced.
  D. the equilibrium is unaffected.

Problem solved:

The correct answer is C. If the temperature of an endothermic forward reaction is raised, products are favored.

16.1.4.2.2 Effects of Temperature on an Exothermic Reaction

Consider the following equilibrium, where the forward reaction is exothermic:

$$R + S \rightleftharpoons U + V$$

We can rewrite this equilibrium as:

$$R + S \rightleftharpoons U + V + heat$$

If the temperature of this system is raised, reactants are favored:

$$\uparrow R + \uparrow S \rightleftharpoons \downarrow U + \downarrow V + \uparrow heat$$

If the temperature of this system is lowered, products are favored:

$$\downarrow R + \downarrow S \rightleftharpoons \uparrow U + \uparrow V + \downarrow heat$$

Please solve this problem:

- The formation of ATP from ADP and inorganic phosphate is an endothermic reaction: $ADP(aq) + P_i(aq) + H^+(aq) \rightarrow ATP(aq) + H_2O(l)$. As body temperature increases, ADP production from ATP:

  A. decreases.
  B. increases.
  C. remains constant.
  D. cannot be determined from the information provided.

Problem solved:

The correct answer is A. To solve this problem, we must recognize that the equilibrium, given the endothermic nature of the forward reaction, may be written:

$$ADP(aq) + P_i(aq) + H^+(aq) + heat \rightleftharpoons ATP(aq) + H_2O(l)$$

Therefore, if the temperature is increased,

$$\downarrow ADP(aq) + \downarrow P_i(aq) + \downarrow H^+(aq) + \uparrow heat \rightleftharpoons \uparrow ATP(aq) + \uparrow H_2O(l)$$

16.2 MASTERY APPLIED: SAMPLE PASSAGE AND QUESTIONS

Passage

The equilibrium constant for the dissolution of one substance into another substance, typically water, is termed the *solubility product constant* and is designated K_{sp}. Since pure solids do not appear in equilibrium expressions, K_{sp} has no denominator. For the dissociation:

$$A_aB_b \rightleftharpoons aA^+ + bB^-$$

the solubility product constant is given by:

$$K_{sp} = [A^+]^a[B^-]^b$$

The solubility of a material is given by its equilibrium concentration in solution. The solubility of A_aB_b can therefore be determined from K_{sp}.

The solubility product constants for selected materials are given in Table 1.

Compound	K_{sp} (at 25°C)
CdS	1.0×10^{-28}
AgI	1.5×10^{-16}
Al(OH)$_3$	2.0×10^{-32}
CuI	5.1×10^{-12}
AgCl	1.6×10^{-10}
BaSO$_4$	1.5×10^{-9}
CaCO$_3$	8.7×10^{-9}
BaCO$_3$	1.6×10^{-9}
PbSO$_4$	1.3×10^{-8}
CaSO$_4$	6.1×10^{-5}
CuSO$_4$	1.9×10^{0}

Table 1

1. Which of the following is the most soluble compound?
   A. PbSO$_4$
   B. CaCO$_3$
   C. CdS
   D. AgCl

2. The solubility of BaSO$_4$ is:
   A. 7.5×10^{-10}
   B. 1.5×10^{-9}
   C. 7.7×10^{-5}
   D. 3.9×10^{-5}

3. The chelator EDTA is sometimes used to treat cases of lead poisoning. EDTA forms a soluble complex with lead(II) which is excreted in the urine:

   $$Pb\text{-}EDTA^{2-} \rightleftharpoons Pb^{2+} + EDTA^{4-}$$

   The equilibrium constant for this reaction is 5.0×10^{-19}. What is the blood concentration of Pb^{2+} after EDTA treatment if $[Pb\text{-}EDTA^{2-}] = 2.0 \times 10^{-4}\ M$ and $[EDTA^{4-}] = 2.5 \times 10^{-2}\ M$?
   A. 4.0×10^{-21}
   B. 2.5×10^{-20}
   C. 6.3×10^{-17}
   D. 1.6×10^{-16}

4. A solution contains Ba^{2+}, Ca^{2+}, Cu^{2+}, and Pb^{2+}. When sulfuric acid is added, the first substance to precipitate will be:
   A. BaSO$_4$
   B. CaSO$_4$
   C. CuSO$_4$
   D. PbSO$_4$

5. The K_{sp} of silver(I) chloride at 100°C is 2.15×10^{-8}. The dissolution of silver(I) chloride is:
   A. exothermic.
   B. endothermic.
   C. neither endothermic nor exothermic.
   D. cannot be determined from the information provided.

6. The chloride ion is infinitely soluble in water. If the solubility product constants for $BaCl_2$, $CuCl_2$, $HgCl_2$, and $PbCl_2$ are 35.8, 73.0, 6.57, and 1.00, respectively, the least soluble cation is:

   A. Ba^{2+}
   B. Cu^{2+}
   C. Hg^{2+}
   D. Pb^{2+}

7. A saturated solution containing silver iodide is added to an equal volume of saturated solution of silver chloride. As a result:

   A. a precipitate of silver chloride will form.
   B. a precipitate of silver iodide will form.
   C. a precipitate of sodium chloride will form.
   D. no precipitate will form.

8. Certain reactions will not proceed without the addition of a catalyst. A catalyst will do all of the following EXCEPT:

   A. increase the rate of the forward reaction.
   B. increase the rate of the reverse reaction.
   C. increase the equilibrium concentration of products.
   D. decrease the activation energy required for an endothermic reaction.

16.3 MASTERY VERIFIED: ANSWERS AND EXPLANATIONS

1. *The correct answer is A.* Since each compound dissociates into two ions, the most soluble compound is the one with the highest K_{sp}: lead(II) sulfate.

2. *The correct answer is D.* Solubility, x, is found from:

$$K_{sp} = [Ba^{2+}][SO_4^{2-}] = [x][x] = x^2$$

From the table, $K_{sp} = 1.5 \times 10^{-9}$. Thus:

$$x = \sqrt{1.5 \times 10^{-9}} = \sqrt{15 \times 10^{-10}} = \sqrt{15} \times \sqrt{10^{-10}} = 3.9 \times 10^{-5}$$

3. *The correct answer is A.* We solve this problem using the expression for K_{eq}:

$$K_{eq} = \frac{\left[EDTA^{4-}\right]\left[Pb^{2+}\right]}{\left[Pb-EDTA^{2-}\right]}$$

Rearranging,

$$\left[Pb^{2+}\right] = \frac{\left[Pb-EDTA^{2-}\right]K_{eq}}{\left[EDTA^{4-}\right]} = \frac{\left(2.0 \times 10^{-4}\right)\left(5.0 \times 10^{-19}\right)}{\left(2.5 \times 10^{-2}\right)} = 4.0 \times 10^{-21}$$

4. *The correct answer is A.* The first substance to precipitate will be the one with the lowest solubility. The substance with the lowest solubility is the substance with the lowest K_{sp}. The substance with the lowest K_{sp} is $BaSO_4$.

5. *The correct answer is B.* The K_{sp} of silver(I) chloride at 25°C is x. At a higher temperature (100°C), the K_{sp} is increased, and more products are formed in the equilibrium:

$$AgCl \rightleftharpoons Ag^+ + Cl^-$$

When accounting for temperature, the equilibrium must be:

$$AgCl + heat \rightleftharpoons Ag^+ + Cl^- \text{ (endothermic)}$$

Thus:

$$\downarrow AgCl + \uparrow heat \rightleftharpoons \uparrow Ag^+ + \uparrow Cl^-$$

6. *The correct answer is D.* $PbCl_2$ has the lowest K_{sp}, and is therefore the least soluble.

7. *The correct answer is B.* Since we are concerned only with concentrations, we are free to choose any volumes we wish. We choose two 1-liter volumes of the saturated solutions. We use the K_{sp}'s of the compounds to find the number of moles in each container before mixing.

$$K_{spAg2} = 1.5 \times 10^{-16} = \left[Ag^+\right]\left[I^-\right] = x^2$$

$$x = 1.2 \times 10^{-8} = \left[Ag^+\right] = \left[I^-\right]$$

$$K_{spAgCl} = 1.6 \times 10^{-10} = \left[Ag^+\right]\left[Cl^-\right] = x^2$$

$$x = 1.2 \times 10^{-5} = \left[Ag^+\right] = \left[Cl^-\right]$$

Now we mix the solutions together and the volume becomes 2 liters. The new concentrations are:

$$\left[Ag^+\right] = \frac{\left(1.2 \times 10^{-8}\right) + \left(1.2 \times 10^{-5}\right)}{2} = 6 \times 10^{-6}$$

$$\left[Cl^-\right] = \frac{1.2 \times 10^{-5}}{2} = 6 \times 10^{-6}$$

$$\left[I^-\right] = \frac{1.2 \times 10^{-8}}{2} = 6 \times 10^{-9}$$

Checking the concentrations against the K_{sp}'s, we have:

$$\left[Ag^+\right]\left[I^-\right] = 3.6 \times 10^{-14} > K_{spAgI} = 1.5 \times 10^{-16}$$

Solid AgI is formed.

$$\left[Ag^+\right]\left[Cl^-\right] = 3.6 \times 10^{-11} < K_{spAgI} = 1.6 \times 10^{-10}$$

No solid AgCl is formed.

Another way to approach this question is to see that when we double the volume, we decrease [I⁻] by a factor of two. Thus we need to increase [Ag⁺] by more than a factor of two in order to get a precipitate. The question then becomes "Does the saturated solution of AgCl have more than three times as much [Ag⁺] as a saturated solution of AgI?"

8. *The correct answer is C.* A catalyst operates by lowering a reaction's activation energy (**Chapter 17**). Once this activation energy is lowered, both the forward *and* reverse reactions in an equilibrium become more favorable. A catalyst does *not* affect the equilibrium of a system nor the equilibrium concentrations; it only moves the system to equilibrium faster.

CHEMICAL REACTIONS III: THERMODYNAMICS

17.1 MASTERY ACHIEVED

17.1.1 THERMODYNAMICS OF CHEMICAL REACTIONS: IN THEORY

17.1.1.1 Basic Definitions and Concepts of Thermodynamics

Thermodynamics is the study of heat and its interconversions with other energy forms. The **system (sys)** is the object under investigation. The **surroundings (surr)** are everything outside the system. The **universe (univ)** is the sum of the system and the surroundings.

An **open** system is a system that allows for the exchange of matter and energy between the surroundings and the system. A **closed** system allows for the exchange of energy only, meaning that mass is conserved within the system. An **isolated** system does not allow for the exchange of anything (matter or energy) between the system and the surroundings. In order for a system to be considered an isolated system it must be a closed system that is neither in mechanical nor thermal contact with the surroundings. While thermodynamics usually focuses on the system, changes in the thermodynamic properties of the surroundings must also be considered.

A variety of functions is used to determine the thermodynamic characteristics of a system. The **state** of a system is characterized by definite values of each of these functions. A **state function** is determined only by the current state of the system, not by the path taken to achieve this state. A **nonstate function** is path-dependent. Common thermodynamic state functions are **pressure, temperature, volume, internal energy, enthalpy, entropy,** and **free energy**. Common thermodynamic nonstate functions include **work** and **heat**. While nonstate functions may be interrelated, state functions are much more co-dependent. Once two or three state functions have been set or determined, the remaining state functions are also set, or may be determined without further measurement.

The **path** that a system takes to reach a given state may be given by a single step or by multiple steps. A **reversible path** is a continuous path that may be reversed at any point to restore the original values of the nonstate functions. An **irreversible path** is characterized by an inability to reverse the direction of the path with the achievement of the original nonstate function values.

The **energy** of a system is a state function that may take many different forms: **mechanical kinetic, mechanical potential, heat, electrical, light, sound, magnetic, chemical,** and others.

Please solve this problem:

- All of the following are thermodynamic state functions EXCEPT:

    A. internal energy.
    B. work.
    C. entropy.
    D. enthalpy.

Problem solved:

The correct answer is B. A state function is determined by the current state of the system and not by the path taken to get to this state. The work performed by, or performed on, a system is dependent on the path.

There are two principal ways by which a system can gain or lose energy: by heat transfer or by work (the two common thermodynamic nonstate functions). Heat transfer occurs only when there is a temperature difference, or gradient, between the two objects (in chemical thermodynamics, these two items are typically the system and the surroundings, but they could be two items within the system itself). In the case of a system with a temperature higher than its surroundings, energy, in the form of heat, is transferred from the system to the surroundings. In the case of a system with a temperature lower than the surroundings, heat is transferred from the surroundings into the system. In the former process, convention dictates that the heat (Q_{sys}) takes a negative value. In the latter process, Q_{sys} takes a positive value. This also implies that Q_{surr} takes a positive value in the former process and that Q_{surr} takes a negative value in the latter process (since energy is conserved in the universe).

We can also denote heat as either Q_{rev} or Q_{irr}, where **rev** indicates a reversible process, and **irr** indicates an irreversible process.

The heat of a reversible process (Q_{rev}) is always greater than the heat of an irreversible process (Q_{irr}).

Thermodynamic work principally takes the form of mechanical work (as in the lifting of an object) or of electrical work (as in a car battery). Work done by the system is negative (less energy is available to the system). Work done by the surroundings upon the system is positive (more energy is available to the system). There are many types of work, but we will focus here on the mechanical work done by expanding gases. The mechanical work done by expanding gases may be represented by the equation:

$$W = P\Delta V$$

where W is work, P is the pressure of the system, and ΔV is the internal volume change undergone by the system.

As was the case for heat, the work performed by a reversible process is always greater than the work performed by an irreversible process.

Please solve this problem:

- Which of the following statements is true for any given change in state?

  I. The heat of an irreversible process is greater than the heat of a reversible process.
  II. The work performed on a system in a reversible process is greater than the work performed on a system in an irreversible process.
  III. The work performed by a system in a reversible process is greater than the work performed by a system in an irreversible process.

  A. I only
  B. II only
  C. III only
  D. II and III only

Problem solved:

The correct answer is D. Both II and III are true, and I is false. The heat (whether given off or gained) in a reversible process is greater than the heat (whether given off or gained) in an irreversible process. Likewise, the work performed in a reversible process is greater than the work performed in an irreversible process, regardless of whether the system is performing work on the surroundings or the surroundings are performing work on the system.

A measure of the internal energy of a system is given by the equation:

$$\Delta U = Q + W$$

where ΔU is the internal energy change of the system, Q is the heat gained by the system and W is the work performed upon the system.

Note that we cannot calculate or measure the exact internal energy (U) of a system. Instead, we must determine **changes** in internal energy, ΔU.

Please solve this problem:

- All of the following are thermodynamic state functions EXCEPT:

  A. heat.
  B. temperature.
  C. pressure.
  D. volume.

Problem solved:

The correct answer is A. Three of the variables of the ideal gas law—pressure, volume, and temperature ($PV = nRT$)—are thermodynamic state functions.

17.1.1.2 Entropy

Entropy is a measure of the disorder of a system. As disorder increases, so too does entropy. As a result, the entropy of a substance in the gaseous state is greater than the entropy of the same substance in the liquid state. Likewise, the entropy of a substance in the liquid state is greater than the entropy of that substance in the solid state.

- Entropy increases as temperature increases.

- Entropy increases in a reaction if that reaction produces more product molecules than it contained reactant molecules.

- Entropy increases when pure liquids and/or pure solids form solutions.

- The entropy of the universe, S_{univ}, always increases.

Please solve this problem:

- All of the following are properties of entropy EXCEPT:

  A. the entropy of the universe increases.
  B. the entropy gained by a system is not equal to the entropy lost by the surroundings.
  C. entropy is an energy term, as are all thermodynamic state functions.
  D. entropy increases with increasing temperature.

Problem solved:

The correct answer is C. Not all thermodynamic state functions are energy terms; examples include entropy, volume, and pressure. Conversely, not all energy terms are state functions; examples of energy terms that are not state functions include work and heat. Choice A is true: The entropy of the universe must increase. Choice B is true: If the entropy gained by a system were equal to the entropy lost by the surroundings (and vice versa), the entropy of the universe (system + surroundings) would remain a constant. Choice D is true.

17.1.1.3 Enthalpy, Endothermic Reactions, and Exothermic Reactions

Enthalpy (H) is a measure of the heat released when pressure is held constant. By definition, the change in enthalpy of a system at constant pressure is given by the equation:

$$\Delta H_{sys} = Q_{sys,p}$$

where ΔH_{sys} is the change in enthalpy of the system, and $Q_{sys,p}$ is the heat absorbed by the system under conditions of constant pressure. As was the case for U, it is not possible to measure or calculate the absolute value of H. ΔH is related to ΔU by the equation:

$$\Delta H = \Delta U + \Delta(PV)$$

- A reaction is termed **endothermic** when ΔH_{sys} is positive.

- A reaction is termed **exothermic** when ΔH_{sys} is negative.

Please solve this problem:

- All of the following are properties of enthalpy EXCEPT:

    A. a positive change in enthalpy indicates that heat is absorbed by the system.
    B. a negative change in enthalpy indicates that heat is lost to the surroundings.
    C. the change in enthalpy of a system is equal to the change in its internal energy
    D. a reaction with a negative change in enthalpy is exothermic, a reaction with a positive change in enthalpy is endothermic.

Problem solved:

The correct answer is C. The change in enthalpy is equal to the change in internal energy of a system only when the work done by a change in pressure and volume is zero.

17.1.1.4 Heats of Formation, Heats of Reaction, and Hess's Law

The **heat of formation** (ΔH_f) of a substance is the enthalpy required for the formation of one mole of that substance from its elements. The standard heat of formation (ΔH_f°) is the change in enthalpy for such a process under standard conditions. Standard thermodynamic conditions are defined as a temperature of 298.15 K (25°C) at a pressure of 1 atm. This should not be confused with **STP (standard temperature and pressure)**, where temperature is defined as 273.15 K (0°C). The ΔH_f° of all elements in their naturally occurring state is defined as zero.

The **heat of reaction** (ΔH°) is given by the sum of the heats of formation of the products minus the sum of the heats of formation of the reactants.

- A positive heat of reaction denotes an **endothermic** reaction.

- A negative heat of reaction denotes an **exothermic** reaction.

Consider the following reaction:

$$H_2(g) + \frac{1}{2} O_2(g) \rightarrow H_2O(g) \qquad \Delta H^\circ = -241.8 \text{ kJ}$$

The heat of formation is taken, by definition, to be zero for both H_2 and O_2, since these are the natural elemental forms of the elements H and O, respectively. Therefore, since the heat of reaction is equal to the heats of formation of the products minus the heats of formation of the reactants, we can say that the heat of formation of $H_2O(g)$ is equal to -241.8 kJ.

Note that the heat of formation of *liquid* water is not the same as the heat of formation of *gaseous* water:

$$H_2(g) + \frac{1}{2} O_2(g) \rightarrow H_2O(g) \rightarrow H_2O(\ell) \qquad \Delta H^\circ = -285.8 \text{ kJ}$$

The extra 44 kJ of enthalpy given off is the result of a transition from the more energetic gaseous form to the less energetic liquid form. This energy is known as the **enthalpy of liquefaction**, or the **enthalpy of condensation**. This and related topics are covered in greater detail in **20.1.2**. Some heats of formation are given in Table 17.1.

Compound	ΔH°_f (kJ/mol)	Compound	ΔH°_f (kJ/mol)
$NH_3(g)$	−46.11	$CH_4(g)$	−74.85
$NH_3(aq)$	−80.29	$C_2H_2(g)$	226.73
$PCl_5(g)$	−374.9	$C_2H_4(g)$	52.26
$PCl_5(s)$	−443.5	$C_2H_6(g)$	−84.86
$C(g)$	716.68	$C_3H_8(g)$	−103.85
$H^+(aq)$	0	$C_4H_{10}(g)$	−126.15
$CO(g)$	−110.53	$C_5H_{12}(g)$	−146.11
$CO_2(g)$	−393.51	$C_6H_{14}(g)$	−198.7
$CO_2(aq)$	−413.80	α-D-glucose(s)	−1,274
$CO_3^{2-}(aq)$	−677.14	β-D-glucose(s)	−1,268
$HCO_3^-(aq)$	−691.99	β-D-fructose(s)	−1,266
$H_2CO_3(aq)$	−699.65	sucrose(s)	−2,222

Heats of Formation for Various Compounds
Table 17.1

Heats of reaction for complex reactions are determined via the use of **Hess' law of constant heat summation**. Consider the following reaction:

$$CO_2(g) + 4\,H_2(g) \rightarrow CH_4(g) + 2\,H_2O(\ell)$$

One method to determine the heat of reaction involves the heats of formation of each reactant and of each product.

For reactants:

- the heat of formation of H_2 is, by definition, zero.

- the heat of formation of $CO_2(g)$ is:

$$C(s) + O_2(g) \rightarrow CO_2(g) \qquad \Delta H^\circ_f = -393.5 \text{ kJ/mol}$$

- Therefore, the heat of formation of the reactants is −393.5 kJ.

For products:

- the heat of formation of $CH_4(g)$ is:

$$C(s) + 2\,H_2(g) \rightarrow CH_4(g) \qquad \Delta H^\circ_f = -74.85 \text{ kJ/mol}$$

- the heat of formation of $H_2O(\ell)$ is –285.8 kJ/mol, as given above.

- Therefore, the heat of formation of the products is:

$$-74.85 + 2(-285.8) = -646.45 \text{ kJ}$$

Thus, the heat of reaction is:

$$-646.45 - (-393.5) = -252.95 \text{ kJ}$$

Please solve this problem:

- The complete combustion of n-butane is given by:

$$C_4H_{10}(g) + \frac{13}{2} O_2(g) \rightarrow 4 CO_2(g) + 5 H_2O(g)$$

The heat of this reaction is:

A. +2,657 kJ
B. +509.15 kJ
C. –509.15 kJ
D. –2,657 kJ

Problem solved:

The correct answer is D. Remember that this is a combustion reaction, which we would expect to be **exothermic**. Also recall that exothermic reactions have *negative* heats of reaction. Therefore, you should have been able to eliminate choices A and B by inspection.

The heat of reaction is given by:

$$\Delta H^\circ_{rxn} = \Delta H^\circ_{f\,(products)} - \Delta H^\circ_{f\,(reactants)}$$

The heat of formation of the products is given by:

$$\Delta H^\circ_{f\,CO_2(g)} \times mol_{CO_2(g)} = (-393.5 \text{ kJ/mol})(4 \text{ mol}) = -1,574 \text{ kJ}$$
$$\Delta H^\circ_{f\,H_2O(g)} \times mol_{H_2O(g)} = (-241.8 \text{ kJ/mol})(5 \text{ mol}) = -1,209 \text{ kJ}$$
$$\Delta H^\circ_p = -2,783 \text{ kJ}$$

The heat of formation of the reactants is given by:

$$\Delta H^\circ_{f\,C_4H_{10}(g)} \times mol_{C_4H_{10}(g)} = (-126.15 \text{ kJ/mol})(1 \text{ mol}) = -126.15 \text{ kJ}$$
$$\Delta H^\circ_{f\,O_2(g)} = 0 \text{ kJ} = 0 \text{ kJ}$$
$$\Delta H^\circ_{f\,(reactants)} = -126.15 \text{ kJ}$$

Therefore, the total heat of reaction is (–2,783 kJ) – (–126.15 kJ) = –2,657 kJ, which is choice D. Choice C could be arrived at by neglecting to multiply the molar heats of formation in Table 17.1 by the stoichiometric coefficients in the balanced equation.

17.1.1.5 Gibbs Free-Energy and Reaction Spontaneity

The **free energy** of a system (or **Gibbs free-energy** of a system) at constant temperature is given by the equation:

$$\Delta G = \Delta H - T\Delta S$$

where all thermodynamic quantities refer to the system, and T is given in kelvin.

The Gibbs free-energy of a system is a measure of the energy available to the system for the performance of useful work. The absolute value of G cannot be calculated, nor can it be measured. As was the case for U and H, we refer to the change in G (ΔG) between two states of the system. Taking a closer look at the equation defining the Gibbs function, we see that ΔG may take either a positive or a negative value, depending upon the signs and magnitudes of ΔH and ΔS.

- When ΔG of a reaction is negative, the reaction is spontaneous in the forward direction.

- When ΔG of a reaction is positive, the reaction is nonspontaneous in the forward direction.

- When ΔG of a reaction is equal to zero, the reaction is at equilibrium.

A reaction with a positive ΔG is termed an **endergonic** reaction. A reaction with a negative ΔG is termed an **exergonic** reaction. Recall that it is ΔH that determines endo- versus exothermicity. All of the possible relationships between ΔG and ΔH, ΔS, and T are shown in Table 17.2.

ΔH	–	T	ΔS	ΔG
+		low	+	+
+		high	+	–
+		low	–	+
+		high	–	+
–		low	+	–
–		high	+	–
–		low	–	–
–		high	–	+

Free Energy Changes
Table 17.2

From these observations it should be clear that only those endothermic reactions that occur at a high temperature with an increase in entropy will occur spontaneously. On the other hand, an exothermic reaction that occurs at high temperature with a decrease in entropy will not be spontaneous. The probability of obtaining a negative entropy at high temperature is not large (recall that a gas possesses more entropy than a liquid and a liquid possesses more entropy than a solid).

Please solve this problem:

- Which of the following statements would serve as useful rules of thumb?

  I. Exothermic reactions at high temperatures will be exergonic.
  II. Exothermic reactions at low temperatures will be exergonic.
  III. Endothermic reactions at low temperatures will be endergonic.
  IV. Endothermic reactions at high temperatures will be endergonic.

  A. I and III only
  B. II and III only
  C. II and IV only
  D. I and IV only

Problem solved:

The correct answer is B. This question is best answered by reference to Table 17.2. You must know the relationships between ΔG, ΔH, ΔS and T to avoid missing easy questions on the MCAT.

17.1.1.6 The Three Laws of Thermodynamics

There are three laws of thermodynamics. The first law states that for any isolated system (as defined in **17.1.1.1**) energy is constant. This law is simply a restatement of the general **principle of conservation of energy**. If we take our system to be the universe, we can state that energy is neither created nor destroyed within our system. In this regard, an isolated system may be thought of as a mini-universe. The equation given in **17.1.1.1** for the internal energy of a system:

$$\Delta U = Q + W$$

is a mathematical statement of the **first law of thermodynamics**.

The **second law of thermodynamics** introduces the concept of entropy. This law states that no cyclic process in which the heat absorbed is completely converted into useful work is possible. This is not to say that natural processes cannot exist that convert heat entirely into work, but no process may exist in which a system is cycled from its point of origin to other points and back to its point of origin, with the heat produced being converted entirely to useful work.

The second law of thermodynamics points directly to the asymmetrical nature of all natural processes. While the first law provides for the conservation of energy, the second law cleaves the first law in half: The second law asserts that even if a forward process converts all of the heat produced into useful work, the reverse process will not do so; similarly, even if a forward process does not convert all of the heat produced into useful work, this does not preempt the reverse process from doing so.

In other words, the entropy of the universe is constantly increasing.

The **third law of thermodynamics** is perhaps the least useful thermodynamic law for the MCAT. This law, in effect, states that absolute zero is unattainable. While you should appreciate the significance of this statement, it probably won't be very useful on any MCAT problems.

Please solve this problem:

- The three laws of thermodynamics do not provide for any of the following EXCEPT:

    A. absolute zero exists and is attainable.
    B. entropy is conserved in the universe
    C. energy is conserved in the universe.
    D. entropy is a thermodynamic state function.

Problem solved:

The correct answer is C. Choice A is false: the third law of thermodynamics posits the existence of absolute zero; however, it also states that the attainment of absolute zero in a finite number of steps is an impossibility. Choice B is false: The second law of thermodynamics shows that the change in entropy of a forward process cannot be equal to the change in entropy of the reverse reaction. If these two quantities were equal, a system could be cycled from one state to another and back without heat loss. If such a cycling were possible, the construction of a perpetual motion machine would also be possible. Choice C is directly provided for by the first law of thermodynamics. While choice D is true, it is not provided for by any of the three laws of thermodynamics.

17.1.2 THERMODYNAMICS OF CHEMICAL REACTIONS: IN PRACTICE

17.1.2.1 Reaction Diagrams, ΔH, and Activation Energy

You can draw reaction diagrams that depict the energy of a reaction system versus the progress of the reaction, called the **reaction coordinate**. The reaction coordinate is often given by the percent of products formed over the percent of reactants remaining. As such, this axis increases from zero on the left (signifying all reactants) to one on the right (signifying all products). The energy coordinate must be examined carefully: Energy may be presented in the form of Gibbs free-energy (G) or enthalpy (H).

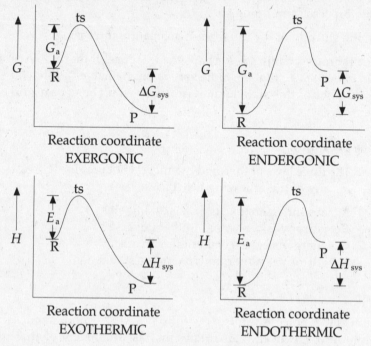

Figure 17.1

In the case of an endergonic or an exergonic reaction, the vertical distance between the energy of the reactants and the energy of the products is a measure of ΔG_{sys}. For exothermic or endothermic reactions, the vertical distance between the energy of the reactants and the energy of the products is a measure of ΔH_{sys}. Additionally, the vertical distance between the reactants and the highest vertical point on the curve is significant. In the case of a graph of free energy versus reaction coordinate, this vertical distance is a measure of the **free energy of activation**, or how much free energy is required to activate, or start, the reaction. In the case of a graph of enthalpy versus reaction coordinate, this vertical distance is a measure of the **enthalpy of activation**, or how much heat is required to activate the reaction. For the MCAT, enthalpy of activation is the activation energy, E_a.

The **transition state (ts)** of a system is the highest energy state that the system achieves during the course of its reaction. At this state, some of the bonds of the reactants are partially broken (elongated), and some of the new bonds that will be in the products have begun to form.

In the case of the exothermic reaction depicted, the transition state is less than halfway along the reaction coordinate. The transition state for the endothermic reaction is more than halfway along the reaction coordinate, which is generally the case in practice. This observation leads us to two conclusions: (1) For exothermic processes, the transition state resembles the reactants more than it resembles the products; (2) for endothermic reactions, the transition state resembles the products more than it does the reactants.

Considering a reversible reaction, we can imagine the reaction diagram for the reverse reaction to be simply the mirror image of the reaction diagram for the forward reaction. From this it is clear that the activation energy is higher in the endothermic direction than in the exothermic direction; thus the transition state in the endothermic direction is more similar to the products than the reactants, while the transition state in the exothermic direction is more similar to the reactants than the products. These are useful concepts to keep in mind when dealing with reaction diagrams.

For the MCAT, you should also be familiar with reaction diagrams of multistep processes. Represented below are typical reaction diagrams for exothermic S_N2 (one-step) and S_N1 (two-step) reactions. (Organic nucleophilic substitution reactions are discussed in detail in Chapter 36.)

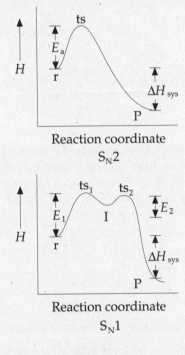

Figure 17.2

The S_N2 reaction diagram is provided merely as a comparison to the S_N1 diagram. The S_N1 diagram has two separate activation energies, labeled E_1 and E_2. The first activation energy is the enthalpy change that is accompanied by a movement from the reactants to the first transition state (ts_1). The second activation energy is the enthalpy change that is accompanied by movement from the reaction intermediate (I) to the second transition state (ts_2). An intermediate in a reaction pathway is an unstable species that has a relatively short lifetime in the reaction mixture compared to the products and the reactants. In terms of a reaction diagram, a trough in the pathway is indicative of an intermediate. The number of steps in an overall reaction is equal to the number of troughs plus one, or alternatively, to the number of peaks (or transition states).

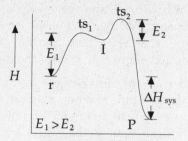

Figure 17.3

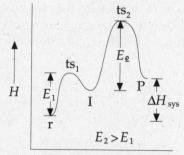

Figure 17.4

The slowest step in a multistep reaction is the **rate-determining step**. The rate-determining step is the step in the reaction diagram that has the greatest *individual* activation energy. The rate-determining step is *not* determined by the step with the highest-energy transition state. In Figure 17.3, you will notice that the second step has the highest-energy transition state, but that the first step has the highest activation energy. For this system, the rate-determining step is the first step. In Figure 17.4, you will notice that the second step has the highest-energy transition state *and* the highest activation energy. For this system, the rate-determining step is the second step.

Please solve this problem:

- The rate-determining step in a reaction sequence is:

    A. the step with the highest activation energy.
    B. the step with the highest energy transition state.
    C. the step which involves the limiting reagent.
    D. all of the above.

Problem solved:

The correct answer is A. Choices B and C are commonly misinterpreted. As explained in the chapter text above, the rate-determining step is the step with the highest individual activation energy. While this may also coincide with the step having the highest-energy transition state, it need not do so. The rate-determining step is the kinetically slowest overall step in a reaction sequence. While the speed of a given step may be affected by the amount of reactants available for the performance of this step, the limiting reagent has little to do with kinetics. The limiting reagent is simply the reagent that gets used up first because there is less of it, not because of the speed of a step that consumes it.

17.1.2.2 Kinetics and Thermodynamic Reaction Energetics

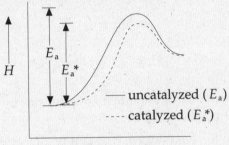

Figure 17.5

Catalysts (**15.1.3**) alter a reaction's pathway. Catalysts cannot alter the reactants nor can they alter the products; therefore, they must alter the transition state(s). A catalyst is employed to reduce the activation energy of a reaction (or a step in a multistep reaction). Therefore, it should be clear that catalysts affect E_a, but they do not affect the ultimate changes in state functions between reactants and products (e.g., ΔH, ΔG). In the reaction diagram depicted in Figure 17.5, the solid line represents the uncatalyzed reaction pathway while the dashed line represents the catalyzed reaction pathway.

Please solve this problem:

- A catalyst causes:
    - **A.** a shift in the equilibrium of a reaction.
    - **B.** a decrease in activation energy of a reaction.
    - **C.** an increase in ΔG.
    - **D.** an decrease in ΔH.

Problem solved:

The correct answer is B. A catalyst affects only the activation energy of a system. A catalyst does not cause the equilibrium of a reaction to shift toward products. The equilibrium mixture of products and reactants in a catalyzed reaction will be identical to the equilibrium mixture of products and reactants in the uncatalyzed reaction. A catalyst affects neither the energy states of the products nor the energy states of the reactants. As a result, a catalyst alters neither ΔG nor ΔH.

17.1.2.3 Reactions at Equilibrium

A reaction may be characterized by its equilibrium constant, K_{eq} (see **16.1.2**). For a reaction, the change in Gibbs free-energy (ΔG) is:

$$\Delta G = \Delta G° + RTlnQ$$

where ΔG is the change in Gibbs free-energy of the reaction at a constant temperature and a constant pressure. $\Delta G°$ is the standard free energy change of the reaction at 298 K and 1 atm.

R is the universal gas constant, T is the temperature at which the reaction is occurring, and Q is given by:

$$Q = \frac{(C)^c (D)^d}{(A)^a (B)^b}$$

For the general reaction:

$$aA + bB \leftrightarrow cC + dD$$

Where (A), (B), (C), and (D) represent the molar concentrations of the respective chemicals at any point in the reaction.

Recall from Chapter 16 that the equilibrium constant of a reaction is temperature-dependent and must be calculated for each temperature.

By definition, $\Delta G = 0$ at equilibrium, giving:

$$\Delta G° = -RT ln K_{eq}$$

From this, we can see that if $\Delta G°$ is negative, then K_{eq} is larger than l; therefore, products are favored. Likewise, if $\Delta G°$ is positive, then K_{eq} is smaller than l, and reactants are favored. In summary:

- If $\Delta G > 0$, then reactants are favored over products.

- If $\Delta G = 0$, then neither reactants nor products are favored.

- If $\Delta G < 0$, then product formation is favored.

Please solve this problem:

- The reaction ATP + H_2O → ADP + phosphate is run at 25°C under atmospheric conditions. Its free energy, $\Delta G°$, is –30 kJ/mol.

    A. The reaction is spontaneous under these conditions, because $\Delta G°$ is negative.
    B. The reaction is nonspontaneous under these conditions, because $\Delta G°$ is negative.
    C. The reaction is at equilibrium under these conditions, because $\Delta G = 0$.
    D. It cannot be said whether this reaction is spontaneous or nonspontaneous under these conditions without knowing the equilibrium constant, K_{eq}.

Problem solved:

The correct answer is A. Since $\Delta G°$ is negative, the reaction is spontaneous.

17.2 MASTERY APPLIED: SAMPLE PASSAGE AND QUESTIONS

Passage

ATP hydrolysis is an important biochemical reaction. The function of ATP is to store energy from food for later use. ATP's ability to store energy is due to its ability to lose a phosphate group by hydrolysis, forming ADP:

$$ATP + H_2O \rightarrow ADP + phosphate$$

Since this reaction is exergonic, it can drive endergonic reactions that might not otherwise occur. At 37°C (body temperature) the thermodynamic values for ATP hydrolysis are $\Delta G = -30$ kJ/mol, $\Delta H = -20$ kJ/mol, and $\Delta S = +34$J/K • mol.

The energy-liberating process in anaerobic organisms is glycolysis. For glycolysis at body temperature, $\Delta G = -218$ kJ/mol and $\Delta H = -120$ kJ/mol. Glycolysis is coupled with the conversion of two ADP molecules into two ATP molecules via the equation:

$$Glucose + ADP + 2\ phosphate \rightarrow$$
$$2\ lactate + 2\ ATP + 2\ H_2O$$

The biosynthesis of sucrose from fructose and glucose has $\Delta G = +23$ kJ/mol. The formation of a peptide bond, which is essential for the production of proteins, directly consumes 17 kJ/mol. However, this latter process is an indirect one that also entails the consumption of three ATP molecules for each peptide bond formed. A moderately small protein contains 150 peptide bonds, a medium-sized protein contains 400 peptide bonds, and a large protein may contain several thousand peptide bonds.

1. The hydrolysis of ATP is:
   A. exergonic and endothermic.
   B. exergonic and exothermic.
   C. endergonic and endothermic.
   D. endergonic and exothermic.

2. The ΔG of the reaction of glucose with ADP and inorganic phosphate to produce lactate, ATP, and water is:
   A. −278 kJ/mol
   B. −218 kJ/mol
   C. −188 kJ/mol
   D. −158 kJ/mol

3. The energy from a mole of ATP molecules hydrolyzed to a mole of ADP molecules is sufficient for the synthesis of how many molecules of sucrose from fructose and glucose?
   A. 7.85×10^{23}
   B. 6.02×10^{23}
   C. 7.85×10^{21}
   D. 6.02×10^{21}

4. The synthesis of a medium-sized protein requires:
   A. 400 ATP molecules.
   B. 627 ATP molecules.
   C. 1,200 ATP molecules.
   D. 1,427 ATP molecules.

5. If the complete aerobic respiration of one glucose molecule produces 38 ATP molecules, and the Gibbs free-energy of combustion of glucose is −2,880 kJ/mol, what is the amount of heat lost in the transformation of one mole of glucose to 38 moles of ATP?
   A. −1,740 kJ
   B. 0 kJ
   C. 1,740 kJ
   D. 2,842 kJ

6. The synthesis of proteins from amino acids and the synthesis of carbohydrates from simple sugars are endergonic processes. This is likely a result of:

A. an overall endothermic process accompanied by a decrease in entropy.

B. an overall endothermic process accompanied by an increase in entropy.

C. an overall exothermic process accompanied by a decrease in entropy.

D. an overall exothermic process accompanied by an increase in entropy.

7. Based on the information in the passage, the process of glycolysis:

A. results in a decrease in entropy.

B. results in an increase in entropy.

C. results in an increase in enthalpy.

D. results in an increase in Gibbs free-energy.

17.3 MASTERY VERIFIED: ANSWERS AND EXPLANATIONS

1. *The correct answer is B.* From the information in the passage, we see that both ΔG and ΔH are negative. Therefore, by definition, this reaction is both exergonic and exothermic.

2. *The correct answer is D.* In this case, we can add the ΔG's:

$$\Delta G_{total} = \Delta G_{glucose} - 2(\Delta G_{ATP}) = -218 \text{ kJ/mol} - [(2)(-30 \text{ kJ/mol})] = -158 \text{ kJ/mol}$$

   From the answer choices, we can see that the assumption of additivity will be valid. We know that since ΔG_{ATP} is negative, ΔG_{ADP} must be positive. For this reason, we can eliminate choice A (which assumes a negative ΔG_{ADP}) and choice B (which assumes $\Delta G_{ADP} = 0$). This leaves only choices C and D. By assuming that $\Delta G_{ADP} = \Delta G_{ATP}$, we can see that choice C has failed to account for the stoichiometric coefficient 2. Therefore, we can eliminate C, and we are left with D.

3. *The correct answer is A.* To solve this problem, we must first recall that Avogadro's number allows us to convert between moles and molecules, and that its value is 6.02×10^{23}. Then we must use the information in the passage that the energy from a mole of ATP molecules is equal to -30 kJ and that the energy required to form a sucrose molecule is $+23$ kJ/mol. Since the energy available in an ATP molecule is larger than the energy required to form a sucrose molecule, we can see that our answer must be larger than Avogadro's number. The only choice that fits this criterion is choice A.

4. *The correct answer is D.* From the passage, we see that the production of a peptide bond requires the input of $+17$ kJ/mol and 3 additional ATP molecules. Since the passage also tells us that the synthesis of a medium-sized protein requires the formation of 400 peptide bonds, we need at least 1,200 ATP's per protein molecule plus the number of ATP's that are necessary to supply the other 17 kJ/mol for each bond. D is the only choice larger than 1,200.

5. *The correct answer is C.* Thirty-eight moles of ATP will store 38 moles $\times$ 30 kJ/mol, or 1,140 kJ of the energy that is released from the glucose. Since the glucose releases 2,880 kJ, the amount of this energy that is stored (and therefore is the amount lost) is $2,880 - 1,140 = 1,740$ kJ.

6. *The correct answer is A.* The formation of an individual bond is an exothermic process, while the breaking of an individual bond is an endothermic process; if this weren't true, the bonds would not have formed in the first place.

   The formation of a peptide linkage requires the breaking of a carbon-oxygen bond and a nitrogen-hydrogen bond, followed by the formation of a carbon-nitrogen bond and an oxygen-hydrogen bond (Chapter 39). This process will be endothermic overall since the strength of the bonds broken is greater than the strength of the bonds formed. Similarly, the synthesis of a carbohydrate involves the formation of bonds that are weaker than the bonds that are broken (Chapter 40).

   As a large molecule is assembled from smaller molecules, the system becomes more ordered: entropy must decrease. The formation of a protein and the formation of a carbohydrate represent two examples of such processes.

7. *The correct answer is B.* From the thermodynamic data given in the passage, we can see that the change in Gibbs free energy associated with this process is negative: Gibbs free energy is decreased. This eliminates choice D.

Since this process occurs at 37°C, we do not have the necessary high-temperature conditions for an exergonic, endothermic reaction (Table 17.2). Therefore, since the reaction is exergonic, it is also exothermic. This eliminates choice C. Since this reaction involves the fragmentation of a large molecule (glucose) into smaller molecules (lactate), we have a condition of increasing entropy. Therefore, we are able to pick choice B over choice A.

CHAPTER 18

SOLUTIONS AND SOLUBILITY

18.1 MASTERY ACHIEVED

18.1.1 SOLUTIONS IN QUALITATIVE TERMS

18.1.1.1 Basic Definitions

A **solution** is a homogeneous mixture of two or more chemical compounds. Solutions may contain materials in any phase (gas, liquid, or solid) mixed with materials in any phase. While gaseous and solid solutions are common, this chapter will focus on solutions in which the liquids are mixed, or liquid is a solvent.

The **solvent** of a solution is the substance into which other chemicals are dissolved. The **solute** of a solution is the compound that is dissolved in the solvent. Sometimes, it is not clear which compound is dissolved; in such cases, the solvent is the compound that is present in the largest quantity, and all other compounds present are considered solutes.

In the pure liquid state, forces exist that stabilize the liquid. In order for a solute to dissolve in a liquid, it must possess similar forces as the solvent. Therefore, substances with similar intermolecular forces will tend to form solutions with one another: like dissolves like. Solutes that have strong attractive forces for a solvent are more soluble in that solvent than solutes with weaker attractive forces for that solvent. Even if the intermolecular forces between solvent molecules are greater than the attractive forces between solvent and solute, dissolution is still possible.

The process of **solvation** occurs when a solute is added to a solvent. As the solute is added, the solvent molecules separate from one another to make room for the solute molecules, and then surround the solute molecules. Solvation depends on the intermolecular forces (Chapter 14) present between the solvent molecules and the solute molecules.

Hydration is the term for the solvation process when the solvent is water. Substances that are water soluble have a high charge density, form hydrogen bonds, or have a large dipole moment. Chemicals with large dipole moments are said to be **polar**.

Please solve this problem:

- Of the following compounds, the LEAST water soluble is:

  A. CH_3OH
  B. CH_3CH_2OH
  C. $CH_3(CH_2)_4CH_2OH$
  D. $CH_3(CH_2)_6CH_2OH$

Problem solved:

The correct answer is D. Polar molecules are water soluble. In each of the four choices, the only polar group is the –OH functionality. As methylene groups (–CH_2–) are added, the dipole moment of the molecule will decrease. Therefore, the molecule with the smallest dipole moment is **1-octanol**.

18.1.1.2 Thermodynamics of Solutions

Solvation is controlled by two different thermodynamic properties: the tendency of a system to seek a minimum energy state and the tendency of a system to maximize entropy. **Heat of solution** is the enthalpy change that occurs when a solute dissolves in a solvent. Heat of solution may be either positive (energy absorbed) or negative (energy released). As with other thermodynamic systems, a **positive heat of solution** indicates an **endothermic solvation** and a **negative heat of solution** indicates an **exothermic solvation**.

An exothermic solvation will result from the dissolution of a solute that has a greater affinity for solvent molecules than for other solute molecules. An endothermic solvation will result from the dissolution of a solute that has a lower affinity for solvent molecules than for other solute molecules. Stated another way, a solution that has a negative heat of solution is lower in energy than the pure solute and the pure solvent. A solution that has a positive heat of solvation is a solution that is higher in energy than the pure states of the solute and the solvent.

When a solution is diluted, there is an associated **heat of dilution**. The heat of dilution of a solution will have the same sign as the heat of solution from the original preparation of the undiluted solution. A solution that has an exothermic heat of solution **must** also have an exothermic heat of dilution. Similarly, a solution that has an endothermic heat of solution **must** also have an endothermic heat of dilution.

Please solve this problem:

- A substance that has a positive enthalpy of solution will also:

    A. exhibit an endothermic heat of dilution and an increased solubility with increasing temperature.
    B. exhibit an endothermic heat of dilution and a decreased solubility with increasing temperature.
    C. exhibit an exothermic heat of dilution and an increased solubility with increasing temperature.
    D. exhibit an exothermic heat of dilution and a decreased solubility with increasing temperature.

Problem solved:

The correct answer is A. Since we are told that the enthalpy of solution is positive, we know that this is an endothermic process. An endothermic enthalpy of solution implies an endothermic heat of dilution. This eliminates choices C and D. An endothermic process is favored by an increase in temperature, while an exothermic process is favored by a decrease in temperature. Therefore, since we are dealing with an endothermic process, solubility will increase with increasing temperature.

18.1.1.3 Relative Concentrations

A solution is **saturated** when no more solute molecules will dissolve in the quantity of solvent available. A solution may become **supersaturated** under certain conditions. A supersaturated solution is an unstable system in which more solute molecules have been dissolved than would normally be possible under normal conditions. This state may have been achieved by preparing the solution at a higher temperature (for an endothermic heat of solution) and then slowly cooling it. A supersaturated solution will eventually stabilize by precipitating out the excess dissolved solute molecules.

A **concentrated solution** is a solution in which there is a relative abundance of solute molecules. A **dilute solution** is a solution in which there is only a relatively small number of solvent molecules. The terms "concentrated" and "dilute" can qualitatively describe the amount of solute in a solution. There are other quantitative expressions for solution concentration such as molarity, normality, molality, and mole fraction. These are discussed in greater detail in **18.1.2.1**.

Please solve this problem:

- A supersaturated solution of sodium thiosulfate is used as a hand warmer. Squeezing a seed crystal of solid sodium thiosulfate into the supersaturated solution causes precipitation of excess solute and the release of heat because:

  A. the enthalpy of solution is negative, and solvation is an exothermic process.
  B. the enthalpy of solution is positive, and solvation is an exothermic process.
  C. the enthalpy of solution is negative, and solvation is an endothermic process.
  D. the enthalpy of solution is positive, and solvation is an endothermic process.

Problem solved:

The correct answer is D. Choices A and C can be eliminated immediately, since a positive enthalpy of solution is an endothermic process and a negative enthalpy of solution is an exothermic process.

We are also told that heat is given off when excess sodium thiosulfate solute precipitates from solution. For a supersaturated solution, equilibrium is reached by precipitation of the excess dissolved solute, and heat is given off when the solute falls out of solution. From this, we conclude that heat must have been absorbed during solvation. Therefore, the enthalpy of solution must be positive, and the process of solvation must be endothermic.

18.1.1.4 Qualitative Solubility

Solubility is the ability of a solute to dissolve in a solvent. The solubility of gases in a liquid solvent is determined using **Henry's law**:

$$P = kC$$

where C is solubility, k is the Henry's law constant for the gas under consideration, and P is the gas pressure, or **partial pressure** of the gaseous solute over the solution. Note that the solubility of a gas is directly proportional to the pressure of that gas above the solution: as pressure is increased, solubility is also increased.

The heat of solution for gases in liquid solvents is almost always negative: as temperature is increased, gas solubility is decreased.

Liquids are said to be **miscible** in other liquids when they are soluble in all proportions. Liquids that do not dissolve in one another are **immiscible**.

Solids that may be dissolved in a liquid solvent to attain a concentration greater than 0.05 M(molarity) are **soluble** in that liquid. Solids that cannot be dissolved in a liquid solvent to attain a concentration greater than 0.01 M are **insoluble** in that liquid. Solids that are soluble between 0.01 M and 0.05 M are **slightly**, or **moderately**, **soluble**.

Some general solubility rules for aqueous solutions can be stated as follows:

- All alkali and ammonium (NH_4^+) compounds are soluble. The alkali metals (**13.1.3.9**) are included in Group 1 (Li^+, Na^+, K^+, Rb^+, Cs^+, Fr^+).

- All acetates (CH_3COO^-), chlorates (ClO_3^-), nitrates (NO_3^-), and perchlorates (ClO_4^-) are soluble.

- All chlorides, except those of Ag^+, Pb^{2+}, Hg_2^{2+}, and Cu^+ are soluble.

- Most sulfates are soluble. Exceptions include Ba^{2+}, Sr^{2+}, Pb^{2+}, Hg^+, and Ag^+.

- All carbonates (CO_3^{2-}), sulfides (S^{2-}), sulfites (SO_3^{2-}), and phosphates (PO_4^{3-}) are insoluble, except those of alkali metals and ammonium.

- Most hydroxides are insoluble. Exceptions include ammonium hydroxide (NH_4OH), alkali metal hydroxides, and barium hydroxide ($Ba(OH)_2$), which are soluble; and some lighter Group 2 (alkaline earth metals) hydroxides, which are slightly soluble.

Please solve this problem:

- Which of the following is LEAST likely to be water soluble?

  A. Na_2CO_3
  B. $CrPO_4$
  C. K_3PO_4
  D. $Ba(OH)_2$

Problem solved:

The correct answer is B. Both Na_2CO_3 and K_3PO_4 contain alkali metals and are water soluble. $Ba(OH)_2$ is soluble, since it is an exception to the rule of insolubility of hydroxides. $CrPO_4$, like most phosphates, is insoluble in aqueous solutions.

18.1.1.5 Factors Affecting Solubility

The solubility of a substance is affected by several factors, including temperature, common ions, and pH.

As discussed earlier, for a system with an endothermic heat of solution, solubility will generally increase with increasing temperature, and will decrease with decreasing temperature. For a system with an exothermic heat of solution, solubility will typically decrease with increasing temperature and increase with decreasing temperature.

The **common ion effect** indicates that the dissolution of a common ion into a solution will decrease the solubility of a solute that contains this ion. Similarly, the removal of the common ion will increase the solubility of the solute.

If a basic or acidic ion is produced in a dissolution process, a change in pH will affect the solubility of this solute. This point will be addressed in greater detail in Chapter 21. For now, let us say that a solute that dissociates into an acidic ion will have enhanced solubility in a solution with a high pH (basic), and diminished solubility in a solution with a low pH (acidic). A solute that dissociates into a basic ion will have enhanced solubility in a solution with a low pH (acidic), and diminished solubility in a solution with a high pH (basic).

Please solve this problem:

- If the pH of an aqueous solution of $NaHCO_3$ is increased, the solubility of $NaHCO_3$ will:

  A. increase.
  B. decrease.
  C. remain unchanged, because sodium bicarbonate does not contain an acidic ion.
  D. remain unchanged, because sodium bicarbonate does not contain a basic ion.

Problem solved:

The correct answer is B. Consider the equilibrium reaction:

$$NaHCO_3(s) \rightleftharpoons Na^+(aq) + HCO_3^-(aq)$$

The bicarbonate ion (HCO_3^-) is a basic ion. In the aqueous solution, the following equilibrium reaction is also occurring:

$$H^+(aq) + HCO_3^-(aq) \rightleftharpoons H_2CO_3(aq)$$

When the pH of this solution is increased, the H^+ concentration is decreased. Therefore,

$$\downarrow H^+ + \uparrow HCO_3^- \rightleftharpoons \downarrow H_2CO_3$$

which leads to,

$$\uparrow NaHCO_3 \rightleftharpoons \downarrow Na^+ + \uparrow HCO_3^-$$

A decrease in [H^+] shifts the second equilibrium reaction to the left, which causes the formation of a greater amount of bicarbonate ion. The increased bicarbonate concentration then causes a shift in the first equilibrium reaction to the left, which indicates decreased solubility of sodium bicarbonate.

18.1.2 SOLUTIONS IN QUANTITATIVE TERMS: CONCENTRATION

In order to determine the quantitative properties of solutions, you must first understand the various ways in which concentration may be expressed. Each of these methods for the expression of concentration is used at different times and for different reasons. You must be familiar with each concentration term.

18.1.2.1 Molarity

The most common quantitative measure of concentration is **molarity** (*M*).

Molarity is defined as:

$$M = \frac{\text{moles of solute}}{\text{liters of solution}}$$

Please solve this problem:

- The molarity of a 750 mL aqueous solution containing 270 grams of glucose ($C_6H_{12}O_6$) is:

  A. 0.36 *M*
  B. 1.0 *M*
  C. 2.0 *M*
  D. 3.6 *M*

Problem solved:

The correct answer is C. Molarity is defined as moles of solute per liter of solution. The number of liters of solution is 0.750 L. In order to find the number of moles of solute, we must convert grams to moles, using the molecular weight of glucose. The molecular weight of glucose is 180 g/mol. Therefore, the number of moles of glucose, *n*, is given by:

$$n = 270 \text{ g} \div 180 \text{ g/mol} = 1.5 \text{ mol}$$

Therefore, molarity is:

$$M = \frac{n}{V} = \frac{1.5 \text{ mol}}{0.750 \text{ L}} = 2 \text{ } M$$

18.1.2.2 Normality

Normality is used almost exclusively when referring to acids and bases, where one is concerned about the number of moles of H^+ or OH^- ions that a compound contains.

$$N = \frac{\text{moles of potential } H^+ \text{ or } OH^-}{\text{liters of solution}}$$

Please solve this problem:

- The normality in acid of a 500 mL aqueous solution of 1 *M* sulfuric acid (H_2SO_4) is:

  A. 1 *N*
  B. 2 *N*
  C. 3 *N*
  D. 8 *N*

Problem solved:

The correct answer is B. The normality of a solution is equal to the number of potential acid particles (H^+) per liter of solution. Since there are two H^+ particles per sulfuric acid molecule, the normality of the solution is 2.

18.1.2.3 Molality

Molality is normally not used unless we are concerned with a colligative property (**18.1.4**). Molality is symbolized by *m*, and is defined as:

$$m = \frac{\text{moles of solute}}{\text{kilograms of solvent}}$$

Note that while both molarity and normality are expressed in terms of volume (liters of solution) in the denominator, molality is expressed in terms of mass (kilograms of solvent). For dilute aqueous solutions, however, molality and molarity are nearly identical, as the density of water is approximately 1 kg per liter.

Please solve this problem:

- The molality of a 300 mL aqueous solution containing 33.3 grams of calcium chloride is:

  A. 1 *m*
  B. 2 *m*
  C. 3 *m*
  D. 4 *m*

Problem solved:

The correct answer is A. The molality is given by:

$$m = \frac{\text{moles of solute}}{\text{kilograms of solvent}}$$

$$\frac{0.3 \text{ mol } CaCl_2}{0.3 \text{ kg } H_2O} = 1 \text{ } m$$

(Note that the density of water is roughly 1 kilogram per liter. Therefore, 0.3 liters of water has a mass of 0.3 kg.)

18.1.2.4 Mole Fraction

The **mole fraction** of a solution is usually of interest only in problems involving gases, or problems concerned with vapor pressure. Mole fraction (X_s, where s is the substance under consideration) is defined as:

$$X_s = \frac{\text{moles of solute (s)}}{\text{total moles of solution}}$$

Please solve this problem:

- An air sample contains 77% nitrogen, 16% oxygen, and 7% carbon dioxide by weight. The mole fraction of oxygen in the air is:

  A. 0.147
  B. 0.160
  C. 0.172
  D. 0.512

Problem solved:

The correct answer is A. To solve this problem, we must first convert the weight percentages to moles. For convenience, assume that this air sample had a mass of 100 g. As such, there are 77 grams of nitrogen, 16 grams of oxygen, and 7 grams of carbon dioxide. Converting to moles:

$$N_2 : \quad \frac{77\ g}{28\ g/mol} = 2.75\ mol\ N_2$$

$$O_2 : \quad \frac{16\ g}{32\ g/mol} = 0.50\ mol\ O_2$$

$$CO_2 : \quad \frac{7\ g}{44\ g/mol} = 0.16\ mol\ CO_2$$

You can add the moles together to get 3.41 mol. From this, the mole fraction of oxygen gas is given by:

$$X_{O_2} = \frac{0.50\ mol\ O_2}{3.41\ total\ moles} = 0.147$$

18.1.3 SOLUBILITY AND SATURATION: K_{sp}

In Chapter 16, we discussed the equilibrium constant, K_{eq}. For the general reaction:

$$aA + bB \rightleftharpoons cC + dD$$

the equilibrium constant is given by:

$$K_{eq} = \frac{[C]^c [D]^d}{[A]^a [B]^b}$$

The solubility product constant, K_{sp}, is the equilibrium constant that results when a solid is in equilibrium with its solution:

$$A_aB_b(s) \rightleftharpoons aA(aq) + bB(aq)$$

(Assuming A_aB_b is an ionic solute, A is the cation and B is the anion.)

Recall that pure liquids and pure solids do not appear in equilibrium expressions. Since A_aB_b is a pure solid, it does not affect the equilibrium constant, which then reduces to:

$$K_{eq} = K_{sp} = [A]^a[B]^b$$

Note that K_{sp} will never have a denominator.

K_{sp} is the solubility product constant for a substance; it is *not* the solubility of that substance. Solubility is the amount of substance (expressed in grams) that may be dissolved in a unit volume of solution. Solubility may be calculated from a known value of K_{sp}, or vice versa.

For example, assume that it is known that the solubility of A_2B is 1×10^{-2} moles per liter of solution. We may now calculate K_{sp}.

From the equilibrium expression:

$$A_2B(s) \rightleftharpoons 2A^+(aq) + B^{2-}(aq)$$

we see that for every one A_2B that is dissolved, two A^+ and one B^{2-} go into solution.

$$A_2B(s) \rightleftharpoons 2A^+(aq) + B^{2-}(aq)$$
$$x \qquad 2x \qquad x$$

Knowing that solubility, x, is 1×10^{-2} M, and employing the equilibrium expression for this reaction:

$$K_{sp} = [A]^2[B] = [2x]^2[x] = [4x^2][x] = 4x^3 = (4)(1 \times 10^{-2})^3 = 4 \times 10^{-6}$$

Similarly, if K_{sp} is known, solubility may be determined.

Please solve this problem:

- The K_{sp} of aluminum hydroxide is 3.7×10^{-15} at 25°C. The solubility of aluminum hydroxide at this temperature is:

  A. 9.3×10^{-16} M
  B. 3.7×10^{-15} M
  C. 6.1×10^{-8} M
  D. 1.1×10^{-4} M

Problem solved:

The correct answer is D. The equilibrium expression for aluminum hydroxide is given by:

$$Al(OH)_3 \rightleftharpoons Al^{3+} + 3OH^-$$
$$x \qquad x \qquad 3x$$

Therefore, the solubility product constant, K_{sp}, is given by:

$$K_{sp} = [Al^{3+}][OH^-]^3 = [x][3x]^3 = 27x^4$$

Since we are told that $K_{sp} = 3.7 \times 10^{-15}$, this becomes:

$$27x^4 = 3.7 \times 10^{-15}$$

or,

$$x = \text{approx. } 1.1 \times 10^{-4} M$$

18.1.4 COLLIGATIVE PROPERTIES

18.1.4.1 Definitions

A **colligative property** is a property that depends only on the number of particles present in solution and **not** on the identity of those particles. Colligative properties are only valid for aqueous solutions when the total concentration of particles (molality) is equal to or less than $0.5\ m$. The four most important colligative properties for the MCAT are discussed in the following sections.

When a substance is solvated, one of three processes occurs. These processes are summarized below:

Process	Effective Number of Particles
Simple solvation, no dissociation	Equal to the molality of the solution
Partial or complete dissociation	Greater than the molality of the solution
Aggregate formation	Less than the molality of the solution

Table 18.1

Most organic molecules are simply solvated by water, without dissociation or aggregation. Examples of molecules that are simply solvated include methanol, ethanol, glucose, and fructose.

Ionic compounds dissociate upon dissolving in water. Solutes that dissociate into constituent ions are **electrolytes**. **Strong electrolytes** dissociate completely or nearly completely, while **weak electrolytes** dissociate only slightly. Examples of strong electrolytes include salts of the alkali metals (Group 1) and of ammonium, some salts of the alkaline earth metals, all nitrates, chlorates, perchlorates, and acetates. Examples of weak electrolytes include weak acids and bases (Chapter 21), such as carbonic acid, phosphoric acid, acetic acid, and ammonia.

Some organic and ionic compounds with large ions of multiple charges aggregate upon solvation. Organic compounds that exhibit strong hydrogen bonding, or other strong intermolecular forces, tend to dimerize. Large ions from ionic compounds form ion pairs; as concentration of solute is increased, probability of ion pair formation increases.

Please answer this question:

- Which of the following would be expected to exhibit the highest change in the colligative properties of a dilute aqueous solution, given equal concentrations of each?

  A. Glucose
  B. Sodium chloride
  C. Potassium phosphate
  D. Silver(II) iodide

Question answered:

The correct answer is C. Glucose will not dissociate in water, therefore it consists of only one piece. Sodium chloride dissociates into two pieces. Silver(II) iodide dissociates into three pieces. Potassium phosphate dissociates into four pieces. The compound that dissociates into the largest number of pieces will have the greatest effect on the colligative properties of water. Therefore, the answer is potassium phosphate.

18.1.4.2 Vapor Pressure

The **vapor pressure** of a pure liquid is lowered by the addition of a nonvolatile solute. The vapor pressure of a liquid is the pressure exerted by its vapor at the liquid-gas interface when the liquid and vapor are at equilibrium. A high vapor pressure indicates a volatile liquid. A low vapor pressure indicates a nonvolatile liquid. When the pressure exerted by a liquid (the vapor pressure) is equal to the pressure of the gas above that liquid, the liquid will boil. When a solute is added to a liquid, solute particles reduce the tendency of solvent particles to escape into the vapor phase. It is this momentary escape into the gas phase by the individual liquid molecules that is responsible for the vapor pressure of the liquid.

The lowering of vapor pressure that is experienced by a liquid in which a nonvolatile solute is dissolved is given by **Raoult's law:**

$$p_i = X_i p_i^\circ$$

where p_i is the **vapor pressure of the solvent i above the solution i**, X_i is the **mole fraction of the solvent i**, and p_i° is the **vapor pressure of the pure solvent i**.

Please solve this problem:

- The vapor pressure of pure water is 0.3 atm at 300 K. Calculate the vapor pressure above a solution prepared from 360 grams of water and 90 grams of glucose ($C_6H_{12}O_6$) at 300 K.

  A. 0.32 atm
  B. 0.30 atm
  C. 0.29 atm
  D. 0.26 atm

Problem solved:

The correct answer is C. To solve this problem, we must use Raoult's law:

$$p_{H_2O} = X_{H_2O} p_{H_2O}^\circ$$

where,

$$p_{H_2O}^\circ = 0.3 \text{ atm}$$

and

$$X_{H_2O} = \frac{(360 \text{ g } H_2O)\left(\dfrac{1 \text{ mol}}{18 \text{ g}}\right)}{(360 \text{ g } H_2O)\left(\dfrac{1 \text{ mol}}{18 \text{ g}}\right) + (90 \text{ g } C_6H_{12}O_6)\left(\dfrac{1 \text{ mol}}{180 \text{ g}}\right)}$$

$$X_{H_2O} = \frac{20 \text{ mol}}{20 \text{ mol} + 0.5 \text{ mol}} = \frac{20}{20.5} = 0.976$$

Therefore,

$$p_{H_2O} = X_{H_2O} p_{H_2O}^\circ = (0.976)(0.3 \text{ atm}) = 0.29 \text{ atm}$$

18.1.4.3 Boiling Point Elevation

The boiling point of a pure liquid is elevated by the addition of a nonvolatile solute; this follows from the effect of solute on vapor pressure (**18.1.4.2**). The boiling point of a substance is defined as the temperature at which the vapor pressure of the substance is equal to atmospheric pressure. Since vapor pressure is lowered by the addition of nonvolatile solute, the solution will require a greater temperature before its vapor pressure is equal to atmospheric pressure. The **boiling point elevation** that is observed in a solution is given by:

$$\Delta T_b = K_b m$$

where ΔT_b is the boiling point elevation (boiling point of the solution minus boiling point of the pure solvent), K_b is the **boiling point elevation constant** (which is a constant for each solvent, $K_b(H_2O) = 0.52°C/m$), and m is the **molality of dissolved particles**.

Please solve this problem:

- The normal boiling point of pure water is 373.15 K. Calculate the boiling point of a solution prepared from 360 grams of water and 106 grams of sodium carbonate (Na_2CO_3), $K_b = 0.52°C/m$.

    A. 368.82 K
    B. 373.15 K
    C. 375.93 K
    D. 377.48 K

Problem solved:

The correct answer is D. To solve this problem, we must first determine the molality of the sodium carbonate solution:

From the equilibrium expression:

$$Na_2CO_3 \rightleftharpoons 2Na^+ + CO_3^{2-}$$

we see that there are three components to each sodium carbonate unit.

$$\frac{(3)(106 \text{ g Na}_2CO_3)\left(\dfrac{1 \text{ mol Na}_2CO_3}{106 \text{ g Na}_2CO_3}\right)}{0.360 \text{ kg H}_2O} = 8.33 \text{ } m$$

Using the boiling point elevation equation:

$$\Delta T_b = K_b m$$

$$\Delta T_b = (0.52)(8.33), \text{ or } 4.33 \text{ K}$$

Since the boiling point is elevated, the boiling point of this solution is equal to:

$$373.15 \text{ K} + 4.33 \text{ K} = 377.48 \text{ K}$$

18.1.4.4 Freezing Point Depression

The freezing point of a pure liquid is depressed by the addition of a solute. The freezing point of a substance is defined as the point at which the attractive forces between the molecules are just great enough to cause a phase change from the liquid state to the solid state. Since solvent molecules are forced to be further apart in a solution than in the pure liquid state, it follows that a lower temperature will be required to reach the point at which the solvent molecules exert sufficient attractive forces upon one another to induce the formation of a solid state. The **freezing point depression** that is observed in a solution is given by:

$$\Delta T_f = K_f m$$

where ΔT_f is the **freezing point depression** (freezing point of the pure solvent minus freezing point of the solution), K_f is the **freezing point depression constant** (which is a constant for each solvent, $K_f(H_2O) = 1.86°C/m$), and m is the **molality of dissolved particles**.

Please solve this problem:

- The normal freezing point of pure water is 273.15 K. Calculate the freezing point of a solution prepared from 1800 grams of water and 106 grams of sodium carbonate (Na_2CO_3), $K_f = 1.86° \text{ C}/m$.

  A. 270.04 K
  B. 272.12 K
  C. 273.15 K
  D. 276.26 K

Problem solved:

The correct answer is A. To solve this problem, we must first determine the molality of the sodium carbonate solution:

From the equilibrium expression:

$$Na_2CO_3 \rightleftharpoons 2\,Na^+ + CO_3^{2-}$$

we see that there are three components to each sodium carbonate unit.

$$\frac{(3)(106\ \text{g Na}_2\text{CO}_3)\left(\dfrac{1\ \text{mol Na}_2\text{CO}_3}{106\ \text{g Na}_2\text{CO}_3}\right)}{1.800\ \text{kg H}_2\text{O}} = 1.67\ m$$

Using the freezing point depression equation:

$$\Delta T_f = K_f m = (1.86)(1.67) = 3.11\ \text{K}$$

Since the freezing point is depressed, the freezing point of this solution is equal to:

$$273.15\ \text{K} - 3.11\ \text{K} = 270.04\ \text{K}$$

18.1.4.5 Osmotic Pressure

Osmosis is the spontaneous process by which solvent molecules (but not solute molecules) pass through a semipermeable membrane along a concentration gradient. **Osmotic pressure** is the excess hydrostatic pressure created on the more concentrated side of a semipermeable membrane due to osmosis. Because a greater concentration of solvent molecules is initially present on the dilute side of the membrane, more solvent molecules will collide with the membrane per unit time on this side. Therefore, more solvent molecules will pass from the dilute side to the concentrated side than from the concentrated side to the dilute side. This process will continue until equilibrium is reached. The pressure exerted on the membrane when equilibrium is reached is the osmotic pressure. The osmotic pressure of a solution is increased by the addition of solute.

Osmotic pressure is given by the equation:

$$\pi = \frac{n}{V}RT$$

where π is the osmotic pressure, n is the number of moles of particles dissolved, R is the gas constant, T is the absolute temperature, and V is the volume of the solution. Since

$$M = \frac{n}{V}$$

We can rewrite the equation for osmotic pressure as:

$$\pi = MRT$$

Also, since molarity and molality may be considered to be identical for dilute aqueous solution, this may be written:

$$\pi = mRT$$

Please solve this problem:

- Calculate the osmotic pressure of a 0.1 M solution of barium hydroxide at 300 K, $R = 0.0821$ L•atm/mol•K.

  A. 0.25 atm
  B. 2.46 atm
  C. 4.93 atm
  D. 7.39 atm

Problem solved:

The correct answer is D. To solve this problem, we must first convert molarity of the solution into molality of dissolved particles. Given the equilibrium expression:

$$Ba(OH)_2 \rightleftharpoons Ba^{2+} + 2OH^-$$

we see that barium hydroxide dissociates into three components. Therefore, the total molality of dissolved particles is $(0.1\ M)(3) = 0.3\ m$. Using the equation for osmotic pressure, we get:

$$(0.3\ m)(0.0821\ L•atm/mol•K)(300\ K) = 7.39\ atm$$

18.2 MASTERY APPLIED: SAMPLE PASSAGE AND QUESTIONS

Passage

Colligative properties are properties of a substance that depend only upon the number of particles involved, not upon the chemical nature of these substances. Colligative properties, such as boiling point elevation, freezing point depression, and osmotic pressure, may be used to determine the molecular weight of an unknown chemical compound.

Boiling point elevation is given by the equation:

$$\Delta T_b = K_b m$$

where ΔT_b is the observed elevation in boiling point, K_b is the boiling point elevation constant for the solvent (tabulated in the table below), and m is the molality of the solution. Since molality is defined as the number of moles of dissolved particles per kilogram of solvent, for a chemical sub-stance that does not dissociate in solution, molality is equal to the number of moles of solute per kilogram of solvent. Once the number of moles has been determined, calculation of the molecular weight is easily accomplished: (mass of unknown added to solution) ÷ (moles of unknown).

The equation for freezing point depression takes a form similar to that for boiling point elevation:

$$\Delta T_f = K_f m$$

where ΔT_f is the observed depression in freezing point, K_f is the freezing point depression constant for the solvent, and m is the molality of the solution. Molecular weight of an unknown is found in a manner analogous to that employed for boiling point elevation data.

Solvent	Normal Boiling Point (°C)	$K_b(°C/m)$	Normal Freezing Point (°C)	$K_f(°C/m)$
benzene	80.1	2.53	5.5	4.90
water	100.0	0.52	0	1.86
acetic acid	117.9	3.07	16.6	3.90
phenol	181.8	3.56	43.0	7.40

1. Assuming that boiling point and freezing point may be determined with equal accuracy, the most accurate measure of the molecular weight of a solute would come from a measurement of the:

   A. boiling point elevation of water.
   B. boiling point elevation of benzene.
   C. freezing point depression of phenol.
   D. freezing point depression of water.

2. The smallest boiling point elevation is demonstrated by a 0.1 M solution of:

   A. sodium chloride in water.
   B. glucose in benzene.
   C. glucose in phenol.
   D. glucose in acetic acid.

3. The solution with the lowest freezing point is:

   A. 50 g sodium chloride in 1 kg water.
   B. 360 g glucose in 1 kg water.
   C. 50 g sodium chloride in 1 kg phenol.
   D. 360 g glucose in 1 kg phenol.

4. A solution is prepared from 100 grams of an unknown material and 1 kg water. This solution has a boiling point of 101.8°C at 1 atm. The identity of the unknown material is most likely:

   A. NaCl
   B. $Ba(OH)_2$
   C. NH_4NO_3
   D. $C_6H_{12}O_6$

5. Two solutions containing equal molar quantities of an unknown material are prepared, using water and acetic acid as solvents. The aqueous solution has a freezing point of –4.65°C. The acetic acid solution has a freezing point of 9.58°C. The best explanation for this difference is that:

   A. the unknown material dissociated equally in the two solvents.
   B. the unknown material dissociated to a greater extent in water than in acetic acid.
   C. the unknown material dissociated to a greater extent in acetic acid than in water.
   D. the unknown material aggregated in water, but it did not aggregate in acetic acid.

6. An aqueous glucose solution has a boiling point of 101.44°C at 1 atm. The approximate ratio of water to glucose, by mass, is:

   A. 1:4
   B. 1:2
   C. 2:1
   D. 4:1

7. An aqueous solution has a boiling point of 101.3°C at 1 atm. This solution is cooled to the freezing point. The freezing point is measured as – 4.09°C. The discrepancy between the boiling point elevation and freezing point depression is most likely due to:

   A. the difference in K_b and K_f for water.
   B. the difference in the volume of water at 100°C versus 0°C.
   C. the difference in solubility of the solute at 100°C versus 0°C.
   D. the difference in the solvation process for the solute at 100°C versus 0°C.

18.3 MASTERY VERIFIED: ANSWERS AND EXPLANATIONS

1. *The correct answer is C.* That measurement that will provide the greatest accuracy is the measurement of the solvent that undergoes the greatest change per molal in phase change temperature (either boiling point elevation or freezing point depression). From the table provided, we see that this is the freezing point depression of phenol ($7.40°C/m$).

2. *The correct answer is A.* To solve this problem, we must convert molarity into molality of particles. For choices B, C, and D, molality is equivalent to molarity, since there is no dissociation in any of these solutions. For choice A, each sodium chloride unit will dissociate into two particles in solution, so molality is twice molarity, or $0.2\ m$.

   Next, we must multiply the molalities of the solutions by the boiling point elevation constants of the solvents:

   A: $(0.2\ m)(0.52°C/m) = 0.104°C$
   B: $(0.1\ m)(2.53°C/m) = 0.253°C$
   C: $(0.1\ m)(3.56°C/m) = 0.356°C$
   D: $(0.1\ m)(3.07°C/m) = 0.307°C$

   The smallest boiling point elevation is given by the solution in choice A.

3. *The correct answer is B.* To solve this problem, we must make sure that we solve for freezing point, *not* for freezing point depression.

   A: $\Delta T_f = (1.86°C/m)\dfrac{(50\ g)(2\ particle)}{(58.5\ g/mol)} = 3.18°C$ $\Delta T_f = 0°C - 3.18°C = -3.18°C$

   B: $\Delta T_f = (1.86°C/m)\dfrac{(360\ g)(1\ particle)}{(180\ g/mol)} = 3.72°C$ $\Delta T_f = 0°C - 3.72°C = -3.72°C$

   C: $\Delta T_f = (7.40°C/m)\dfrac{(50\ g)(2\ particle)}{(58.5\ g/mol)} = 12.64°C$ $\Delta T_f = 43°C - 12.64°C = 30.26°C$

   D: $\Delta T_f = (7.40°C/m)\dfrac{(360\ g)(1\ particle)}{(180\ g/mol)} = 14.80°C$ $\Delta T_f = 43°C - 14.80°C = 28.20°C$

   From the above calculations, we see that the solution in choice A provides the lowest freezing point.

4. *The correct answer is A.* From the problem, we see that the solution has a boiling point elevation of $1.8°C$.

   $$\Delta T_f = \frac{(100\ g)(2\ particles)}{(58.5\ g/mol)}(.52°C/m) = 1.8°C$$

5. *The correct answer is B.* A freezing point depression of 4.65°C in water corresponds to a solution that has a molality given by:

$$4.65°C \div 1.86°C/m = 2.5\ m$$

A freezing point of 9.58°C, in acetic acid gives a freezing point depression of

$$16.6°C - 9.58°C = 7.02°C$$

A freezing point depression of 7.02°C in acetic acid corresponds to a solution that has a molality of:

$$7.02°C \div 3.90°C/m = 1.8\ m$$

Therefore, the molality of this substance in water is higher than the molality of this substance in acetic acid.

6. *The correct answer is C.* A boiling point elevation of 1.44°C corresponds to a molality of:

$$1.44°C \div 0.52°C/m = 2.77\ m$$

Since the molecular weight of glucose is 180 g/mol, a molality of 2.77 *m* corresponds to:

$$180\ g/mol \times 2.77\ mol = 498.6$$

This 500 grams of glucose is per kilogram (1000 g) of water, by the definition of molality. Therefore, the ratio of water to glucose is 1000:500, or 2:1.

7. *The correct answer is C.* At the boiling point, the molality of the solution is:

$$1.3°C \div 0.52°C/m = 2.5\ m$$

At the freezing point, the molality of the solution is:

$$4.09°C \div 1.86°C/m = 2.2\ m$$

Therefore, the molality of the solution is higher at the boiling point than at the freezing point.

CHAPTER 19

GASES

19.1 MASTERY ACHIEVED

19.1.1 THE GAS PHASE AND ASSOCIATED PHENOMENA

19.1.1.1 Temperature

Temperature is a function of the **average translational kinetic energy** of the molecule in a system. As the molecular kinetic energy of a system increases, the temperature increases. As the molecular kinetic energy of a system decreases, the temperature decreases. A temperature scale may be either **absolute** or **relative**. The absolute temperature scale you must be familiar with is **Kelvin (K)**. The **Celsius** scale (°C) and the **Fahrenheit** scale (°F) are examples of relative scales. A relative temperature scale chooses two points of known energy and assigns them fixed and convenient values. The Celsius scale fixes the temperature of the freezing point of water at 1 atm as 0°C, and the temperature of the boiling point of water at 1 atm as 100°C. The Fahrenheit scale fixes the temperature of the freezing point of water at 1 atm as 32°F, and the temperature of the boiling point of water at 1 atm as 212°F. The MCAT does not use the Fahrenheit scale, so you don't need to concern yourself with conversions from Celsius to Fahrenheit.

Absolute zero (0 K) is the lowest possible temperature. At this temperature, virtually all movement has ceased. The third law of thermodynamics shows that absolute zero is unattainable (**17.1.1.6**), but it can still be determined with great accuracy. The Kelvin temperature scale is based on the Celsius scale in that one degree Kelvin is equivalent in magnitude to one degree Celsius. Absolute zero on the Celsius scale is –273.15°C, therefore the conversion from Celsius to Kelvin is given by:

$$K = °C + 273.15$$

It is important to notice that this relationship (a temperature increase of 1 K is equivalent to a temperature increase of 1°C) can give rise to traps on the MCAT. Also note that in the questions that follow, the Kelvin to Celsius conversion is rounded to K = °C + 273.

Please solve this problem:

- The rate at which heat is radiated by an object is given by the **Stefan-Boltzmann Law**: $H = Ae\sigma T^4$, where A is surface area, T is temperature of the substance, emissivity (e) is material specific and ranges from 1 for a black body radiator to 0 for a perfect reflector, and σ is 5.6×10^{-8} W/m²K⁴. The rate of heat radiated by a substance at –233°C would be equal to the rate of heat radiated by the same substance at –253°C times:

  A. 0.719
  B. 2
  C. 16
  D. 20

Problem solved:

C is the correct anwer. The key to answering this problem is to realize that the temperature has changed from –253°C to –233°C, but everything else (A, e, and σ) remains constant. Therefore, if we take –253°C as state 1 and –233°C as state 2, we have the following relationship:

$$\frac{H_2}{H_1} = \frac{Ae\sigma T_2^4}{Ae\sigma T_1^4} = \frac{T_2^4}{T_1^4}$$

$$\text{or, } H_2 = \left(\frac{T_2^4}{T_1^4}\right) H_1$$

This reduces the question to "what is the ratio of T_2^4 to T_1^4"? If you leave the temperatures in terms of °C, you will find:

$$\frac{T_2^4}{T_1^4} = \frac{(-233)^4}{(-253)^4} = \frac{2.947 \times 10^9}{4.097 \times 10^9} = 0.719$$

But this is a trap. Convert the temperatures to the Kelvin scale (as the units of σ make necessary). $T_1 = 20$ K and $T_2 = 40$ K, or:

$$\frac{T_2^4}{T_1^4} = \frac{(40)^4}{(20)^4} = \frac{(2)^4 \times (20)^4}{(20)^4} = 2^4 = 16$$

19.1.1.2 Pressure

The **pressure** exerted by a gas is a measure of the **force per unit area** of the total of all the collisions that the moving gas particles have with the walls of their container:

$$P = \frac{F}{A}$$

Pressure depends on the number of **collisions** with the walls, the **velocity** of the colliding gas molecules, and the **mass** of the colliding gas molecules. As each of these factors increase, the pressure increases. The number of collisions with the walls will increase if there is a greater number of molecules, or if the same number of molecules are confined to a smaller volume. The velocity of the colliding gas molecules will increase as temperature (average kinetic energy) increases.

Pressure is measured in the SI units of **pascals (Pa)**.

$$P = \frac{F}{A} = \frac{N}{m^2} = Pa$$

Pressure may also be measured in **atmospheres (atm)**, **millimeters of mercury (mmHg)**, or **torr**.

$$1 \text{ atm} = 760 \text{ mmHg} = 760 \text{ torr} = 1.013 \times 10^5 \text{ Pa}$$

19.1.1.3 STP

Standard temperature and pressure (STP) is defined as 0°C and 760 torr. This is a reference point for the comparison of one gas to another. One mole of an ideal gas at STP occupies a volume of 22.4 liters (or 0.0224 m³ in SI units). It should be noted that gas STP differs from the standard state for thermodynamic functions. The temperature at STP for a gas is 0°C, the temperature of the standard thermodynamic state is 25°C. Both are defined at a pressure of 760 torr, or 1 atm.

19.1.2 KINETIC MOLECULAR THEORY

The **kinetic molecular theory** of gases regards a gas as a collection of point masses in constant chaotic independent motion. There are five basic premises of kinetic molecular theory:

1. Gases are composed of molecules, or particles, which are in **rapid, random translational motion** (straight-line motion). Because these particles have mass and velocity, they possess kinetic energy given by: $KE = \frac{1}{2}mv^2$

2. The particles undergo collisions with the walls of their container and with one another. These collisions are perfectly elastic: There is no loss of kinetic energy during any collision.

3. At any instant in time, the particles are separated by a distance much greater than the size of the particles themselves. Thus, the space occupied by the particles is negligible with regard to the size of the container.

4. There are no attractive nor repulsive forces between the particles.

5. The average kinetic energy of the particles is directly proportional to the absolute temperature of the particles. From the **Maxwell-Boltzmann distribution**: $KE = \frac{3}{2}nRT$, where n = moles of gas particles, R = the Universal Gas Constant, and T = temperature of the gas.

The first statement says that any particle that possesses both mass and velocity will have a kinetic energy given by: $KE = \frac{1}{2}mv^2$.

The second statement says that all collisions are elastic. In practice, perfectly elastic collisions are extremely rare.

The third states that there is no excluded volume. That is, none of the volume of the container is excluded from use by any one gas molecule at any moment in time. This, of course, is not true. The only way this could be true is if only one gas molecule was present in a given volume, or if the gas particles were truly point masses.

The fourth states that all other gas particles do not influence each other except in collisions.

However, as we have seen (**14.1.1**), all molecules will exert either repulsive or attractive forces upon one another (**London dispersion forces**).

The fifth is a statement of the Maxwell-Boltzmann distribution, which is a special case of the equipartition theorem of classical physics. When quantum effects become important, the equipartition theorem, and thus the Maxwell-Boltzmann distribution, fails.

Ideal behavior of gases relies upon the above five premises, so they will be considered valid throughout section **19.1.3**. Deviations from ideality, which are caused by the failure of one or more of the five premises of the kinetic molecular theory, are treated in detail in section **19.1.4**.

19.1.3 THE GAS LAWS

19.1.3.1 Boyle's Law

Boyle's law for ideal gases states that under conditions of constant temperature and with a constant number of moles of gas, the product of pressure and volume is a constant:

$$PV = \text{constant}$$

$$\text{or, } P_1 V_1 = P_2 V_2$$

The subscript 1 refers to initial conditions and the subscript 2 refers to conditions after either a change in volume or a change in pressure. The important relationship to understand from this law is that pressure and volume are inversely proportional:

$$P \propto \frac{1}{V}$$

$$V \propto \frac{1}{P}$$

Please solve this problem:

- A fixed quantity of gas at a temperature of 200°C has a volume of 2 liters and pressure of 2 atm. If the volume is increased to 6 liters, the pressure is:

  A. increased by a factor of nine.
  B. increased by a factor of three.
  C. decreased by a factor of three.
  D. decreased by a factor of nine.

Problem solved:

C is the correct answer. Using Boyle's law:

$$P_2 = \left(\frac{V_1}{V_2}\right) P_1 = \left(\frac{2}{6}\right) P_1 = \frac{P_1}{3}$$

Therefore, P_2 is decreased by a factor of three.

19.1.3.2 Charles's Law

Charles's law establishes the relationship between volume and temperature for ideal gases under conditions of constant pressure and a constant number of moles of gas:

$$\frac{V}{T} = \text{constant}$$

$$\text{or, } V = (\text{constant})(T)$$

$$\text{or, } \frac{V_1}{T_1} = \frac{V_2}{T_2}$$

$$\text{or, } V_1 T_2 = V_2 T_1$$

The important relationship to remember from this law is that temperature and volume are directly proportional:

$$V \propto T$$
$$T \propto V$$

Please solve this problem:

- A fixed quantity of gas at a constant pressure of 10 atm and a temperature of 500 K is heated. If the temperature is increased to 750 K, the gas will occupy a volume that is:

  A. twice the original volume.
  B. one and a half times the original volume.
  C. equal to the original volume.
  D. two-thirds of the original volume.

Problem solved:

B is the correct answer. Using Charles's law:

$$V_2 = \left(\frac{T_2}{T_1} \right) V_1 = \left(\frac{750}{500} \right) V_1 = \left(\frac{1.5T_1}{T_1} \right) V_1 = 1.5 V_1$$

Therefore, V_2 is increased by a factor of one and a half.

19.1.3.3 Gay-Lussac's Law

Gay-Lussac's law includes Charles's law and the relationship between pressure and temperature under conditions of constant volume and a constant number of moles of gas:

$$\frac{P}{T} = \text{constant}$$

$$\text{or, } P = (\text{constant})(T)$$

$$\text{or, } \frac{P_1}{T_1} = \frac{P_2}{T_2}$$

$$\text{or, } P_1 T_2 = P_2 T_1$$

The important relationship to understand from this law is that temperature is directly proportional to pressure and that pressure is, therefore, also directly proportional to temperature:

$$P \propto T$$
$$T \propto P$$

Please solve this problem:

- A fixed quantity of gas at a constant volume and a temperature of 500 K has a pressure of 5 atm. If the temperature is increased to 750 K, the gas will develop a pressure of:

  A. 10 atm
  B. 7.5 atm
  C. 5 atm
  D. 3.33 atm

Problem solved:

The correct answer is B. Using Gay-Lussac's law:

$$P_2 = \left(\frac{T_2}{T_1}\right) P_1 = \left(\frac{750}{500}\right) P_1 = \left(\frac{1.5 T_1}{T_1}\right) P_1 = 1.5 P_1 = 1.5(5 \text{ atm}) = 7.5 \text{ atm}$$

Therefore, P_2 is increased by a factor of one and a half to 7.5 atm.

19.1.3.4 The Combined Gas Law

The **combined gas law** unites the relationships found in Boyle's law, Charles's law and Gay-Lussac's law, for conditions where the number of moles of gas is constant, as:

$$\frac{PV}{T} = \text{constant}$$
$$\text{or, } PV = (\text{constant})(T)$$
$$\text{or, } \frac{P_1 V_1}{T_1} = \frac{P_2 V_2}{T_2}$$
$$\text{or, } P_1 V_1 T_2 = P_2 V_2 T_1$$

Please solve this problem:

- A gas has an initial volume of 5 liters at a temperature of 400 K. If the volume of the same amount of gas is 15 liters at 800 K, the pressure is:

  A. increased by a factor of six.
  B. increased by a factor of one and a half.
  C. decreased by one-third.

D. decreased by five-sixths.

Problem solved:

C is the correct answer. Using the combined gas law:

$$\frac{P_1V_1}{T_1} = \frac{P_2V_2}{T_2}$$

which becomes:

$$P_2 = \frac{P_1V_1T_2}{V_2T_1} = \left(\frac{V_1}{V_2}\right)\left(\frac{T_2}{T_1}\right)P_1 = \left(\frac{5}{15}\right)\left(\frac{800}{400}\right)P_1 = \left(\frac{1}{3}\right)(2)P_1 = \frac{2}{3}P_1$$

Therefore, since the volume change decreases the pressure by a factor of three, and the temperature increases the pressure by a factor of two, the overall effect is a decrease in pressure of one-third.

19.1.3.5 Avogadro's Hypothesis

Avogadro's hypothesis establishes the relationship between the number of moles (n) of gas and volume for ideal gases under conditions of constant pressure and constant temperature:

$$\frac{V}{n} = \text{constant}$$

$$\text{or, } V = (\text{constant})(n)$$

$$\text{or, } \frac{V_1}{n_1} = \frac{V_2}{n_2}$$

$$\text{or, } V_1n_2 = V_2n_1$$

The important relationship to extract from this hypothesis is that volume is directly proportional to number of moles of gas and that number of moles of gas is, therefore, also directly proportional to volume:

$$V \propto n$$

$$n \propto V$$

This hypothesis also asserts that under identical pressure and temperature conditions, the volume taken up by one mole of a gas is equal to the volume taken up by one mole of any other gas.

Please solve this problem:

- Initially a balloon at STP has a volume of 2.24 liters. If the gas in the balloon is allowed to escape until the balloon has a volume of one-tenth the original volume, the total number of moles of gas in the balloon (still at STP) is:

  A. 0.01 mol
  B. 0.1 mol
  C. 1 mol

D. not determinable from the information provided.

Problem solved:

A is the correct answer. From Avogadro's hypothesis, since $n \propto V$, when V decreases by a factor of 10, n must also decrease by a factor of 10. We now know:

$$n_2 = \frac{n_1}{10}$$

But how much was n_1? This we can get from the information that the balloon is at STP. From section **19.1.1.3**, one mole of gas occupies a volume of 22.4 liters at STP. Again using Avogadro's hypothesis:

$$\frac{V_1}{n_1} = \frac{V_{STP}}{n_{STP}}, \text{ therefore, } n_1 = \frac{V_1 n_{STP}}{V_{STP}} = \frac{(2.24)(1)}{(22.4)} = 0.1 \text{ mol}$$

Plugging this back into our first equation:

$$n_2 = \frac{n_1}{10} = \frac{0.1 \text{ mol}}{10} = 0.01 \text{ mol}$$

19.1.3.6 The Ideal Gas Law and the Gas Constant

Avogadro's hypothesis may be incorporated into the combined gas law to give the following relationship:

$$\frac{PV}{nT} = \text{constant}$$

This constant, since it holds for any ideal gas, is called the **universal gas constant** and is symbolized by R. Thus,

$$\frac{PV}{nT} = R$$

or, $PV = nRT$

In SI units, the value of R is given by:

$$R = \frac{PV}{nT} = \frac{(Pa)(m^3)}{(mol)(K)} = \frac{\left(\frac{N}{m^2}\right)(m^3)}{(mol)(K)} = \frac{(N \cdot m)}{(mol)(K)} = \frac{J}{(mol)(K)}$$

If we consider conditions of STP (**19.1.1.3**), we can numerically solve for R:

$$R = \frac{PV}{nT} = \frac{(1.01325 \times 10^5 \text{Pa})(0.0022414 \text{m}^3)}{(1 \text{mol})(273.15 \text{K})} = 8.314 \frac{J}{(mol)(K)}$$

You don't need to memorize the value of the universal gas constant; it will be provided on the MCAT.

Under conditions of low pressure and high temperature, the ideal gas law holds for most gases. Deviations from the ideal occur at low temperatures and at high pressures (conditions that tend to favor the formation of a liquid phase from the gas phase), and these deviations are the subject of the next section (19.1.4).

Please solve this problem:

- A sample of gas has a volume of 100 ml at 35°C and 740 torr. The gas constant, R, is 0.0821 L•atm/mol•K. The volume of the same quantity of gas at STP is:

  A. 114 ml
  B. 106 ml
  C. 100 ml
  D. 86 ml

Problem solved:

D is the correct answer. First we must convert all units into the units given for R:

$$V = 100 \text{ ml} = 0.100 \text{ L}$$

$$T = 35°C = 308 \text{ K}$$

$$P = 740 \text{ torr} = 0.974 \text{ atm}$$

Then, using the ideal gas law to solve for the initial number of moles:

$$n = \frac{PV}{RT} = \frac{(0.974 \text{ atm})(0.100 \text{ L})}{(0.0821 \text{ L} \cdot \text{atm/mol} \cdot \text{K})(308 \text{ K})} = 0.00385 \text{ mol.}$$

Finally, we solve for the final volume using the STP values of P = 1 atm and T = 273 K:

$$V_{STP} = \frac{nRT_{STP}}{P_{STP}} = \frac{(0.00385 \text{ mol})(0.0821 \text{ L} \cdot \text{atm/mol} \cdot \text{K})(273 \text{ K})}{1 \text{ atm}} = 0.086 \text{ L} = 86 \text{ ml}$$

As an alternative to performing all these calculations (which would have to be done on the MCAT without a calculator), we could instead set the ideal gas law for the initial conditions equal to the ideal gas law for the final conditions:

$$\frac{P_1 V_1}{n R T_1} = \frac{P_2 V_2}{n R T_2}$$

Rearrange to solve for V_2:

$$V_2 = \frac{P_1 n R T_2 V_1}{P_2 n R T_1} = \left(\frac{P_1}{P_2} \right) \left(\frac{n}{n} \right) \left(\frac{R}{R} \right) \left(\frac{T_2}{T_1} \right) V_1$$

Eliminate the unity terms:

$$V_2 = \left(\frac{P_1}{P_2} \right) \left(\frac{T_2}{T_1} \right) V_1$$

We must then recognize that since P_1 is 740 torr and P_2 is 760 torr, the ratio of P_1 to P_2 must be less than unity. Similarly, since T_2 is 273 K and T_1 is 308 K, the ratio of T_2 to T_1 must also be less than unity, therefore $V_2 < V_1$ and the answer must be D.

19.1.4 DEVIATIONS FROM IDEALITY

19.1.4.1 Deviations in Pressure

As temperature is decreased in a gas, the individual gas particles have decreasing kinetic energy (as seen in premise 5 of the kinetic molecular theory). As a result, the velocity of the particles is decreased, which leads to a higher probability of inelastic collisions (violation of premise 2). Molecules that are moving at a slower velocity are also more likely to feel the attractive or repulsive forces of other gas molecules in the container (violation of premise 4). Any, or all, of these factors will lead to the measurement of an actual pressure that is less than the pressure calculated from the ideal gas law. *The actual pressure exerted by a gas is always less than or equal to the pressure calculated by the ideal gas law.*

19.1.4.2 Deviations in Volume

As the pressure of a gas is increased, the volume occupied by the individual gas particles themselves becomes more important. As pressure goes up, the volume in which gas particles move goes down. Therefore, the average separation between any two gas molecules must also decrease (violation of premise 3). Individual gas molecules now occupy a more significant amount of the total volume. Thus, there is an **excluded volume**, which is the volume occupied by the gas molecules themselves. The actual volume of the gas is equal to the volume of the container plus the excluded volume. *The actual volume occupied by a gas is always greater than or equal to the volume calculated by the ideal gas law.*

19.1.4.3 van der Waals's Equation

The results of the above two sections are summarized by the **van der Waals' equation**:

$$\left(P + \frac{an^2}{V^2}\right)(V - nb) = nRT$$

It is not important to memorize this equation, but you should be familiar with the form. The $\frac{an^2}{V^2}$ term is a correction factor for the presence of intermolecular forces and the nb term is a correction factor that accounts for the excluded volume. The constants a and b are specific to individual gases. Employing the van der Waals equation, we see that the relationship between ideal pressure (P_I) and actual pressure (P_A) is given by:

$$P_I = P_A + \frac{an^2}{V^2}$$

and that the relationship between ideal volume (V_I) and actual volume (V_A) is given by:

$$V_I = V_A - nb$$

Please solve this problem:

- When a gas deviates from ideal gas values, the pressure and volume measured will be related to the values calculated from the ideal gas law by which of the following?

  A. Both measured values will be higher than the calculated values.

  B. The measured pressure will be higher, the measured volume will be lower.

  C. The measured pressure will be lower, the measured volume will be higher.

  D. Both measured values will be lower than the calculated values.

Problem solved:

C is the correct answer. This is a simple application of the van der Waals equation. If you did not answer this question correctly, you should reread section **19.1.4**.

19.1.5 MIXTURES OF GASES

19.1.5.1 Dalton's Law

The key to understanding gaseous mixtures is to assume that each individual gas behaves as if no other gases are present. In terms of number of moles (n), it is obvious that the presence of other gases does not affect this value. In terms of temperature, each individual gas will have an average kinetic energy that is directly proportional to the temperature: each gas will have the same distribution of energies as each other gas, and these will be independent of the presence of the other gases. Since we can assume that, under ideal conditions, all gas molecules occupy no volume, the presence of other gases in a container with a gas will not affect the volume of the container that is available to this gas. Pressure is affected by the presence of other gases. Since pressure is a measure of the force of gas particle collisions against the walls of the container, it stands to reason that each gas of a mixture will contribute only part of the total pressure on the container walls (since all gases collide with the walls).

Dalton's law of partial pressures sets forth the relationship between the total pressure exerted by the mixture and that part of the pressure that is due to a given gas in the mixture. This law states that the pressure exerted by a mixture of gases behaving ideally is equal to the sum of the pressures exerted by the individual gases:

$$P_T = P_A + P_B$$

where P_T is the total pressure exerted by a mixture of gas A and gas B, P_A is the pressure that gas A would exert alone under the same conditions in the same volume, and P_B is the pressure that gas B would exert alone. Putting this relationship into the ideal gas law yields:

$$P_T = \frac{(n_A + n_B)RT}{V}$$

where n_A and n_B are the number of moles of gas A and gas B, respectively. Put another way, the partial pressure exerted by gas A is equal to the product of the total pressure exerted by the mixture and the mole fraction of gas A that is present in the mixture:

$$P_A = X_A P_T$$

where X_A is the mole fraction of gas A, which is given by:

$$X_A = \frac{n_A}{n_T} = \frac{n_A}{n_A + n_B}$$

Vapor pressure is a special case of Dalton's law that applies to gases in contact with a liquid. In this case, some molecules of the liquid will escape into gas phase and contribute to the total gas pressure. The partial pressure so exerted by the liquid (by molecules that have escaped into the gas phase) is the vapor pressure of the liquid. The vapor pressure of a liquid is dependent on its temperature.

Please solve this problem:

- The vapor pressure of water at 296 K is 0.0275 atm. The value of the gas constant is 0.0821 L•atm/mol•K. If 500 ml of oxygen is collected over a bath of water at a temperature of 296 K and a pressure of 0.5135 atm, the weight of the oxygen collected will be:

  A. 32.00 g.
  B. 3.2 g.
  C. 0.32 g.
  D. 0.032 g.

Problem solved:

C is the correct answer. To solve this problem, we must realize that the ideal gas law may also be written:

$$PV = \left(\frac{m}{MW}\right)RT$$

since moles, n, is equal to mass (in grams) divided by molecular weight (in g/mol). We must also realize that the term P in the above equation refers to the partial pressure of oxygen, which is given by Dalton's law of partial pressures:

$$P_T = P_A + P_B$$

Taking A as oxygen and B as the water vapor, we can solve for P_A:

$$P_{O_2} = P_T - P_{H_2O} = 0.5135 - 0.0275 = 0.486 \text{ atm}$$

Plugging this and the other known values into the ideal gas law, we get:

$$m = \frac{PV(MW)}{RT} = \frac{(.486 \text{ atm})(.5 \text{ L})(32 \text{ g/mol})}{(0.0821 \text{ L} \cdot \text{atm/mol} \cdot \text{K})(296 \text{ K})} = 0.32 \text{ g}$$

Alternatively, if we had realized that the temperature given is approximately STP temperature and that the given pressure is approximately one-half of STP pressure, we could reason that our volume is approximately twice STP volume. Twice STP volume for one mole of gas is 44.8 liters. Using Avogadro's hypothesis, we could solve:

$$n_{O_2} = \left(\frac{V_{O_2}}{2V_{STP}}\right)n_{STP} = \left(\frac{.486 \text{ L}}{44.8 \text{ L}}\right)(1 \text{ mol}) \approx 0.01 \text{ mol}$$

From this, our approximate O_2 mass must be closest to 0.32 g—therefore the answer is C.

19.1.5.2 Raoult's Law

Raoult's law describes a relationship similar to Dalton's law, observed in certain ideal solutions. Raoult's law asserts that the vapor pressure exerted by a component of a liquid mixture is equal to the product of the vapor pressure of the pure component and the mole fraction of that component in the *liquid* phase:

$$P_{soln} = X_{solv}P_{solv}^*$$

where $P_{A(v)}$ is the vapor pressure exerted by liquid component A, $X_{A(\ell)}$ is the mole fraction of A in the liquid phase, and $P_{A(v)}^*$ is the vapor pressure of pure A. In the case of a nonvolatile solute dissolved in a solvent, the vapor pressure of the solution can be calculated from: $P_{soln} = X_{solv}P_{solv}^*$ where:

$$P_{soln} = \text{vapor pressure of solution}$$
$$X_{solv} = \text{mol fraction of solvent}$$
$$P_{solv}^* = \text{vapor pressure of pure solvent.}$$

Please solve this problem:

- The vapor pressure of water at 300 K is 0.3 atm. Calculate the vapor pressure above a solution prepared from 360 g of water and 106 g of sodium carbonate, Na_2CO_3.

A. 0.315 atm
B. 0.300 atm
C. 0.286 atm
D. 0.235 atm

Problem solved:

C *is the correct answer.* To solve this problem, we must first convert all terms given in grams to moles:

$$\text{moles } H_2O = \frac{360 \text{ g}}{18 \text{ g/mol}} = 20 \text{ mol}$$

$$\text{moles glucose} = \frac{180\,g}{180\,g/mol} = 1\,mol$$

Then we apply Raoult's law:

$$P_{soln} = X_{H_2O}P_{H_2O}^* = \left(\frac{20\,mol}{20\,mol + 1\,mol}\right)(0.300\,atm) = \left(\frac{20}{21}\right)(0.300\,atm) = 0.286\,atm$$

19.1.6 DIFFUSION AND EFFUSION OF GASES: GRAHAM'S LAW OF DIFFUSION

Diffusion is the movement of a gas through space, while **effusion** is the movement of a gas under pressure through a small hole. An example of effusion is the escape of air through the walls of a balloon along the pressure gradient as the balloon slowly deflates. The mathematics of diffusion and effusion are the same. Remember that premise 1 of the kinetic molecular theory (**19.1.2**) provided for gas molecules with an average kinetic energy of $KE = \frac{1}{2}mv^2$. Rewriting to solve for velocity, we get:

$$v = \sqrt{\frac{2KE}{m}}$$

from which come the two proportionalities:

$$v \propto (KE)^{1/2}$$

$$v \propto \left(\frac{1}{m}\right)^{1/2}$$

Remembering that kinetic energy is directly proportional to absolute temperature, which is premise 5 of the kinetic molecular theory (**19.1.2**), we can also write:

$$v \propto T^{1/2}$$

Any two gases at the same temperature will have identical average kinetic energies:

$$KE_1 = KE_2$$

$$\text{or, } \tfrac{1}{2}m_1v_1^2 = \tfrac{1}{2}m_2v_2^2$$

Therefore:

$$\frac{v_1^2}{v_2^2} = \frac{m_2}{m_1}$$

$$\frac{v_1}{v_2} = \sqrt{\frac{m_2}{m_1}}$$

The above relation is an expression of **Graham's law of diffusion**. According to Graham's law, for any two gas molecules of unequal mass at an identical temperature, the lighter molecule will have a higher velocity (or rate of diffusion) than the heavier molecule.

Please solve this problem:

- An oxygen molecule at 500 K has:

  A. sixteen times the velocity of a hydrogen molecule at 500 K.

  B. one-sixteenth the velocity of a hydrogen molecule at 500 K.

  C. four times the velocity of a hydrogen molecule at 500 K.

  D. one-fourth the velocity of a hydrogen molecule at 500 K.

Problem solved:

D is the correct answer. Using Graham's law of diffusion:

$$\frac{v_{O_2}}{v_{H_2}} = \sqrt{\frac{m_{H_2}}{m_{O_2}}} = \sqrt{\frac{2 \text{ g/mol}}{32 \text{ g/mol}}} = \sqrt{\frac{1}{16}} = \frac{1}{4}$$

19.2 MASTERY APPLIED: SAMPLE PASSAGE AND QUESTIONS

Passage

Since an ideal gas is not subjected to intermolecular forces, an ideal gas will never liquefy. Any real gas, however, will liquefy if subjected to a sufficiently high pressure and a significantly low temperature. A necessary condition of liquefaction is that the kinetic energy of the molecules be reduced enough that the attractive forces between molecules predominate. Because the relationship of kinetic energy, given by the Maxwell-Boltzmann distribution:

$$KE = \tfrac{3}{2}nRT,$$

does not depend on pressure, but only upon temperature, there is, for any gas, a critical temperature above which the gas will not liquefy, regardless of the pressure applied. The pressure necessary to liquefy a gas at its critical temperature is called the critical pressure.

The critical temperature of a gas depends on its intermolecular forces. A gas with high intermolecular forces will liquefy more easily and, thus, will have a higher critical temperature. In general, polar gases may be expected to have higher critical temperatures than nonpolar gases. Among nonpolar gases, higher molecular weight gases will be expected to have higher critical temperatures than lower molecular weight gases, as shown in Table 1.

GAS	Critical Temperature (K)	Critical Pressure (atm)	Critical Volume (ml/mol)
H_2O	647	217.7	56
NH_3	406	111.5	72
HCl	324	81.6	81
CO_2	304	72.9	94.0
O_2	155	49.7	73
Ar	151	48.0	75.3
N_2	126	33.5	90.1
H_2	33	12.8	65
He	5	2.3	57.8

Table 1

If liquefaction occurs at precisely the critical temperature there is no surface between the gas phase and the liquid phase during the liquefaction process. The absence of this visible phase separation (the meniscus) is indicative of a liquid volume, after the liquefaction, that is equal to the gaseous volume prior to the liquefaction. This volume is the critical volume.

1. When liquefaction occurs at the critical point of a substance the absence of a meniscus is most likely due to:
   A. the gas phase and the liquid phase having equal densities.
   B. the gas phase having a density higher than that of the liquid phase.
   C. the absence of a gas phase.
   D. the absence of a liquid phase.

2. According to the passage:
   A. helium would be correctly predicted to have a critical temperature lower than that of hydrogen.
   B. hydrogen would be correctly predicted to have a critical temperature lower than that of helium.
   C. helium would be incorrectly predicted to have a critical temperature lower than that of hydrogen.
   D. hydrogen would be incorrectly predicted to have a critical temperature lower than that of helium.

3. The universal gas constant is 0.0821 L•atm/mol•K. From Table 1, which of the following is behaving most ideally at its critical point?
   A. Ar
   B. N_2
   C. H_2
   D. He

4. The critical temperature of dimethyl ether is 126.9°C, while that of ethanol is 243°C. This could be due to all of the following EXCEPT:

A. dimethyl ether experiences lesser intermolecular forces than does ethanol.

B. ethanol tends to ionize in the gaseous state.

C. dimethyl ether does not experience hydrogen bonding.

D. ethanol has a higher boiling point than does dimethyl ether.

5. Which of the following could NOT be converted to a liquid at room temperature?

A. H_2O

B. CO_2

C. H_2

D. It cannot be determined from the information given.

6. An unknown gas with a molecular weight of 30 g/mol is determined to be nonpolar. Its critical temperature is most likely:

A. 165 K.

B. 140 K.

C. 115 K.

D. 90 K.

19.3 MASTERY VERIFIED: ANSWERS AND EXPLANATIONS

1. *A is the correct answer.* Based on information in the last paragraph of the passage, the gas phase prior to liquefaction and the liquid phase after liquefaction occupy equal volumes. Since mass is conserved in the liquefaction process, and density is given by:

$$\rho = \frac{m}{V}$$

the densities must also be equal. If B were true, there would still be a meniscus between the phases but the gas would be on the bottom of the container rather than the liquid. C and D are incorrect since during any liquefaction process there must be both gas and liquid present until the process is complete.

2. *D is the correct answer.* According to the passage, nonpolar molecules are expected to show a linear relationship between molecular weight and critical temperature. Helium has a molecular weight of 4 g/mol. Hydrogen gas has a molecular weight of 2 g/mol. From this, we would predict that helium would have the higher critical temperature. This eliminates choices A and C, which predict a higher critical temperature for hydrogen. From Table 1, we see that a lower critical temperature is observed for helium than is observed for hydrogen. Although we would have predicted that hydrogen would have had the lower critical temperature from the passage, Table 1 clearly shows this to be incorrect; therefore the answer is D.

3. *D is the correct answer.* We answer this question by using the information in Table 1, and the ideal gas law in the form:

$$\frac{PV}{nT} = R$$

The table gives us values for T, P, and V/n for each gas. Solving for R for each gas (after converting the volumes from milliliters to liters):

$$R_{Ar} = \frac{(48.0 \text{ atm})(0.0753 \text{ L/mol})}{(151 \text{ K})} = 0.0239 \text{L} \cdot \text{atm/mol} \cdot \text{K}$$

$$R_{N_2} = \frac{(33.5 \text{ atm})(0.0901 \text{ L/mol})}{(126 \text{ K})} = 0.0240 \text{L} \cdot \text{atm/mol} \cdot \text{K}$$

$$R_{H_2} = \frac{(12.8 \text{ atm})(0.0635 \text{ L/mol})}{(33 \text{ K})} = 0.0246 \text{L} \cdot \text{atm/mol} \cdot \text{K}$$

$$R_{He} = \frac{(2.3 \text{ atm})(0.0578 \text{ L/mol})}{(5 \text{ K})} = 0.0266 \text{L} \cdot \text{atm/mol} \cdot \text{K}$$

Since we know that $R = 0.0821$ L$\cdot$atm/mol$\cdot$K, the gas behaving most ideally is that gas with a calculated value of R closest to this ideal value, which is helium.

4. *B is the correct answer.* Dimethyl ether does not experience hydrogen bonding with itself, and so it has lesser intermolecular interactions than ethanol, which will hydrogen bond with other molecules of ethanol. Therefore, both A and C are true. Ethanol has a higher boiling point than dimethyl ether because of these hydrogen bonds. As pointed out in question 2, the passage suggests that materials with higher boiling points will also have higher critical temperatures. Therefore choice D is true. Choice B is false, substances do not tend to ionize simply by passing from one phase to another.

5. *C is the correct answer.* Room temperature is approximately 295 K. Referring to Table 1, we see that the critical temperatures of water and carbon dioxide are both above room temperature; whereas the critical temperature of hydrogen gas is below room temperature. The definition of critical temperature is that temperature above which a liquid will not form, regardless of the pressure applied. As we know, water is a liquid at room temperature and atmospheric pressure: A is obviously incorrect. Carbon dioxide (dry ice) does not have a liquid phase at room temperature (under atmospheric pressure conditions). However, since room temperature is below the critical temperature of carbon dioxide, there is a pressure at which carbon dioxide would become a liquid, with a temperature of 295 K. Since room temperature is well above the critical temperature of hydrogen gas, it is clear that hydrogen gas cannot be a liquid at room temperature: hydrogen gas cannot become a liquid above 33 K.

6. *B is the correct answer.* From the passage, nonpolar gases will tend to show a direct relationship between molecular weight and critical temperature. Since our unknown gas has a molecular weight of 30 g/mol, we would expect it to have a critical temperature between the nonpolar gas O_2 (MW = 32 g/mol) and the nonpolar gas N_2 (MW = 28 g/mol). B is the only answer choice between 153 K and 126 K, the critical temperatures of oxygen gas and nitrogen gas, respectively.

CHAPTER 20

PHASE CHANGES

20.1 MASTERY ACHIEVED

20.1.1 CHANGING PHASES: SOLID, LIQUID, GAS

20.1.1.1 Phases and Their Dependence on Temperature and Pressure

Within a system, all matter that has a particular set of properties is said to be in a **phase**. On the MCAT, you need only concern yourself with single component systems when considering phases. The phases available to a system are the **gas** phase (g), the **liquid** phase (ℓ), and the **solid** phase (s). In certain cases, a pure substance may adopt more than one crystalline structure in the solid phase; for example, diamond and graphite are two different solid phases of carbon.

In MCAT terms:

- The gas phase of a material is characterized by the ability of the material to take the shape of the container that holds it and the ability of the material to expand to fill the available volume.

- The liquid phase of a material is characterized by the ability of the material to conform to the shape of the container that holds it, but an inability of the material to expand to fill the available volume.

- The solid phase of a material is characterized by an inability of the material to conform to the shape of the container that holds it and an inability of the material to expand to fill the available volume.

Whether a substance exists in the solid, liquid, or gas phase depends primarily on temperature and pressure. As temperature is increased under conditions of constant pressure, a substance will move from the solid phase to the liquid phase. As temperature is further increased, the substance will move from the liquid phase to the gas phase, following Charles' Law (**19.1.3.2**): as temperature is increased, volume is increased.

To summarize:

- Under conditions of high temperature and/or low pressure, the gas phase will be favored over the liquid phase, and the liquid phase will be favored over the solid phase.

- Under conditions of low temperature and/or high pressure, the solid phase will be favored over the liquid phase, and the liquid phase will be favored over the gas phase.

Please solve this problem:

- A substance exists in the gas phase at room temperature at atmospheric conditions. If the pressure is doubled and the temperature is halved, the substance will:

   A. remain in the gas phase.
   B. become a liquid.
   C. become a solid.
   D. it is impossible to tell the final phase of the material from the information given.

Problem solved:

The correct answer is D. Unless we know the pressures and temperatures of the phase changes of this substance, we cannot say with certainty in which phase the substance will be. An increase in pressure and a reduction in temperature favor the formation of a liquid or solid phase. However, the question is whether we have increased the pressure and lowered the temperature enough to cause a phase change to occur. We cannot tell.

20.1.1.2 The Available Phase Changes

The change in phase that occurs when a solid becomes a liquid is called **melting**. The opposite of melting is **freezing**.

When a liquid becomes a gas, this process is called **boiling**, or **vaporization**. The opposite of boiling is **condensing**.

Under appropriate conditions, such as carbon dioxide (dry ice) at room temperature and atmospheric pressure, it is possible for a substance to skip the liquid phase altogether. Such a process—the direct conversion of a solid to a gas—is called **sublimation**. The direct conversion from a gas phase to a solid phase, without an intervening liquid phase, is **deposition**.

Please solve this problem:

- The opposite of sublimation is:

   A. freezing.
   B. vaporization.
   C. deposition.
   D. condensation.

Problem solved:

The correct answer is C. Sublimation is the process whereby a solid is transformed directly into a gas, without an intervening liquid phase. Deposition is the process whereby a gas is transformed directly into a solid, without an intervening liquid phase.

20.1.2 THE THERMODYNAMICS OF PHASE CHANGES

There are six possible phase changes: **melting, vaporization, sublimation, deposition, condensation**, and **freezing**. The first three changes involve a change from a lower energy state to a higher energy state; the second three involve a change from a higher energy state to a lower energy state.

Since energy is always conserved, the transition from a phase or state that contains more energy to a phase or state that contains less energy must involve the release of energy; it must be **exothermic**. Deposition, condensation, and freezing are all exothermic processes.

Conversely, a transition from a phase or state that contains less energy to a phase or state that contains more energy requires the input of energy. Such a process is **endothermic**. Melting, vaporization, and sublimation are endothermic processes.

Associated with each phase change is an increase or decrease in enthalpy. The enthalpy of the phase change from solid to liquid is termed the **heat of fusion**. The heat of fusion, ΔH_{fus}, of any substance at constant temperature and pressure normally takes a positive value, since melting (fusion) is an endothermic process, and any endothermic process will have a positive value of ΔH. Since energy is conserved in forward and reverse processes, the negative of the heat of fusion is the enthalpy change associated with freezing.

The enthalpy change associated with the phase change from liquid to gas is called the **heat of vaporization**. The heat of vaporization, ΔH_{vap}, of any substance at constant temperature and pressure normally takes a positive value, since vaporization is an endothermic process, and any endothermic process will have a positive value of ΔH. The negative of the heat of vaporization is the enthalpy change associated with condensation.

The enthalpy change associated with the phase change from a solid directly to a gas is called the **heat of sublimation** (ΔH_{sub}). As was the case for heat of fusion and heat of vaporization, heat of sublimation at constant temperature and pressure normally takes a positive value for any substance, since sublimation is an endothermic process. The negative of the heat of sublimation is the enthalpy change associated with deposition.

Please solve this problem:

- The heat of fusion is:

    A. positive, because melting is an exothermic process.
    B. positive, because melting is an endothermic process.
    C. negative, because melting is an exothermic process.
    D. negative, because melting is an endothermic process.

Problem solved:

The correct answer is B. Heat of fusion refers to the heat that must be supplied to a substance to make it melt. When heat must be supplied to a reaction, that reaction is termed endothermic.

Had this question asked about the process of solidification, heat would have been given off, leading to a negative ΔH, or an exothermic process.

20.1.3 CALCULATING WITH HEAT: AT AND AWAY FROM PHASE CHANGES

20.1.3.1 Comparing Heat During and Away From a Phase Change

During a phase change, there is no change in temperature. For example, when solid water is heated from –5°C to +5°C, the temperature of the system changes until the melting point of water is reached (0°C). At this point, even though heat is being supplied, the temperature of the water does not change. All the energy being supplied to the system is used to convert the solid water into liquid water. It is not until the phase change is complete that the temperature again begins to rise. In this regard: energy added to a system at a time other than at a phase change will induce a change in temperature in the system. Energy added to a system during a phase change will *not* induce a change in temperature. Molecular kinetic energy is directly related to temperature (see **19.1.2**). Therefore, when temperature is increased, molecular kinetic energy is also increased. When a system gains energy without an increase in temperature, the system must be gaining potential energy.

- When a system is not undergoing a phase change, the heat added to that system adds to the kinetic energy of the molecules of that system.

- When a system is undergoing a phase change, the heat added to that system adds to the potential energy of the molecules of that system.

The converse of these two postulates is also true:

- When a system is not undergoing a phase change, the heat released by that system diminishes the kinetic energy of the molecules of that system.

- When a system is undergoing a phase change, the heat released by that system diminishes the potential energy of the molecules of that system.

Please solve this problem:

- As water is cooled slowly from 5°C to –5°C, it will undergo a phase change from the liquid state to the solid state, and:

    A. the kinetic energy of the water molecules will increase, and the potential energy will decrease.
    B. the kinetic energy of the water molecules will decrease, and the potential energy will increase.
    C. both the kinetic energy and the potential energy of the water molecules will increase.
    D. both the kinetic energy and the potential energy of the water molecules will decrease.

Problem solved:

The correct answer is D. As the temperature is lowered, the molecules of that system will contain less kinetic energy. Recall that kinetic energy is directly proportional to temperature. The phase change from a liquid to a solid is an exothermic process; heat is given off. When energy is given off in the form of heat, there must be less potential energy in the system, since energy is conserved.

20.1.3.2 Heat Away From a Phase Change

When a system is not undergoing a phase change the heat absorbed by the system is given by:

$$q = mc\,\Delta T$$

where:

q is the heat absorbed

m is the mass of the substance under consideration where c is the specific heat.

c is the specific heat capacity of the substance in this particular phase

ΔT is the change in temperature observed

We are familiar with all these variables, except specific heat capacity, c.

Specific heat is the heat capacity of a substance per unit mass. As can be seen from the above equation, **Specific heat** has the units of energy per mass per temperature:

$$c = \frac{q}{\Delta T} = \frac{J}{kg \bullet K} \text{ or } \frac{J}{kg°C} \text{ or } \frac{cal}{g \bullet °C} \text{ or } \frac{kcal}{kg \bullet °C}$$

Calories (cal) are a unit of energy. One calorie is defined as the amount of heat energy that must be supplied to one gram of liquid water at 25°C to raise the temperature of the water 1°C. Therefore, the specific heat of liquid water is defined as 1 cal/g•°C.

Please solve this problem:

- The specific heat of liquid water is 4.18 J/°C•g. The heat required to raise the temperature of 10 grams of liquid water from a temperature of 20°C to 50°C is:

  A. 125.4 J
  B. 836.0 J
  C. 1254.0 J
  D. 2090.0 J

Problem solved:

The correct answer is C. Employing the formula:

$$q = mc\,\Delta T$$

where:

$m = 10$ g

$c = 4.18$ J/°C•g

$\Delta T = 50°C - 20°C = 30°C$

$$q = (10 \text{ g})(4.18 \text{ J/°C} \bullet \text{g})(30°C) = 1254 \text{ J}$$

20.1.3.3 Heat During a Phase Change

To calculate the heat of a phase change, we only need to know how much material is undergoing the change and the magnitude of the change of enthalpy that is associated with this change for this substance. As stated in **20.1.2**, each substance has a heat of fusion, heat of vaporization, and heat of sublimation. The opposite of each of these is heat of freezing, heat of condensation, and heat of deposition, respectively. The formula for calculating the amount of heat that is either absorbed (fusion, vaporization, or sublimation) or given off (freezing, condensation, or deposition) is given by:

$$q = m \Delta H$$

where q is the heat, m is the mass, and ΔH is the enthalpy of the phase change in the units of energy per mass. The uses of this equation are summarized in Table 20.1.

Phase Change	Formula
melting (solid to liquid)	$q = m\Delta H_{fus}$
vaporizing (liquid to gas)	$q = m\Delta H_{vap}$
subliming (solid to gas)	$q = m\Delta H_{sub}$
freezing (liquid to solid)	$q = m(-\Delta H_{fus})$
condensing (gas to liquid)	$q = m(-\Delta H_{vap})$
depositing (gas to solid)	$q = m(-\Delta H_{sub})$

Table 20.1

Please solve this problem:

- How much heat must be supplied to slowly lower the temperature of one gram of water from 120°C to −10°C? (Assume that the water is initially in the gas phase, passes through the liquid phase, and ends up in the solid phase. The specific heat of gaseous water is 1.87 J/°C·g. The specific heat of liquid water is 4.18 J/°C·g. The specific heat of solid water is 2.03 J/°C·g. The heat of fusion of water is 333.8 J/g. The heat of vaporization of water is 2259 J/g.)

A. 0 J
B. 476.4 J
C. 2592.8 J
D. 3068.5 J

Problem solved:

The correct answer is A. You should be careful not to fall for traps like this on the MCAT. No heat must be *supplied* in order for this process to take place: heat must be *removed*! Had the question been "how much heat must be removed...," the answer would have been D, based on the following:

120°C to 100°C:	$q = mc\,\Delta T$	=	$(1\text{ g})(1.87\text{ J}/°C\cdot g)(20°C)$	=	37.4 J
at 100°C:	$q = m\,\Delta H_{vap}$	=	$(1\text{ g})(2259\text{ J}/g)$	=	2259.0 J
100°C to 0°C:	$q = mc\,\Delta T$	=	$(1\text{ g})(4.18\text{ J}/°C\cdot g)(100°C)$	=	418.0 J
at 0°C:	$q = m\,\Delta H_{fus}$	=	$(1\text{ g})(333.8\text{ J}/g)$	=	333.8 J
0°C to -10°C:	$q = mc\,\Delta T$	=	$(1\text{ g})(2.03\text{ J}/°C\cdot g)(10°C)$	=	20.3 J
Therefore, total q is given by:		q_{total}		=	3068.5 J

20.1.4 THE PHASE CHANGE DIAGRAM

The phase changes of a substance may be represented graphically in a variety of ways, two of which will be used on the MCAT. The first of these is the **phase change diagram**, shown below. The second is the phase diagram, or P-T diagram, which is covered in the next section (**20.1.5**).

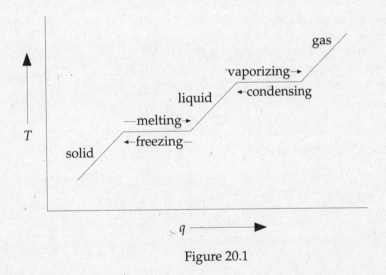

Figure 20.1

The phase change diagram is useful for graphical depiction of many things. All of the horizontal lines denote the amount of heat energy that is added or released during a change in phase. Horizontal components of the graph are given by the formula:

$$q = m\,\Delta H$$

Therefore, the length of such a line divided by the mass under consideration gives a value for ΔH.

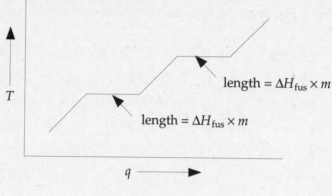

Figure 20.2

Non-horizontal components of the phase change diagram represent the thermodynamics of a system that is not undergoing a phase change; these portions of the graph are given by the equation:

$$q = mc \Delta T$$

Since the slope of a line is defined as:

$$\text{slope} = \frac{\Delta Y}{\Delta X} = \frac{\text{rise}}{\text{run}}$$

we can see that since $X = q$, and $Y = T$, the slope of the line is given by:

$$\text{slope} = \frac{\Delta T}{\Delta q}$$

Rearranging the equation for heat, we get:

$$\frac{q}{\Delta T} = mc, \text{ or}$$

$$\frac{1}{\text{slope}} = mc, \text{ since } mc = C$$

$$\text{slope} = \frac{1}{C}$$

where C is the heat capacity for the exact amount of substance being considered.

Therefore, from a phase change diagram, we can calculate the heat capacity of each phase.

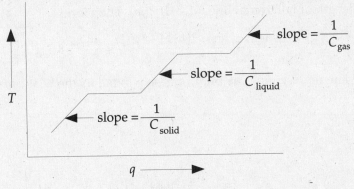

Figure 20.3

You should be aware that each phase change diagram is calculated for a specific constant pressure. If pressure is changed, the phase change diagram must also be changed.

Please solve this problem:

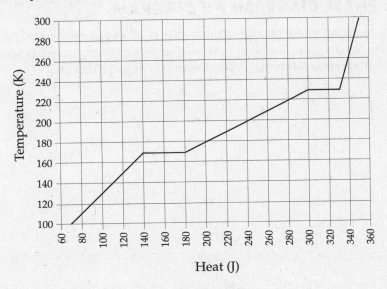

Figure 20.4

- Referring to the phase change diagram (Figure 20.4), which was derived experimentally from a 5 g sample of an unknown substance, the heat of fusion of this substance and specific heat capacity of the liquid phase are:

  A. $\Delta H_{fus} = 40 \text{ J/g}$, and $C_{liquid} = 0.4 \text{ J/K} \cdot g$
  B. $\Delta H_{fus} = 40 \text{ J/g}$, and $C_{liquid} = 0.5 \text{ J/K} \cdot g$
  C. $\Delta H_{fus} = 8 \text{ J/g}$, and $C_{liquid} = 0.4 \text{ J/K} \cdot g$
  D. $\Delta H_{fus} = 8 \text{ J/g}$, and $C_{liquid} = 0.5 \text{ J/K} \cdot g$

Problem solved:

The correct answer is C. The distance of the phase transition from a solid to a liquid gives us the heat of fusion: length of horizontal line = $(\Delta H_{fus})(m)$. Therefore,

$$\Delta H_{fus} = \frac{\text{length of line}}{m} = \frac{(180\text{ J} - 140\text{ J})}{5\text{ g}} = \frac{40\text{ J}}{5\text{ g}} = 8\text{ J/g}$$

The slope of the line representing the liquid phase will tell us the heat capacity of the liquid:

$$c = \frac{1}{m(\text{slope})}$$

where,

$$\text{slope} = \frac{\Delta T}{\Delta q} = \frac{(230\text{ K} - 170\text{ K})}{(300\text{ J} - 180\text{ J})} = \frac{60\text{ K}}{120\text{ J}} = 0.5\text{ K/J}$$

Therefore,

$$c = \frac{1}{(0.5\text{ K/J})(5\text{ g})} = \frac{1}{2.5\text{ K}\cdot\text{g/J}} = 0.4\text{ J/K}\cdot\text{g}$$

20.1.5 THE PHASE DIAGRAM: P-T DIAGRAM

A second way to depict phase changes graphically is in a **phase diagram**. The usual axes for such a diagram are pressure and temperature. For this reason, phase diagrams are often referred to as **P-T diagrams**. A typical phase diagram is depicted below:

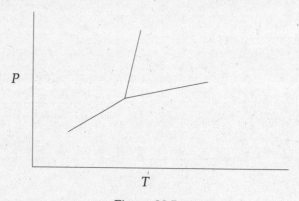

Figure 20.5

Under conditions of sufficiently high temperature or sufficiently low pressure, we would expect to find any substance in the gas phase. Therefore, the region to the far right bottom of a phase diagram represents the gas phase.

Under conditions of sufficiently low temperature or sufficiently high pressure, we would expect to find any substance in the solid phase, so the region to the far left top of a phase diagram represents the solid phase.

Liquids exist under conditions of moderate temperature or moderate pressure, so the middle region of a phase diagram represents the liquid phase.

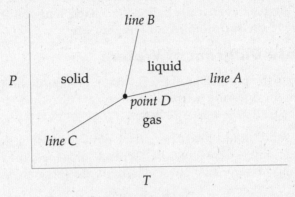

Figure 20.6

The lines in a phase diagram represent the boundaries between two phases. Above *line A*, the substance is in the liquid phase. Below *line A*, the substance is in the gas phase. Along *line A*, the liquid and the gas phases are in equilibrium.

To the left of *line B*, the substance is in the solid phase. To the right of *line B*, the substance is in the liquid phase. Along *line B*, the solid and the liquid phases are in equilibrium.

Above *line C*, the substance is in the solid phase. Below *line C*, the substance is in the gas phase. Along *line C*, the solid and the gas phases are in equilibrium.

Point *D* lies at the point at which all three phases are in equilibrium. This point is referred to as the triple point. There is no way to get back to this point after a decrease in temperature, other than by increasing the temperature. Likewise, there is no way to return to this point after a decrease in pressure, other than by raising the pressure.

Please solve this problem:

- A phase diagram is most likely constructed experimentally by:

    A. changing both temperature and pressure simultaneously from one data point to the next.

    B. changing temperature slowly at several constant pressure readings.

    C. changing pressure slowly at several constant temperature readings.

    D. changing one variable—either temperature or pressure—while holding the other variable constant.

Problem solved:

The correct answer is C. While choice D makes sense in theory, in practice, it is much easier to vary temperature at a constant pressure than to vary pressure at a constant temperature. This is particularly true in the gas phase, where a gas will cool via an effect (known as the Joule-Thomson effect) as pressure is released.

While it is not important for you to understand the Joule-Thomson effect for the MCAT, it is important that you understand basic experimental design. Common sense dictates that it is easier to control temperature than pressure. For example, the air coming out of a balloon feels cooler than the surrounding air, even if the balloon has had plenty of time to equilibrate its internal gas temperature to the surrounding air temperature.

20.1.5.1 The Phase Diagram of Water

For a typical substance, the phase boundary between the liquid and the solid phases has a positive slope; for water, the opposite is true. For a typical substance, the solid phase is denser than the liquid phase; for water the opposite is true.

The significance of a solid/liquid phase boundary with a negative slope is that as pressure is increased, the freezing point is depressed. In a typical substance, the freezing point is increased with increasing pressure. Two phase diagrams are shown below:

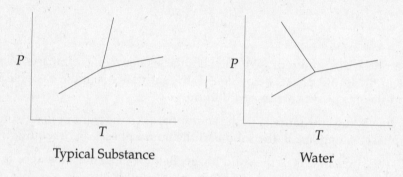

Typical Substance   Water

Figure 20.8

Please solve this problem:

- As the pressure on a sample of water is increased, the melting point of the water:

  A. decreases, as is expected for "normal" substances.

  B. decreases, contrary to what is expected for "normal" substances.

  C. increases, as is expected for "normal" substances.

  D. increases, contrary to what is expected for "normal" substances.

Problem solved:

The correct answer is B. From our knowledge of phase diagrams, we can see that the solid/liquid phase boundary line depicts melting point versus pressure. From our phase diagrams of water and "normal" substances above, we can see that as the pressure in a sample of water is increased, the melting point decreases; whereas, for "normal" substances, the opposite is true: as pressure increases, melting point increases.

In a typical substance, the solid phase expands upon melting. In water, the solid phase contracts on melting. In other words, for most materials, the solid phase is more dense than the liquid phase. In water, the liquid phase is more dense than the solid phase.

20.1.5.2 Substances with More than One Solid Form

Certain substances exist in more than one solid form. Examples include the graphite and diamond forms of carbon, and the S_4 and S_8 forms of sulfur. The phase diagram of sulfur is given below:

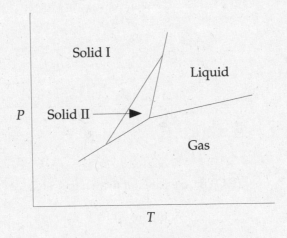

Figure 20.9

20.1.6 THE TRIPLE POINT AND CRITICAL POINT

As mentioned previously (20.1.5), **the triple point** of a substance is the point, defined by a specific temperature and a specific pressure, at which all three phases of the substance exist at equilibrium. A slight decrease in temperature from the triple point will often lead to entrance into the solid phase. A slight increase in temperature will lead to entrance into the gas phase. A small increase in pressure will lead to the formation of the liquid or solid phase. A slight decrease in pressure will lead to entrance into the gas phase.

If the triple point of a substance occurs at a pressure greater than 1 atm (atmospheric pressure), the substance will sublimate under atmospheric conditions and an appropriate change in temperature. Such is the case for carbon dioxide, which has a triple point at 216.8 K and 5.11 atm.

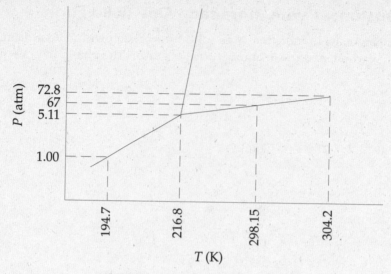

(NOTE: Axes are not drawn to scale.)

Figure 20.10

The triple point should not be confused with the **critical point**. The triple point is where all three phases exist in equilibrium. The critical point of a substance is the temperature above which there is no phase boundary between the liquid and the gas phases (**19.2**). The minimum pressure that is required to convert the gas to its liquid at the critical temperature is the critical pressure of that substance. The critical values of carbon dioxide are given on the above graph (T_c = 304.2 K, P_c = 72.8 atm).

Note that, in a phase diagram, the liquid/gas phase boundary cannot be extrapolated above the critical temperature. By definition, there is no way to distinguish between these two phases above this temperature.

Please solve this problem:

- A substance has a triple point at 300 K and 760 torr. Under conditions of atmospheric pressure at sea level, this substance:

    A. is a liquid at room temperature.
    B. is a solid at room temperature.
    C. is a gas at room temperature.
    D. sublimates at room temperature.

Problem solved:

The correct answer is B. Since room temperature is 298 K, this represents a decrease in temperature from the triple point. As pointed out above, if pressure is held constant, a decrease in temperature from the triple point of a substance will lead to the formation of a solid phase. Since 760 torr is atmospheric pressure at sea level, there is no change in pressure from the triple point pressure to atmospheric pressure.

20.2 MASTERY APPLIED: SAMPLE PASSAGE AND QUESTIONS

Passage

Campers and military personnel routinely carry freeze-dried foods because these foods are lightweight. Additionally, bacteria cannot grow or reproduce in the total absence of moisture that is afforded by freeze-dried items. Freeze-dried foods may be quickly reconstituted simply by adding water to them. The technique of freeze-drying can be applied to almost any substance that contains water. Biologists often freeze-dry tissue cultures in order to preserve them for later research.

Freeze-drying takes advantage of the phase properties of water. In the process of freeze-drying, a sample is first cooled to a temperature below the freezing point of water such that all of the water solidifies. Next, the sample is placed in a chamber to which a vacuum pump is attached. The pump serves to lower the pressure in the chamber below the vapor pressure of ice, such that all of the ice sublimates. Once the water is in the gaseous state, it is evacuated from the chamber by the vacuum pump.

This process has many advantages over traditional drying methods which rely on boiling off the unwanted water. The heat necessary to remove all the water from a sample usually results in damage to the sample itself, especially with regard to most flavor agents in foods. The majority of the chemicals responsible for the flavor of food are esters, which decompose at high temperatures.

The triple point of water exists at a temperature of 0.01°C and a pressure of 0.006 atm. The critical temperature and pressure of water are 374.2°C and 218 atm, respectively. The triple point of carbon dioxide exists at a temperature of 216.8 K and a pressure of 5.11 atm. The critical temperature and pressure of carbon dioxide are 31.1°C and 72.8 atm, respectively. The sublimation point of carbon dioxide at 1 atm is 195 K.

1. A liquid that is surrounded by a gaseous medium, such as the atmosphere, will boil when:
   A. the density of the liquid is equal to the density of the surrounding gas.
   B. the heat capacity of the liquid is equal to the heat capacity of the surrounding gas.
   C. the vapor pressure of the liquid is equal to the pressure of the surrounding gas.
   D. the kinetic energy of the molecules of the liquid is equal to the kinetic energy of the molecules of the surrounding gas.

2. One plausible explanation for the difference in triple points of carbon dioxide and water is:
   A. carbon dioxide has a higher molecular weight than water.
   B. carbon dioxide is a linear molecule, water is bent.
   C. carbon dioxide participates in hydrogen bonds with water molecules in the air, which cause it to sublimate.
   D. carbon dioxide cannot form hydrogen bonds with itself, unlike water.

3. A mixture of 0.5 moles of carbon dioxide vapor and 0.5 moles of water vapor are held in a 35-liter container at atmospheric pressure. The temperature of the container is:
   A. 426 K
   B. 373 K
   C. 293 K
   D. 273 K

4. If the same mixture is confined to a volume of 12 liters, at a temperature of 150 K:

   A. the water will liquefy, the carbon dioxide will remain a gas.
   B. the water will solidify, the carbon dioxide will liquefy.
   C. the water will solidify, the carbon dioxide will remain a gas.
   D. both will solidify.

5. A refrigerator freezer removes heat from the air inside the refrigerator. This heat is absorbed in the phase transition from liquid to gas of the refrigerant. A compressor is then employed to reconvert the gas to a liquid so that it may be recirculated. The boiling and freezing points of the refrigerant relate in what way to the boiling and freezing points of water?

   A. The boiling point of water is lower than the boiling point of the refrigerant.
   B. The freezing point of water is higher than the boiling point of the refrigerant.
   C. The boiling point of water is lower than the freezing point of the refrigerant.
   D. The freezing point of water is lower than the freezing point of the refrigerant.

6. Which of the following statements is true?

   A. Sublimation occurs when the critical pressure is greater than atmospheric pressure.
   B. Sublimation occurs when the triple point pressure is greater than atmospheric pressure.
   C. Deposition occurs when the critical pressure is lower than atmospheric pressure.
   D. Deposition occurs when the triple point pressure is lower than atmospheric pressure.

7. The pressure that must be achieved in a freeze-drier to remove all water is:

   A. 4.56 atm
   B. less than 4.56 atm
   C. 4.56 torr
   D. less than 4.56 torr

20.3 MASTERY VERIFIED: ANSWERS AND EXPLANATIONS

1. *C is the correct answer.* When the vapor pressure of a liquid is equal in pressure to the pressure of the surrounding gas, the liquid will boil. When the density of a liquid is equal to the density of its own gas phase, it is at or above the critical point and cannot distinguish between the gas and liquid phases, so the term "boil" becomes meaningless. If the surrounding gas is a substance other than that which we wish to boil, we cannot directly compare the two substances' densities for any meaningful information about the boiling point of the liquid.

   Heat capacity is the ability of a substance, in a particular phase, to absorb heat. The heat capacity of a liquid can be equal to the heat capacity of the same substance, or another substance, in the gas phase. Again, comparing heat capacities tells us nothing about the boiling point of the liquid.

   If the kinetic energy of the molecules of the liquid were equal to the kinetic energy of the molecules of the surrounding gas, we could only conclude that the two phases are at the same temperature. We cannot say anything about whether or not the liquid will boil unless we know what the liquid is and what the temperature is.

2. *D is the correct answer.* Choices A and B are true, but they do not offer an explanation of the difference in triple points of carbon dioxide and water. The strength of hydrogen bonds in water is responsible for the peculiarities of water, including its high freezing temperature and low triple point pressure.

3. *A is the correct answer.* Employing the ideal gas law:

$$T = \frac{PV}{nR} = \frac{(1 \text{ atm})(35 \text{ L})}{(1 \text{ mol})(0.082 \text{ L} \cdot \text{atm}/\text{mol} \cdot \text{K})} = \frac{35}{0.082} \text{K} = 426 \text{ K}$$

   Choice B is the boiling point of water under atmospheric conditions. Since we know that the water is in the gas phase at atmospheric pressure, we must have a temperature higher than 373 K.

4. *D is the correct answer.* In order to solve this problem, we must first compute the pressure in the vessel:

$$P = \frac{nRT}{V} = \frac{(1 \text{ mol})(0.082 \text{ L} \cdot \text{atm}/\text{mol} \cdot \text{K})(150 \text{ K})}{12 \text{ L}} = 1.02 \text{ atm}$$

   From this, and the phase transition points of water and carbon dioxide, we can determine the phase of each. This eliminates choice A:

$$H_2O: T_b = 373 \text{ K}$$

$$T_f = 273 \text{ K}$$

   The temperature of the vessel is below the freezing point of water; therefore, water is a solid under these conditions:

$$CO_2: T_s = 195 \text{ K}$$

   Since carbon dioxide sublimates at this temperature at 1 atm, freezing point is meaningless, and the liquid phase is not an option. This eliminates choice B.

   The temperature of the vessel is below the sublimation point of carbon dioxide; carbon dioxide must also exist in the solid phase. This eliminates choice C, leaving only D.

5. *B is the correct answer.* For the freezer compartment of a refrigerator to work, it must cool the air in the freezer to a temperature below the freezing point of water.

   If the freezing point of water was lower than the freezing point of the refrigerant, we would freeze our refrigerant before we froze any water. This would be a problem, since we want the refrigerant to alternate between the liquid and gas phases, so that it can continue to circulate through our system. We must be concerned only with the boiling point of the refrigerant and the freezing point of water.

   If the freezing point of water were lower than the boiling point of the refrigerant, we might still have been able to cool the air in the refrigerator, but we would have been unable to make ice.

6. *B is the correct answer.* Choice B is the definition of the conditions that are necessary for sublimation to occur, as stated in **20.1.6**. While this may lead one to believe that D is also true, having a triple point pressure that is lower than atmospheric pressure is not sufficient to cause deposition.

7. *D is the correct answer.* First, we must convert the critical pressure, given in the passage as 0.006 atm, to torr:

$$1 \text{ atm} = 760 \text{ torr}$$

$$0.006 \text{ atm} = 4.56 \text{ torr}$$

   Freeze-drying works by sublimating water. From a knowledge of phase diagrams, we understand that for sublimation to occur, we must be in a region of the phase diagram that allows us to cross a solid/gas phase boundary. Such a boundary can only exist at pressures lower than the triple point pressure. (See Figure 20.6, *line C*, in section **20.1.5**.)

CHAPTER 21

ACID-BASE CHEMISTRY

21.1 MASTERY ACHIEVED

21.1.1 BASIC CONCEPTS AND DEFINITIONS

21.1.1.1 Ionization of Water, pH, and pOH

Under any conditions of hydrogen ion concentration (pH), water is subject to the ionizing equilibrium:

$$H_2O(l) \rightleftharpoons H^+(aq) + OH^-(aq)$$

This is called the autoionization of water. The equilibrium expression for the autoionization of water is:

$$K_w = [H^+][OH^-] = 1 \times 10^{-14}$$

From this expression and the equilibrium equation, we can see that, in the absence of outside influence, the concentration of hydrogen ions must be equal to the concentration of hydroxide ions. Therefore, $[H^+] = [OH^-] = 1 \times 10^{-7} M$. Although the ion product constant for water, K_w, was obtained for pure water, it is valid for any aqueous solutions at 25°C.

This is one of the most important relationships in all chemistry, since it establishes the inverse relationship between $[H^+]$ and $[OH^-]$ for all dilute ($< 1 M$) aqueous solutions.

To summarize:

- *When $[H^+] = [OH^-]$, a solution is neutral.*

- *When $[H^+] > [OH^-]$, a solution is acidic.*

- *When $[H^+] < [OH^-]$, a solution is basic.*

- *$[H^+][OH^-] = 1 \times 10^{-14}$.*

The pH scale provides a convenient method of expressing the relative acidity (or basicity) of dilute aqueous solutions. The pH of a solution is defined as:

$$pH = \log \frac{1}{[H^+]}$$

which may also be written:

$$pH = -\log[H^+]$$

Likewise, the pOH of a solution is defined as:

$$pOH = \log\frac{1}{[OH^-]}$$

or:

$$pOH = -\log[OH^-]$$

Expressing the ion product constant equation in terms of pH and pOH, we see that:

$$-\log(K_w) = (-\log[H^+]) + (-\log[OH^-]) = -\log(1 \times 10^{-14})$$

or,

$$pH + pOH = 14$$

Therefore, once we have determined the pH (or pOH) of a solution, the pOH (or pH) is given as 14 – pH (or pOH). The pH of a solution with a pOH of 8.2 is 14 – 8.2 = 5.8.

Restating the basic definitions of neutrality, acidity, and basicity in terms of pH and pOH:

- *When pH = 7 (pOH = 7), a solution is neutral.*

- *When pH < 7 (pOH > 7), a solution is acidic.*

- *When pH > 7 (pOH < 7), a solution is basic.*

- *pH + pOH = 14.*

To summarize, as pH increases, $[H^+]$ decreases, and as pOH increases, $[OH^-]$ decreases.

The pH ranges for some common substances are provided in Table 21.1.

Substance	pH Range
human stomach	1.0 – 2.0
human urine	4.8 – 8.4
human saliva	6.5 – 7.5
human blood plasma	7.3 – 7.5
hot salsa	1.5 – 2.5
soft drinks	2.0 – 4.0
vinegar	2.4 – 3.4
tomatoes	4.0 – 4.4
beer	4.0 – 5.0
cow's milk	6.3 – 6.6
household ammonia	11.0 – 12.0

Table 21.1

A pH of 4 corresponds to an $[H^+]$ of 1×10^{-4} M. A pH of 5 corresponds to an $[H^+]$ of 1×10^{-5} M. A pH of 4.2 corresponds to a $[H^+]$ between 1×10^{-4} M and 1×10^{-5} M, or 6.3×10^{-5} M.

Please solve this problem:

- The pH of a solution with $[H^+]$ of 2.7×10^{-7} is:

    A. 2.7
    B. 6.2
    C. 6.6
    D. 7.6

Problem solved:

The correct answer is C. pH = –log [H⁺]. Because the H⁺ concentration has an exponent of –7 we know: $6 < pH \leq 7$. This alone is enough to eliminate choices A, B, and D. Note that [H⁺] is always given as follows: $n \times 10^{-X}$.

When:

$n = 1$	$X = pH$
$n = 3.17$	$X - 0.5 = pH$
$1 < n < 3.17$	$X - 0.5 < pH < X$
$10 > n > 3.17$	$X - 0.5 > pH > X - 1$

21.1.1.2 Arrhenius Definition of Acid and Base

The classical definition of acids and bases is attributed to Svante Arrhenius. According to the Arrhenius definitions, an **Arrhenius acid** is a substance that contains hydrogen and produces H⁺ in solution, and an **Arrhenius base** is a substance that contains hydroxyl groups and produces OH⁻ in solution. In broader terms, an acid is a substance that increases the concentration of hydrogen ions in solution, and a base is a substance that increases the concentration of hydroxide ions in solution. As such, an acid lowers the pH of a solution, and a base raises the pH of a solution.

Acids and bases may be categorized as strong acids, weak acids, strong bases, and weak bases. Strong acids and strong bases completely ionize in dilute aqueous solutions. Weak acids and weak bases only slightly ionize in dilute aqueous solutions. A solution of a strong acid or strong base will predominantly contain the ions of that acid or base, rather than the acid or base molecule. A solution of a weak acid or base will predominantly contain the complete acid or base molecule, rather than the ions.

Please solve this problem:

- An Arrhenius acid is:

    A. a proton donor.
    B. an electron pair acceptor.
    C. a hydrogen atom source.
    D. a hydrogen ion source.

Problem solved:

The correct answer is D. This is the definition of an acid in terms of Arrhenius' theory for acids and bases.

21.1.1.3 Brønsted–Lowry Definition of Acid and Base

In 1923 Brønsted and Lowry independently expanded upon the Arrhenius definition of acids and bases. The **Brønsted-Lowry acid** is a *proton* (H^+) *donor*, while the **Brønsted-Lowry base** is a *proton acceptor*. According to the Brønsted-Lowry theory, an acid-base reaction is a reaction that involves the transfer of a proton from a proton donor (an acid) to a proton acceptor (a base).

Any substance that can be either a proton donor or a proton acceptor is an **amphoteric** substance within the Brønsted-Lowry definitions. Since water can act as either an acid or as a base, it is called amphoteric.

An acid-base neutralization reaction is defined by Brønsted-Lowry theory as a reaction in which an acid and a base react to form water.

Please solve this problem:

- A Brønsted-Lowry base is:

   A. an electron pair donor.
   B. a proton acceptor.
   C. a hydrogen ion source.
   D. a proton donor.

Problem solved:

The correct answer is B. A base is defined as a proton acceptor, according to Brønsted-Lowry theory. Choice D is the definition of an acid according to this theory.

21.1.1.4 Conjugate Acid/Base Pairs

In terms of the Brønsted-Lowry acid-base theory, the complete ionization of a strong acid in water is an example of an acid-base reaction:

$$HCl + H_2O \rightarrow H_3O^+ + Cl^-$$

In this instance, water served as a base, and hydrochloric acid is the acid. In the reaction of any acid or any base, another base or acid is generated. In the above example, H_3O^+ is the acid generated from the base, H_2O. And Cl^- is the base generated from the acid HCl. These "pairs" of acids and bases are termed **conjugate acid/base pairs**. The above ionization reaction involves two conjugate acid/base pairs: HCl/Cl^- and H_3O^+/H_2O. Conjugate acid/base pairs differ only by a single proton. The possible general forms of conjugate acid/base pairs are: HA/A^- and HB^+/B.

We can say that Cl^- is the conjugate base of HCl, and the hydronium ion (H_3O^+) is the conjugate acid of water; but, we could have also said that HCl is the conjugate acid of Cl^-, and water is the conjugate base of the hydronium ion (H_3O^+).

The conjugate base of a strong acid is a weak base. The conjugate base of a weak acid is a strong base. Likewise, the conjugate acid of a strong base is a weak acid, and the conjugate acid of a weak base is a strong acid.

Please solve this problem:

- All of the following are conjugate acid/base pairs EXCEPT:

    A. H_3O^+/H_2O
    B. H^+/OH^-
    C. H_2O/OH^-
    D. H_4O^{+2}/H_3O^+

Problem solved:

The correct answer is B. While choice D lists a highly improbable pair, it still fits the criteria—conjugate acid/base pairs must differ only by a single proton. H^+ and OH^- do *not* differ only by a proton, and so they are *not* a conjugate acid/base pair.

21.1.1.5 Lewis Definition of Acid and Base

In 1923 (the same year that the Brønsted-Lowry theory was proposed), G. N. Lewis developed the most comprehensive theory of acids and bases. A **Lewis acid** is defined as an *electron pair acceptor*, while a **Lewis base** is defined as an *electron pair donor*. Note that these definitions do not imply that the electron pair must be completely transferred from the base to the acid, only that the Lewis base is willing to share one of its electron pairs with a Lewis acid.

A **neutralization reaction** is defined by Lewis acid-base theory as a reaction in which an acid and a base form a coordinate covalent bond. A coordinate covalent bond is a bond in which both of the electrons that make up the bond are originally furnished by one atom, the Lewis base.

Please solve this problem:

- A neutralization reaction is:
  A. a reaction between an acid and a base.
  B. a reaction between an acid and a base to form water.
  C. a reaction between an acid and a base that results in the formation of a coordinate covalent bond.
  D. possibly any of the above answer choices.

Problem solved:

The correct answer is D. A neutralization reaction is a reaction between an acid and a base, so choice A is true; a neutralization reaction in Brønsted-Lowry terms is a reaction between an acid and a base to form water, so choice B is true; and a neutralization reaction in Lewis terms is a reaction between an acid and a base that results in the formation of a coordinate covalent bond, so choice C is also true.

21.1.1.6 Strong and Weak Acids: Equilibrium Constants

For the ionization of an acid in water, the equilibrium is:

$$HA + H_2O \rightarrow H_3O^+ + A^-$$

Recalling that pure liquids (such as water) do not appear in the equilibrium expression, the equilibrium constant may be rewritten as an **acid ionization constant**, K_a, expression:

$$K_a = \frac{[H_3O^+][A^-]}{[HA]}$$

Likewise, for the ionization of a base in water, the equilibrium is:

$$B + H_2O \rightarrow HB^+ + OH^-$$

Once again, since water does not appear in the equilibrium expression, the equilibrium constant may be rewritten as a **base ionization constant**, K_b, expression:

$$K_b = \frac{[HB^+][OH^-]}{[B]}$$

As the strength of an acid increases, the concentration of the acid, [HA], becomes negligible, and the acid ionization constant, K_a, approaches infinity. Similarly, as the strength of a base increases, the concentration of unionized base, [B], becomes negligible, and the base ionization constant, K_b, approaches infinity. In other words, a higher value of K_a implies a stronger acid and a higher value of K_b implies a stronger base. A strong acid has a K_a greater than 10^{-2}, and a strong base has a K_b greater than 10^{-2}.

Acid strengths are also given in pK_a's. A pK_a is the negative log of K_a: a low pK_a (less than 2) indicates a strong acid, and a high pK_a indicates a weak acid; a low pK_b (less than 2) indicates a strong base, and a high pK_b indicates a weak base.

For *any* conjugate acid/base pair in a dilute aqueous solution:

$$K_a K_b = K_w$$

And, just as

$$pH + pOH = pK_w = 14$$

$$pK_a + pK_b = 14$$

for any conjugate acid/base pair in a dilute aqueous solution.

The pK_a's of common acids and pK_b's of common bases are given in Tables 21.2 and 21.3.

Acid	pK_a
HCN	9.22
Acetic acid	4.75
Benzoic acid	4.19
HF	3.14
HNO_2	3.29

Table 21.2

Base	pK_b
Triethylamine	3.00
Diethylamine	3.51
AgOH	3.96
Benzylamine	4.67
NH_4OH	4.75

Table 21.3

Please solve this problem:

- What is the pH of a 0.10 M aqueous solution of HCN?

    A. 3.16
    B. 5.11
    C. 7.16
    D. 9.16

Problem solved:

The correct answer is B. To solve this problem, we must consider the equilibrium:

$$HCN \rightleftharpoons H^+ + CN^-$$

where, using the pK_a given for HCN in Table 21.2:

$$K_a = \frac{[H^+][CN^-]}{[HCN]} = \frac{[x][x]}{[0.10 - x]} = 10^{-pK_a} = 10^{-9.22} = 6.02 \times 10^{-10}$$

Given the small value of K_a, it is safe to consider x as negligible compared to 0.10, so the acid ionization constant expression simplifies to:

$$K_a = 6.02 \times 10^{-10} = \frac{x^2}{0.10}$$

or,

$$x^2 = 6.02 \times 10^{-11}$$

From which,

$$x = [H^+] = 7.7 \times 10^{-6}$$

Therefore,

$$pH = -\log [H^+] = -\log [7.0 \times 10^{-6}] = 5.11$$

21.1.2 TITRATION

21.1.2.1 A Mixture of an Acid and a Base

When a strong acid and a base or a strong base and an acid are placed in the same container, a neutralization reaction occurs:

$$HA + BOH \rightarrow H_2O + B^+ + A^-$$

This reaction will continue to produce water and salt until either the acid (HA) or the base (BOH) is consumed. When there is an excess of acid in solution, the base will be entirely consumed in the neutralization reaction, and the solution will be acidic. When there is an excess of base in solution, the acid will be entirely consumed, and the solution will be basic. When the quantity of acid is equal to the quantity of base, the solution is completely neutralized and has a pH of 7.

Please solve this problem:

- What is the pH of a 100 ml aqueous solution containing 0.10 mol HCl and 0.07 mol NaOH?

    A. 0.52
    B. 4.52
    C. 8.52
    D. 12.52

Problem solved:

The correct answer is A. To solve this problem, we must recognize that we have an excess of 0.03 mol of the strong acid HCl. This translates to an excess of 0.03 mol H^+. Therefore, the hydrogen ion concentration is given by:

$$[H^+] = 0.03 \text{ mol} \div 0.100 \text{ L} = 0.3 \, M$$

Therefore,

$$pH = -\log [H^+] = -\log [0.3] = 0.52$$

21.1.2.2 Acid/Base Titrations

In section **21.1.2.1**, we only considered a mixture of a fixed amount of acid with a fixed amount of base. A **titration** is the gradual addition of a base to an acid or the gradual addition of an acid to a base. (Base to acid is the usual manner in which MCAT questions are phrased.)

As base is added to acid, the pH of the solution rises, until all the acid has been consumed, and excess base is present. A typical acid-base titration curve is shown in Figure 21.1.

21.1.2.3 Equivalence Point: Titration of a Strong Acid

In a titration, the point at which the acid has been neutralized by base is referred to as the **equivalence point**. This point is indicated on Figure 21.2.

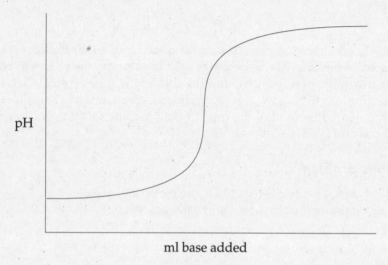

Figure 21.1

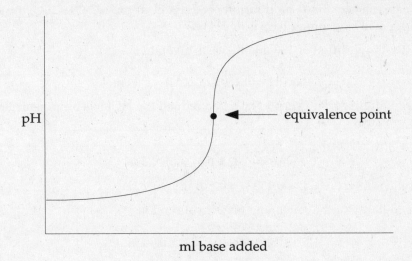

Figure 21.2

The equivalence point of a titration curve is the point at which exactly one equivalent of base has been added for one equivalent of acid. At any point in a titration curve prior to the equivalence point, the pH may be calculated from the concentration of acid. At any point after the equivalence point, the pH is determined by the excess base present.

Consider the following questions: 100 ml of 0.2 M hydrochloric acid, a strong acid, is titrated with 0.2 M sodium hydroxide, a strong base. What is the pH after (a) 50 ml, (b) 100 ml, and (c) 150 ml of NaOH have been added?

The initial conditions of this titration are (0.100 L)(0.2 M) = 0.02 mol HCl and 0.00 mol NaOH.

(a) The pH after the addition of 50 ml of base is given by:

$$NaOH = (0.050 \text{ L})(0.2 \text{ } M) = 0.01 \text{ mol}$$

Since 1 HCl is neutralized for every 1 NaOH added, 0.01 mol HCl have been neutralized.

This leaves:
$$0.02 - 0.01 = 0.01 \text{ mol HCl}$$

The total volume is now 0.100 L + 0.050 L = 0.150 L.

Therefore, the molarity of the remaining HCl solution is:

$$0.01 \text{ mol} \div 0.150 \text{ L} = 0.067 \text{ } M$$

Since the HCl is completely ionized, this gives us an [H⁺] of 0.067 M, from which:

$$pH = -\log [H^+] = -\log [0.067] = 1.17$$

(b) The pH after the addition of 100 ml of base is given by:

$$NaOH = (0.100 \text{ L})(0.2 \text{ } M) = 0.02 \text{ mol}$$

Since 1 HCl is neutralized for every 1 NaOH added, 0.02 mol HCl have been neutralized. We are at the equivalence point.

While the equivalence point of a titration need not be at pH = 7 (**21.1.2.4**), the equivalence point of a strong acid by a strong base is at pH = 7.

(c) The pH after the addition of 150 ml of base is given by:

$$NaOH = (0.150 \text{ L})(0.2 \text{ } M) = 0.03 \text{ mol}$$

Since 1 HCl is neutralized for every 1 NaOH added, all the HCl has been neutralized and excess NaOH remains.

This leaves:

$$0.03 - 0.02 = 0.01 \text{ mol NaOH}$$

The total volume is now 0.100 L + 0.150 L = 0.250 L.

Therefore, the molarity of the remaining NaOH solution is:

$$0.01 \text{ mol} \div 0.250 \text{ L} = 0.04 \text{ } M$$

Since the NaOH is completely ionized, this gives us a $[OH^-]$ of 0.04 M, from which:

$$pOH = -\log [OH^-] = -\log [0.04] = 1.40$$

Therefore,

$$pH = 14 - pOH = 14 - 1.40 = 12.60$$

Please solve this problem:

- The pH at the equivalence point of the titration of a strong acid with a strong base is:

  A. less than 7.
  B. equal to 7.
  C. greater than 7.
  D. possibly any one of the above answer choices.

Problem solved:

The correct answer is B. By definition, the pH at the equivalence point of the titration of a strong acid with a strong base is equal to 7, because both the strong acid and the strong base ionize completely in water. The equivalence point is the point at which $[H^+] = [OH^-]$, which, as we saw in **21.1.1.1**, is defined as pH = 7.

21.1.2.4 Titration of a Weak Acid

The titration of a weak acid by a strong base is vastly different from the titration of a strong acid by a strong base: the equivalence point is not equal to pH = 7, but is determined by the pK_a of the weak acid. Also, the solution is buffered prior to the equivalence point (**21.1.3**). Consider the titration of 100 ml of a 0.100 M solution of acetic acid ($K_a = 1.8 \times 10^{-5}$) with a 0.100 M solution of sodium hydroxide. What is the pH (a) before the titration, and after (b) 50 ml, (c) 100 ml, and (d) 150 ml of NaOH have been added?

(a) the pH of the solution prior to the titration must be calculated from the equilibrium expression:

$$CH_3COOH \rightleftharpoons H^+ + CH_3COO^-$$

which gives:

$$K_a = \frac{[H^+][CH_3COO^-]}{[CH_3COOH]}$$

Considering the equilibrium expression:

	CH_3COOH	$\rightleftharpoons$	H^+	+	CH_3COO^-
initially	0.100 M		0		0
change	$-x$		$+x$		$+x$
at equilibrium	0.100 $-x$ M		x		x

Therefore, at equilibrium:

$$K_a = \frac{[H^+][CH_3COO^-]}{[CH_3COOH]} = \frac{[x][x]}{[0.100 - x]} = 1.8 \times 10^{-5}$$

We may safely consider x to be very small relative to 0.100; therefore, the equilibrium expression becomes:

$$1.8 \times 10^{-5} = \frac{[x][x]}{[0.100]} = \frac{x^2}{0.100}$$

Therefore,

$$x^2 = 1.8 \times 10^{-6}$$

So,

$$x = 1.34 \times 10^{-3} = [H^+]$$

And,

$$pH = -\log[H^+] = -\log[1.34 \times 10^{-3}] = 2.87$$

(b) the pH of the solution after the addition of 50 ml of 0.100 M NaOH must also be calculated from the equilibrium expression:

	CH_3COOH	$\rightleftharpoons$	H^+	+	CH_3COO^-
initially	0.010 mol		0		0
change	-0.005 mol		$+x$		$+0.005$ mol
at equilibrium	0.005 mol		x		0.005 mol

Therefore, after the addition, the molarity of CH_3COOH is:

$$0.005 \text{ mol} \div 0.150 \text{ L} = 0.033 \text{ } M$$

And, the molarity of CH_3COO^- is also:

$$0.005 \text{ mol} \div 0.150 \text{ L} = 0.033 \text{ } M$$

Therefore,

$$K_a = \frac{[H^+][CH_3COO^-]}{[CH_3COOH]} = \frac{[x][0.033]}{[0.033]} = 1.8 \times 10^{-5}$$

Therefore, the equilibrium expression becomes:

$$[H^+] = x = K_a = 1.8 \times 10^{-5}$$

Therefore,

$$pH = -\log[H^+] = -\log[1.8 \times 10^{-5}] = 4.74$$

(c) the pH of the solution after the addition of 100 ml of 0.100 M NaOH is given by:

	CH_3COOH	$\rightleftharpoons$	H^+	+	CH_3COO^-
initially	0.010 mol		0		0
change	−0.010 mol		+x		+0.010 mol
after addition	0.000 mol		x		0.010 mol

The molarity of CH_3COO^- is:

$$0.010 \text{ mol} \div 0.2 \text{ L} = 0.05 \text{ } M$$

In this case, we must consider the base ionization constant expression:

$$K_b = \frac{[CH_3COOH][OH^-]}{[CH_3COO^-]} = \frac{K_w}{K_a} = \frac{1 \times 10^{-14}}{1.8 \times 10^{-5}} = 5.6 \times 10^{-10}$$

	CH_3COO^-	$\rightleftharpoons$	OH^-	+	CH_3COOH
initially	.05M		0		0
change	$-x$		$+x$		$+x$
at equilibrium	.05$M - x$		x		x

Therefore,

$$K_b = \frac{[CH_3COOH][OH^-]}{[CH_3COO^-]} = \frac{[x][x]}{[0.05 - x]} = 5.6 \times 10^{-10}$$

We may safely consider x to be very small relative to 0.050, therefore, the equilibrium expression becomes:

$$5.6 \times 10^{-10} = \frac{[x][x]}{[0.050]} = \frac{x^2}{0.050}$$

Therefore,

$$x^2 = (5.6 \times 10^{-10})(0.050) = 2.8 \times 10^{-11}$$

So,

$$x = 5.29 \times 10^{-6} = [OH^-]$$

And,

$$pOH = -\log [OH^-] = -\log [5.29 \times 10^{-6}] = 5.28$$

$$pH = 14 - pOH$$

$$pH = 8.72$$

(d) Since NaOH is a much stronger base than the acetate ion, we can ignore the OH-contribution made by the acetate ion once we are beyond the equivalence point. The pH after the addition of 150 ml of base is calculated in a manner identical to that for the titration of a strong acid:

$$NaOH = (0.150 \text{ L})(0.1 \, M) = 0.015 \text{ mol}$$

Since 1 CH_3COOH is neutralized for every 1 NaOH added, all the CH_3COOH has been neutralized and excess NaOH remains.

This leaves:

$$0.015 - 0.01 = 0.005 \text{ mol NaOH}$$

The total volume is now 0.100 L + 0.150 L = 0.250 L.

Therefore, the molarity of the remaining NaOH solution is:

$$0.005 \text{ mol} \div 0.250 \text{ L} = 0.02 \ M$$

Since the NaOH is completely ionized, this gives us a [OH⁻] of 0.02 M, from which:

$$\text{pOH} = -\log [\text{OH}^-] = -\log [0.02] = 1.70$$

Therefore,

$$\text{pH} = 14 - \text{pOH} = 14 - 1.70 = 12.30$$

Please solve this problem:

- The pH at the equivalence point of the titration of a strong acid with a weak base is:

  A. less than 7.
  B. equal to 7.
  C. greater than 7.
  D. possibly any one of the above answer choices.

Problem solved:

The correct answer is A. Since the acid, unlike the base, will dissociate completely in solution, the pH, even in the presence of equivalent amounts of the acid and the base, will favor the acid. To solve this problem mathematically, implement the scenario for case (c) above, substituting K_b for K_a and K_a for K_b.

21.1.2.5 Indicators and the End Point

It is often convenient to use a chemical that changes color when the equivalence point of a titration is reached. Such a chemical is called an **indicator**. The point at which the titration is stopped (because the indicator has changed color) is called the **end point**.

Some common indicators are given in Table 21.4.

Indicator	pH range
methyl violet	0.0 to 1.6
malachite green	0.2 to 1.8
Congo red	3.0 to 5.0
methyl orange	3.1 to 4.4
methyl red	4.4 to 6.2
phenolpthalein	8.2 to 10.0

Table 21.4

An indicator is titrated by the base, following the equation:

$$HIn^+ + OH^- \rightarrow In + H_2O$$

where HIn^+ and In indicate the two forms of the indicator—one that is protonated and one that is deprotonated. Each form of the indicator appears as a different color in aqueous solution. When the color change is noticed, we know that the indicator is being titrated, indicating that the equivalence point of the acid has been reached. Figure 21.3 shows the appropriate pH range within which an indicator should operate for the given acid.

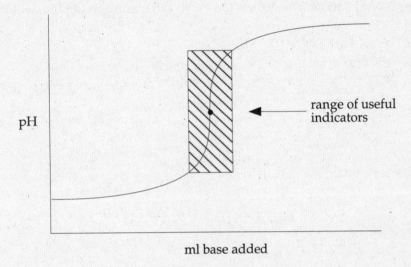

ml base added

Figure 21.3

An indicator color change signifies the end point of a titration, as mentioned above. In the best-case scenario, the end point will equal the equivalence point for the acid being titrated. Remember that the equivalence point is the point at which the amount of base is exactly equal to the amount of acid. Therefore, the closer our end point (the point at which we stop adding base) is to the equivalence point, the more accurate our titration will be.

Please solve this problem:

- An acid has a pK_a of 1.8×10^{-5}. The appropriate indicator to use when titrating a $0.1\ M$ solution of this acid with $0.1\ M$ potassium hydroxide is:

  A. methyl red.
  B. malachite green.
  C. Congo red.
  D. phenolphthalein.

Problem solved:

The correct answer is D. To solve this problem, we must first recognize that this is a weak acid being titrated by a strong base. Therefore, at the equivalence point, an equilibrium defined by K_b is in effect:

$$K_b = \frac{[BH][OH^-]}{[B^-]} = \frac{K_w}{K_a} = \frac{1 \times 10^{-14}}{1.8 \times 10^{-5}} = 5.6 \times 10^{-10}$$

At the equivalence point, an equal volume of base has been added to the acid so the volume has doubled. The concentration of B^- is equal to half the original concentration of acid. The B^- concentration is 0.05 M. The expression for K_b (after simplifying the denominator) becomes:

$$5.6 \times 10^{-10} = \frac{x^2}{0.05}$$

So,

$$x^2 = 2.8 \times 10^{-11}$$

And,

$$x = [OH^-] = 5.3 \times 10^{-6}$$

Therefore,

$$pOH = -\log [5.3 \times 10^{-6}] = 5.28$$

And,

$$pH = 14 - 5.28 = 8.72$$

Of the answer choices, the indicator that operates best in the pH range 8.2 to 10.0, is phenolpthalein.

21.1.2.6 Polyprotic Acids

A **polyprotic acid** is an acid that contains more than one acidic proton. Sulfuric acid (H_2SO_4) is an example of a **diprotic acid**. Phosphoric acid (H_3PO_4) is an example of a **triprotic acid**. When dealing with polyprotic acids, it is important to remember that each proton will have a different K_a and, therefore, each proton will be titrated separately. An example of a titration curve for a triprotic acid is shown in Figure 21.4.

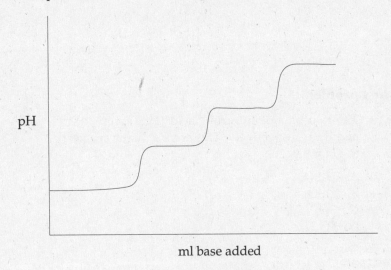

Figure 21.4

Note that since there are three acidic protons to be titrated, there are three equivalence points in the titration curve. The first equivalence point corresponds to the equilibrium:

$$H_3A \rightleftharpoons H^+ + H_2A^-$$

the acid ionization constant expression for which is:

$$K_{a1} = \frac{[H^+][H_2A^-]}{[H_3A]}$$

The second equivalence point corresponds to the equilibrium:

$$H_2A^- \rightleftharpoons H^+ + HA^{2-}$$

the acid ionization constant expression for which is:

$$K_{a2} = \frac{[H^+][HA^{2-}]}{[H_2A^-]}$$

And the third equivalence point corresponds to the equilibrium:

$$HA^{2-} \rightleftharpoons H^+ + A^{3-}$$

the acid ionization constant expression for which is:

$$K_{a3} = \frac{[H^+][HA^{3-}]}{[HA^{2-}]}$$

Please solve this problem:

- The two pK_as of sulfurous acid (H_2SO_3) are 1.81 and 6.91, respectively. The predominant species at pH = 9 is:

  A. H_2SO_3
  B. HSO_3^-
  C. SO_3^{2-}
  D. H^+

Problem solved:

The correct answer is C. At a pH of 9, the hydrogen ion concentration is 1×10^{-9}. It is not likely that a concentration of this magnitude is indicative of a *predominant* species, so choice D is eliminated. At a pH of 1.81, the titration of the first acidic proton is halfway complete and, at a pH of 9, there is not likely to be a measurable quantity of H_2SO_3 left. Therefore, choice A is eliminated. At a pH of 6.91, the titration of the second acidic proton is halfway complete; at this point $[HSO_3^-] = [SO_3^{2-}]$. Therefore, for any pH greater than 6.91, $[SO_3^{2-}] > [HSO_3^-]$, eliminating choice B and leaving only choice C.

21.1.3 BUFFERS

A **buffer** is composed of a weak acid and its conjugate base salt, or a weak base and its conjugate acid salt. A buffer is designed to resist a change in pH when an external acid or base is added to the solution. The acid component of a buffer system neutralizes added base, while the base component of a buffer system neutralizes added acid.

The equilibrium expressions for a buffer system comprised of the weak acid, acetic acid (CH_3COOH), and its conjugate base salt, sodium acetate ($CH_3COO^-Na^+$), are:

$$CH_3COOH \rightleftharpoons H^+ + CH_3COO^-$$

and

$$CH_3COO^-Na^+ \rightleftharpoons Na^+ + CH_3COO^-$$

The pH of a buffered solution is calculated using the Henderson-Hasselbach equation:

$$pH = pK_a + \log \frac{[A^-]}{[HA]}$$

where the pK_a is that for the acid component of the buffer system, $[A^-]$ is the concentration of the conjugate base, and [HA] is the concentration of the acid. When $[A^-] = [HA]$, this reduces to:

$$pH = pK_a$$

When the concentration of the buffer solution far exceeds the concentration of acid or base to be added, the ratio $[A^-]$ to [HA] will not be strongly affected and, thus, the pH will remain relatively stable.

Buffers are most effective in a pH range that is near the pK_a of the acid component. A good rule to follow is that a buffer will be effective in the range:

$$pK_a - 1 < pH < pK_a + 1$$

Written another way:

$$pH = pK_a \pm 1$$

Please solve this problem:

- All of the following acid-base pairs are examples of buffers EXCEPT:

    A. HF/NaF
    B. H_2CO_3/$NaHCO_3$
    C. CH_3CO_2H/$NaCH_3CO_2$
    D. HCl/NaCl

Problem solved:

The correct answer is D. A buffer system is a mixture of a weak acid and its conjugate base salt, or a weak base and its conjugate acid salt. All of the choices give examples of weak acids and their conjugate base salts *except* choice D. HCl is a strong acid. Given the strength of the H–F bond and the capacity of fluorine to engage in hydrogen bonds, HF is *not* a strong acid. Compare the hydrohalogen acids:

HF: $pK_a = 3.14$

HCl: $pK_a = -6$

HBr: $pK_a = -9$

HI: $pK_a = -9.5$

21.2 MASTERY APPLIED: SAMPLE PASSAGE AND QUESTIONS

Passage

The suitability of a buffer made of components of a polyprotic system can be estimated from a distribution curve, which shows the variation in the percentage of each species with pH.

For the general triprotic system, the equilibria are:

$$H_3A \rightleftharpoons H^+ + H_2A^-$$

$$H_2A^- \rightleftharpoons H^+ + HA^{2-}$$

$$HA^{2-} \rightleftharpoons H^+ + A^{3-}$$

The ionization constant expressions are:

$$K_{a1} = \frac{[H^+][H_2A^-]}{[H_3A]}, \text{ and } K_{b1} = \frac{[H_3A][OH^-]}{[H_2A^-]}$$

$$K_{a2} = \frac{[H^+][HA^{2-}]}{[H_2A^-]}, \text{ and } K_{b2} = \frac{[H_2A^-][OH^-]}{[HA^{2-}]}$$

$$K_{a3} = \frac{[H^+][H^{3-}]}{[HA^{2-}]}, \text{ and } K_{b3} = \frac{[HA^{2-}][OH^-]}{[A^{3-}]}$$

And the distribution curve is:

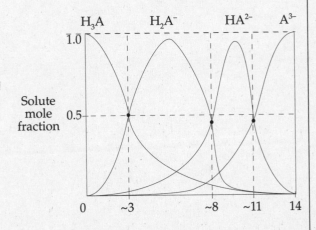

1. A buffer pair for a pH of 11 is:
   A. H_3A/H_2A^-
   B. H_3A/HA^{2-}
   C. H_2A^-/HA^{2-}
   D. HA^{2-}/A^{3-}

2. The K_b of H_2A^- is approximately:
   A. 1×10^{-4}
   B. 1×10^{-6}
   C. 1×10^{-8}
   D. 1×10^{-12}

3. Point x represents:
   A. the pH of the endpoint of the titration of H_3A with base.
   B. halfway to the equivalence point of the titration of H_3A with base.
   C. the pH of the equivalence point of the titration of H_3A with base.
   D. the pH of the equivalence point of the titration of H_2A^- with acid.

4. To monitor the titration of 0.1 M H_2A^- with a 0.1 M solution of strong base, the best indicator to use is one that changes color in the range:
   A. 6.8 to 7.8
   B. 7.8 to 8.8
   C. 8.8 to 9.8
   D. 10.8 to 11.8

5. What is the predominant species when the hydrogen ion concentration is 3.17×10^{-12} ?
   A. H_3A
   B. H_2A^-
   C. HA^{2-}
   D. A^{3-}

6. Benzoic acid has a pKa of 4.19. Ranked in order of acidity:

   A. benzoic acid > H_3A > H_2A^- > HA^{2-} > A^{3-}

   B. H_3A > benzoic acid > H_2A^- > HA^{2-} > A^{3-}

   C. H_3A > H_2A^- > benzoic acid > HA^{2-} > A^{3-}

   D. H_3A > H_2A^- > HA^{2-} > benzoic acid > A^{3-}

7. When 1,000 ml of 0.1 M H_2A^- is mixed with 500 ml of 0.1 M H_3A. The resulting pH is:

   A. 9.65

   B. 7.65

   C. 5.65

   D. 3.3

21.3 MASTERY VERIFIED: ANSWERS AND EXPLANATIONS

1. *The correct answer is D.* The answer is taken directly from the distribution curve. At pH = 11, the two predominant species are HA^{2-} and A^{3-}.

2. *The correct answer is B.* The pK_a of H_2A^- is approximately 8 (from the graph). Using the relationship $pK_w = pK_a + pK_b$, where $pK_w = 14$, we see that $pK_b = 6$. Therefore, $K_b = 1 \times 10^{-6}$.

3. *The correct answer is B.* Point x represents the point at which $[H_3A] = [H_2A^-]$. Using the Henderson-Hasselbach equation:

$$pH = pK_a + \log\frac{[A^-]}{[HA]}$$

we see that the log term reduces to zero (log 1 = 0), and we are left with $pH = pK_a$. The point at which this is true is halfway to the equivalence point.

4. *The correct answer is C.* By definition, the equivalence point is where all the acid is neutralized. In the case it is where all H_2A^- has turned to HA^{2-}. From the graph we see that HA^{2-} is 100% at about 9.5. Thus C is the best answer. Note that in reality there exists a negligible amount of H_2A^- at the equivalence point.

5. *The correct answer is D.* When $[H^+] = 3.17 \times 10^{-12}$, pH = 11.5. The predominant species at pH = 11.5 is A^{3-}, as seen from the distribution curve.

6. *The correct answer is B.* From the distribution curve data: $pK_{a1} = 3$, $pK_{a2} = 8$, and $pK_{a3} = 11$. Therefore, benzoic acid, with a pK_a of 4.19, is less acidic than H_3A, but more acidic than H_2A^-.

7. *The correct answer is D.* To solve this problem, we must use the Henderson-Hasselbach equation:

$$pH = pK_a + \log\frac{[A^-]}{[HA]}$$

We also can quickly calculate the final concentrations of H_3A and H_2A^-:

$$[H_3A] = \frac{0.05 \text{ mol}}{(1.000 \text{ L} + 0.500 \text{ L})} = 0.0333 \text{ } M$$

$$[H_2A] = \frac{0.1 \text{ mol}}{(1.000 \text{ L} + 0.500 \text{ L})} = 0.0667 \text{ } M$$

Thus:

$$pH_a = pK_a + \log\frac{[H_2A]}{[H_3A]}$$
$$= 3 + \log 2$$
$$= 3 + .3$$
$$pH = 3.3$$

CHAPTER 22

ELECTROCHEMISTRY

22.1 MASTERY ACHIEVED

22.1.1 REVIEW OF REDOX

22.1.1.1 The Half Reaction

As was discussed in Chapter 15, an **oxidation** cannot happen without a concomitant **reduction**. In this regard, we may consider an **oxidation–reduction reaction (redox)** as consisting of two **half reactions**: a half reaction representing an oxidation and a half reaction representing a reduction.

Oxidation is a loss of electrons. Reduction is a gain of electrons. Since an electron carries a charge of negative one, a single electron oxidation will increase the oxidation state by $-(-1)$, or $+1$. Similarly, a single electron reduction will decrease the oxidation state by $+(-1)$, or -1.

An oxidation half reaction takes the form:

$$M^{c+} \rightarrow M^{(c+n)+} + ne^-$$

for example:

$$Fe^{2+} \rightarrow Fe^{3+} + e^-$$

A reduction half reaction takes the form:

$$M^{c+} + ne^- \rightarrow M^{(c-n)+}$$

for example:

$$Al^{3+} + 3e^- \rightarrow Al^0$$

An **oxidizing agent**, or oxidant, is an agent that oxidizes. An oxidizing agent oxidizes another species by accepting electrons from that species. By accepting these electrons, the oxidizing agent is reduced.

A **reducing agent**, or reductant, is an agent that reduces. A reducing agent reduces another species by giving up electrons to that species. By giving up these electrons, the reducing agent is oxidized.

Please solve this problem:

- In the reaction $2Li + 2H_2O \rightarrow 2LiOH + H_2$:

  A. Li^+ is the oxidizing agent, and H^+ is the reducing agent.
  B. H^+ is the oxidizing agent, and Li is the reducing agent.
  C. Li^+ is the oxidizing agent, and H_2 is the reducing agent.
  D. H_2 is the oxidizing agent, and Li^+ is the reducing agent.

Problem solved:

B is the correct answer. The half reactions for this redox equation are:

$$2Li \rightarrow 2Li^{+1} + 2e^-$$

$$2H^+ + 2e^- \rightarrow H_2$$

From these, we see that lithium metal is oxidized to lithium(I) and two protons are reduced to hydrogen gas. Therefore, H^+ is the oxidizing agent (the agent that caused the oxidation of lithium), and lithium is the reducing agent (the agent that caused the reduction of H^+).

22.1.1.2 Redox Couples

As we have previously stated, a redox reaction consists of a pair of half reactions: one oxidation reaction and one reduction reaction. These half reactions are reversible. The direction in which a given half reaction proceeds is determined by the half reaction with which it is allowed to react.

For instance, consider the half reaction:

$$Cu^{2+} + 2e^- \rightarrow Cu^0$$

If zinc metal is coupled with Cu^{2+}, the zinc metal is oxidized, and the copper(II) is reduced, since zinc(II) is a weaker oxidizing agent than Cu^{2+}:

$$Zn^0 + Cu^{2+} \rightarrow Zn^{2+} + Cu^0$$

However, iron(III) is a stronger oxidizing agent than copper(II). When copper metal is placed in a solution of Fe^{3+}, the copper metal is oxidized, and the iron(III) is reduced:

$$2Fe^{3+} + Cu^0 \rightarrow 2Fe^{2+} + Cu^{2+}$$

Given the reversibility of half reactions, it is often convenient to refer to **redox couples**—a couple consists of an oxidized form and a reduced form of a given species. The three redox couples referred to above are: Cu^{2+}/Cu, Zn^{2+}/Zn and Fe^{3+}/Fe^{2+}. Note that redox couples are written: oxidized form/reduced form. In many ways, redox couples are analogous to acid/conjugate base or base/conjugate acid pairs (Chapter 21).

Please solve this problem:

- The redox couples involved in the reaction
  $3Cu + 8HNO_3 \rightarrow 3Cu(NO_3)_2 + 4H_2O + NO$ are:

  A. Cu/Cu^{2+}, N^{5+}/N^{2+}
  B. Cu^{2+}/Cu, N^{5+}/N^{2+}
  C. Cu/Cu^{2+}, N^{5+}/N^{2+}
  D. Cu^{2+}/Cu, N^{2+}/N^{5+}

Problem solved:

B is the correct answer. Redox couples must always be written as **oxidized form/reduced form**, so you should have been able to eliminate choices A, C, and D by inspection. B is the only answer choice with both the copper couple and the nitrogen couple written in the correct form.

22.1.2 ELECTROCHEMISTRY DEFINITIONS

An **electrode** is the interface in an electrochemical cell at which the electron transfer in a redox reaction occurs. This does not imply, however, that the electrode is either oxidized or reduced. An **inert electrode** does **not** take part in the reaction: it simply facilitates the **electron transfer** process, or provides a site for deposition of a reacting chemical. An **active electrode** does take part in the redox reaction. As a result, an active electrode is either used up or augmented during the reaction. In redox reactions, there must be a minimum of two electrodes. The **anode** is the electrode at which **oxidation** occurs. The **cathode** is the electrode at which **reduction** occurs. One can remember these relationships through use of the simple vowel-vowel, consonant-consonant mnemonic:

c̲athode = r̲eduction;   a̲node = o̲xidation

At the anode, electrons are transferred into the circuit. At the cathode, electrons are taken from the circuit. The circuit is a metal wire or other substance that connects the electrodes to one another, and allows the transfer of electrons.

Please solve this problem:

- The definition of a cathode is:

  A. the negative electrode in an electrochemical cell.
  B. the positive electrode in an electrochemical cell.
  C. the electrode at which oxidation occurs in an electrochemical cell.
  D. the electrode at which reduction occurs in an electrochemical cell.

Problem solved:

D is the correct answer. Choice C is the definition of an anode. As we will see below, the cathode is the positive electrode in certain circumstances (galvanic cells) and the negative electrode in other circumstances (electrolytic cells).

22.1.3 REDUCTION POTENTIAL, VOLTAGE, AND SPONTANEITY

22.1.3.1 Reduction Potentials and Oxidation Potentials

In order to determine the direction in which an oxidation-reduction equilibrium will run, we must have a means of quantifying half reactions. The most common method for quantification is the **reduction potential**. The sign and magnitude of a reduction potential tell how easily a species is reduced. The reduction potentials of some common species are given in Table 22.1.

Reduction	$E°$ (volts)	$\Delta G°$ (kJ)
$Li^+ + e^- \longrightarrow Li(s)$	−3.05	294.3
$K^+ + e^- \longrightarrow K(s)$	−2.93	282.7
$H_2(g) + 2e^- \longrightarrow 2H^-$	−2.25	434.3
$Al^{3+} + 3e^- \longrightarrow Al(s)$	−1.66	480.6
$Cr^{3+} + e^- \longrightarrow Cr^{2+}$	−0.41	39.6
$Pb^{2+} + 2e^- \longrightarrow Pb(s)$	−0.13	25.1
$2H^+ + 2e^- \longrightarrow H_2(g)$	0.00	0.0
$Cu^{2+} + 2e^- \longrightarrow Cu(s)$	+0.34	−65.6
$Cu^+ + e^- \longrightarrow Cu(s)$	+0.52	−50.2
$I_2 + 2e^- \longrightarrow 2I^-$	+0.54	−104.2
$Fe^{3+} + e^- \longrightarrow Fe^{2+}$	+0.77	−74.3
$Ag^+ + e^- \longrightarrow Ag(s)$	+0.80	−77.2
$Br_2 + 2e^- \longrightarrow 2Br^-$	+1.09	−210.4
$O_2(g) + 4H^+ + 4e^- \longrightarrow 2H_2O$	+1.23	−474.8
$Cr_2O_7^{2-} + 14H^+ + 6e^- \longrightarrow 2Cr^{3+} + 7H_2O$	+1.33	−770.1
$Cl_2 + 2e^- \longrightarrow 2Cl^-$	+1.36	−262.5
$MnO_4^- + 8H^+ + 5e^- \longrightarrow Mn^{2+} + 4H_2O$	+1.49	−718.9
$MnO_2 + 4H^+ + 2e^- \longrightarrow Mn^{2+} + 4H_2O$	+1.61	−310.7
$F_2 + 2e^- \longrightarrow 2F^-$	+2.87	−553.9

Reduction Potentials of Common Species

Table 22.1

Table 22.1 gives data both in terms of **voltage** ($E°$) and in terms of **standard Gibbs free energy** ($G°$). Recall (Chapter 17) that a negative $\Delta G°$ denotes a spontaneous reaction. Therefore, a positive $E°$ also denotes a spontaneous reaction. Those reactions in the above table with a negative $\Delta G°$ (or positive $E°$) are expected to proceed to the right. Those reactions with a positive $\Delta G°$ (or negative $E°$) are expected to be nonspontaneous, or to proceed to the left.

Please solve this problem:

- Using the data in Table 22.1, the most easily oxidized species given below is:

    A. Mn^{2+}
    B. Fe^{2+}
    C. Al
    D. Li

Problem solved:

D is the correct answer. Note the following four reduction potentials:

Reduction	$E°$ (volts)
$Li^+ + e^- \longrightarrow Li(s)$	−3.05
$Al^{3+} + 3e^- \longrightarrow Al(s)$	−1.66
$Fe^{3+} + e^- \longrightarrow Fe^{2+}$	+0.77
$MnO_4^- + 8H^+ + 5e^- \longrightarrow Mn^{2+} + 4H_2O$	+1.49

Table 22.2

In a reduction potential table, reductions will always be listed from the most negative $E°$ to the most positive $E°$. All you have to recognize is that the substances on the left of the reaction are being reduced, and the substances on the right are being oxidized. Using the four-item table above, in order from most easily reduced to least easily reduced, we see that: $Mn^{7+} > Fe^{3+} > Al^{3+} > Li^+$. Likewise, the most easily oxidized substance to the least easily oxidized substance is: $Li > Al > Fe^{2+} > Mn^{2+}$. Therefore, in a table of reduction potentials, the most easily reduced species may be found on the bottom left, and the least easily reduced species may be found on the top left. Similarly, the most easily oxidized species is found on the top right, and the least easily oxidized species is found on the bottom right.

Note that while it is customary to report **reduction potentials**, we also could have reported the above data as **oxidation potentials**. Table 22.3 shows the oxidation potentials for the four half reactions of the halogens given in Table 22.1.

Oxidation	$E°$ (volts)	$\Delta G°$ (kJ)
$2I^- \rightarrow I_2 + 2e^-$	−0.54	+104.2
$2Br^- \rightarrow Br_2 + 2e^-$	−1.09	+210.4
$2Cl^- \rightarrow Cl_2 + 2e^-$	−1.36	+262.5
$2F^- \rightarrow F_2 + 2e^-$	−2.87	+553.9

Oxidation Potentials for Halogens
Table 22.3

Note that while the half reaction for the reduction of F_2 is spontaneous (negative $\Delta G°$, positive $E°$), the half reaction for the oxidation of F^- is nonspontaneous (positive $\Delta G°$, negative $E°$). It should be clear that oxidation half reactions are simply the reverse of the corresponding reduction half reactions. It should also be clear that the oxidation potential of a half reaction is simply the negative of the reduction potential for that half reaction.

Please solve this problem:

- Using the data from Table 22.3, the strongest oxidizing agent within the halogen family is:

  A. F_2
  B. F^-
  C. I^-
  D. I_2

Problem solved:

A is the correct answer. Remember that an oxidizing agent is reduced. This changes the problem to, "Which member of the halogen family is most easily reduced?" To have reduction potentials, we need to reverse the direction of the reactions given in Table 22.3, as well as reverse the sign of $E°$. The most positive $E°$ indicates the most easily reduced species, which is F_2.

22.1.3.2 The Electromotive Force

A **standard potential**, or **electromotive force (emf)**, is represented by $E°$. In a redox reaction, there is a movement of electrons from the substance being oxidized to the substance being reduced. This current arises from a **voltage**, which can be measured. In order to predict the efficacy of a redox pair, it is easier to refer to a table such as 22.1 than to perform an experiment. But since the reactions given in the table are half reactions, we must have a standard half reaction (or half cell) to which we may compare these half reactions. For electrochemistry, the **standard conditions** are: **1 molar** in any solute (for instance, Cu^{2+}); **1 atm** for any gas; and **25°C**. The **standard half cell** is the **hydrogen electrode**:

$$2H^+(aq, 1\ M) + 2e^- \rightarrow H_2(g, 1\ atm)$$

By definition, the emf of the hydrogen half cell is taken as $E° = 0$ V.

Once a half reaction has been compared to the hydrogen half cell under standard conditions, its behavior, relative to each other half reaction that has also been compared to the hydrogen half cell, may be predicted. Table 22.1 is a tabulation of such comparisons to the hydrogen half cell.

Since emf will be altered by changes in **concentration** (for solutes), **pressure** (for gases), and **temperature**, all emfs recorded at nonstandard conditions are represented by E. For emfs at nonstandard conditions, the temperature and concentration (or pressure) must also be given.

Much like Hess' law (**17.1.1.4**) allowed the summation of enthalpies of formation, the emfs of half reactions may also be summed to produce a **cell emf**.

$Pb^{2+} + 2e^- \rightarrow Pb(s)$	$E° = -0.13$
$2I^- \rightarrow I_2 + 2e^-$	$E° = -0.54$

$Pb^{2+} + 2I^- \rightarrow Pb(s) + I_2$	$E° = -0.67$

Note: The most common error made on the MCAT is the multiplication of half reaction emfs by stoichiometric coefficients.

Never multiply an emf by a stoichiometric coefficient! Electromotive forces are independent of the total amount of material present, and depend only on concentration.

For example, consider the following balanced redox reaction:

$$14H^+ + Cr_2O_7^{2-} + 6Fe^{2+} \rightarrow 2Cr^{3+} + 6Fe^{3+} + 7H_2O$$

This reaction comes from the half reactions:

$$Cr_2O_7^{2-} + 14H^+ + 6e^- \rightarrow 2Cr^{3+} + 7H_2O \qquad\qquad E° = +1.33$$

and

$$6 \times (Fe^{2+} \rightarrow Fe^{3+} + e^-) \qquad\qquad E° = -0.77$$

The total emf for this reaction is $E° = +0.56$, **not** -3.26. By incorrectly using stoichiometric coefficients in this example, not only would you predict the wrong numerical answer for this redox equation, but you would also incorrectly predict that this reaction is nonspontaneous.

Please solve this problem:

- Using the data from Table 22.1, the emf for the redox reaction between manganese(II) oxide (MnO), potassium dichromate ($K_2Cr_2O_7$), and nitric acid (HNO_3) in water to produce chromium(III) nitrate ($Cr(NO_3)_3$), permanganic acid ($HMnO_4$), and potassium oxide (K_2O) is:

  A. -0.16 V
  B. -2.29 V
  C. -2.82 V
  D. -15.59 V

Problem solved:

A is the correct answer. The balanced equation for this reaction is:

$$6MnO + 5K_2Cr_2O_7 + 30HNO_3 \rightarrow 10Cr(NO_3)_3 + 6HMnO_4 + 5K_2O + 12H_2O$$

To solve this problem, you must recognize those species that undergo a change in oxidation state. Manganese changes from a +2 oxidation state to a +7 oxidation state, and chromium changes from a +6 oxidation state to a +3 oxidation state. All other species remain unchanged in oxidation state. Therefore, manganese is oxidized, and chromium is reduced. Using Table 22.1, we see:

Reduction/Oxidation	$E°$ (volts)
$Cr_2O_7^{2-} + 14H^+ + 6e^- \rightarrow 2Cr^{3+} + 7H_2O$	+1.33
$Mn^{2+} + 4H_2O \rightarrow MnO_4^- + 8H^+ + 5e^-$	-1.49
Total	-0.16

Table 22.4

22.1.3.3 Cell Diagrams

A **cell diagram** is the standard way to represent the half reactions in a redox reaction. By convention, the anode is given on the left, and the cathode is given on the right:

$$Fe^{2+}(aq) \,\|\, Fe^{3+}(aq) \,\|\, Cr_2O_7^{2-}(aq) \,\|\, Cr^{3+}(aq)$$

In a cell reaction, if the conditions are other than standard, the state (gas, liquid, solid, aqueous) and the concentration may be shown in parenthesis:

$$Fe^{2+}(aq, 0.5\ M) \,\|\, Fe^{3+}(aq, 0.5\ M) \,\|\, Cr_2O_7^{2-}(aq, 0.9\ M) \,\|\, Cr^{3+}(aq, 0.9\ M)$$

The double vertical line represents a salt bridge, or other ion conduit, through which ions are transferred from one half reaction to the other. Salt bridges are discussed in detail in section **22.1.4**.

The order of listing reactants and products in a cell diagram is:

oxidation reactant | oxidation product | reduction reactant | reduction product

Please solve this problem:

- The cell diagram for the reaction:

$$6MnO + 5K_2Cr_2O_7 + 30HNO_3 \rightarrow 10Cr(NO_3)_3 + 6HMnO_4 + 5K_2O + 12H_2O$$

  is given by:

  A. $Cr^{6+}(aq) \,\|\, Cr^{3+}(aq) \,\|\, Mn^{2+}(aq) \,\|\, Mn^{7+}(aq)$
  B. $Cr^{3+}(aq) \,\|\, Cr^{6+}(aq) \,\|\, Mn^{2+}(aq) \,\|\, Mn^{7+}(aq)$
  C. $Mn^{2+}(aq) \,\|\, Mn^{7+}(aq) \,\|\, Cr^{6+}(aq) \,\|\, Cr^{3+}(aq)$
  D. $Mn^{7+}(aq) \,\|\, Mn^{2+}(aq) \,\|\, Cr^{6+}(aq) \,\|\, Cr^{3+}(aq)$

Problem solved:

C is correct. This is the same redox reaction referred to in the problem in **22.1.3.2**. In that section, we saw that manganese is oxidized from +2 to +7, and that chromium is reduced from +6 to +3. Using the rules for writing cell diagrams (oxidation reactant | oxidation product | reduction reactant | reduction product), the correct answer must be C. Choices B and D are incorrect, since B depicts two oxidations and D depicts two reductions. Choice A would be correct if it were reversed.

22.1.4 GALVANIC CELLS

A **galvanic**, or **voltaic**, cell was first used to demonstrate the validity of the electron transfer occurring in a redox reaction. Consider the reaction of dichromate with iodine:

$$14H^+ + Cr_2O_7^{2-} + 6I^- \rightarrow 2Cr^{3+} + 3I_2 + 7H_2O$$

This reaction was chosen because it is easy to follow visually. Initially, a solution containing the dichromate ion will be orange. After the reduction to chromate, the solution will be green. Likewise, a solution containing iodide (I^-) will be colorless; however, a solution containing I_2 will be yellow-brown.

If a solution of potassium iodide is poured into an orange-colored potassium dichromate solution (which also contains sulfuric acid, H_2SO_4, as a proton source), the reaction mixture becomes green. The color of the iodine is masked by the green of the chromium(III). While simple chemical tests will indicate that the green color is indeed due to chromium(III) and that iodine (I_2) is also present in the resultant solution, we do not have direct proof of an electron exchange process. A galvanic cell provides such a direct proof.

Suppose that instead of mixing our two solutions, we connect them via a platinum wire connected to a **galvanometer** (to detect current), as shown below. Platinum is chosen, since it will not react with either of our initial solutions. The galvanometer will indicate a flow of electrons from one solution to the other.

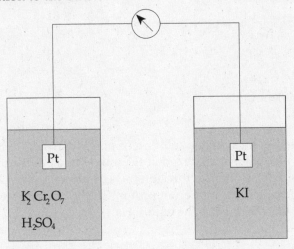

Please solve this problem:

- In the above diagram, there is no flow of electrons. Why?

Problem solved:

Initially, electrons flow from one solution to the other. A salt bridge is necessary to sustain the flow of electrons. In the solution containing the iodide, some of the iodide ions contact the platinum wire and electrons flow to the wire, thus becoming oxidized to iodine:

$$2I^- - 2e^- \rightarrow I_2$$

These electrons are then transferred through the wire to the solution containing the dichromate ion. Some of the dichromate ions accept these electrons and are reduced to chromate ions:

$$Cr_2O_7^{2-} + 14H^+ + 6e^- \rightarrow 2Cr^{3+} + 7H_2O$$

However, this process cannot continue. A consumption of the iodide ions in the oxidation vessel will leave an excess of positively charged potassium ions in this vessel. This build-up of positive charge will prevent the further release of electrons from the remaining iodide ions. Eliminating this excess positive charge is done by using a salt bridge.

A **salt bridge** is a link between the oxidation and reduction vessels that allows for the passage of the counter ions in each of the vessels. These counter ions must not be reactive under the conditions of either half reaction, and they should be highly soluble in the solution medium. A complete galvanic cell for the redox reaction of iodide and dichromate is depicted below:

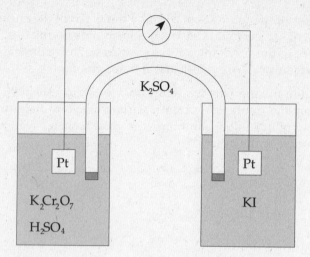

The salt bridge consists of an aqueous solution of potassium sulfate held into a U-tube by plugs of glass wool. As the iodide is oxidized at the anode, the build-up of positive charge is alleviated by the flow of potassium ions through the salt bridge to the cathodic vessel. Similarly, we recognize that a consumption of protons in the cathode reaction leaves an excess of negatively charged sulfate ions from the equilibria:

$$H_2SO_4 \rightleftharpoons H^+ + HSO_4^-$$

$$HSO_4^- \rightleftharpoons H^+ + SO_4^{2-}$$

To alleviate this build-up of negative charge in the cathodic vessel, sulfate flows through the salt bridge to the anodic vessel. The flow of the potassium ions and the sulfate ion maintain a charge balance in the reaction vessels and allow the redox reactions to proceed, thereby producing a measurable current in the galvanometer.

Because of the need for platinum electrodes in this galvanic cell, the cell diagram is slightly more complicated than those illustrated above (22.1.3.3):

$$Pt \mid I^-, I_2 \mid Cr_2O_7^{2-}, H^+, Cr^{3+} \mid Pt$$

A galvanic cell is a spontaneous redox cell. That is, a galvanic cell may be employed to produce a current (which results from the voltage) for the performance of useful work.

In a galvanic cell:

- the redox reaction is spontaneous

- the cell creates an electron flow

- oxidation occurs at the anode

- reduction occurs at the cathode

- the cathode is the positive electrode

- the anode is the negative electrode

- electrons flow from the anode to the cathode

Please solve this problem:

- The redox reaction which occurs in a galvanic cell:

   A. is nonspontaneous, requiring an electric current from anode to cathode.

   B. is spontaneous, creating an electric current from anode to cathode.

   C. is nonspontaneous, requiring an electric current from cathode to anode.

   D. is spontaneous, creating an electric current from cathode to anode.

Problem solved:

D is the correct answer. By definition, an electrochemical cell is galvanic if the redox reaction is spontaneous. This definition eliminates choices A and C. To decide between choices B and D, one must remember that current flows in the opposite direction of electron flow: a galvanic cell creates a flow of electrons from the anode to the cathode, and a current flow from cathode to anode.

22.1.5 ELECTROLYTIC CELLS

We saw in **22.1.4** that a galvanic cell uses a spontaneous redox reaction to produce an electrical current. In an **electrolytic cell**, we are concerned with driving nonspontaneous redox reactions by supplying an electrical current.

Electroplating is an important application of electrolysis. This technique is often employed to improve the appearance and durability of metal objects. For example, a thin film of chromium is applied over steel automobile bumpers to improve appearance and to retard corrosion of the underlying steel. Silver plating is common on eating utensils. The typical apparatus for electroplating a fork is shown below:

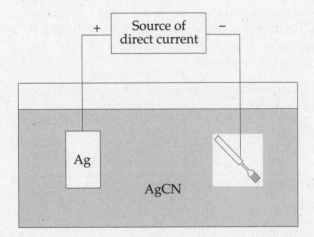

In this example, a direct current is supplied to the system from an external source. The silver bar is the anode and the fork is the cathode. At the anode, the silver is oxidized to furnish Ag^+ ions to the solution. At the cathode, the Ag^+ ions in solution are reduced to silver metal, which adheres to the surface of the fork. The half reactions are:

Anode: $Ag(s) - e^- \rightarrow Ag^+$
Cathode: $Ag^+ + e^- \rightarrow Ag(s)$

The purpose of the **external current source** is to supply electrons to the cathode for the reduction process. The oxidation process at the anode then supplies electrons to the external current source, so the process may continue. As time passes, silver metal from the anode is transferred to the cathode. You should note that electron flow in an electrolytic cell is confined to the wires attaching the anode and cathode to the external current source. Electrons do not flow through the electrolytic medium.

In an electrolytic cell:

- the redox reaction is nonspontaneous*

- the cell requires an electron flow*

- oxidation occurs at the anode

- reduction occurs at the cathode

- the anode is the positive electrode*

- the cathode is the negative electrode*

- electrons flow from the anode to the cathode

- current flows from the cathode to the anode

Items marked with asterisks differ from the case of a galvanic cell.

Please solve this problem:

- The electrolysis of brine (concentrated aqueous sodium chloride) is important for the production of hydrogen gas, chlorine gas, and sodium hydroxide. The overall reaction within the electrolytic system is:

$$2H_2O + 2NaCl \rightarrow H_2 + Cl_2 + 2NaOH$$

The half reaction occurring at the cathode is:

A. $2Cl^- - 2e^- \rightarrow Cl_2$
B. $2Na^+ + 2e^- \rightarrow 2Na$
C. $2H_2O \rightarrow 2H_2 + O_2$
D. $2H_2O + 2e^- \rightarrow H_2 + 2OH^-$

Problem solved:

D is the correct answer. Inspection of the choices leads to the immediate elimination of both B and C. Choice B is eliminated, since no sodium metal is produced in the electrolysis of brine. Choice C is eliminated, since no oxygen gas is produced in the electrolysis of brine. Choice A represents an oxidation, choice D represents a reduction. D must be correct, since, by definition, oxidation occurs at the anode, and reduction occurs at the cathode, regardless of the type of cell.

22.1.6 A COMPARISON OF GALVANIC AND ELECTROLYTIC CELLS

Table 22.5, shown below, summarizes the similarities and differences between electrolytic and galvanic cells:

	Galvanic	Electrolytic
type of redox reaction	spontaneous	nonspontaneous
electron flow	created	supplied
site of oxidation	anode	anode
site of reduction	cathode	cathode
positive electrode	cathode	anode
negative electrode	anode	cathode
flow of electrons	anode to cathode	anode to cathode
flow of current	cathode to anode	cathode to anode

Table 22.5

22.1.7 CONCENTRATION CELLS

A **concentration cell** is a galvanic cell in which the cathodic half reaction and the anodic half reaction are the same reaction but opposite directions. It is possible to sustain such a cell by differing the concentrations between the two electrode vessels. Below is an example of a concentration cell employing differing concentrations of silver(I) with silver electrodes is shown below:

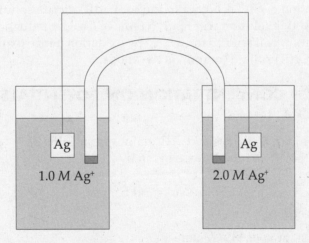

In this cell, the redox couple in each case is Ag^+/Ag. Since the vessel on the right contains a higher concentration of Ag^+, it is the more positive electrode, and is, therefore, the cathode. Since this is an example of a galvanic cell, we see that the half reaction for the right vessel will be:

$$Ag^+ + e^- \rightarrow Ag(s)$$

while the half reaction for the left vessel (anode) will be:

$$Ag(s) \rightarrow Ag^+ + e^-$$

The cell diagram for this cell is given by:

$$Ag(s) \,\|\, Ag^+ (aq, 0.10\ M) \,\|\, Ag^+ (aq, 2.0\ M) \,\|\, Ag(s)$$

Please solve this problem:

- A concentration cell is formed between a one liter aqueous solution containing 125 g $Cu(NO_3)_2$ and a one liter aqueous solution containing 100 g $CuSO_4$. Using Le Châtelier's principle, predict which solution will be the anode.

  A. The copper(II) nitrate solution
  B. The copper(II) sulfate solution
  C. These two solutions will not form a concentration cell.
  D. These solutions will form a concentration cell, but it cannot be determined which will be the anode.

Problem solved:

B is the correct answer. To solve this problem, we must first determine the molarity of Cu^{2+} ions in each solution:

$$125\text{ g Cu(NO}_3)_2 \div 187.5\text{ g/mol} = 0.667\text{ mol} \div 1\text{ L} = 0.667\ M$$

$$100\text{ g CuSO}_4 \div 159.5\text{ g/mol} = 0.627\text{ mol} \div 1\text{ L} = 0.627\ M$$

Since the concentration of Cu^{2+} is higher in the copper(II) nitrate solution, Le Châtelier's principle indicates that this solution will tend to remove Cu^{2+} by reduction, while the copper(II) sulfate solution will tend to form Cu^{2+} by oxidation. Since oxidation always occurs at the anode, the copper(II) sulfate solution is the anode.

22.1.8 EFFECT OF CONCENTRATION ON POTENTIALS: THE NERNST EQUATION

In a quick comparison of $E°$ values and $\Delta G°$ values from Table 22.1, we can see that the relationship between these two quantities is given by:

$$\Delta G° = -nFE°$$

where n = moles of electrons

and F = Faraday's constant = 96,485 C/mole

For nonstandard conditions:

$$\Delta G = -nFE$$

Also from **17.1.2.3**, ΔG is given by:

$$\Delta G = \Delta G^\circ + RT\ln Q$$

where Q is the reaction coefficient.

Substituting for ΔG and ΔG°, and then dividing by -nF we arrive at:

$$E = E^\circ - \frac{RT}{nF}\ln Q$$

Using the relationship between natural log (ln) and log base ten (log), we see that

$$E = E^\circ - 2.303\frac{RT}{nF}\log Q$$

This is the **Nernst equation**.

The Nernst equation is used to calculate E at conditions other than standard, since R and F are constants, and Q, T and n can be determined.

The Nernst equation can also be used to calculate the equilibrium constant, K_{eq}, for electrochemical systems at equilibrium under standard conditions. For a system under standard conditions, T is 298 K, and by definition, $E = 0$ at equilibrium. Therefore, the Nernst equation reduces to:

$$E^\circ = (2.303)\frac{RT}{nF}\log K_{eq} = \frac{(2.303)(8.314)(298)}{n(96,485)}\log K_{eq} = \frac{0.0592}{n}\log K_{eq}$$

Please solve this problem:

- Using the problem from **22.1.7**, the value of E is:

    A. − 0.795 V
    B. − 0.795 mV
    C. +0.795 mV
    D. +0.795 V

Problem solved:

C is the correct answer. Using the Nernst equation:

$$E = E^\circ - (2.303)\frac{RT}{nF}\log Q = E^\circ - \frac{0.0591}{n}\log Q$$

$E^\circ = 0$ (since the half reactions are the same)

$n = 2$ (since the half reaction involves a two-electron transfer)

$$Q = \frac{\left[Cu^{2+}(\text{anode})\right]}{\left[Cu^{2+}(\text{cathode})\right]} = \frac{0.627}{0.667} = 0.940$$

$$\log Q = \log(0.940) = -0.0269$$

$$E = E^\circ - \frac{0.0591}{n}\log Q$$

$$= 0 - \left(\frac{0.0591}{2}\right)(-0.0269) = 7.95 \times 10^{-4}\,V$$

$$= 0.795\,mV$$

22.2 MASTERY APPLIED: SAMPLE PASSAGE AND QUESTIONS

Passage

Electricity may be generated in an electrochemical cell, termed a **galvanic**, or **voltaic cell**. Such a cell uses a spontaneous oxidation-reduction reaction. The total **electromotive force (emf)** available from the cell is the sum of the electromotive force of the oxidation half reaction and the electromotive force of the reduction half reaction.

Cell emf is related to the Gibbs free energy change of the cell by:

$$\Delta G° = -nFE°$$

where n is the number of moles of electrons transferred in the reaction, and

$$F = 96,500 \text{ C/mole.}$$

Therefore, like ΔG, cell emf is a measure of the spontaneity of the oxidation-reduction reaction occurring within a cell. Examples of standard reduction potentials (emfs) are given in Table 1.

Reduction	$E°$(volts)	$\Delta G°$ (kJ)
$Li^+(aq) + e^- \longrightarrow Li(s)$	−3.05	294.3
$K^+(aq) + e^- \longrightarrow K(s)$	−2.93	282.7
$H_2(g) + 2e^- \longrightarrow 2H^-(aq)$	−2.25	434.3
$Al^{3+}(aq) + 3e^- \longrightarrow Al(s)$	−1.66	480.6
$Cr^{3+}(aq) + e^- \longrightarrow Cr^{2+}(aq)$	−0.41	39.6
$Pb^{2+}(aq) + 2e^- \longrightarrow Pb(s)$	−0.13	25.1
$2H^+(aq) + 2e^- \longrightarrow H_2(g)$	0.00	00.0
$Cu^{2+}(aq) + 2e^- \longrightarrow Cu(s)$	+0.34	−65.5
$Cu^+(aq) + e^- \longrightarrow Cu(s)$	+0.52	−50.2
$I_2(aq) + 2e^- \longrightarrow 2I^-(aq)$	+0.54	−104.2
$Fe^{3+}(aq) + e^- \longrightarrow Fe^{2+}(aq)$	+0.77	−74.3
$Ag^+(aq) + e^- \longrightarrow Ag(s)$	+0.80	−77.2

Standard Reduction Potentials
Table 1

The electrochemical cell in which zinc metal reacts with aqueous copper(II) ions is termed the Daniell cell. The reaction in a Daniell cell is given by:

$$Zn(s) + Cu^{2+}(aq) \rightarrow Zn^{2+}(aq) + Cu(s)$$

The emf of a Daniell cell is +1.10 V.

Another example of the use of electrochemical cells is the nickel-cadmium (or NiCad) rechargeable battery. The half reactions associated with this system are:

Anode:

$$Cd(s) + 2OH^-(aq) \rightarrow Cd(OH)_2(s) + 2e^-$$

$$E° = +0.761 \text{ V}$$

Cathode:

$$NiO_2(s) + 2H_2O(l) + 2e^- \rightarrow Ni(OH)_2(s) + 2OH^-(aq)$$

$$E° = +0.490 \text{ V}$$

1. Which of the following is the strongest reducing agent?
   A. $K(s)$
   B. $Cr^{2+}(aq)$
   C. $H_2(g)$
   D. $Fe^{2+}(aq)$

2. Which of the following cells would produce the galvanic cell with the largest emf?
   A. $Al \mid Al^{3+} \mid Li^+ \mid Li$
   B. $K \mid K^+ \mid Al^{3+} \mid Al$
   C. $Ag \mid Ag^+ \mid Li^+ \mid Li$
   D. $Cr^{2+} \mid Cr^{3+} \mid Fe^{3+} \mid Fe^{2+}$

3. What is the emf of the reduction of $Zn^{2+}(aq)$ to zinc metal?

   A. −1.10 V
   B. −0.76 V
   C. −0.58 V
   D. +0.76 V

4. How much voltage is supplied by a NiCad battery after it is 75 percent discharged?

   A. 1.251 V
   B. 0.938 V
   C. 0.413 V
   D. 0.313 V

5. NiCad batteries can be recharged by being run as electrolytic cells. During the recharging process, the reaction at the anode is:

   A. $Cd + 2OH^- \rightarrow Cd(OH)_2 + 2e^-$

   B. $NiO_2 + 2H_2O + 2e^- \rightarrow Ni(OH)_2 + 2OH^-$

   C. $Cd(OH)_2 + 2e^- \rightarrow Cd + 2OH^-$

   D. $Ni(OH)_2 + 2OH^- \rightarrow NiO_2 + 2H_2O + 2e^-$

6. In a Daniell cell, the Lewis acid is:

   A. Zn^{2+}
   B. Cu
   C. Zn
   D. Cu^{2+}

7. What is the power associated with a Daniell cell that is connected to a circuit with a total resistance of 6 Ω?

   A. 0.183 W
   B. 0.202 W
   C. 6.60 W
   D. 7.26 W

8. To achieve the maximum voltage from a two-cell system, a scientist should:

   A. attach two Daniell cells in parallel.
   B. attach two Daniell cells in series.
   C. attach two NiCad cells in parallel.
   D. attach two NiCad cells in series.

22.3 MASTERY VERIFIED: ANSWERS AND EXPLANATIONS

1. *A is the correct answer.* The strongest reducing agent is the species that is most easily oxidized. The most easily oxidized species is the product of the least favorable reduction. The least favorable reduction of the four answer choices is the reduction of K^+ to form solid potassium. Therefore, the most easily oxidized species is $K(s)$.

2. *B is the correct answer.* Using the data from the table in the passage, we can calculate the cell emfs for each cell diagram. Cell diagrams are written: oxidation reactant | oxidation product | reduction reactant | reduction product. So, to find cell emf, we must reverse the sign of the emf listed in the table for the oxidation half reaction, and add it to the emf listed in the table for the reduction half reaction.

   choice A: (+1.66) + (−3.05) = −1.39 V

   choice B: (+2.93) + (−1.66) = +1.27 V

   choice C: (−0.80) + (−3.05) = −3.85 V

   choice D: (+0.41) + (+0.77) = +1.18 V

   The question asked for the **galvanic** cell with the largest emf. Choices A and C are not galvanic cells. The emf of the cell given in choice B is larger than the emf of the cell given in choice D, so the correct answer is B.

3. *B is the correct answer.* From the emf given for the Daniell cell and the emf of the reduction of Cu^{2+}, we can immediately find the emf for the oxidation of $Zn(s)$:

$$1.10 - 0.34 = +0.76$$

   The question asks for the emf of the reduction of Zn^{2+}, so we reverse the sign:

$$-0.76 \text{ V}$$

4. *A is the correct answer.* A cell's voltage remains constant, or almost constant, until just before it dies. A battery that has 25 percent of its life left, will have a voltage that is very close to its standard potential.

5. *D is the correct answer.* A galvanic cell runs in reverse in an electrolytic cell. For any cell, the reaction at the anode is oxidation. Thus B and C are wrong. The reaction in either choice takes place at the anode in the galvanic cell and, thus, does not occur in the electrolytic cell.

6. *D is the correct answer.* A Lewis acid is an electron pair acceptor. We can see from the reaction equation given in the passage that Cu^{2+} accepts an electron pair from Zn. Choice A is also a Lewis acid; but in this cell, it is a product, not a reactant.

7. *B is the correct answer.* Using Ohm's law and the power law:

$$V = IR \quad \text{and} \quad P = IV$$

we can rearrange to get:

$$P = (I)(V) = \left(\frac{V}{R}\right)(V) = \left(\frac{V^2}{R}\right)$$

Therefore,

$$P = \left(\frac{V^2}{R}\right) = \frac{(1.10\ V)^2}{6\ \Omega} = \frac{1.21\ V^2}{6\ \Omega} = 0.202\ W$$

8. *D is the correct answer*. To solve this problem, we must first recognize that our NiCad batteries have a larger emf than the Daniell cell, so, we can immediately eliminate choices A and B. This reduces the problem to the question of whether we will double our voltage by putting two voltage sources in parallel or by putting these voltage sources in series. Using only knowledge of circuits from everyday life, we can state emphatically, "In series!" Why? How do you put batteries into a flashlight?

CHAPTER 23

EUKARYOTIC CELLS

23.1 MASTERY ACHIEVED

23.1.1 THE CELL MEMBRANE

You should familiarize yourself with the principal features of the eukaryotic cell which, in outline include:

- a cell wall;

- a cell membrane;

- the cytoplasm, in which organelles are housed;

- a nucleus, separated from the remainder of the cell by a **nuclear membrane.**

The **cell wall** is a carbohydrate-containing structure which is found on the cells of most organisms. Where the cell wall is present, it is the outermost structure of the cell. All cells, whether or not they have a cell wall, possess a **cell membrane**, which is composed primarily of protein and phospholipid. Plant cells possess a cell wall; animal cells do not.

You should be familiar with the **fluid mosaic model** of the cell membrane. According to this model, phospholipids comprise the bulk of the membrane and are arranged in a bilayer surrounding the cell. The hydrophobic lipid "tails" of the phospholipids point toward the inside of the membrane, while the hydrophilic phosphate "heads" point toward the surrounding, aqueous medium. One surface of the membrane faces the cell cytoplasm, and the other faces the extracellular space.

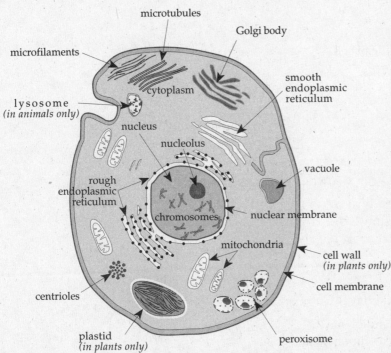

microtubules

Golgi body

microfilaments

cytoplasm

smooth endoplasmic reticulum

lysosome
(in animals only)

nucleus

nucleolus

vacuole

rough endoplasmic reticulum

chromosomes

nuclear membrane

mitochondria

cell wall
(in plants only)

cell membrane

centrioles

plastid
(in plants only)

peroxisome

Prototypical Eukaryotic Cell
Figure 23.1

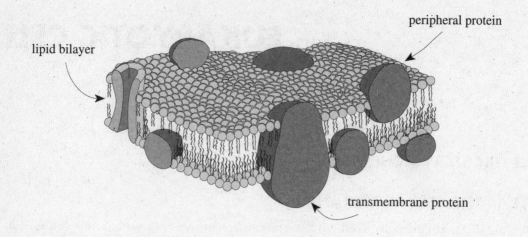

Fluid Mosaic Model of the Cell Membrane
Figure 23.2

Associated with the membrane are proteins. Those proteins that are embedded in one of the two surfaces of the membrane are called **peripheral proteins**. Those that penetrate completely through the membrane are called **transmembrane proteins**. Proteins that are contained entirely within the membrane are known as **integral proteins**.

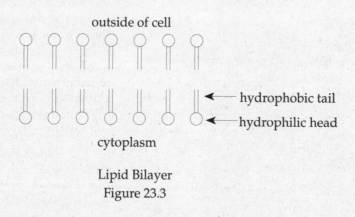

Lipid Bilayer
Figure 23.3

Please solve this problem:

- The phospholipid bilayer features:

    A. fat soluble components.
    B. water soluble components.
    C. both A and B.
    D. neither A nor B.

Problem solved:

C is the correct answer. The cell membrane is composed primarily of protein and phospholipid. The phospholipid molecules have fat-soluble and water-soluble components.

Please solve this problem:

- The hydrophobic moieties of the cell membrane's phospholipid molecules are oriented:

    A. toward the inner portion of the membrane.
    B. toward the external environment surrounding the membrane.
    C. both A and B.
    D. neither A nor B.

Problem solved:

A is the correct answer. The hydrophobic tails of each phospholipid molecule within the cell membrane are oriented so that they face one another, and have no significant contact with the intracellular or extracellular environments. The cell's internal and external environments are water rich and therefore tend to repel the hydrophobic moieties.

Please solve this problem:

- The typical animal cell contains all of the following EXCEPT:

    A. a cell wall.
    B. a mitochondrion.
    C. microtubules.
    D. a discrete nucleus.

Problem solved:

A is the correct answer. The cell wall is a feature of plant cells *only*. The outermost layer of an animal cell is the cell membrane, which is composed of protein and phospholipid.

23.1.1.1 Regulation of the Cell's Internal Environment

23.1.1.1.1 PASSIVE TRANSPORT OF IONS AND MOLECULES

The cell membrane is permeable to some substances and impermeable to others. It can also regulate the degree to which it is permeable to certain substances. Therefore, the cell membrane is **semipermeable**, or **selectively permeable**. Since the cell membrane determines, by and large, which substances enter the cell and which do not, it is said to exert regulatory control over the cell's internal environment.

Certain substances can pass through the membrane freely. These substances will move from an area where they are more concentrated to an area where they are less concentrated through the process of **simple diffusion**. When a substance diffuses it is said to be moving down its **concentration gradient**. A substance will diffuse down its concentration gradient until its concentration is the same everywhere within the system. Because the cell membrane is mostly lipid, lipid-soluble substances are soluble in the membrane and will pass through it in whichever direction the substance's concentration gradient dictates.

The cell does not have to expend any energy in this process; diffusion therefore occurs **passively**. Other substances to which the cell membrane is freely permeable include small, uncharged molecules such as oxygen and carbon dioxide. Water can also diffuse through the cell membrane.

There are a few other terms pertaining to diffusion and concentration that you should be familiar with:

• **Osmosis** refers to the tendency of a solvent to move down its own concentration gradient. Usually, osmosis is used to describe the diffusion of water. As with any type of diffusion, osmosis is a passive process. **Osmotic pressure** describes the strength of the force compelling water to move. The more concentrated the solute is in a particular place in a system, the less concentrated the water, and the greater the osmotic pressure driving the water towards that part of the system.

• A solution is **hypertonic** if it is more concentrated than another solution to which it is being compared. Conversely, a **hypotonic** solution is less concentrated than another solution. If the inside of a cell were hypertonic relative to the extracellular space (which would mean that the extracellular space is hypotonic), osmotic pressure would cause water to move into the cell from the outside.

Please solve this problem:

• Which of the following is NOT true of cell membranes?

A. They regulate the cell's internal environment.
B. They can alter their permeability to certain substances.
C. They are universally permeable.
D. They can mediate diffusion.

Problem solved:

C is the correct answer. The cell membrane helps the cell to maintain homeostasis by regulating the movement of substances into and out of the cell. A is a restatement of this fact. B and D describe ways in which this is accomplished. Answer choice C is untrue.

Please solve this problem:

• Passive diffusion occurs because:

A. Solutes tend to spread evenly throughout a solution.
B. Cells expend energy to make it occur.
C. Cell membranes are permeable only to certain substances.
D. The internal environment of a cell is self-regulating

Problem solved:

A is the correct answer. As noted in the text, passive diffusion does not require the expenditure of energy by the cell. It relies on the tendency of a solute to become distributed evenly throughout a solution by moving down its concentration gradient. Answer choice C is true, but it does not answer the question.

Please solve this problem:

Table 23.1 lists the approximate ion concentrations found in the axon cytoplasm and in the blood of the squid.

Ion	Axon cytoplasm concentration (mmol/L)	Blood concentration (mmol/L)
K^+	397	20
Na^+	50	437
Cl^-	40	556
Ca^{++}	0.4	10

Table 23.1

- Assuming that the axon cell membrane is permeable only to potassium (K^+), sodium (Na^+), and calcium (Ca^{++}), and that no cellular energy is available for transport, which of the following ion movements presented is most consistent with the data set forth in the table?

  A. Potassium flows out of the blood into the axon cytoplasm.
  B. Sodium does not flow in either direction across the axon cell membrane.
  C. Chloride flows from the blood into the axon cytoplasm.
  D. Calcium flows from the blood into the axon cytoplasm.

Problem solved:

D is the correct answer. Calcium's relative concentrations—0.4 mmol/L in the axon cytonplasm, 10 mmol/L in the blood—indicate that it will flow from the blood into the axon cytoplasm. Option A is incorrect because it suggests that potassium would move from a region of lower concentration (20 mmol/L in the blood) to one of higher concentration (397 mmol/L in the axon cytoplasm). This movement would require the expenditure of energy; it cannot occur passively. Option B is incorrect because sodium's relative concentrations (50 mmol/L in the axoplasm; 437 mmol/L in the blood) dictate that sodium flow from the blood into the axon cytoplasm. Option C is wrong because the question establishes that the axon cell membrane is not permeable to chloride.

Please solve this problem:

- If two solutions, X and Y, are separated by a membrane, and X has higher solute concentration than does Y, it may be concluded that:

  A. X is hypotonic to Y.
  B. Y is hypotonic to X.
  C. solvent will move from X to Y.
  D. solute will move from Y to X.

Problem solved:

B is the correct answer. The question depends upon the meaning of the term "hypotonic," which describes a solution with a solute concentration less than that of some other solution. Since solution X has a higher solute concentration, Y is hypotonic to X. Such movement (if any) as might occur would depend on the permeability properties of the membrane interposed between the two solutions. In any event, it could not be expected that solvent should move from the hypertonic to the hypotonic region nor that solute should move from the hypotonic to the hypertonic region. The natural tendencies would dictate just the opposite.

Please solve this problem:

- Which of the following correctly characterizes osmotic pressure?

    A. It tends to move solute from a hypotonic to a hypertonic region.
    B. It tends to move solute from a hypertonic to a hypotonic region.
    C. It tends to move solvent from a hypotonic to a hypertonic region.
    D. It tends to move solvent from a hypertonic to a hypotonic region.

Problem solved:

C is the correct answer. Osmotic pressure tends to promote the movement of solvent from regions of greater concentration of solvent to regions of lower concentration of solvent. In other words, it is the driving force that causes water to move down its concentration gradient. Options A and B are incorrect because they refer to the movement of solute, not solvent. Note that a solute does tend to move from hypertonic to hypotonic regions, but the term "osmotic pressure" is generally reserved for the tendency of concentration gradients to promote the movement of solvent.

Please solve this problem:

- Which of the following terms most closely approximates the meaning of the phrase "selective permeability"?

    A. Hypotonicity
    B. Hypertonicity
    C. Osmotic pressure
    D. Semipermeability

Problem solved:

D is the correct answer. "Selective permeability" is closely related in its meaning to "semipermeability." Each term can be used to describe a membrane that is permeable to some substances and not to others.

Please solve this problem:

- Which of the following describes a form of passive diffusion?

    A. Semipermeability
    B. Osmosis
    C. Hypertonicity
    D. Hypotonicity

Problem solved:

B is the correct answer. Osmosis refers, in essence, to the passive diffusion of solvent. Passive diffusion, generally, is the process by which solute or solvent moves down its concentration gradient. Osmosis is the specialized term applied to the passive movement of solvent.

23.1.1.1.2 FACILITATED AND ACTIVE TRANSPORT OF IONS AND MOLECULES

Passive diffusion is but one of several mechanisms of transmembrane transport. Others include **facilitated diffusion** and **active transport**. Facilitated diffusion refers to the movement of certain lipid insoluble substances, these having little ability to cross the lipid bilayer without mediation by specialized mechanism. Facilitated diffusion proceeds with the help of **protein channels**. Protein channels are transmembrane proteins that allow small charged particles, like K^+, to travel into the cell from the outside.

Like passive diffusion, facilitated diffusion follows a substance's concentration gradient. The mechanism does not overcome unfavorable gradients; it overcomes obstacles of solubility. Like passive diffusion, it does *not* require the cell to expend energy.

Active transport is an active process that requires ATP (the cell's "energy currency"). It permits movement against a substance's concentration gradient. The MCAT candidate should be careful to distinguish between active transport, passive diffusion, and facilitated diffusion. Active transport requires the expenditure of energy by the cell, whereas the other two processes do not. You should also further recall that energy is required when the cell needs to move substances against their concentration gradients.

Facilitated diffusion is largely mediated by the cell membrane's protein components. You should regard the membrane's protein components as allowing the cell to vary and adjust its permeability. You should also regard the cell membrane and its phospholipid bilayer as a fluid, dynamic entity whose specialized structure permits it to govern the transport of materials across the cell membrane.

Please solve this problem:

- Under the conditions of saturation, an increased concentration gradient does not promote greater net movement of solute across a membrane. It is observed that the condition impairs the movement of substances that depend on facilitated diffusion but not of those that depend on passive diffusion. How might the observation be explained?

Problem solved:

The problem asks the test-taker to examine the implications of saturation as it relates to the mechanisms of facilitated diffusion. Facilitated diffusion makes use of membrane proteins to transport a solute across a cell. When few solute molecules are being transported, few of the available transport proteins are engaged. A higher number of available solute molecules for transport will lead to increased rate of transport. However, as increasing numbers of solute molecules become available for transport across the membrane, all existing transport proteins eventually become active so that none are available for binding *additional* solute. This creates the condition of saturation.

Please solve this problem:

- The sodium-potassium pump ($Na^+ - K^+$ pump) is a means by which the cell maintains a fixed internal concentration of sodium and potassium ions. The pump continuously forces sodium ions out of the cell and draws potassium ions inward. For every two potassium ions drawn inward, however, three sodium ions are moved outward. A transmembrane protein facilitates this "ion exchange." Based on your knowledge of equilibria, would you speculate that the sodium-potassium pump is active? Assuming that the cell membrane is permeable to both sodium and potassium ions, predict the events that would occur if the pump were to suddenly cease operation.

Problem solved:

The problem asks that the student apply his or her understanding of transmembrane flow and equilibrium as it relates to intracellular and extracellular ion concentrations. In order to continuously expel sodium and take in potassium the cell must expend energy, since the activity contravenes prevailing concentration gradients. The pump itself produces and maintains the concentration gradients against which it operates: one in which sodium concentration is higher on the outside of the cell than on the inside and the other in which potassium concentration is higher on the inside of the cell than on the outside. The process demands energy, which is supplied by ATP. The pump defies the natural tendency for solute concentrations to equilibrate. If it were to cease operating, the natural tendencies would manifest. Sodium would flow passively down its concentration gradient and enter the cell. Potassium would flow passively down its concentration gradient and exit the cell.

23.1.1.1.3 ENDOCYTOSIS: PINOCYTOSIS AND PHAGOCYTOSIS

Endocytosis is a process by which cells can ingest particles larger than an ion or molecule. In this process a small region of the lipid bilayer located near the target particle **invaginates**, surrounding the target. The invaginating portion of the lipid bilayer eventually pinches off to create a **vesicle**, which harbors the particle within the cell's interior. Endocytosis of liquids or small particles is termed **pinocytosis**, whereas **endocytosis** of larger particles, like bacteria or foreign matter, is termed **phagocytosis**. **Receptor-mediated endocytosis** involves the ingestion of specific particles after they bind to specific protein receptors.

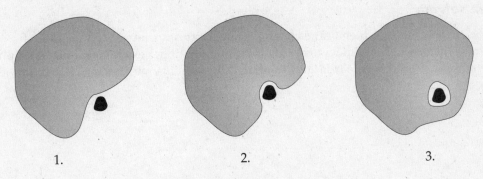

1.   2.   3.

Endocytosis of Substance by Cell

Figure 23.4

Please solve this problem:

- Which of the following pairs of phenomena demonstrates a set : subset relationship?

  A. Pinocytosis : phagocytosis
  B. Endocytosis : phagocytosis
  C. Vesicle formation : endocytosis
  D. Expulsion : pinocytosis

Problem solved:

B is the correct answer. Through endocytosis, cells can engulf relatively large particles or molecules. In the process the cell *forms* a vesicle, but endocytosis does not constitute a subset of vesicle formation. Both phagocytosis and pinocytosis are forms of endocytosis, one concerning the ingestion of large particles and the other concerning the ingestion of fluid matter or small particles. Phagocytosis, therefore, is a subset of endocytosis.

Please solve this problem:

- Which among the following does NOT play a role
  in the process of endocytosis?

  A. Vesicle formation
  B. Pinching off of the membrane
  C. Membrane channel
  D. Invagination

Problem solved:

C *is the correct answer.* A membrane channel is an entity associated with facilitated transport, not endocytosis. Endocytosis involves invagination, vesicle formation, and pinching off the membrane. The process is largely mediated by proteins within the cell membrane.

23.1.1.1.4 CELLULAR ADHESIONS

While cells can be viewed as discrete living entities, those of the human body are organized into tissues. **Cellular adhesions** serve to join cells together in various ways. In general, there are three types of cellular adhesions: tight junctions, gap junctions, and desmosomes.

Tight junctions link the cell membranes of adjacent cells together to form a barrier. There is no intercellular space at a tight junction. Tight junctions are important in maintaining the structural integrity of the surface of the small intestine; they form the barrier that keeps the contents of the small intestine from leaking out between cells.

Gap junctions link the cytoplasms of adjacent cells together, and small particles, such as ions, can flow through them freely. They consist of protein channels that form a bridge between the two cells. Gap junctions are important in heart muscle contraction; they allow the heart's electrical signals to be passed quickly from cell to cell.

Desmosomes are plaque-like proteins embedded in the cell membrane to which the cytoskeleton is attached. Also anchored at these points are filaments that join adjacent cells. Desmosomes are responsible for the structural integrity of most tissues in the human body.

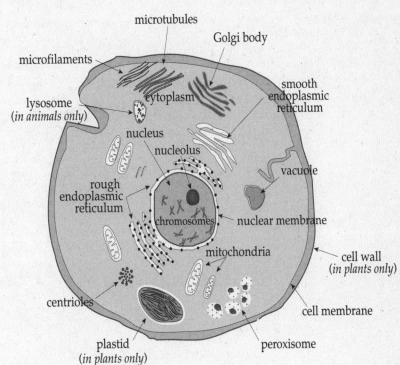

Prototypical Eukaryotic Cell
Figure 23.5

23.1.1.2 Eukaryotic Cell Organelles

23.1.1.2.1 THE CELL MEMBRANE, ENDOPLASMIC RETICULUM, AND GOLGI APPARATUS

You should be familiar with the structure and function of the principal organelles of the eukaryotic cell.

The **endomembrane system** of the cell consists of the outer membrane, located at the cell periphery; the **endoplasmic reticulum**, found throughout the cell cytoplasm; and the **nuclear membrane**, which encloses the cell nucleus. The network of channels that comprises the endoplasmic reticulum (ER) is of two types: **rough endoplasmic reticulum** (rough ER) and **smooth endoplasmic reticulum** (smooth ER). Rough ER is found in close association with granules called **ribosomes**, which function in protein synthesis. *Rough ER constitutes a principal site of cellular protein synthesis*, and its ribosomes are intimately involved in that process.

Smooth ER is devoid of ribosomes; smooth ER does not participate in protein synthesis but is involved in lipid synthesis and drug detoxification.

The **Golgi apparatus** is a specialized derivative of the endoplasmic reticulum, consisting of a series of flattened **sacs** rather than channels. It is responsible for packaging and transporting proteins to the cell surface, where they are either expelled into the extracellular space or incorporated into the cell membrane. This transport is accomplished through **vesicles**, which pinch off from the Golgi and migrate to the cell surface. They then fuse with the cell membrane and release their contents through the process of **exocytosis**.

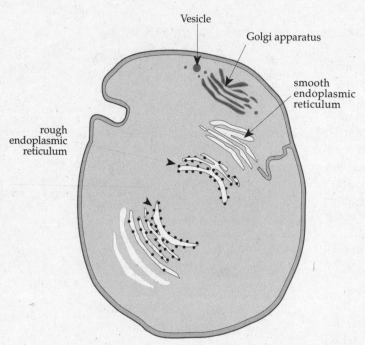

Membrane Structures of a Eukaryotic Cell

Figure 23.6

Please solve this problem:

- Among the following, which site is most closely associated with protein synthesis in the eukaryotic cell?

    A. The smooth endoplasmic reticulum
    B. The rough endoplasmic reticulum
    C. The nuclear membrane
    D. The Golgi apparatus

Problem solved:

B is the correct answer. The question asks the student to associate protein synthesis with the appropriate cellular organelle. Protein synthesis occurs on ribosomes, which may exist associated with endoplasmic reticulum, thus forming rough endoplasmic reticulum. (They may also float freely in the cytoplasm.)

Please solve this problem:

- Which among the following is a true statement regarding the Golgi apparatus?

    A. It functions in secretion.
    B. It functions in protein synthesis.
    C. It is a derivative of the nuclear membrane.
    D. It carries ribosomes on its surface.

Problem solved:

A is the correct answer. The Golgi apparatus is a derivative of the endoplasmic reticulum. It does not carry ribosomes. (Ribosomes, if attached to an organelle, are attached to endoplasmic reticulum to form rough endoplasmic reticulum.) The Golgi apparatus forms vesicles that contain secretory proteins, which are then expelled from the cell via the process of exocytosis.

23.1.1.2.2 Peroxisomes, Lysosomes, Mitochondria, and Plastids

The term "vesicle" applies to a number of structures including the two already mentioned: those that arise during endocytosis and those that arise from the Golgi apparatus. **Peroxisomes** and **lysosomes** are vesicles as well. Peroxisomes contain catalase, an enzyme relevant to the processing of hydrogen peroxide. Lysosomes harbor hydrolytic enzymes that digest foreign particles and senescent (aged) organelles. **Vacuoles** constitute spaces or vacancies within the cytoplasm. Often they are fluid-filled. In protozoans, vacuoles function to expel wastes or excess fluid.

Mitochondria are double-membraned organelles that mediate the synthesis of ATP (adenosine triphosphate), the molecule associated with energy storage, and commonly termed the cell's "energy currency." The **inner mitochondrial membrane** is folded into convolutions called **cristae**. The interior of the inner mitochondrial membrane is termed the **matrix**. The Krebs cycle and oxidative phosphorylation occur within the mitochondria. These processes produce the bulk of the ATP generated in **aerobic** (oxygen-using) organisms. **Glycolysis** is a precursor step to these processes and itself produces some quantity of ATP. It does not occur in the mitochondria. Indeed, **anaerobic** organisms, which lack mitochondria, can and do conduct glycolysis, but conduct neither the Krebs cycle nor oxidative phosphorylation. Processes that depend on the mitochondria are aerobic; glycolysis is not. The student will address cellular respiration and mitochondrial structure and function in greater detail when studying the chapter pertaining to cellular energy.

Plastids, found almost solely in plant cells, contain **pigment** and function in **photosynthesis** as well as in other cellular processes. The most abundant of the plastids are **chloroplasts**, which contain the green pigment **chlorophyll**.

Please solve this problem:

- Autolysis refers to the process by which the cell digests its own structures. Cell death allows the release of material normally sequestered within membrane-bound enclosures. The release of these materials brings on autolysis. Which of the following organelles most likely releases the substances that mediate autolysis?

    A. Plastid
    B. Mitochondrion
    C. Lysosome
    D. Vacuole

Problem solved:

C is the correct answer. The question calls on the test-taker to identify a cellular organelle that harbors is degradative enzymes. You should recall that lysosomes contain hydrolytic enzymes that digest, among other things, senescent cellular components. Plastids are found in plant cells and do not function in autolysis. Mitochondria function in ATP production. Vacuoles are spaces in the cell cytoplasm that may contain, among other materials, water, food, or wastes.

Please solve this problem:

- Which of the following organelles plays the most direct role in the maintenance of concentration gradients across the cell membrane?

  A. Vesicle
  B. Mitochondrion
  C. Golgi apparatus
  D. Smooth endoplasmic reticulum

Problem solved:

B is the correct answer. Maintaining a concentration gradient requires the expenditure of energy. ATP, which serves as the source of energy for this and other active processes, is synthesized in the mitochondria

23.1.1.2.3 CHROMOSOMES AND THE NUCLEOLUS

Chromosomes, composed of DNA (deoxyribonucleic acid) and proteins, bear the cell's genetic material and reside within the nucleus. Also located in the nucleus is an organelle called the **nucleolus**. It is the site of formation of ribosomal ribonucleic acid (rRNA), which functions in the translation of the genetic code. (Later chapters will discuss rRNA more fully.)

23.1.1.2.4 CILIA AND FLAGELLA

Cilia and **flagella** are associated with cellular locomotion but, depending on the cell site, they may serve other functions as well. In the human airway, cilia serve to propel foreign particles toward the throat, from which they can be expelled or swallowed. In the paramecium, they serve as means of locomotion. The flagellum comprises the tail of a sperm cell and confers motility so that the sperm may reach and fertilize the ovum. Both cilia and flagella are composed of a structured arrangement of **microtubules**.

23.1.1.2.5 MICROTUBULES, MICROFILAMENTS, AND CENTRIOLES

Microtubules, as just noted, are the structural basis of cilia and flagella. They are also the main component of **centrioles**. The centriole functions during cell division, assisting in the formation of the **mitotic spindle**. Microtubules are also found in the cytoplasm, where they serve as a quasi-skeletal structure for the cell itself (**cytoskeleton**). Microtubules are principally formed of a protein termed **tubulin**. **Microfilaments**, also found in the cytoplasm, serve as a second element of the cytoskeleton. Microfilaments are composed of the protein **actin**. They also function in cellular movement.

Please solve this problem:

- All of the following structures contain microtubules EXCEPT:

  A. the cytoskeleton.
  B. the mitotic spindle.
  C. cilia.
  D. the nucleolus.

Problem solved:

D is the correct answer. You should be mindful of the multiple functions performed by microtubules and be aware also that they are largely composed of the protein tubulin. Singly or in groups, microtubules provide the cell and some cell components with form and rigidity. They form the structural basis of the cytoskeleton, cilia, flagella and the mitotic spindle (which functions during cell division). The nucleolus does not contain microtubules.

Please solve this problem:

- Microtubules and microfilaments are composed primarily of:

  A. phospholipid.
  B. carbohydrate.
  C. protein.
  D. mucopolysaccharide.

Problem solved:

C is the correct answer. Microtubules are composed of the protein tubulin, and microfilaments of the protein actin.

Please solve this problem:

- In chronic obstructive pulmonary disease (COPD), the patient suffers, among other difficulties, an inability to expel mucosal secretion from the airway. Which cellular component is most likely dysfunctional?

  A. The nucleolus.
  B. The cilia.
  C. The centriole.
  D. The mitotic spindle.

Problem solved:

B is the correct answer. Cilia may participate in cellular locomotion and, depending on the site of the cells on which they are located, other functions as well. In the human airway they serve to remove secretions and thus to keep the airway free of obstruction. The nucleolus is located in the nucleus and is the site of the formation of rRNA; the centriole functions in the formation of the mitotic spindle. Neither serves to mediate the expulsion of secretions from the human airway.

23.2   MASTERY APPLIED: SAMPLE PASSAGE AND QUESTIONS

Passage

Two principal organelles of eukaryotic cells are mitochondria and chloroplasts. Mitochondria are found in nearly all eukaryotic cells, and chloroplasts are found in higher plant cells. Both organelles are double-membraned structures that enable the cell to synthesize ATP by way of a series of biochemical reactions. In mitochondria the energy source is food molecules; in chloroplasts the source is radiant energy from the sun.

The evolutionary origins of these organelles are not precisely known. The *endosymbiont theory* maintains that primitive prokaryotic organisms engulfed aerobic bacteria and entered into a symbiotic relationship with them. The high oxygen content of the atmosphere enabled the aerobic bacteria to provide the anaerobic organisms with energy. The primitive organism in turn provided the bacteria with shelter and protection. Chloroplasts, according to this theory, are descendants of cyanobacteria. The following are two evolutionary biologists' views on the symbiotic theory. One argues in favor of the theory; the other argues against it.

Biologist 1

The symbiotic theory explains why mitochondria and chloroplasts show so many similarities to prokaryotic organisms today. Like free-living prokaryotes, these organelles possess their own DNA and reproduce by binary fission. Furthermore, these organelles are of similar size and shape as prokaryotes. The respiratory apparatus of the cell is located only in the mitochondria; without the mitochondria the cell could not conduct respiration. Many bacteria also have respiratory capabilities, strikingly similar in their mechanism to those of mitochondria.

Biologist 2

Eukaryotes could not have evolved by way of symbiotic arrangement between a prokaryotic anaerobe and an aerobic bacterium. Mitochondria and chloroplasts differ significantly from present-day bacteria. Not only is the quantity of their DNA quite small compared to that of bacteria, but all of the molecules required for their structure must be produced and imported from the rest of the cell.

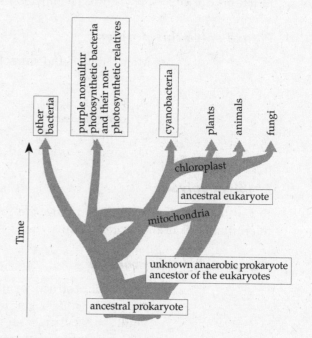

Figure 1

1. If Biologist 1 is correct, then the relationship that ancestral organisms had with aerobic bacteria is an example of:

    A. commensalism.
    B. parasitism.
    C. mutualism.
    D. socialism.

2. Which of the following observations provides the LEAST support for the viewpoint of Biologist 1?

   A. An amoeba exists that does not possess mitochondria but instead harbors aerobic bacteria in a symbiotic relationship.
   B. Some present-day eukaryotic cells contain cyanobacteria.
   C. Chloroplasts carry out photosynthesis in the same manner as do cyanobacteria.
   D. Different eukaryotic cells share in common a number of different organelles that do not occur in prokaryotes.

3. Which of the following processes would be undertaken by a cell in the process of engulfing a bacterium in a symbiotic relationship?

   I. Pinocytosis
   II. Phagocytosis
   III. Endocytosis

   A. II only
   B. III only
   C. I and II only
   D. II and III only

4. Among the following, which explanation would best reconcile the differences in perspectives taken by Biologists 1 and 2?

   A. Mitochondria and chloroplasts represent only two of many different organelles and compartmentalized structures that reside in eukaryotic cells.
   B. Mitochondria and chloroplasts both contain a double membrane which differs in its molecular makeup from the membrane that surrounds the nucleus.
   C. Mitochondria and chloroplasts may have originated as symbiotic organisms that evolved to become gradually more dependent on their hosts.
   D. Mitochondria and chloroplasts are shown to contain circular DNA, and while bacteria contains comparatively more DNA, its DNA is also circular.

5. A eukaryotic cell that had its mitochondria removed would be capable of carrying out:

   A. only glycolysis, which is an anaerobic process.
   B. only glycolysis, which is an aerobic process.
   C. only glycolysis and the Krebs cycle.
   D. only the Krebs cycle and oxidative phosphorylation, which are both aerobic.

6. Biologist 2 argues against the symbiotic theory based on which of the following criteria?

   A. Mitochondria and chloroplasts evolved from the ingestion of two different bacterial types.
   B. Mitochondria and chloroplasts rely on different energy sources to produce ATP.
   C. Mitochondria and chloroplasts do not contain DNA whereas bacteria do.
   D. Mitochondria and chloroplasts are not entirely self-sufficient organelles.

7. The folded portion of the inner membrane of mitochondria is termed the:

   A. endoplasmic reticulum.
   B. grana.
   C. cristae.
   D. plasma membrane.

8. If Biologist 1 is correct, which of the following organisms have a reproductive strategy in common with mitochondria?

   A. Bacteria
   B. Fungi
   C. Viruses
   D. Bacteriophages

23.3 MASTERY VERIFIED: ANSWERS AND EXPLANATIONS

1. *C is the correct answer.* The passage states that both members of the symbiotic relationship enjoyed a benefit. Hence the correct answer choice must denote a mutually beneficial relationship. Mutualism describes just such a symbiotic relationship. Two organisms living in mutualistic alliance confer some gain on each other. Commensalism defines a symbiotic relationship in which one member benefits and the other experiences neither benefit nor harm. Parasitism defines a symbiotic relationship in which one member benefits and the other is harmed. Socialism does not constitute a type of symbiosis.

2. *D is the correct answer.* That eukaryotic cells share a variety of organelles represents a true statement, but tends neither to support nor refute the viewpoint at issue. The statement in choice A furnishes evidence of the symbiotic relationship in which Biologist 1 believes. The statement set forth in choice B also support's Biologist 1's thesis: it provides evidence that eukaryotic cells can form a symbiotic relationship with cyanobacteria, consistent with the biologist's view on the origin of chloroplasts. If chloroplasts did arise from cyanobacteria, similarities in their structure and/or function would be expected. Choice C, therefore, also lends support to the thesis.

3. *D is the correct answer.* Pinocytosis, a form of endocytosis, involves cellular ingestion of liquid or small particles. Since the question refers to the ingestion of an entire bacterium, item I is not an accurate statement. Phagocytosis pertains to the ingestion of a foreign particle(s), which might include a bacterium, so item II is true. Phagocytosis is, in fact, a type of endocytosis and so item III is true as well.

4. *D is the correct answer.* The statement in choice D meaningfully addresses the apparent discrepancies noted by Biologists 1 and 2.

   Choice A sets forth a true statement that does not, however, tend to reconcile the conflicting views. Choice B also makes a true statement, but also fails to harmonize the differences between the theories. Choice C, too, offers a true statement. Indeed, it tends to support the view of Biologist 1, but fails to make any point that would bridge the conceptual gap between Biologists 1 and 2.

5. *A is the correct answer.* Glycolysis, an anaerobic process, occurs in the cellular cytoplasm. In the absence of mitochondria the cell would still be able to conduct glycolysis. Glycolysis is not an aerobic process, which fact renders choice B incorrect. Although glycolysis can occur in a cell that lacks mitochondria, the Krebs cycle cannot. The Krebs cycle takes place within the mitochondria. Choice C, therefore, is incorrect. Both the Krebs cycle and oxidative phosphorylation are aerobic processes that occur in the mitochondria. If the mitochondria are absent, these processes cannot occur. Choice D is wrong.

6. *D is the correct answer.* The statement forms a part of Biologist 2's argument. Although choice A makes a correct statement, it does not provide a correct answer since it fails to advance Biologist 2's viewpoint. Neither does it represent the criteria upon which she based her conclusion. Choice B also sets forth a true statement, but it neither advances the argument nor represents criteria on which the argument is based. Choice C sets forth a false statement. Both bacteria and the two organelles in question contain DNA. True *or* false, the statement plays no role in Biologist 2's argument.

7. *C is the correct answer.* Cristae are the numerous infoldings of the inner membrane of mitochondria. Enzymes necessary to carry out oxidative phosphorylation are located

7. *C is the correct answer*. Cristae are the numerous infoldings of the inner membrane of mitochondria. Enzymes necessary to carry out oxidative phosphorylation are located there. The endoplasmic reticulum (ER) is a membrane network that winds its way through the cytoplasm of the cell. Rough ER features ribosomes that function in protein synthesis. Smooth ER carries no ribosomes. Grana refer to flattened stacks of membranes that contain chlorophyll; they are located in the chloroplasts of photosynthesizing plants. The plasma membrane is a selectively permeable membrane that encloses the cell cytoplasm; it is found at the periphery of the cell.

8. *A is the correct answer*. Biologist 1 states that mitochondria reproduce by binary fission. The correct answer, then, must describe an organism that reproduces in the same manner. A bacterium reproduces by binary fission. It always divides by splitting into two daughter cells. As will be discussed in subsequent chapters, a fungus can reproduce sexually or asexually. When it undergoes sexual reproduction, two haploid gametes fuse to become a diploid. A fungus can undergo asexual reproduction by either budding (breaking off a small portion of itself) or producing spores (which are disseminated from a specialized structure). A virus reproduces by injecting its nucleic acid into a host cell and causing the host cell to produce multiple copies of its nucleic acid as well as protein coats to enclose the nucleic acid. (That too will be discussed in subsequent chapters.) A bacteriophage is a virus that uses a bacterium as its host. It reproduces in the same way as do all viruses: it appropriates its host's genetic machinery to create multiple copies of itself.

CHAPTER 24

THE GENETIC MATERIAL: DEOXYRIBONUCLEIC ACID

24.1 MASTERY ACHIEVED

24.1.1 CHROMOSOMES AND DNA IN OVERVIEW

Within the nucleus of a eukaryotic cell are housed the chromosomes, which contain the cell's heritable material. Organisms vary in the number of chromosomes they possess; humans possess 46 chromosomes, or 23 pairs of **homologous** chromosomes, and each member of a pair of homologues is similar, but not identical, to the other member of the pair. Each human receives one set of 23 from his or her mother and one from his or her father. A cell that posseses both sets of homologues is called **diploid**; a cell that contains only one set is termed **haploid**. Chromosomes are composed of **deoxyribonucleic acid** (DNA) and protein. It is the DNA that contains the blueprints for the construction of the cell's proteins. These blueprints are organized into **genes**, and each gene contains the blueprint for one protein.

Please solve this problem:

- Would an organism of higher complexity be expected to contain more, or less, total DNA than one of lower complexity?

Problem solved:

The problem calls on the student to speculate and to draw sensible inferences. Since the chromosomes contain DNA and DNA directs protein synthesis, increased DNA content allows for the synthesis of more proteins. The cell or organism with a relatively larger number of structural and enzymatic proteins is likely to show greater complexity. The student should note that greater DNA content increases cellular and organismic complexity notwithstanding the fact that in all cells a significant portion of DNA has no known function. Ongoing research, however, continues to disclose the function of DNA segments whose purpose was previously unknown.

24.1.2 STRUCTURAL ARRANGEMENT OF DNA

Prokaryotic genetic material consists of a single, circular DNA molecule that floats free in the cytoplasm. The DNA of eukaryotes, on the other hand, is organized in complex ways that allow the extremely long DNA molecules to fit within the nucleus and yet retain structural integrity. This structure also facilitates accurate replication of the genetic material. This organization invovles the wrapping of the DNA around **histone proteins** in a complex arrangement. Part of this arrangement involves the formation of eight-histone units known as **nucleosomes**.

Please solve this problem:

- The complex packaging of the human chromosome within the nucleus allows for:

    A. mixing of genetic information between and among gene segments.
    B. proper reproduction of chromosomes.
    C. enzyme synthesis within the nucleus.
    D. efficient packaging of the nucleolus.

Problem solved:

B is correct. The cells of complex organisms, like those of the human being, have very long chromosomes. In order for the chromosomes to (a) fit, physically, within the nucleus, and (b) undergo accurate reproduction, they must be packed efficiently.

Please solve this problem:

- Histones are composed of:

    A. ribonucleic acid.
    B. nitrogen and phosphate.
    C. base pairs.
    D. protein.

Problem solved:

D is correct. Histones are proteins around which deoxyribonucleic acid is "wrapped" in its complex packaging structure. The student should associate the term "histone" with the protein component of the chromosome.

24.1.3 COMPOSITION AND ARRANGEMENT OF DNA: DEOXYRIBOSE, PHOSPHATE GROUPS, AND NUCLEOTIDE BASE PAIRS

Each strand of a double-stranded DNA molecule is composed of two functional regions: (1) the **backbone**, which consists of alternating phosphate groups and **deoxyribose** sugar molecules are bonded to each other through **phosphodiester** bonds; and (2) a **variable region**, consisting of one of four different **nitrogenous bases**. The backbone gives the DNA molecule its structure, while the order of the nitrogenous bases along the backbone conatins the cell's genetic information.

Please solve this problem:

- In terms of its principal function, the variable section of DNA carries:

  A. the molecule's structural backbone.
  B. the genetic information.
  C. the histones.
  D. the nucleosomes.

Problem solved:

B is correct. DNA consists of a sugar-phosphate backbone and a variable portion. The variable portion carries the cell's genetic information.

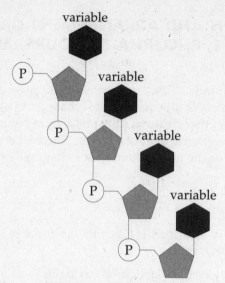

DNA: Sugar-Phosphate
Backbone and Variable Portion

Figure 24.2

The nitrogenous bases of the DNA molecule's variable portion are categorized (by structural similarities) as *purines* and *pyrimidines*. Two bases belong to each category. The purine bases are *adenine* (A) and *guanine* (G). The pyrimidine bases are *thymine* (T) and *cytosine* (C). The structure of each base is shown below.

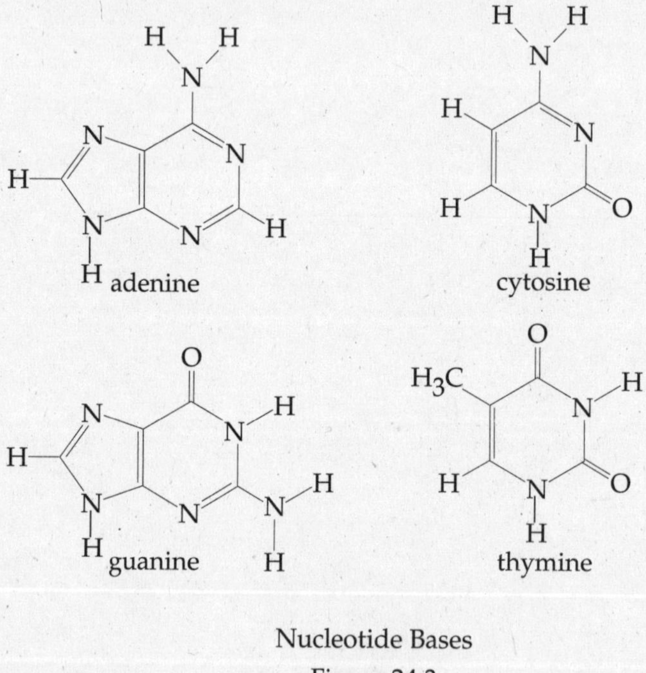

Nucleotide Bases

Figure 24.3

One nitrogenous base together with a deoxyribose molecule and a phosphate group forms a *nucleotide*. Nucleotides are the building blocks of DNA.

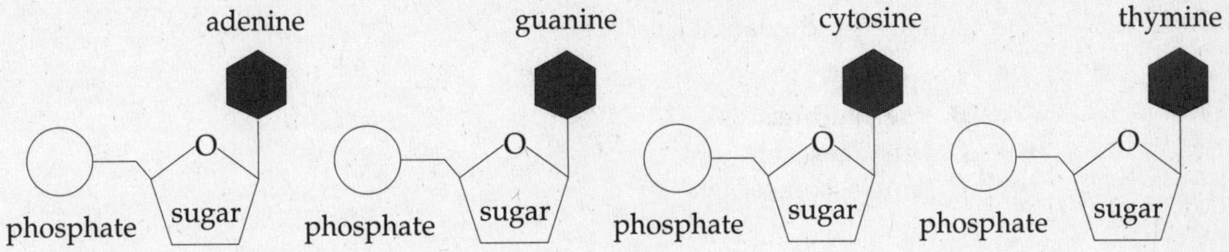

adenine   guanine   cytosine   thymine

phosphate   sugar   phosphate   sugar   phosphate   sugar   phosphate   sugar

Nucleotides

Figure 24.4

In forming the DNA molecule, the nucleotide units are assembled in a stablilized orientation that produces a molecule with a ladder-like appearance. The completed DNA molecule is **double-stranded**. Two strands of DNA are aligned next to one another so that their sugar-phosphate backbones form the outer borders of the molecule, and their bases are positioned at the molecule's interior. The two strands, each facing the other, are **complementary**. One base from each strand forms a **matched base pair** with the base opposite to it. Bases are paired according to the following rules: adenine (A) pairs with thymine (T), and cytosine (C) pairs with guanine (G). The test-taker should note that *a pyrimidine base is always paired with a purine base.*

Base pairs are joined by **hydrogen bonds**, which do not offer the strength of true covalent bonds, but by their large number impart an impressive strength and support to the DNA molecule (just as they produce, for the water molecule, a high degree of surface tension). Furthermore, the ease with which hydrogen bonds break and form generally confers a degree of resiliency to a biological molecule. Adenine and thymine pairs contain two hydrogen bonds while guanine and cytosine pairs contain three.

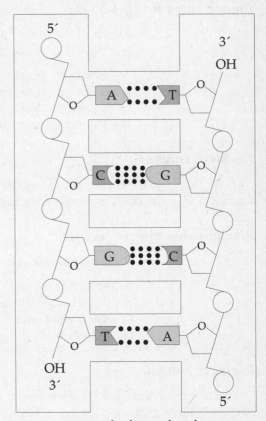

•••• = hydrogen bonds

Base-Pairing of a
Double-Stranded
DNA Molecule

Figure 24.5

Please solve this problem:

- Adenine and guanine are:

    A. purines.
    B. pyrimidines.
    C. histones.
    D. nucleosomes.

Problem solved:

A is correct. Adenine and guanine are nitrogenous bases that belong to the purine category. Histones are protein components of the chromosome that play a role in structural support. Nucleosomes represent discrete packaging units within the chromosome. They are not *functional* units.

Please solve this problem:

- Which of the following represents a correct base pairing within a DNA molecule?

    A. Adenine - guanine
    B. Adenine - cytosine
    C. Cytosine - thymine
    D. Thymine - adenine

Problem solved:

D is correct. In the formation of base pairs a purine always bonds with a pyrimidine. More specifically, in the DNA molecule adenine bonds to thymine, and cytosine bonds to guanine.

Please solve this problem:

- Matched bases within a base pair are linked by:

    A. nonpolar covalent bonds.
    B. polar covalent bonds.
    C. hydrogen bonds.
    D. ionic bonds.

Problem solved:

C is correct. Within the DNA molecule, matched bases are linked by hydrogen bonds. Although these are not so strong as any of the other bonds listed in the answer choices, their large number affords the DNA molecule significant structural integrity and support.

Please solve this problem:

- Which of the following correctly characterizes a DNA molecule?

    A. It is devoid of carbohydrate.
    B. It consists of two complementary strands.
    C. It is composed of phospholipid.
    D. It is single stranded.

Problem solved:

B is correct. DNA is a double-stranded molecule. Each strand is the complement of the other. DNA contains carbohydrate; deoxyribose is a sugar which means that it is a carbohydrate. The molecule is not composed of phospholipid. Phospholipid is the substance of which cell membranes are principally composed.

As just noted, each strand of a double-stranded DNA molecule is the *complement* of the other. Because of the rules of base-pairing, the sequence of bases arranged on one strand dictates the sequence of matching bases situated on the complementary strand. (The rules of base pairing arise partly from *steric hindrance*, or size restrictions regarding the structure of the different bases and the spaces available to them.) Hence, a region of one DNA strand that reads:

guanine, cytosine, adenine, adenine, and cytosine

—will correspond to a complementary strand bearing the sequence:

cytosine, guanine, thymine, thymine, and guanine.

Please solve this problem:

- If one strand of a DNA molecule shows the base sequence A G A T, its complementary strand will show the sequence:

    A. C C T A
    B. A A G A
    C. T C T A
    D. C T T G

Problem solved:

C is correct. According to the DNA base-pairing rules, adenine (a purine) pairs with thymine (a pyrimidine) and cytosine (a purine) pairs with guanine (a pyrimidine). Therefore the sequence: adenine-guanine-adenine-thymine pairs with the sequence: thymine-cytosine-thymine-adenine.

24.1.4 ORIENTATION OF NUCLEOTIDE STRANDS

The two strands of the DNA molecule coil around an axis to form a **double helix**. The double helical structure of DNA was discovered in 1953 by James Watson and Francis Crick in an experiment involving **x-ray diffraction** images of DNA photographed by Rosalind Franklin and Maurice Wilkins. Watson and Crick's discovery of the helical structure of DNA enabled scientists to further their understanding of gene function on a molecular level. Most significantly, it allowed them to elucidate the mechanism by which the DNA molecule replicates.

A significant component of the Watson and Crick model (since confirmed through biochemical analysis) concerns the **antiparallel orientation** of the nucleotide strands. On a given DNA molecule, the two complementary strands run in opposite directions. One strand runs in the *five prime to three prime direction* (5´→3´), and its complement runs in the *three prime to five prime direction* (3´→5´). Convention requires that, for any strand, bases be *listed in the five prime to three prime* (5´→3´) direction. (The directional numbers refer to the numbered carbons in the deoxyribose sugar.) The bond linking two nucleotides is called a **phosphodiester bond**.

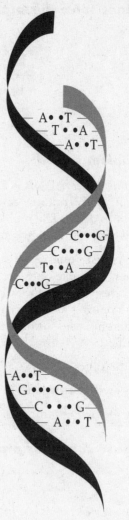

DNA: The Double Helix

Figure 24.6

Please solve this problem:

- Which of the following properly describes the antiparallel structure of a DNA molecule?

  A. Base-pairing rules require that purines pair with pyrimidines and pyrimidines with purines.

  B. Complementary strands show opposite orientation in terms of their 3´ and 5´ carbon ends.

  C. Each complementary strand has a 3´ carbon at its bottom end and a 5´ carbon at its top end.

  D. Complementary strands will not bond unless bases are matched purine to purine and pyrimidine to pyrimidine.

Problem solved:

B is correct. Antiparallelism refers to the orientation of the two sugar-phosphate backbones with respect to each other in a DNA molecule. Specifically, it refers to the manner in which each such backbone is oriented as to its 3´ and 5´ carbon ends. The 3´ end of one strand is associated with the 5´ end of the complement. Choice A makes a true statement, but one that does not refer to antiparallelism. Choice C makes reference to the 3´ and 5´ ends, but it does not make a true statement.

Please solve this problem:

- Among the following, the discovery of the double helix was most significant in that it:
  - **A.** highlighted the importance of the three-dimensional structure of biological molecules.
  - **B.** resulted from the first meaningful use of x-ray diffraction.
  - **C.** allowed for productive study of chromosome reproduction.
  - **D.** fully elucidated the rules of base-pairing.

Problem solved:

C is correct. The Watson and Crick experiment did use the x-ray diffraction technique but it did not originate it. Among the listings in options A–D, the most significant is that listed in C. The elucidation of the double helix allowed subsequent investigators to explore the mechanism through which a chromosome reproduces itself.

24.1.5 CHROMOSOME REPRODUCTION

Chromosome reproduction requires the *replication of DNA.* DNA replication is initiated with the "unwinding" of the double helix by DNA *helicase enzymes* and subsequent "unzipping" and separation of the complementary strands.

Each resulting **parent strand** of DNA serves as the **template** from which a new complement is ultimately synthesized. An **RNA primer** is required for initiation of DNA synthesis. **DNA polymerases** are crucial for the synthesis of a new DNA strand: they function to align appropriate bases opposite the template strand. *Nucleotides are added to the 3' end of the* growing DNA strand. Each original parent strand produces an exact copy of its own complement. Each newly synthesized DNA strand is secured to the parent strand that generated it by the formation of *hydrogen bonds between bases* and **phosphodiester bonds** between the sugar and phosphate groups of the backbone.

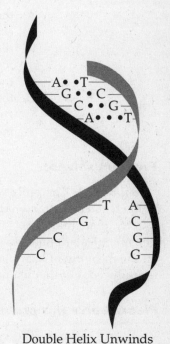

Double Helix Unwinds

Figure 24.7

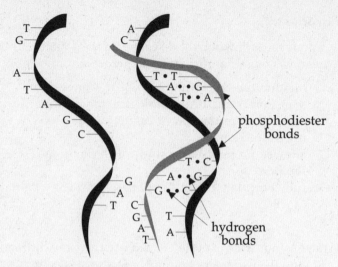

Template Produces New DNA Strand

Figure 24.8

Please solve this problem:

- In DNA replication, the term "template" refers to:

    A. the role of enzymes in "unwinding" the molecule to be reproduced.
    B. the role of the parent strand in directing the formation of a new complementary strand.
    C. the elongation of a growing DNA strand.
    D. the phosphodiester bonding that secures the sugar-phosphate backbone of a new DNA molecule.

Problem solved:

B is correct. The process of chromosomal reproduction involves DNA replication. As noted in the text, each strand of the molecule to be replicated is called a "parent strand" and serves as a template that directs the production of a complementary strand. In choice D, phosphodiester bonds do secure the sugar-phosphate backbone but that does not bear directly on the meaning of "template." In choice A, enzymes do "unwind" the molecule to be reproduced, but that phenomenon also lacks any direct relationship to the term "template."

Please solve this problem:

- The synthesis of the daughter strand is accomplished most directly by:

    A. a helicase enzyme.
    B. a polymerase enzyme.
    C. a phospholipid-protein backbone.
    D. hydrogen bonding between base pairs.

Problem solved:

B is correct. As noted in the text, DNA polymerases serve in the synthesis of daughter DNA strands. The helicase enzymes are involved in the "unwinding" of the original DNA molecule to be replicated. Phospholipid does not form a part of the DNA molecule's structure. Although bases within a base pair are joined by hydrogen bonds, the joining of paired bases is less relevant to the actual creation of a new strand than is the functioning of DNA polymerose enzymes.

24.1.5.1 Semiconservative Replication

DNA replicates through a **semiconservative mechanism:** Each daughter strand is a complement of the parent strand that serves as its template. At the end of the replication process, two double-stranded molecules of DNA are formed. Each double-stranded DNA molecule contains one daughter (new) strand and one parent (old) strand.

Please solve this problem:

- An experiment is conducted in which the DNA molecules of *E. coli* are labeled with a heavy isotope of nitrogen (^{15}N) in order to make them denser than ordinary DNA. The *E. coli* is then transferred to a medium containing only the common isotope of nitrogen (^{14}N). What would be the expected distribution of ^{15}N and ^{14}N in the *E. coli's* DNA molecules after the first episode of DNA replication? What would be the likely distribution after the second episode of replication?

Problem solved:

The question requires you to apply the principle of semiconservative replication to an experimental situation involving two successive episodes of DNA synthesis. The experimental conditions presented in the question provide that the parent DNA is labeled with the heavy isotope of nitrogen, and that when the parent DNA undergoes replication, its daughter strands will not contain the heavy isotope.

You can determine, based on the principles of semiconservative replication, that the first episode of replication yields two hybrid double-stranded DNA molecules, each composed of one daughter strand (containing normal ^{14}N isotope) and one parent strand (containing heavy ^{15}N isotope). The answer to part one of the question, then, is that both isotopes would be evenly distributed in the two DNA molecules after one episode of replication. (Indeed, the technique of density-gradient equilibrium sedimentation would reveal a single band of DNA whose density is registered at the halfway mark between the respective densities of the ^{15}N and ^{14}N strands, implying that the parent molecule composed solely of ^{15}N no longer existed; nor would there be evidence of a daughter DNA molecule composed solely of ^{14}N DNA.)

You can then conclude, logically, that the next episode of replication will yield four DNA molecules that, according to the rules of semiconservative replication, can be thus characterized: (a) two hybrid DNA molecules containing one heavy isotope (^{15}N) parent strand and one normal isotope (^{14}N) daughter strand, and (b) two normal isotope (^{14}N) DNA molecules, each one containing one strand of ^{14}N parent DNA and one strand of ^{14}N daughter DNA. The answer to part two of the question, then, is that two of the four resulting DNA molecules consist of 50% ^{15}N and 50% ^{14}N DNA, while the remaining two DNA molecules consist solely of ^{14}N DNA. (Density-gradient equilibrium sedimentation here reveals two bands of DNA, one band showing a density midway between those of ^{15}N and ^{14}N, and the other band showing a density matching that of ^{14}N.)

24.1.5.2 Leading and Lagging Strands

DNA synthesis originates at specific sites—the **origins of replication**—and proceeds bidirectionally from those sites at **replication forks** that run in opposite directions. As mentioned earlier, the *overall direction of DNA synthesis must be from 5′ to 3′* (the only direction in which DNA polymerases can link nucleotides). To reconcile this limitation with the fact that bidirectional DNA synthesis includes the unacceptable 3′ to 5′ direction (because the strands are antiparallel to each other), the cell synthesizes small fragments of DNA in the 5′ to 3′ direction on one of the strands. These fragments, called the **Okazaki fragments**, are then connected. The strand that is composed of small fragments of discontinuous DNA is termed the **lagging strand**; the daughter strand that grows continuously in the 5′ to 3′ direction is known as the **leading strand**.

24.1.6 TRANSCRIPTION: THE PROCESS OF RNA PRODUCTION

DNA is capable of directing the synthesis of **ribonucleic acid** (RNA) in a process known as **transcription**. *Both RNA and DNA are nucleic acids*, but they are different in the following ways: (1) RNA is *single-stranded* as opposed to double-stranded; (2) RNA contains the sugar *ribose in place of deoxyribose*; and (3) RNA contains the nitrogenous base *uracil in place of thymine*. As in replication, synthesis of RNA begins with the unwinding and separation of the DNA strands, *only one* of which will serve as the template for production of RNA. Nitrogenous bases for the new RNA strand will align at the DNA template according to the base-pair rules that apply to DNA synthesis, as already discussed. There is, however, a modification that arises from the fact that the RNA molecule does not contain the pyrimidine thymine; it contains uracil instead. Each adenine base on the DNA template is paired with a uracil base (not a thymine base) on the daughter RNA molecule. The enzyme RNA polymerase is required for both initiation and elongation of a daughter RNA strand. The resulting RNA strand has a *sequence complementary to the DNA template*.

There are, in fact, 3 forms of RNA: **ribosomal RNA** (rRNA), **transfer RNA** (tRNA), and **messenger RNA** (mRNA). DNA serves as the template for the synthesis of each. Once each type of RNA is produced, it leaves the nucleus and enters the cytoplasm of the cell, where it plays a part in protein synthesis.

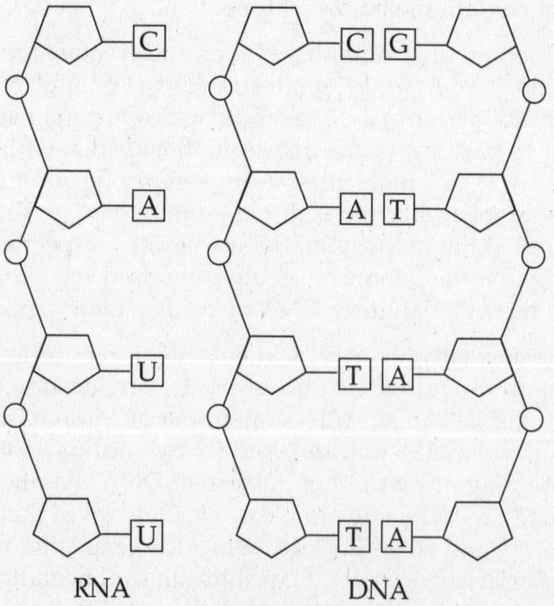

Figure 24.9

Please solve this problem:

- What are the principal differences between deoxy-ribonucleic acid (DNA) and ribonucleic acid (RNA)?

Problem solved:

Three principal factors distinguish DNA from RNA: (1) DNA is double-stranded while RNA is single-stranded; (2) DNA contains the sugar deoxyribose while RNA contains the sugar ribose; and (3) DNA contains the nitrogenous base thymine while RNA contains the base uracil.

Please solve this problem:

- What is the sequence of the mRNA molecule transcribed from a DNA template with the base sequence 5´ – T A G C G G C T T A – 3´

Problem solved:

5´ – T A G C G G C T T A – 3´
3´ – A U C G C C G A A U – 5´

Messenger RNA has a base sequence that is complementary to that of the DNA template from which it was transcribed. According to the rules of base-pairing for RNA, for any given section of template DNA, each thymine in DNA is matched with an adenine in RNA, each adenine in DNA is matched with a uracil in RNA, each guanine in DNA is matched with a cytosine in RNA, and each cytosine in DNA is matched with a guanine in RNA. By convention, base sequences are listed in the five prime to three prime direction of any DNA or RNA molecule under dicussion. Thus the answer is : 5´ – UAAGCCGCUA – 3´

Please solve this problem:

- Discuss the principal similarities and differences between DNA synthesis and RNA synthesis.

Problem solved:

Similarities

- The direction of synthesis in both processes is from five prime to three prime.

- The base sequence of each newly synthesized strand is the complement of the base sequence of its parent strand.

- Both use DNA as their template.

- Both require polymerase enzymes for the synthesis of the daughter strand.

Differences

- RNA synthesis does not require the use of a primer in order to begin.

Please solve this problem:

- How are DNA polymerases and RNA polymerase similiar? How are they different?

Problem solved:

DNA polymerases and RNA polymerase are similar in that each is required to catalyze the elongation of the developing nucleic acid strand in replication and transcription, respectively. Their differences lie in the fact that RNA polymerase does not require a primer to initiate synthesis of the RNA chain, while DNA polymerase do (they require RNA primer).

24.1.7 TRANSLATION

You should be prepared to (a) differentiate between the separate processes of replication (DNA synthesis), transcription (RNA synthesis), and translation (protein synthesis), and (b) understand the mechanisms by which each process occurs. (The student should also bear in mind the sites at which each of these processes occur.)

Translation is the process of protein synthesis. The "blueprint" for the protein is encoded in mRNA. The process is more fully detailed in **24.1.7.1** and **24.1.7.2**. The mRNA is generated, it should be recalled, from DNA. Amino acids are the structural units of protein, as nucleotides are the structural units of DNA. There are, however, some twenty amino acids from which proteins are generally assembled. Amino acids have the general structure of a carboxyl group (COOH), an amino group (NH_2), a hydrogen atom (H), and a variable group, designated an R group, all of which are linked to a carbon atom. An R group may contain a variety of side chains. The R group of a given amino acid, then, affords the amino acid its identity and specificity.

Please solve this problem:

- Translation refers to:

  A. the replication of mRNA from tRNA and rRNA.
  B. the formation of multiple forms of RNA from a single DNA template, with base-pairing analogous to that of DNA synthesis.
  C. the assembly of R groups that govern the identity and properties of amino acid moieties.
  D. the association of amino acids in accordance with the order dictated by a cell's DNA molecule.

Problem solved:

D is correct. Translation refers to the generation of polypeptide chains (which are composed of amino acid subunits). The alignment and assembly of the amino acids to be joined are governed directly by an mRNA molecule sent from the nucleus to the ribosome. The mRNA molecule, in turn, is generated by transcription according to the base sequence of the analogous DNA molecule. It is, therefore, the DNA base sequence that ultimately governs protein synthesis. It is true that R groups differ among the amino acids, but that phenomenon has no relation to translation.

24.1.7.1 Roles of mRNA and Ribosomes in Protein Synthesis

Messenger RNA's name reflects the molecule's role in bringing information from the nucleus of the cell to the cytoplasm. The mRNA conveys its message in the form of three-nucleotide units called *codons*. On entering the cytoplasm, mRNA binds to specific mRNA-**binding sites** of a ribosome. The ribosome provides a binding site for mRNA and transfer RNA (tRNA), both of which participate in protein synthesis. Ribosomes also contain ribosomal RNA (rRNA). Ribosomes may be found free in the cytoplasm or attached to the endoplasmic reticulum (rough ER).

The ribosome (termed *70S in prokaryotes* and *80S in eukaryotes*) is composed of *two subunits*: a *large subunit* (termed 50S in prokaryotes and 60S in eukaryotes) and a *small subunit* (termed 30S in prokaryotes and 40S in eukaryotes). The numerical terms for the ribosome and its subunits derive from their respective rates of sedimentation under centrifugation (which is why the numbers by which they are designated do not sum arithmetically). The ribosome contains *two tRNA binding sites*: the *A (aminoacyl)* site and the *P (peptidyl)* binding site. These sites play an important role in the translation of mRNA, as is discussed below.

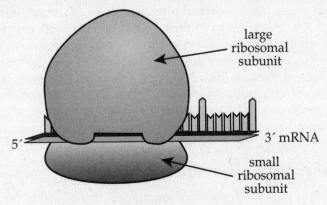

Ribosome containing small and large subunit
at mRNA molecule

Figure 24.10

Each of the codons carried by mRNA specifies a particular amino acid, according to the **genetic code**. The genetic code refers to the correspondence between codons in messenger RNA and the amino acid each codon codes for within a polypeptide. Significantly, the *genetic code is universal*, it does not change from organism to organism. Each of the 64 codons in the code is associated with only one of the 20 amino acids. The code, therefore, is redundant. It offers more than one codon per amino acid. Because of its redundancy, the code is said to be **degenerate**.

Please solve this problem:

- The genetic code refers to:

    A. the mRNA codons and their correspondence to exactly one amino acid.

    B. the set of enzymes that facilitate the flow of information from chromosome to ribosome to protein molecule.

    C. the base-pairing rules that permit replication of DNA and transcription of RNA.

    D. the molecular information stored within a particular amino acid sequence.

Problem solved:

A is correct. The genetic code refers to sequences of mRNA subunits that code for amino acids to be bonded together to form protein molecules. The code is degenerate, meaning that it features more codons than amino acids. Thus, while each codon codes for exactly one amino acid, more than one codon codes for the same amino acid.

Please solve this problem:

- Genetic information flows from DNA to RNA to protein molecule. Identify and define the processes that facilitate the flow of information.

Problem solved:

The question tests your understanding of the processes of transcription and translation—the mechanisms through which genetic information residing in the DNA molecules is conveyed to other areas of the cell in order to direct specific cellular activities. Transcription is the process by which RNA is synthesized from a DNA template. Because the RNA is made of base pairs that are complementary to those of the DNA template strand, it carries information from the DNA molecule by virtue of its sequence. Translation is the process by which protein is synthesized from an mRNA template. Because a protein is produced from amino acids whose identity and order are dictated by the sequence of bases associated with the RNA molecule, the protein reflects the information carried by the RNA molecule. Various proteins (including enzymes) produce the myraid traits of a cell and also facilitate diverse and numerous cellular activities.

24.1.7.2 Role of tRNA in Protein Synthesis

Transfer RNA (tRNA) is equipped with two functional sites of which the test-taker should take note. One site is the **anticodon**, which serves as the mRNA template recognition site. The tRNA's anticodon recognizes its complement sequence of triplet bases on the mRNA transcript. The transfer RNA molecule's second functional site is its amino acid attachment site. Each amino acid is associated with a particular transfer RNA; the amino acid attachment site of a tRNA molecule is highly specific for only one type of amino acid.

Transfer RNA binds mRNA at its complementary region, so that the tRNA anticodon associates with the mRNA codon. By binding the mRNA this way, the tRNA brings into position its attached amino acid, aligning it so that the amino acid encoded by the next codon may be placed adjacent to it. Additional tRNA molecules arrive at the mRNA molecule in an order that corresponds to the base sequences and codons of the mRNA molecule. Each tRNA brings its attached amino acid molecule and transfers it to the growing polypeptide chain. Each amino acid is added to the carboxyl end of the one preceding it in the order of synthesis.

Translation occurs in three phases: an **initiation phase**, an **elongation phase**, and a **termination phase**. Initiation of protein synthesis requires a specific tRNA molecule named **formylmethionyl-tRNA** (f-methionyl tRNA; in eukaryotes the initiator tRNA carries methionine). F-methionyl tRNA transports formyl-methionine to the smaller (30S) subunit of the ribosome, where it is required as initiator of protein synthesis. F-methionyl tRNA recognizes the initiating codon AUG on the mRNA. The initiator formyl-methionyl-tRNA binds to the 30S ribosome subunit at the ribosome's peptidyl (P) site, forming a 30S initiation complex composed of: (a) the 30S subunit of the ribosome, (b) the formylmethionyl-tRNA, and (c) the mRNA. The larger 50S subunit of the ribosome then joins the initiation complex to form a 70S initiation complex. (In eukaryotes the process is the same but the ribosome molecule is slightly larger; as noted earlier, the small subunit is 40S, the large subunit is 60S and the two together are 80S.) GTP provides the energy necessary for the complex to form.

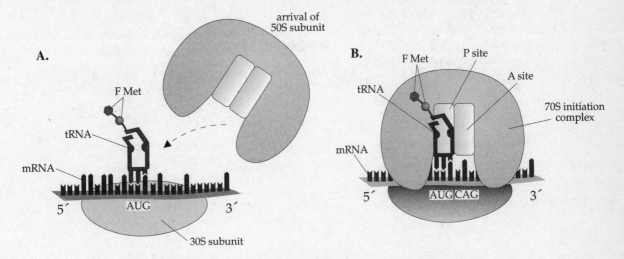

Initiation Complex Formed in Prokaryote at Onset of Translation

Figure 24.11

Please solve this problem:

- What triplet of bases constitutes the anticodon of formylmethionyl-tRNA?

Problem solved:

The anticodon of f-methionyl tRNA is UAC. This question asks the student to apply his or her understanding of the relationship between codon and anticodon and of base pair rules. F-methionyl tRNA recognizes the mRNA start codon AUG; the tRNA's anticodon must be composed of the triplet that is complementary to the triplet AUG. According to base-pairing rules for RNA, adenine pairs with uracil, uracil pairs with adenine, and guanine pairs with cytosine.

The 70S initiation complex facilitates elongation of the peptide chain. The P site is occupied with the f-methionyl tRNA, and the A site is vacant. Binding of the P site by f-methionyl tRNA ensures that the tRNA's anticodon aligns with the codon of the mRNA, establishing the **reading frame** for all subsequent events. Elongation then occurs, and individual amino acids are added to the methionine residue already present.

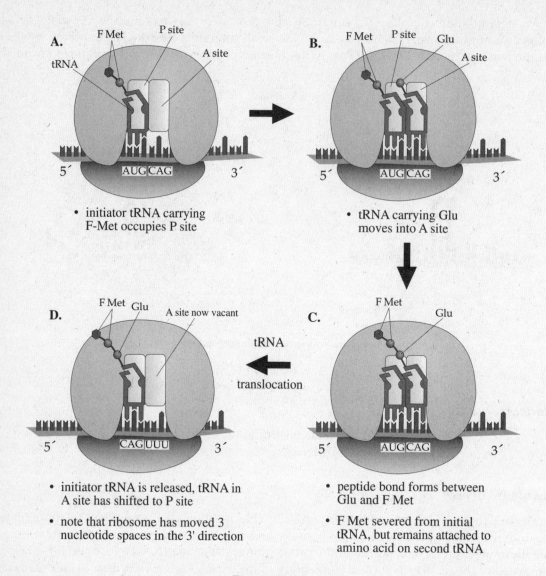

A.
tRNA
F Met   P site   A site
• initiator tRNA carrying
  F-Met occupies P site

B.
F Met   P site   Glu   A site
• tRNA carrying Glu
  moves into A site

C.
F Met   Glu
• peptide bond forms between
  Glu and F Met
• F Met severed from initial
  tRNA, but remains attached to
  amino acid on second tRNA

D.
F Met   Glu   A site now vacant
tRNA
translocation
• initiator tRNA is released, tRNA in
  A site has shifted to P site
• note that ribosome has moved 3
  nucleotide spaces in the 3' direction

Figure 24.12

Each cycle of the elongation phase proceeds according to the following series of events. Next to the initiator tRNA, an incoming tRNA molecule specific to the codon carried by the mRNA molecule arrives at the **A site** of the ribosome. The specific tRNA carries its designated amino acid. Occupation of the A site promotes the association of the two adjacent amino acids by a peptide bond. The bond that connected f-methionine (or methionine, in the case of eukaryotes) to the initiator tRNA is broken. However, the f-methionine remains connected to the new amino acid by the peptide bond. The release of the f-methionine from the initiator tRNA frees the initiator tRNA from the **P site**, and it moves into the cytoplasm to bond with another f-methionine. The ribosome then moves three nucleotides along the mRNA molecule, shifting the tRNA carrying the two amino acids from the A site to the P site. The movement of mRNA through the ribosome—*in the 5′ to 3′ direction*—aligns the next mRNA codon with the ribosome's available A site. The shift of the tRNA from the A site to the P site frees the A site so that the next tRNA molecule can attach to the next codon. This process is termed *translocation*. Translocation requires the hydrolysis of GTP.

The elongation cycle just described is repeated for each amino acid that is added to the chain of peptides.

Termination of translation involves a codon signal similiar to that needed for initiation. While the initiation codon is AUG, the termination codon may be one of three nucleotide triplets: UAG, UAA, or UGA. Stop codons are unusual in that they have *no tRNA complement* with which to pair. In this way the genetic code provides a built-in mechanism for terminating protein synthesis: when a stop codon is aligned at the A site of the ribosome, no matching tRNA can fill the A site and protein elongation is arrested. Release factors disengage the completed polypeptide carried by the tRNA in the P site, and the ribosome dissociates into large and small subunits, ready to begin the process anew.

Please solve this problem:

- The antibiotic actinomycin D binds tightly to double-stranded DNA, preventing separation into its component strands. Which of the following can most reasonably be expected to immediately result from the introduction of actinomycin D into a cell?

  A. The arrest of protein synthesis
  B. The arrest of RNA synthesis
  C. Both A and B
  D. Neither A nor B

Problem solved:

B is correct. The question describes an experimental situation in which DNA is prevented from separating into individual strands. It prompts you to consider the effect of this situation in light of relevant mechanisms of protein and RNA synthesis. Since the antibiotic prevents the DNA from functioning properly as a template, RNA synthesis (transcription) would not occur. However, RNA transcripts that already exist in the cell are *not* prevented from directing protein synthesis in their usual manner. Transcription would be arrested but translation would continue.

Please solve this problem:

- Specify the site of origin, basic molecular structure, and overall role in translation, of the following three types of RNA:

  (a) messenger RNA (mRNA);
  (b) ribosomal RNA (rRNA); and
  (c) transfer RNA (tRNA)

Problem solved:

(a) Messenger RNA (mRNA) is formed in the *nucleus* of the cell and travels from the nucleus to the cytoplasm. Messenger RNA is a single-stranded structure composed of a sugar-phosphate backbone and nucleotides that code for the synthesis of specific proteins. In the cytoplasm mRNA binds to the small subunit of a ribosome in preparation for translation. The information carried in the mRNA is read in nucleotide triplets, which are called codons. Each codon codes for a specific amino acid. The mRNA dictates the order of amino acids in the formation of a protein.

(b) Ribosomal RNA (rRNA) is formed in the *nucleolus* (a specialized structure within the nucleus) and enters the cytoplasm. It is a component of the ribosome, a two-part structure consisting of a small subunit and a large subunit. The ribosome provides a binding site for mRNA and tRNA during protein synthesis and participates in the process itself. Messenger RNA binds to the small subunit of a ribosome in preparation for protein synthesis, forming a complex. After tRNA joins the complex, the large subunit of the ribosome does the same. At this point, the ribosome is fully assembled around the mRNA, allowing for the initiation of protein synthesis.

Another structural feature of the ribosome is that it contains two tRNA binding sites: the P site and the A site. The P site holds the tRNA that carries the growing polypeptide chain; the A site is aligned with codons on the mRNA and provides a binding site for incoming tRNA molecules and their associated amino acids. Ribosomes move along the mRNA molecule in the five prime to three prime (5´→3´) direction.

(c) Transfer RNA (tRNA) is synthesized in the *nucleus* and travels into the cytoplasm. It is a *clover-shaped molecule* containing an mRNA recognition site (the anticodon) and an amino acid binding site that is specific for one amino acid (there are twenty biologically significant amino acids). Each amino acid is associated with a tRNA molecule containing a specific anticodon. Specific tRNAs and their associated amino acids arrive one at a time at the ribosome. Which tRNAs will bind to the mRNA depends on the codon of the mRNA at that site. The tRNA whose anticodon matches the codon of the mRNA at the ribosome will bind to the site and eventually release its associated amino acid. Without its amino acid, the tRNA molecule will leave the ribosome and be recycled. This process is repeated until the polypeptide (protein) specified by the mRNA transcript is fully assembled.

24.2 MASTERY APPLIED: SAMPLE PASSAGE AND QUESTIONS

Passage

Chromosome abnormalities in an embryo can result in either spontaneous abortions (miscarriages), or serious disorders, such as trisomy 21 (Down's syndrome) and the fragile X syndrome. Chromosomal abnormalities may be due to either a structural defect or a numeric defect. A standard technique for examining human chromosomes employs phytohemagglutinin, which is derived from the red bean. Added to a small quantity of anticoagulated blood, it engenders agglutination and stimulates the division of lymphocytes. Microtubule inhibitors can then be employed to halt mitosis, and metaphase chromosomes can be observed for any alterations in number and/or structure.

Another common technique used to examine chromosomes is Giemsa banding (G-banding). Trypsin is added to chromosome preparations and the chromosomes are then stained with Giemsa to produce a pattern of light and dark bands. Each chromosome can be identified by its unique banding pattern. This banding method results in the resolution of approximately 350-550 bands per haploid set of chromosomes. A single band represents about 5×10^6 to 10×10^6 base pairs of DNA. Each band represents a range of genes, from a few to many. A gene may involve 10^3 base pairs to over 2×10^6 base pairs. Improvements to the Giemsa technique now permit observation of chromosomes in prometaphase. The advantage of this is that chromosomes in prometaphase are more extended than those in metaphase, which allows the band resolution to be more refined. The improved technique is associated with the definition of over 850 bands.

Banding reveals the substructure of a chromosome and allows each chromosome to be identified unequivocally. Chromosomes are defined by their size, band pattern and morphology (shape and structural characteristics); this last includes the positioning of their centromere (see Figure 1). The centromere is the point of constriction of the metaphase chromosome and its position is constant for a specific chromosome. The centromere divides the chromosome into two arms. Metacentric chromosomes have their centromeres positioned near the center of the two arms, while submetacentric chromosomes have centrosomes located in between the two arms, somewhat more distant from the center. Acrocentric chromosomes have centromeres positioned near one end of the two arms; often these chromosomes show satellites positioned above a thin stalk. Another useful piece of information is the number of chromosomes present. Once chromosomes have been sorted according to the criteria listed above, they are arranged in a karyotype, a sequential ordering of metaphase chromosomes based on length and position of centromere.

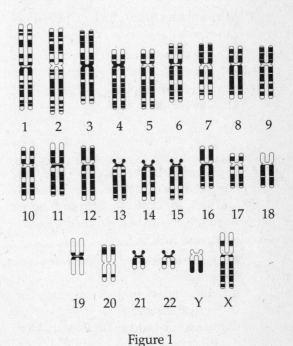

Figure 1

1. Which of the following reveals a chromosomal abnormality resulting from a numerical defect?

    I. A karyotype showing a total of 46 chromosomes.

    II. A karyotype showing a total of 22 sets of autosomes.

    III. A karyotype showing a total of 69 chromosomes.

    A. II only
    B. III only
    C. I and III only
    D. II and III only

2. The inhibitor used to arrest mitosis prevented the occurrence of which stages of cell division?

    A. Metaphase and prophase.
    B. Anaphase and telophase.
    C. Telophase, anaphase, and prophase.
    D. Metaphase, anaphase, prophase, and telophase.

3. Microtubules form which of the following structures during mitosis?

    A. The centrosomes
    B. The centrioles
    C. The mitotic spindle
    D. The chromosomes

4. A geneticist in the process of assembling the karyotype of a cell based on stained metaphase chromosomes would assess all of the following characteristics EXCEPT:

    A. the number of chromosomes present.
    B. the individual sizes of the chromosomes.
    C. the comparative condensed states of a chromosome.
    D. the location of centromeres on the chromosomes.

5. Might chromosome banding of a mitotic chromosome be expected to identify sections of chromosomes that have been exchanged between chromosomes?

    A. Yes, because banding allows each specific chromosome to be identified unequivocally.
    B. Yes, because banding patterns vary from individual to individual.
    C. No, because banding does not reveal the substructure of a given chromosome.
    D. No, because banding only reveals the size and number of chromosomes.

6. The improved staining technique mentioned in the passage takes advantage of which of the following mitotic events?

    A. Chromosomes begin to condense during prophase and are still incompletely condensed at prometaphase.
    B. Chromosomes begin to condense during metaphase and at prometaphase have not yet condensed.
    C. Chromosomes have not yet begun to condense at prometaphase or metaphase.
    D. Chromosomes do not condense until after anaphase, when cytokinesis is completed.

7. Research has shown that chromosomal abnormalities are found in fifty percent of spontaneously aborted fetuses, compared to a five-percent rate in stillborns. These data indicate that:

A. chromosomal aberrations are spontaneously eliminated in 55% of conceptions.

B. loss of chromosomally abnormal zygotes typically occurs early in gestation.

C. ninety-five percent of live-borns will have chromosomal abnormalities.

D. viability of offspring decreases as gestation proceeds.

8. Among the following, which metaphase chromosome depicted in Figure 1 is acrocentric?

A. Chromosome 3
B. Chromosome 7
C. Chromosome 14
D. The X chromosome

24.3 MASTERY VERIFIED: ANSWERS AND EXPLANATIONS

1. *B is the correct answer.* Human cells feature a total of 46 chromosomes in their nucleus. Statement I does not relate to a numeric chromosomal abnormality. Human cells do not normally have a total of 69 chromosomes. A genotype of 69 chromosomes however, indicates triploidy, a numeric chromosomal aberration. Humans have a total of 22 sets of autosomes and 1 set of sex chromosomes (XX for a female, XY for a male). Choice II therefore does not substantiate a numerical chromosomal abnormality. The correct answer option includes statement III and excludes the other two.

2. *B is the correct answer.* The microtubule inhibitor used to inhibit mitosis yielded metaphase chromosomes. The stages of mitosis are, in sequential order, prophase, metaphase, anaphase, and telophase. Halting the cell division at metaphase circumvented anaphase and telophase, which would have followed metaphase.

3. *C is the correct answer.* The mitotic spindle forms between the cell division stages of prophase and metaphase; it consists of microtubules and other components. The spindle spans the cell. The centrosomes are the two poles from which the microtubules emanate, not microtubules as themselves, choice A suggests. Similarly, in B, the centrioles are located at the two poles from which the microtubules emanate but are not microtubules. (Centrioles are at the center of the centrosomes.) D is wrong because the chromosomes are composed only of DNA and protein.

4. *C is the correct answer.* As described in the passage, karyotype is determined by four characteristics: the number of chromosomes present, their individual sizes, the location of their centromeres, and the banding pattern of individual chromosomes.

5. *A is the correct answer.* A change in chromosome content would be detected using the method described. In B, variations from individual to individual, even if verifiable, would not address the question of a translocation between one individual's chromosomes. C and D are incorrect because banding does reveal the substructure of a given chromosome; it also reveals more than the size and number of chromosomes.

6. *A is the correct answer.* Duplicated chromosomes begin to condense during prophase; by prometaphase they are still slightly extended compared to their status at metaphase. Chromosomes begin to condense at prophase, which precedes prometaphase and metaphase.

7. *B is the correct answer.* The data suggest that embryos with chromosomal abnormalities are spontaneously rejected early in development rather than later in development. Choice A is incorrect because chromosomal aberrations are permanent. Choice C is nonsensical and is calculated to cause the student to account for the remaining 95% of stillborns whose conditions are not described. Organisms that are not viable tend to be rejected early in gestation rather than later in gestation. Choice D, therefore, is incorrect.

8. *C is the correct answer.* Chromosome 14 is acrocentric: its centromere is positioned toward the end of the chromosome arms and it shows the characteristic satellites described in the passage. Chromosome 3 is metacentric: its centromere is located at the center of the two chromosome arms. Chromosome 7 is submetacentric: its centromere is located in between the two chromosome arms some distance from the center; this makes C wrong. The X chromosome (one of the sex chromosomes) is also submetacentric: its centromere is located in between the two chromosome arms some distance from the center. Choice D is not correct.

CHAPTER 25

PERPETUATION OF THE SPECIES—THE BIOLOGY OF REPRODUCTION

25.1 MASTERY ACHIEVED

25.1.1 HOMOLOGY, DIPLOIDY, AND HAPLOIDY

To understand the reproduction of cells and multicellular organisms, you must understand the terms **homology**, **diploidy**, and **haploidy** (also called **monoploidy**). In the human, all cells other than the **germ cells** (i.e., sperm and ova) contain 46 chromosomes, or 23 homologous pairs. **Diploid** is the state in which every chromosome of a cell has a homologue. The diploid state is also designated "2N."

If one chromosome were removed from each of the 23 pairs in a diploid human cell, the cell would be left with 23 chromosomes in total. Each of the 23 chromosomes would lack a homologous counterpart, and the cell would be termed "haploid." For any organism the number of chromosomes in a haploid cell is one-half the number of chromosomes in a diploid cell. The haploid condition is designated "1N."

Please solve this problem:

- If a cell is diploid, then:

    A. each of its chromosomes contains four strands of nucleic acid.
    B. each of its chromosomes has a homologous counterpart.
    C. it contains two nuclei.
    D. its nucleus contains single-stranded DNA.

Problem solved:

B is the correct answer. The diploid state describes a cell in which all chromosomes possess homologous pairs. The haploid state describes a cell whose chromosomes do not have homologues. Regardless of whether a cell is diploid or haploid, its chromosomes are composed of double-stranded DNA; choices A and D are incorrect. Choice C is incorrect as well; the diploid cell does not contain two nuclei.

Please solve this problem:

- If, for a given organism, the diploid (2N) number is 24, the haploid number (1N) is:

  A. 48
  B. 18
  C. 12
  D. 9

Problem solved:

C is the correct answer. A haploid cell has one-half the number of chromosomes found in a diploid cell. A haploid cell's chromosomes do not have homologous counterparts. A diploid human cell has 46 chromosomes or 23 homologous pairs. A haploid human cell (such as a sperm cell or an ovum) contains a total of 23 chromosomes.

25.1.2 CELLULAR REPRODUCTION

Cells reproduce through the process of **mitosis**. The period of the cell's life cycle between mitotic divisions is called **interphase**. Interphase has three subphases: (1) the G_1 **phase**, also called the **gap phase**, (2) the **S phase**, also called the **synthesis phase**, and (3) the G_2 **phase**. During the S phase the cell reproduces its genome in preparation for division. Mitosis involves **nuclear division**. **Cytoplasmic division** is also called **cytokinesis**.

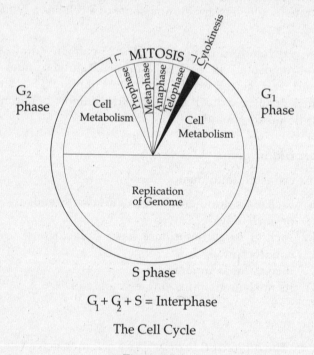

The Cell Cycle

Figure 25.1

Please solve this problem:

- The cell cycle phase associated with the replication of the cell's genome is:

    A. the S phase of interphase.
    B. mitosis.
    C. the G_2 period of interphase.
    D. cytokinesis.

Problem solved:

A is the correct answer. The cell's genome is replicated during the S phase of the cell cycle. The G_2 portion of interphase represents the second gap phase. Mitosis involves nuclear division. Cytokinesis refers to the division of the cytoplasm (as opposed to the division of the nucleus).

25.1.2.1 Replication of the Genome

During the S phase of interphase all 23 pairs of the cell's chromosomes replicate. When replication is complete, each chromosome has a duplicate. Each pair of duplicates is joined by a **centromere**. The two duplicate chromosomes are at this stage called **sister chromatids**.

Please solve this problem:

- Sister chromatids are:

    A. homologous to one another.
    B. identical to one another.
    C. unrelated to one another.
    D. produced during the G_1 phase of the cell cycle

Problem solved:

B is the correct answer. Sister chromatids are produced through DNA replication and are therefore identical to one another. They are produced during the S phase, not the G_1 phase; choice D is incorrect.

25.1.2.2 Mitosis

Interphase is followed by mitosis, a process that is customarily divided into four phases, **prophase, metaphase, anaphase, and telophase** and results in division of the nucleus. Mitosis is followed by the division of the cytoplasm, called cytokinesis.

During prophase the chromosomes condense to the point that they are visible under the light microscope as an X-shaped structure. The **nucleolus** slowly disappears. Centrioles move to opposite poles of the cell. Star-shaped fibers called **aster fibers** form around the centrioles. Microtubules give rise to a mitotic spindle, which spans the cell from pole to pole. The nuclear membrane begins to dissolve.

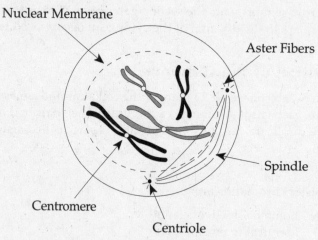

The Cell at Prophase of Mitosis

Figure 25.2

The beginning of metaphase is termed **prometaphase** and is marked by complete dissolution of the nuclear membrane. **Kinetochore fibers** associated with the centromeres interact with the mitotic spindle, producing movement of chromosomes. At metaphase proper, the chromosomes align on the **metaphase plate** so that centromeres lie in a plane along an axis at the cell's midpoint. The kinetochore fibers help to align and maintain the chromosomes on the metaphase plate.

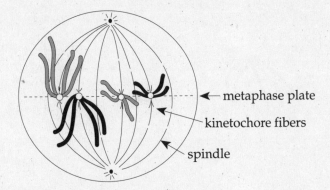

The Cell at Metaphase of Mitosis

Figure 25.3

During anaphase, sister chromatids separate (as a result of the splitting of the centromere) and move toward opposite poles of the cell along the path marked by the spindle apparatus. With the separation of sister chromatids, each chromatid is called a **daughter chromosome**.

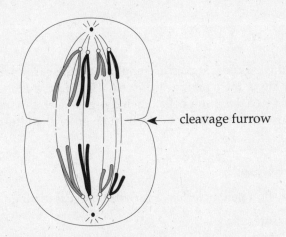

The Cell at Anaphase of Mitosis

Figure 25.4

At telophase the daughter chromosomes are positioned at opposite poles of the cell and the kinetochore fibers disappear. A nuclear membrane forms around each set of daughter chromosomes. The chromosomes decondense and are no longer visable by light microscopy. Nucleoli then reappear; mitosis and nuclear division are complete.

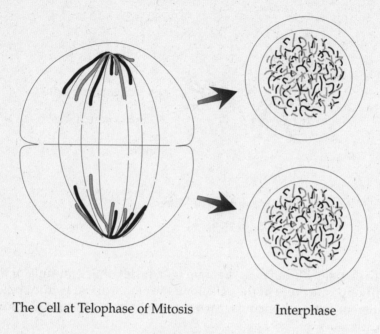

The Cell at Telophase of Mitosis   Interphase

Figure 25.5

Cytokinesis begins during the last part of anaphase or the early part of telophase. A **cleavage furrow** forms along the equator of the cell. The furrow deepens until it ultimately divides the cell, forming two daughter cells. Each daughter cell possesses a diploid number of single-stranded chromosomes. The daughter cells then enter the interphase period of the cell cycle.

Please solve this problem:

- Development of a cleavage furrow occurs during:

    A. interphase.
    B. prophase.
    C. metaphase.
    D. cytokinesis.

Problem solved:

D is the correct answer. The cleavage furrow develops around the periphery of the cell toward late anaphase or early telophase. However, the development of the cleavage furrow is the beginning of cytokinesis, which makes D the best answer. It initiates the division of the parent cell into two daughter cells. The daughter cells normally receive approximately equal amounts of cytoplasm and an equal inventory of organelles.

Please solve this problem:

- Which of the following stages involve(s) a change in chromosome density?

  A. Prophase alone
  B. Interphase alone
  C. Prophase and telophase
  D. Anaphase and telophase

Problem solved:

C is the correct answer. At prophase the chromosomes condense and become visible under the light microscope. At telophase, the process is reversed: chromosomes decondense and disappear.

25.1.3 REDUCTION DIVISION: MEIOSIS

Reduction division refers to the generation by a diploid parent cell of haploid daughter cells. Reduction division is accomplished by meiosis and is the basis of **gametogenesis** (as discussed below). Like mitosis, meiosis involves nuclear division and cytokinesis. Nuclear division in meiosis embodies four stages bearing the same names as those in mitosis: prophase, metaphase, anaphase, and telophase. Meiosis, however, involves *two* divisions instead of one. The first meiotic division consists of prophase I, metaphase I, anaphase I, and telophase I; the second meiotic division entails prophase II, metaphase II, anaphase II, and telophase II.

25.1.3.1 The First Meiotic Division

The first phase of the first meiotic division is termed prophase I. Prophase I follows interphase, during which the cell duplicates its chromosomes. As in mitosis, chromosomes condense during prophase I, the nucleolus begins to disassemble and disappear, and centrioles move to opposite poles of the cell. Aster fibers form around the centrioles. The mitotic spindle forms and spans the cell from pole to pole. The nuclear membrane begins to dissolve.

Prophase I differs from mitotic prophase in that *homologous pairs* of duplicated chromosomes align in close proximity to one another, forming **tetrads**. The association of homologous pairs of duplicated chromosomes to form the tetrad is termed **synapsis**.

The close proximity between homologous chromosomes during synapsis frequently leads chromatids from one homologue to physically bind with chromatids from the other homologue. The site at which binding occurs is called the **chiasma**. Chromatids may break at the chiasma. When this happens, the resulting segments may change places with one another, in a process called **crossing over**. Crossing over produces a physical exchange of chromatid segments between sections of homologous chromatids. The process causes each chromatid to lose a component of its own DNA and to acquire in its place a corresponding section of DNA from its homologue. Crossing over, therefore, is a form of **genetic recombination** that is specific to meiosis.

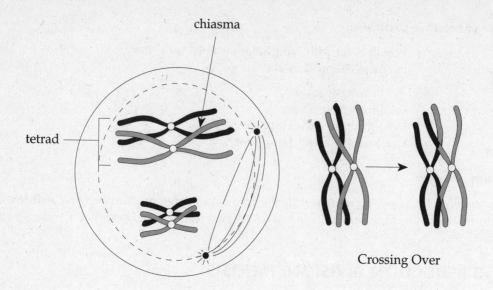

Synapsis and Crossing Over During Meiosis I

Figure 25.6

*Mei*otic metaphase I differs from *mi*totic metaphase in that *pairs* of homologous chromosomes (instead of *single* chromosomes) align on the spindle apparatus. That is, **tetrads** (composed of four chromatids) align along the spindles. By comparison, in mitotic metaphase a double-stranded chromosome composed of *two* sister chromatids aligns on the metaphase plate.

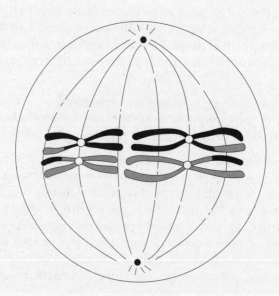

Alignment of Chromosome Pairs on Metaphase Plate
During Metaphase I of Meiosis

Figure 25.7

In meiotic anaphase I, homologous chromosome pairs separate and move to opposite poles of the cell. *Centromeres, however, do not split.* The two chromatids belonging to a chromosome remain attached. Each pole of the cell, therefore, contains one double-stranded chromosome from each pair of homologous chromosomes.

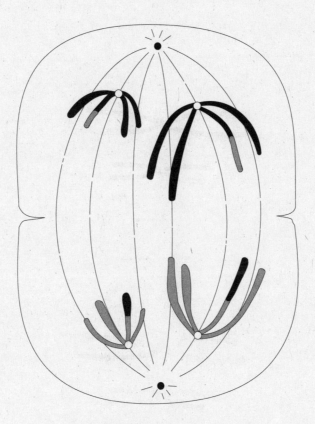

The Cell at Anaphase of Meiosis I

Figure 25.8

At meiotic telophase I, the chromosomes form two clusters at either end of the cell. The cell cytoplasm divides, leaving two daughter cells, each with genetic material from *only one* member of each pair of homologous chromosomes.

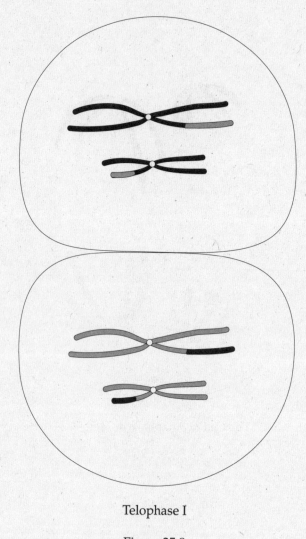

Telophase I

Figure 25.9

Please solve this problem:

- Which of the following is associated with meiotic prophase I, but not with mitotic prophase?

   A. Spindle formation
   B. Double-stranded chromosomes
   C. Condensed chromosomes
   D. Tetrad formation

Problem solved:

D is the correct answer. During mitotic prophase, chromosomes consisting of two sister chromatids align along the spindle fibers, without associating with their homologues. During meiotic prophase I, each chromosome aligns along the spindle fibers at the metaphase plate in association with its homologue, forming the four-chromatid tetrad. The formation of tetrads and the subsequent separation of homologous pairs without the splitting of centromeres provides each daughter cell with the genetic information from only one homologue of each chromosomal pair.

Spindle formation, condensed chromosomes, and the existence of sister chromatids are found during both mitotic and meiotic prophases.

Please solve this problem:

- Which of the following most completely characterizes the process of crossing over?

   A. Genetic material is exchanged between homologous chromosomes during synapsis.
   B. Duplicated chromosomes pair with their duplicated homologues.
   C. A chiasma is formed.
   D. A nuclear division during which each daughter cell receives the genetic material from only one chromosome of each homologous pair.

Problem solved:

A is the correct answer. Crossing over is associated with the process of synapsis, which occurs during meiotic prophase. Homologous chromosomes associate and exchange portions of their DNA. The result is an exchange of the genetic material and, consequently, genetic recombination. Choice B characterizes tetrad formation, a prelude to crossing over, and choice D characterizes the first meiotic division. The chiasma (choice C) is the site at which crossing over begins. Thus choice C does not characterize the process fully.

Please solve this problem:

- Which of the following correctly distinguishes mitosis from the first division of meiosis?

   A. After the first meiotic division, each daughter cell possesses a full complement of genetic material; after mitosis, they do not.
   B. After mitosis, each daughter cell possesses a full complement of genetic material; after the first meiotic division, they do not.
   C. After mitosis, each daughter cell possesses duplicated chromosomes; after meiosis, they do not.
   D. After the first meiotic division, each daughter cell possesses chromosomes that are organized into tetrads; after mitosis, they do not.

Problem solved:

B is the correct answer. The daughter cells produced by the first meiotic division do not have a full complement of genetic material. Because homologues separate while their centromeres remain intact, each daughter cell receives only *one* member of each homologous chromosomal pair. The absence of the other member of the homologous pair means that each daughter receives half of the full parental genome.

Each of the daughter cells produced by mitosis, on the other hand, receives one copy of each member of each chromosome; it receives the full parental genome. Choices A and C are wrong because they reverse the truth. Choice D is incorrect as well; during meiosis, tetrads separate during anaphase I. The tetrad does not exist within the daughter cells.

25.1.3.2 The Second Meiotic Division

Each daughter cell that arises from the first meiotic division has half of the full complement of chromosomes, but it has two copies of that half. The two copies of each chromosome are joined by a centromere. During the second meiotic division, each daughter cell undergoes prophase II, metaphase II, anaphase II, and telephase II in much the same manner as a cell that undergoes mitosis. At anaphase II, centromeres divide and the two chromatids are pulled to opposite poles of the cell. Cytokinesis follows and two daughter cells result, each of which has one of the four chromatids from each original tetrad. Because the process just described occurs in each of the two daughter cells produced in the first meiotic division, a total of four daughter cells are produced. Each of the four daughter cells produced by meiosis is haploid.

25.1.4 MITOSIS AND MEIOSIS: THE FUNDAMENTAL DIFFERENCES

Mitosis generates two diploid daughters and meiosis generates four haploid daughters. The difference in ploidy and number of daughter cells arises from an initial difference in the alignment of chromosomes on the spindle apparatus and in the subsequent separation of chromosomes to form new daughter nuclei. In mitosis, chromosomes align without pairing with their homologues. Centromeres then divide and each daughter is provided with one copy of *all* chromosomes. In the first meiotic division, chromosomes align on the spindle apparatus in association with their homologues. Centromeres do not then divide. Rather, homologues separate and each daughter cell is provided with two copies of one-half the original genome. That is, each receives two copies of only one member of each homologous pair.

Each daughter then undergoes the second meiotic division, in which centromeres divide. Each daughter produces two new daughters (for a total of four daughters). Each daughter cell has one copy of one member of each homologous pair.

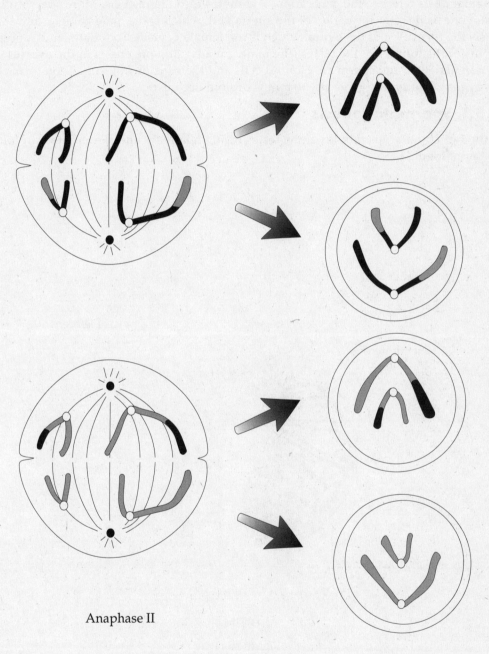

Anaphase II

Telophase II

Anaphase II and Telophase II of Meiosis

Figure 25.10

25.1.5 GAMETOGENESIS: REPRODUCTION OF THE SEX CELLS

Gametogenesis refers to the generation of **gametes** through meiosis. More specifically, **spermatogenesis** denotes formation of the **sperm cell**, which is the male gamete, and **oogenesis** the formation of the **ovum**, which is the female gamete. Spermatogenesis occurs in the **seminiferous tubules** of the **testes** (the **male gonads**), and oogenesis in the **ovaries** (the **female gonads**). Ova and sperm are haploid cells and their fusion at fertilization forms the diploid **zygote**. The zygote gives rise to a new diploid organism.

25.1.5.1 Spermatogenesis

Within the seminiferous tubules of the testes reside relatively undifferentiated diploid cells called **spermatogonia**.

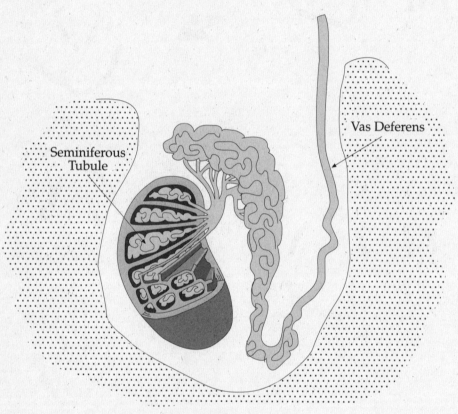

Testis

Figure 25.11

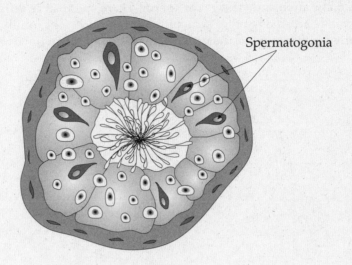

Cross-section View of a Seminiferous Tubule

Figure 25.12

Some spermatogonia enlarge and undergo genome replication to become **primary spermatocytes**, which then undergo a first meiotic division to yield two **secondary spermatocytes**. Each secondary spermatocyte then undergoes a second meiotic division to produce two haploid **spermatids**. Each diploid spermatogonium thus produces four haploid spermatids.

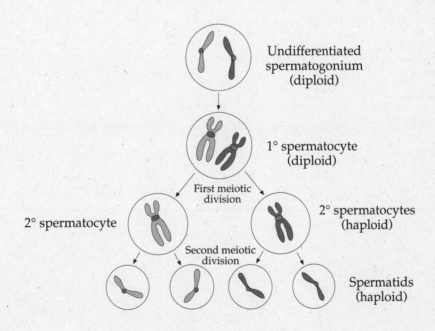

Spermatogenesis

Figure 25.13

Spermatids are immature sperm cells which travel to the **epididymus**, a coiled tube that serves as the site of maturation and storage for sperm. There spermatids differentiate into mature sperm that will bear, among other structures, a **flagellum** for motility and an **acrosome** filled with degradative enzymes which facilitate penetration of the ovum during fertilization.

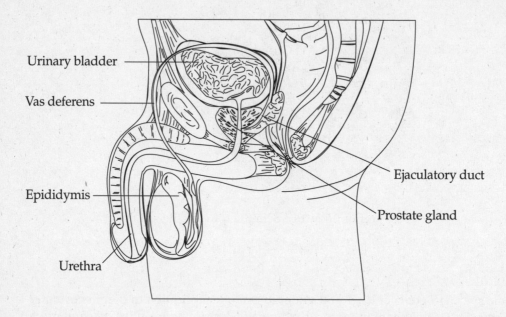

From the epididymus the mature sperm enters first the **vas deferens**, then the **ejaculatory duct**, and finally the **urethra**, which runs through the **penis** to the outside of the body.

Please solve this problem:

- Which of the following correctly orders the structures through which sperm cells travel?

  A. Epididymus, vas deferens, ejaculatory duct, seminiferous tubule, urethra
  B. Vas deferens, epididymus, ejaculatory duct, seminiferous tubule, urethra
  C. Seminiferous tubule, epididymus, vas deferens, ejaculatory duct, urethra
  D. Ejaculatory duct, seminiferous tubule, vas deferens, epididymus, urethra

Problem solved:

C is the correct answer. Newly formed spermatozoa travel first through the seminiferous tubule, then through the epididymus, then through the vas deferens, the ejaculatory duct, and the urethra. A flagellum affords a sperm cell the motility it needs to reach the ovum, and acrosomal enzymes assist it in penetrating the ovum during fertilization.

Please solve this problem:

- Which of the following human cells is haploid?

  A. Spermatogonium
  B. Primary spermatocyte
  C. Spermatid
  D. Zygote

Problem solved:

C is the correct answer. Spermatogenesis begins with the spermatogonium, a diploid cell. After it enlarges and undergoes replication of its genome it becomes a primary spermatocyte, which is also diploid. The primary spermatocyte undergoes a first and second meiotic division to generate four spermatids, which are haploid cells. The spermatids mature to become spermatozoa. The fusion of a spermatozoan with an ovum (a haploid cell) produces a zygote, which is diploid.

25.1.5.2 Oogenesis

Oogenesis produces a single mature haploid ovum. The process begins in the ovary, where a diploid **oogonium** begins meiosis to produce a **primary oocyte**. The primary oocyte undergoes a first meiotic division. Unlike the first meiotic division that accompanies spermatogenesis, this division divides cytoplasm unequally between the progeny, producing one larger and one smaller daughter cell. The larger one is called a **secondary oocyte**, and the smaller a **polar body**. The secondary oocyte undergos a second meiotic division. The polar body may or may not divide; if it does, it produces two new polar bodies, each haploid. The secondary oocyte produces two daughter cells, which are also haploid. When the secondary oocyte undergoes the second meiotic division, it again allocates cytoplasm unequally, producing one small haploid polar body and one large haploid ovum. The net products of oogenesis, then, are two or three small haploid polar bodies, which degenerate, and one large haploid ovum.

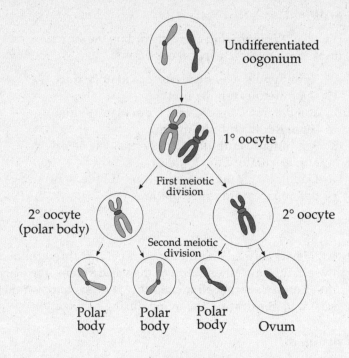

Oogenesis

Figure 25.15

Please solve this problem:

- Which of the following correctly orders the cell types that arise during oogenesis?

    A. Secondary oocyte, primary oocyte, oogonia, ovum
    B. Primary oocyte, secondary oocyte, oogonia, ovum
    C. Ovum, primary oocyte, secondary oocyte, oogonia
    D. Oogonia, primary oocyte, secondary oocyte, ovum

Problem solved:

D is the correct answer. The undifferentiated oogonium becomes the primary oocyte, which produces secondary oocytes and then the ovum. In the course of oogenesis, as many as three polar bodies are generated.

Please solve this problem:

- Which of the following does NOT apply to a polar body?

    A. It is small in relation to an ovum.
    B. It arises as a by-product of oogenesis.
    C. It is diploid.
    D. It degenerates.

Problem solved:

C is the correct answer. Meiosis generates four haploid cells from one diploid cell. In the case of oogenesis the first meiotic division allocates cytoplasm unequally, yielding two progeny of unequal size. The smaller of the two is a polar body. The larger progeny, a secondary oocyte, undergoes a second meiotic division which yields a relatively large ovum and a relatively small polar body, both haploid. The polar bodies degenerate. Choices A, B, and D make true statements. Choice C does not.

Please solve this problem:

- Which of the following correctly distinguishes spermatogenesis from oogenesis?

    A. Spermatogenesis yields haploid cells; oogenesis does not.
    B. Spermatogenesis produces four functional cells; oogenesis does not.
    C. Spermatogenesis produces a gamete; oogenesis does not.
    D. Spermatogenesis occurs in the gonads; oogenesis does not.

Problem solved:

B is the correct answer. Spermatogenesis and oogenesis both lead to the production of gametes. Each occurs in the gonads: oogenesis occurs in the ovaries (the female gonads) and spermatogenesis occurs in the testes (the male gonads). Both processes produce haploid gametes. Spermatogenesis produces four functional haploid cells; oogenesis, however, produces only one functional haploid cell and as many as three polar bodies, which degenerate. The disparate products of oogenesis result from unequal allocation of cytoplasm during the first and second meiotic divisions of the oocyte.

25.1.6 OVULATION, FERTILIZATION, AND IMPLANTATION

The mature ovum is surrounded by supporting cells. Together, the ovum and supporting cells compose a **follicle**. During **ovulation** a given follicle in one of the two ovaries ruptures, releasing the ovum, which then enters the **fallopian tube**. The fallopian tube connects the ovaries and the **uterus**, and is normally the site of fertilization.

The ovum is surrounded by an outer and an inner membrane, termed the **corona radiata** and **zona pellucida**, respectively. During **fertilization,** the sperm releases *degradative enzymes* from its *acrosome*, located at its head. These degrade the corona radiata and zona pellucida. Fertilization is complete when sperm and ovum nucleii have fused to form the zygote, a single diploid cell. The zygote travels to the uterus, where it implants in the **endometrial tissue** in a process known as **implantation**.

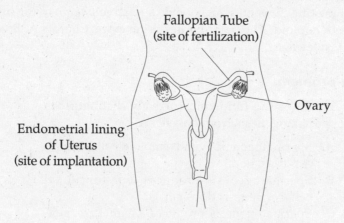

Sites of Fertilization and Implantation
in the Female Reproductive System

Figure 25.16

The **placenta**, a complex mix of embryonic and maternal tissue, develops at the site of implantation. The placenta is the site of the transfer of nutrients from mother to fetus as well as waste products from fetus to mother.

Please solve this problem:

- Which of the following is a false statement?

  A. The site of fertilization is the uterus.
  B. The site of implantation is the uterine wall.
  C. The placenta functions to exchange wastes and nutrients between the embryo and the mother.
  D. Enzymes derived from the acrosome of the sperm facilitate the sperm's penetration of the zona pellucida and corona radiata.

Problem solved:

A is the correct answer. Fertilization occurs in the fallopian tube. The penetration of the ovum's outer layers is facilitated by degradative enzymes, which are stored in the acrosome of the sperm. The resulting zygote implants in the uterine wall. The placenta forms from a combination of maternal and embryonic tissue and functions in the exchange of nutrients and waste products between the embryo and the mother.

25.2 MASTERY APPLIED: SAMPLE PASSAGE AND QUESTIONS

Passage

The process of fertilization allows the transmission to the offspring of genes that are contributed by both parents. Fusion of the genetic material of the sperm and egg—the male and female gametes, respectively—initiates a series of reactions in the egg cytoplasm that marks the beginning of the development of a new organism. Crucial to the success of fertilization is a species-specific recognition between sperm and egg. The egg governs the entry of sperm. Only one sperm can ultimately fertilize the egg.

A mature sperm cell possesses a haploid nucleus containing tightly compressed DNA, a flagellum for propulsion, and an acrosomal vesicle containing enzymes that facilitate entry of the nucleus into the egg. A modified lysozome, the acrosomal vesicle is derived from the Golgi apparatus. Enzymes within it digest proteins and complex sugars, enabling the sperm to penetrate the outer layers of the egg.

In sea urchins (the best-studied animal model of fertilization), globular actin molecules lie between the nucleus and the acrosomal vesicle in sperm. These molecules are proteins that polymerize to project a finger-like process in early fertilization during the acrosome reaction.

The egg also contains a haploid nucleus and is much larger than a sperm cell. Unlike sperm, the egg has vast reserves of cytoplasm containing proteins, ribosomes, tRNA, mRNA and morphogenic factors needed to facilitate the development of a new organism. The morphogenic factors govern the differentiation of cells.

The plasma membrane surrounds the egg cytoplasm. During fertilization the plasma membrane regulates the flow of ions and is capable of fusing with the sperm plasma membrane. Directly above the plasma membrane is the vitelline envelope—a glycoprotein membrane critical to species-specific binding of sperm. In mammals it is thickened and called the *zona pellucida*. Mammals also have the *corona radiata*, a layer of ovarian follicular cells responsible for providing nutrients to the egg at the time of ovulation. Sea urchin eggs contain an outer layer of jelly which the acrosomal enzymes must penetrate to reach the inner membrane layers.

An investigator wished to determine the location of a sperm protein called *bindin* during fertilization in order to observe when it promotes species-specific binding between sperm and egg. He conducted two experiments using the Mediterranean sea urchin, *Toxopneustes lividus*.

The first experiment was conducted as follows:

Step 1:

Rabbit anti-bindin (an antibody) was produced by injecting purified sea urchin bindin into rabbits.

Step 2:

The rabbit anti-bindin was then bound to sea urchin sperm that had undergone the acrosomal reaction.

Step 3:

Unbound antibody was washed off and the sperm were exposed to swine antibodies that were capable of binding to rabbit antibodies. The swine antibodies were covalently linked to peroxidase enzymes, allowing peroxidase to be deposited wherever bindin occurred.

The peroxidase enzymes were able to produce an electron-dense precipitate upon reaction with diaminobenzidine (DAB) and hydrogen peroxide (H_2O_2). The precipitate indicates the location of bindin on the sperm.

Results:

The precipitate was found to be localized on the surface of the entire acrosomal process. (See Figure 1.)

A second experiment was performed in the same manner as the first except that in Step 2 the sperm had not yet undergone the acrosome reaction. No bindin was detected on the sperm surface in this trial.

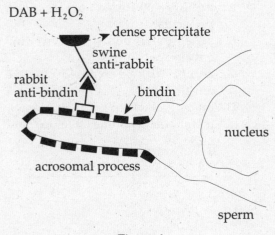

Figure 1

1. A frog egg would contain all of the following EXCEPT:

    A. morphogenic factors.
    B. a vitelline membrane.
    C. a plasma membrane.
    D. the corona radiata.

2. In the sea urchin egg, cortical granules that lie beneath the plasma membrane are homologous to the acrosomal vesicle of sperm. Which of the following characteristic(s) most likely apply (applies) to both structures?

    I. Both are derived from the Golgi apparatus.
    II. Both contain large stores of mRNA and tRNA.
    III. Both contain proteolytic enzymes.

    A. I only
    B. III only
    C. I and II only
    D. I and III only

3. Which of the following undergoes cleavage?

    A. A diploid cell in the S phase of its cell cycle.
    B. A haploid cell at the onset of gametogenesis.
    C. A diploid zygote just after fertilization.
    D. A haploid gamete just after implantation.

4. On the basis of the results of Experiments I and II, the researcher would be most justified in concluding that:

    A. bindin is virtually identical in function to egg cortical granules.
    B. bindin promotes species-specific binding of egg and sperm after the acrosomal reaction.
    C. rabbit anti-bindin caused bindin to localize on the acrosomal process.
    D. rabbit anti-bindin caused the sperm in experiment I to undergo the acrosomal reaction.

5. Under normal conditions in humans, the egg is fertilized in which of the following reproductive structures?

    A. The ovary
    B. The fallopian tubes
    C. The uterus
    D. The corpus luteum

6. Which of the following statements is (are) true with regard to Experiment II?

 I. Rabbit anti-bindin did not bind to bindin.
 II. Diaminobenzidine and hydrogen peroxide did not react with peroxidases to yield a precipitate.
 III. Swine anti-rabbit did not bind to rabbit anti-bindin.

A. I only
B. II only
C. I and III only
D. I, II, and III

7. The bond that links swine antibodies to peroxidase enzymes in Experiments I and II is most similar in character to all of the following EXCEPT:

A. the bond that links hydrogen and oxygen within a single water molecule.
B. the bond that links hydrogen and oxygen among water molecules.
C. the bond that links one amino acid to the next in a polypeptide.
D. the bond that links a third phosphate group to adenosine diphosphate in ATP.

8. Based on the information in the passage, if an experimenter wished to directly observe the aggregation of bindin molecules on a sea urchin egg in a laboratory, she would expose isolated bindin molecules to:

A. an egg stripped of its zona pellucida.
B. an egg stripped of its vitelline envelope.
C. an egg with an exposed vitelline envelope.
D. an egg with an intact plasma membrane, vitelline envelope, and outer jelly coat.

25.3 MASTERY VERIFIED: ANSWERS AND EXPLANATIONS

1. *D is the correct answer.* The corona radiata only exists in mammalian eggs; it is not present in amphibian egg. Choice A is incorrect; the passage states that morphogenic factors in eggs provide for differentiation of cells during development of the organism. Choice B is incorrect as well: the vitelline membrane of the egg, located above the plasma membrane, allows for species-specific binding of sperm. Choice C is wrong because the plasma membrane is common to all eggs; it encloses the cytoplasm.

2. *D is the correct answer.* The passage states that the acrosomal vesicle derives from the Golgi apparatus. Since cortical granules are homologous to the acrosomal vesicle, they too must derive from the Golgi apparatus. Statement I is accurate. According to the passage, only the egg contains mRNA and tRNA stores. Furthermore, these are located in the cytoplasm, not in the cortical granules. Statement II is inaccurate. The passage states that the acrosomal vesicle contains enzymes that break down proteins (proteolytic enzymes). Since cortical granules are homologous to (similar to) acrosomes, they too should contain proteolytic enzymes. Statement III is accurate.

3. *C is the correct answer.* Fertilization produces the zygote and triggers cleavage, a series of rapid and successive cell divisions that take place without an increase in size of the initial zygote. Choice A is incorrect because the S phase is the period during which DNA is replicated in the nucleus of the cell. Choice B, too, is incorrect. Gametogenesis entails a series of cell divisions that ultimately generate the gametes—the egg and sperm. Choice D is wrong because haploid gametes do not implant.

4. *B is the correct answer.* The passage states that bindin is responsible for mediating species-specific recognition of egg and sperm; the experiments showed that bindin was localized only on the acrosomal process. Choice A is incorrect because egg cortical granules are similar to—but not identical to—the acrosomal vesicle, which contains proteolytic enzymes. Choice C is wrong as well. Rabbit anti-bindin's only function is to attach to any bindin that is present. It does not influence where bindin is located. Choice D is wrong because rabbit anti-bindin only serves to attach to any bindin present on sperm. It does not determine whether the acrosomal reaction will proceed.

5. *B is the correct answer.* The fallopian tubes are the site of fertilization of the egg by a sperm. Choice A is incorrect; the ovary releases the egg at the time of ovulation. Choice C is wrong because the egg has already been fertilized when it implants in the uterus. Choice D, too, is wrong. The corpus luteum is the remains of the follicle from which the egg is released at the time of ovulation.

6. *D is the correct answer.* Because bindin was not present on sperm in Experiment II, rabbit anti-bindin failed to bind to it. Statement I is accurate. Statements II and III are accurate as well. When unbound rabbit anti-bindin was washed off during Step 3, all of the rabbit anti-bindin was removed, since no bindin was available for attachment. When swine antibodies were then introduced, no rabbit anti-bindin remained for them to bind. Because the swine antibodies could not bind rabbit anti-bindin at binding sites, they did not deposit peroxidases, which would have reacted with DAB and H_2O_2 to form precipitate. (The diagram also indicates this sequence: if bindin is removed from the acrosomal process, then no reactions that would occur subsequently are possible.)

7. *B is the correct answer.* The passage states that the bond linking swine antibodies to peroxidase enzymes is covalent. The correct answer describes a bond that is *not* covalent. Water molecules are linked to one another by hydrogen bonds. A hydrogen bond is a weak, noncovalent bond created by the polarity of the bonds in a water molecule. Choice A is incorrect because the bond that links hydrogen to oxygen *within* a single water molecule is covalent. Choice C, too, is incorrect: within a polypeptide, one amino acid is linked to the next by a peptide bond, which is covalent. Choice D is wrong because it, too, describes a covalent bond—that between inorganic phosphate and adenosine diphosphate.

8. *C is the correct answer.* The vitelline envelope is the site at which bindin attaches to the egg. Furthermore, the vitelline envelope must be accessible to isolated bindin molecules. (The acrosomal vesicle, which contains enzymes capable of penetrating the outer egg layer, is absent in this experiment.) Choice A is wrong because, according to the passage, only mammalian eggs possess a zona pellucida. Choice B is wrong because, according to the passage, the vitelline envelope is the site of species-specific binding of bindin and egg. The investigator will observe the protein attaching to the egg only if the envelope is present. Choice D, too, is incorrect. Bindin molecules bind to, but do not penetrate, the outer jelly coat. Without the addition of acrosomal enzymes, bindin would not gain access to the vitelline envelope.

CHAPTER 26

THE DEVELOPING ORGANISM

26.1 MASTERY ACHIEVED

26.1.1 EMBRYOLOGY IN OVERVIEW

This chapter will enable the student to identify and order the developmental stages and processes the early embryo passes through. In sequential order these are **zygote**, **cleavage**, **morulation**, **blastulation**, **gastrulation**, **germ layer formation**, and **neurulation**. The student will also learn to define and relate terms associated with these stages, including **morphogenesis**, **determination**, **differentiation**, and **induction**. Finally, the student will learn to associate a mature organ or tissue with the embryonic germ layer from which it is derived.

26.1.2 DEVELOPMENTAL STAGES OF THE EARLY EMBRYO

26.1.2.1 Transitional States from Zygote through Gastrula

The developmental process begins with the fertilized zygote, which is produced from the fusion of the **female gamete** (the **ovum**) and the **male gamete** (the **sperm**). Both gametes are **haploid**; their fusion yields a **diploid** zygote. Once the zygote is formed, it enters into a series of rapid cell divisions called **cleavage**. Each mitotic division that occurs during cleavage doubles the cell count, but the organism does not increase in size initially. When the developing organism consists of approximately 32 cells it is called a **morula**. Cleavage continues, and the morula takes the shape of a hollow ball, called a **blastula** (the **blastocoele** is its fluid-filled center). The blastula, still hollow, next invaginates during **gastrulation** to form the **gastrula**. Invagination marks the beginning of morphogenesis, or "the genesis of form."

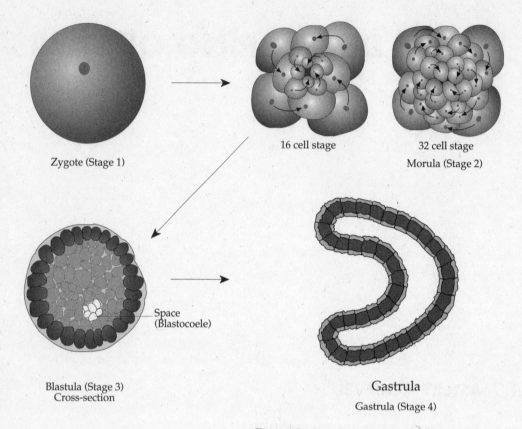

Zygote (Stage 1)

16 cell stage

32 cell stage
Morula (Stage 2)

Space
(Blastocoele)

Blastula (Stage 3)
Cross-section

Gastrula

Gastrula (Stage 4)

Figure 26.1

Please solve this problem:

- What are the names of the male and female gametes? Is either haploid? Diploid? What is the
  name of the entity they produce through fusion?
  Is it haploid or diploid?

Problem solved:

The male gamete is the sperm and the female gamete is the ovum. Each contains the
haploid number of chromosomes; upon fusion during fertilization they produce the diploid
zygote.

Please solve this problem:

- After a period of cleavage what is the developing organism first called?

    A. Morula
    B. Gastrula
    C. Zygote
    D. Gamete

Problem solved:

A is the correct answer. Cleavage is a series of rapid mitotic divisions that begin after fertilization of the ovum by a sperm cell. Each division produces a doubling of the number of cells present, but does not increase the volume of the initial zygote. During cleavage, the developing organism is called first the morula, and then the blastula. The blastula contains hundreds of cells surrounding a hollow, fluid-filled center.

26.1.2.2 Derivation of Ectoderm, Endoderm, and Mesoderm

Through morphogenesis, the invaginated gastrula generates three distinct **germ cell layers**, called the **ectoderm** (the outer cell layer), **endoderm** (the inner cell layer), and **mesoderm** (the middle cell layer). The creation of these organized layers is directed by the developing embryo's genes.

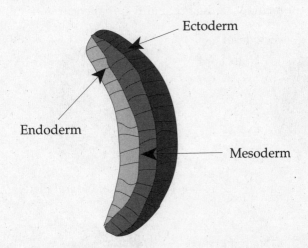

Please solve this problem:

- The outermost germ cell layer is the:

    A. epiderm.
    B. mesoderm.
    C. endoderm.
    D. ectoderm.

Problem solved:

D is the correct answer. Germ cell layer formation creates *three* layers; the outermost is the ectoderm. "Epiderm" is not a germ cell layer.

Please solve this problem:

- Ectoderm, endoderm, and mesoderm develop as a result of:

  A. maternal intervention.
  B. programming within the genome.
  C. random orientation.
  D. sex-linked determination.

Problem solved:

B is the correct answer. The formation of the three germ cell layers is genetically coded.

26.1.2.3 Neural Plate Formation

Once gastrulation is complete and the three germ cell layers have been established, **neurulation** occurs. A portion of the mesoderm forms a tube-like structure called the **notochord**. The notochord induces a thickening of the ectoderm directly above it. The thickened ectoderm forms the **neural plate**. Invagination causes it to assume a tubular shape and form the **neural tube**, a precursor to the brain and spinal cord.

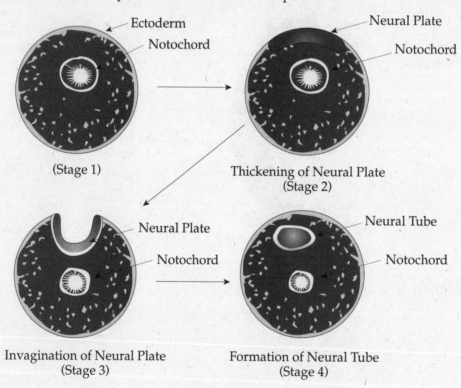

Stages of Neurulation
Figure 26.3

Please solve this problem:

- Neurulation occurs just after:

  A. morulation.
  B. gastrulation.
  C. fertilization.
  D. morphogenesis.

Problem solved:

B is the correct answer. Neurulation, the formation of the neural tube, occurs just after gastrulation.

Please solve this problem:

- The invagination of the neural plate directly produces:

  A. the notochord.
  B. the brain.
  C. the neural tube.
  D. the spinal column.

Problem solved:

C is the correct answer. Neurulation involves formation of the notochord, which causes the development of the neural plate, which, upon invagination, becomes the neural tube. The neural tube *ultimately* gives rise to the brain and spinal cord.

Please solve this problem:

- Trace the development of an embryo from zygote through neurula.

Problem solved:

The question tests your mastery of the sequential stages of embryological development. The zygote undergoes cleavage to become first a morula (a cluster of 32 cells), then a blastula (a fluid-filled ball of hundreds of cells), then a gastrula (formed through invagination of the blastula), and then a neurula, at which stage the neural tube is formed through invagination of the neural plate.

26.1.3 REQUIRED TERMINOLOGY

26.1.3.1 Induction, Determination, and Differentiation

Neurulation illustrates the process of **induction**, whereby development of one region of tissue is influenced by the tissues that surround it. The notochord releases chemical factors, called *inducers*, which activate certain genes in the ectodermal tissue. The products of the activated genes cause the tissue to undergo the process of neurulation. Induction is a common mechanism in development; it does not only occur during neurulation.

Differentiation is the process whereby a cell becomes more specialized. The cells of the gastrula become *differentiated* when the three germ layers are formed. It is thereafter possible to distinguish a mesodermal cell from an ectodermal cell, for example. It is no longer possible, however, for a mesodermal cell to *become* an ectodermal cell, at least under normal conditions. A mesodermal cell is now **determined** to become part of an organ that develops from the mesoderm. As development continues, a particular mesodermal cell will become determined to develop into one mesodermal organ and not another. Determination is the process whereby the number of possible tissue types a cell could conceivably become is progressively limited.

Differentiation and determination are closely related concepts. As a cell becomes more differentiated, its fate becomes more determined. A heart muscle cell can be *differentiated* from a stomach chief cell. Sometime during the process of development, the heart muscle cell was *determined* to become a heart muscle cell; it was no longer possible that the cell's progeny would be part of the stomach. (Cancer cells appear able to reverse the differentiation process.)

Please solve this problem:

- Induction may result in all of the following EXCEPT:

    A. cell movement.
    B. cell genome rearrangement.
    C. cell proliferation.
    D. cellular differentiation.

Problem solved:

B is the correct answer. In a developing organism, induction refers to the influence that one set of cells has on another nearby set. This influence can produce cell movement or determine the development of a cell group, but it cannot alter the genome.

26.1.4 GERM-LAYER ORIGINS OF ORGANS

The germ layers formed during gastrulation constitute the source of all of the organs and tissues of the body. The endoderm gives rise to the inner linings of the esophagus, the stomach, and the small and large intestines. It also gives rise to organs that are anatomic outgrowths of the digestive tract, such as the pancreas, gall bladder, and liver. The endoderm also gives rise to the inner linings of the respiratory tract. The ectoderm is the source of the epidermis, the eye, and the nervous system. The mesoderm is the origin of the connective tissue, the heart, blood cells, the urogenital system, as well as parts of many other internal organs.

Please solve this problem:

- The lining of the digestive tract and the lungs, as well as the liver and the pancreas are formed from which germ cell layer?

Problem solved:

All of these develop from the endoderm.

Please solve this problem:

- All of the following structures arise from the ectoderm EXCEPT:

  A. the outer layer of the skin.
  B. the nervous system.
  C. the excretory system.
  D. the structures of the eye.

Problem solved:

C is the correct answer. The outer layer of the skin, the nervous system, and the structures of the eye derive from ectoderm. The excretory system derives from mesoderm.

Please solve this problem:

- The retina develops from the same germ cell layer as does the:

  A. brain.
  B. trachea.
  C. heart.
  D. pancreas.

Problem solved:

A is the correct answer. The eye, epidermis, and all structures of the central nervous system develop from ectoderm. The retina, being part of the eye, develops from ectoderm, as does the brain.

Please solve this problem:

- Which of the following structures derives from the same germ cell layer as the heart?

  A. Liver
  B. Spinal cord
  C. Bone
  D. Eye

Problem solved:

C is the correct answer. The heart derives from mesoderm as do all structures other than (a) eye, epidermis, and nervous tissues (which develop from ectoderm) and (b) the inner linings of digestive organs and the respiratory tract, as well as the accessory organs to the digestive system (all of which derive from the endoderm). Heart and bone (among many other tissues and organs) derive from mesoderm.

Please solve this problem:

- Which of the following does NOT derive from mesoderm?

  A. Arteries and arterioles
  B. Veins, venules, and capillaries
  C. Muscles and associated connective tissues
  D. Inner linings of the lungs

Problem solved:

D is the correct answer. The structures named in options A, B, and C derive from mesoderm. Once again, all tissues and organs derive from mesoderm except (a) the ectodermal structures: epidermis, eye, and nervous tissue and (b) the endodermal structures: inner linings of the digestive tract and the respiratory tract, and the accessory digestive organs.

26.2 MASTERY APPLIED: SAMPLE PASSAGE AND QUESTIONS

Passage

The developing embryo arises from a series of mitotic divisions by the zygote. The gene content of each cell is identical throughout development, but as development proceeds the genetic material's potential expression becomes increasingly restricted. Determination refers to the process that limits the number of cell types an embryonic cell might become. Two separate mechanisms lead to determination in a developing embryo's cells. The first is cytoplasmic segregation. Egg cytoplasm contains determinative molecules; during cleavage the zygote's cytoplasm is segregated into cells with unequal biochemical content. The second mechanism is embryonic induction, in which the interaction of cells (or tissues) with one another affects the development of one or both groups of cells. Differentiated cells express certain genes of their genome while other genes in their genome remain unexpressed. The differentiated cell takes on the characteristics of a specific cell type.

In order to test the reversibility of determination, the following experiment was conducted. The egg cell of a *Rana pipiens* (leopard frog) was selected. (The leopard frog is a diploid organism.) The egg nucleus was removed and the enucleated egg was then pricked with a sterile glass needle to initiate parthenogenetic activation. (Parthenogenesis is the production of offspring without fertilization.) A nucleus from a donor *Rana pipiens* cell was then introduced into the enucleated oocyte using a micropipette. Results of the experiment are shown in Figure 1. Most blastula nuclei, when transplanted, were able to orchestrate the development of a fully formed tadpole. When the experiment was repeated using nuclei from cells derived from increasingly later stages of development, a pronounced decrease in the number of fully formed tadpoles was observed.

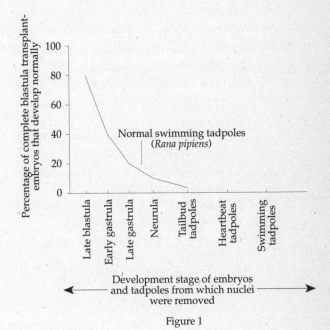

Figure 1

1. The nervous tissue, eye, and epidermis all derive from:

   A. the ectoderm.
   B. the mesoderm.
   C. the endoderm.
   D. the mesenchyme.

2. The decreasing percentage of viable tadpoles produced from nuclear transplants after the early gastrula stage (Figure 1) can most likely be explained by:

   A. a decrease in the genetic content of the transplanted nucleus.
   B. a shift in function of donor nuclei from regulation to temporary dormancy.
   C. an increase in nuclear instability due to decreasing levels of cell regulation.
   D. a decrease in genomic potential for expression due to increasing determination and differentiation.

3. A researcher interested in observing all of the mechanisms involved in determination would most benefit by observing cells in which of the following stages?

A. The fertilization stage only
B. The neurulation stage onwards
C. The gastrulation stage only
D. The cleavage stage onwards

4. According to the information in the passage, cleavage results in:

A. unequal distribution of nuclei to daughter cells.
B. unequal distribution of determinative factors to daughter cells.
C. reduced gene content in daughter cells.
D. increased size compared to that of the initial zygote.

5. Pricking the cell with a sterile needle in the experiment served the same purpose as:

I. fusion of the egg nucleus by a sperm nucleus.
II. penetration of the egg by a sperm.
III. attachment of sperm cells to receptors located on the egg's outer layer

A. I only
B. II only
C. III only
D. I and II only

6. Which of the following experiments does NOT provide evidence of embryonic induction?

A. A section of mesoderm removed during gastrulation was placed directly beneath ectoderm from another gastrulating embryo that would normally develop into epidermis. The underlying ectoderm thickened and formed a section of neural tube.
B. Cells comprising the apical ectodermal ridge (AER) were removed from the developing limb bud of a chick. The limb development ceased.
C. The optic vesicle of the embryonic eye was experimentally positioned close to a region of head ectoderm that would normally form epidermis. The region of ectoderm developed into skin.
D. Dermis from the whiskered region of the snout of a mouse was placed close to embryonic chick epidermis. The chick epidermis formed feather buds arranged in a pattern typical of mouse whiskers.

7. Would the nucleus provided by the *Rana pipiens* donor cell have been haploid or diploid?

A. Diploid, because the experimental oocyte received a nucleus from a developing organism.
B. Diploid, because the donor cell that provided the nucleus was a germ cell.
C. Haploid, because the donor nucleus did not undergo fusion with the oocyte nucleus.
D. Haploid, because the oocyte already contained a haploid genome.

26.3 MASTERY VERIFIED: ANSWERS AND EXPLANATIONS

1. *A is the correct answer.* The ectoderm, one of the three germ cell layers formed after gastrulation, gives rise to all three structures listed. The mesoderm, another of the germ cell layers, gives rise to such organs as the connective tissue (bone, muscle, cartilage, and skin), the urinary system, the urogenital system, the heart, blood vessels, and blood cells of the circulatory system, and the inner linings of body cavities. The endoderm, the third germ cell layer, generates the inner linings of (a) the digestive tract (including the pancreas, gall bladder, and liver) and (b) the respiratory tract. Mesenchyme are migrating embryonic cells associated with morphogenic changes of cell clusters.

2. *D is the correct answer.* As development progresses, cells undergo differentiation. Differentiation restricts the cell's ability to express all of its genomic potential. Differentiated cells cannot direct the development of a complete organism. Gene content does not change during development; genes are not lost. (The cell's ability to *express* certain of its genes is impaired.) Choice A, therefore, is incorrect.

   Choice B is incorrect because cell nuclei do not become temporarily dormant during later stages of development. Instead they become more limited in the number of genes that they can express. Choice C is incorrect in both its implications: cell nuclei do not become unstable, and a cell is not subject to reduced regulation as development progresses.

3. *D is the correct answer.* The cleavage stage marks the unequal distribution of cytoplasmic determinants into cells. This stage and those that follow create the developmental pathways that lead to determination and differentiation. Once the germ cell layers are produced, embryonic induction may be observed. Choice A is incorrect because fertilization precedes determination of any sort. Choice B is incorrect as well. Neurulation and subsequent stages would provide information about embryonic induction mechanisms but would not reveal the role played by egg cytoplasmic determinants from the cleavage stage forward. The three germ layers are formed during gastrulation, which sets the stage for subsequent cell and tissue interactions. The researcher would have to observe subsequent stages. Furthermore, the researcher would once again be deprived of information concerning the influence of egg cytoplasm determinants. For these reasons, choice C is not correct.

4. *B is the correct answer.* The passage states that determinative factors in the egg cytoplasm are unequally distributed during cleavage. Mitosis gives rise to daughter cells bearing the same ploidy as that of the egg cell. The passage does not imply otherwise, so choice C is not correct. Cleavage involves a series of rapid cell divisions. The total amount of cytoplasm of the original zygote remains the same and the resulting mass of cells is the same size as was the zygote. The passage does not suggest otherwise, so choice D is incorrect. All viable cells possess a nucleus, so choice A is incorrect.

5. *B is the correct answer.* Only choice II is an accurate statement. The needle prick was a substitute for the penetration of the egg by a sperm cell. The penetration initiates a series of fertilization reactions in the egg, such as the release of cortical granules. In this experiment the egg nucleus was removed and replaced with a donor cell nucleus. The needle prick would not be an adequate substitute for the insertion of genomic material. For these reasons, choice I is not an accurate statement. Attachment of sperm cells to the receptor sites available on the outer egg surface does not cause cell division; choice III, therefore, is not an accurate statement.

6. *C is the correct answer*. Embryonic induction involves the influential interaction of one tissue or cell group on another. The influence results in a developmental outcome in the influenced cell group that otherwise would not have occurred. The correct answer choice will show an *absence* of inductive effect. Choice C is correct because it indicates that induction did *not* take place. Specifically, ectoderm that was to become epidermis (skin) did develop into epidermis, even though it was in close proximity to a transplanted optic vesicle. Choice A reflects evidence of induction; mesoderm that was to become epidermis became neural tube as a result of induction. Choice B reflects induction as well: removal of the AER caused cessation of limb development. AER, therefore, likely influences limb development. Similarly, choice D reflects evidence of induction; mouse snout dermis caused embryonic chick dermis to deviate from normal feather bud pattern to display a characteristic mouse whisker pattern instead.

7. *A is the correct answer*. The frog is a diploid organism. Because the oocyte was enucleated (the nucleus was removed) before the donor nucleus was introduced, the donor nucleus had to be diploid, as the egg cell would have been *after* fertilization. If it were otherwise, the organism would not have pursued a normal developmental course. Also, since the donor nucleus had come from an organism that had developed normally so far (the youngest nucleus came from a late blastula), the nucleus had to be diploid, by the same line of reasoning. Choice B is incorrect because a germ cell is haploid and could not, therefore, have supplied the diploid nucleus. Choice C is a false statement; the donor cell had to be diploid. (It is true, however, that the donor nucleus did not undergo fusion with the oocyte.) Choice D is incorrect because the donor cell had to be diploid, not haploid. Furthermore, the oocyte's haploid genome had been removed prior to introduction of the donor nucleus.

CHAPTER 27

MICROBIOLOGY: BACTERIA, VIRUSES, AND FUNGI

27.1 MASTERY ACHIEVED

27.1.1 BACTERIA

27.1.1.1 Identifying Features

Bacteria are single-celled organisms that typically contain an outer **cell wall**, a **cell membrane**, and a single **circular-shaped chromosome** in the cytoplasm. Because a bacterium is a **prokaryotic** organism it lacks a nucleus and shows, generally, a more primitive organization than that of a eukaryotic cell. Bacteria lack membrane-bound organelles such as the endoplasmic reticulum, mitochondria, the nuclear membrane, and Golgi bodies.

Differences in the composition of the bacterial cell wall allow the classification of bacterial species as **Gram positive** or **Gram negative**. A species is Gram positive if it absorbs Gram's dye and Gram negative if it does not.

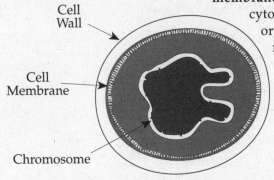

Cell Wall

Cell Membrane

Chromosome

Bacterium with its Chromosome

Figure 27.1

You should be familiar with three types of bacteria, categorized by shape: **bacilli**, **cocci**, and **spirilla**. Bacilli are rod-shaped. There is an enormous variety of bacilli. They cause, among other diseases, tuberculosis, leprosy, plague, and cholera. Cocci are ovoid, or round-shaped. Again, there are a great many types of cocci. The illnesses they produce include gonorrhea, pneumonia, and scarlet fever. Spirilla, the third bacteria category, have a helical or spiral shape. Among other diseases, they cause rat-bite fever.

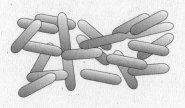

Bacilli

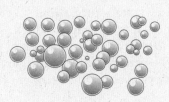

Cocci

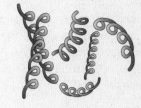

Spirilla

Figure 27.2

Please solve this problem:

- Bacilli are:

    A. bacteria with a round or ovoid shape.
    B. bacteria with a rodlike shape.
    C. viruses with a spiral shape.
    D. fungi with a spiral shape.

Problem solved:

B is the correct answer. Bacilli are rod-shaped bacteria.

Please solve this problem:

- Cocci are:

    A. bacteria with a round or ovoid shape.
    B. bacteria with a rodlike shape.
    C. bacteria with a spiral shape.
    D. fungi with a spiral shape.

Problem solved:

A is the correct answer. Cocci are bacteria with a round or ovoid shape.

Please solve this problem:

- Spirilla are:

    A. bacteria with a round or ovoid shape.
    B. bacteria with a rod shape.
    C. bacteria with a spiral shape.
    D. fungi with a spiral shape.

Problem solved:

C is the correct answer. Spirilla are spiral-shaped bacteria.

27.1.1.2 Bacterial Reproduction

The growth cycle of a bacterium is markedly rapid. A bacterium replicates its DNA and divides into two daughter cells of approximately equal size. This process is termed **binary fission**. Because each instance of division produces two bacteria, *bacterial population growth is exponential,* and if population size is plotted against time, the resulting curve will be *logarithmic.* If a first generation has a population of one bacterium, the seventh has a population of $2^6 = 64$ bacteria.

A bacterium may acquire a different genome from that of its parents through one of three recombinant processes. These are (1) **transformation**, (2) **conjugation**, and (3) **transduction**. You should be able to recognize the mechanism by which each event transpires. Transformation involves the addition and incorporation of genetic material into a bacterium's genome from its surrounding. The genetic material it receives may be prokaryotic or eukaryotic. In relation to its genetic content, the recipient bacterium cell is said to be

transformed. Conjugation is, in some rudimentary ways, analogous to mating in animals. A **plasmid**, called the **F (fertility) factor**, facilitates the transfer of DNA from one bacterium to another. The third recombinant mechanism is transduction, in which a *virus* transfers DNA from one bacterium to another.

Please solve this problem:

- Which of the following recombinant processes is dependent on the F factor plasmid?

    A. Transduction
    B. Translocation
    C. Conjugation
    D. Transformation

Problem solved:

C is correct. Conjugation involves the direct transfer of genetic material from one bacterium to another. The transfer is mediated by a plasmid called the F factor.

Please solve this problem:

- Which of the following recombinant processes is carried out by a virus?

    A. Transduction
    B. Translocation
    C. Conjugation
    D. Transformation

Problem solved:

A is correct. Transduction involves the transfer of genetic material from one bacterium to another, with a virus acting as the carrier.

Please solve this problem:

- Which of the following does NOT constitute a recombinant process among bacteria?

    A. Transduction
    B. Translocation
    C. Conjugation
    D. Transformation

Problem solved:

B is correct. The three recombinant processes observed among bacteria are transduction, conjugation, and transformation.

Please solve this problem:

- Which of the following represents the incorporation of genetic material into a bacterial genome that is not necessarily from a bacterium?

   A. Transduction
   B. Translocation
   C. Conjugation
   D. Transformation

Problem solved:

D is correct. Transformation is a recombinant process in which a bacterium acquires genetic material that is not necessarily a bacterium. The cell might, indeed, be prokaryotic or eukaryotic.

27.1.2 VIRUSES

27.1.2.1 Identifying Features

There is some debate as to whether or not viruses are alive. They lack all organelles as well as most features normally associated with cells. Viruses have just two primitive cellular attributes: (1) an outer coat, or **capsid**, made of protein, and (2) a **core** of **nucleic acid**, contained within the coat. The nucleic acid may be DNA or RNA, depending on the virus. On that basis, viruses may be broadly classified as **RNA viruses** or **DNA viruses**.

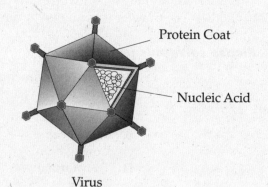

Virus
Figure 27.3

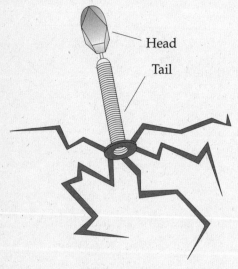

Bacteriophage
Figure 27.4

You should be familiar, in particular, with the **bacteriophage**, a type of virus that, in addition to the capsid and nucleic acid core, possesses a **tail fiber**. The bacteriophage infects bacteria; the tail fiber facilitates infection by allowing the virus to attach itself to the bacterial **host**.

27.1.2.2 Viral Reproduction

Viral reproduction is a four-stage process. In the first stage, the virus binds to its host (the cell to be infected). **Receptors** found on the host's cell membrane facilitate the attachment of viral protein coat molecules. Viruses are **host-specific organisms**, meaning that in selecting their hosts, they depend on the presence of receptors to which they attach. Most viruses are capable of infecting only a relatively small number of organisms.

After the virus attaches to its host, it injects its contents into the host's cytoplasm. At this point, two general processes might take place. If the virus is **lytic**, it will then appropriate the cell's reproductive machinery to make copies of its own nucleic acids and proteins. The proteins and nucleic acid combine to form new viral particles, which then leave the cell, often by *lysing*, or bursting, the cell. If the virus is **lysogenic**, its nucleic acid becomes incorporated into the host's genome. At this point, the virus is called a **prophage** or a **provirus**, depending on the type of virus. The viral DNA is then replicated along with the host's genome. Under certain conditions, the viral DNA emerges from the host's genome and resumes the lytic life cycle.

Please solve this problem:

- Most viruses are very host-specific because:

    A. the viral capsid is composed of protein.
    B. a virus has no cellular organelles.
    C. viral nucleic acid might be DNA or RNA, depending on the virus.
    D. the attachment to the host involves the host's cell surface receptors.

Problem solved:

D is correct. To state that a virus is host-specific is to state that any one virus will infect only a limited number of host cell types. Whether the virus will or will not infect a given host is determined by the host's cell membrane receptors. If a given host has the receptors that will allow a given virus to attach, then viral infection by that virus is possible. Host cell receptors, therefore, create the specificity. Choices A, B, and C are accurate statements, but they do not answer the question.

Please solve this problem:

- Which of the following precedes the replication of viral nucleic acid?

    A. Attachment to host cell receptors
    B. Replication of capsid protein
    C. Host cell lysis
    D. Assembly of viral progeny

Problem solved:

A is correct. The question requires that the student understand the sequence associated with viral reproduction: attachment, injection, replication of nucleic acid and capsid protein, assembly of new viruses, and lysis of the host. In terms of the processes listed in Choices A-D, the appropriate order is A,B,D,C. Replication of viral nucleic acid occurs after A but either before or simultaneously with B.

Please solve this problem:

- Which of the following would be the most un-likely to occur after a virus has reproduced and its progeny have left the host cell?

  A. New infection by progeny virus of new host cells
  B. Reproduction of the original host cell itself
  C. Symptomatic disease in the organism to which the original host cell belonged
  D. Death of the organism to which the orignal host cell belonged

Problem solved:

B is correct. In the final stage of viral reproduction the host cell often undergoes lysis (bursting); it is destroyed. It cannot itself undergo reproduction thereafter. Choices B, C, and D refer to processes that do at least represent possibilities. The newly produced viruses might go on to infect new host cells and, moreover, if infection is repeated and widespread (as it often is), the virus might cause symptomatic disease (like the common cold) or death (from, for example, poliomyelitis).

Please solve this problem:

- Which of the following distinguishes a bacterioph-age from other viruses?

  A. The presence of mitochondria
  B. The presence of a protein capsid
  C. The presence of RNA in the nucleic acid core
  D. The presence of a tail fiber

Problem solved:

D is correct. The bacteriophage possesses the two structures that characterize the prototypical virus—a protein capsid and a nucleic acid core—and then a third, the tail fiber, which facilitates attachment to a bacterial cell. (Viruses that lack a tail fiber nonetheless attach themselves to their target hosts. They make direct attachment between the capsid and host cell membrane receptors.)

27.1.3 FUNGI

27.1.3.1 Identifying Features

Fungi are primarily haploid organisms whose cells are eukaryotic. They contain a cell wall, composed largely of **chitin**, and organelles. A fungus can be **unicellular** or **multicellular**. Yeasts, for example, are unicellular fungi. **Molds**, **mushrooms**, and **mildews** are multicellular fungi. The fungal nucleus is surrounded by a **nuclear membrane**. The principal distinguishing feature of many multicellular fungi is the *absence of a partition between what would otherwise be separate cells*. In a sense, such multicellular fungi are simply composed of a large number of cells enclosed within one cell wall. Viewed another way, the organism can be thought of as a single cell with multiple nuclei. When viewed this way, fungi can be considered **multinucleate**.

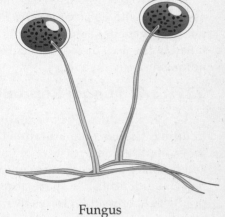

Fungus
Figure 27.5

Please solve this problem:

- Which one of the following does NOT possess a cell wall?

    A. A bacterium
    B. A plant cell
    C. A fungal cell
    D. A viruses

Problem solved:

D is correct. Bacteria, plant cells, and fungi do possess cell walls. Viruses do not; they are contained within a protein capsid. Indeed, the cell walls of bacteria promote the categorization of species according to Gram staining. Some bacteria are Gram positive and others are Gram negative. A plant cell's cell wall is composed of cellulose, whose thickness and rigidity protect the cell against osmotic swelling and injury. Fungi possess cell walls that are in most cases extremely rigid and are composed primarily of chitin (which also comprises the exoskeletons of many insects).

Please solve this problem:

- Which among the following possesses such organelles as the endoplasmic reticulum, Golgi bodies, mitochondria, and a nuclear membrane?

    A. Viruses
    B. Prokaryotic cells
    C. Bacteria
    D. Fungi

Problem solved:

D is correct. Fungi possesses membrane-bound nuclei and other organelles ordinarily associated with eukaryotic cells. Prokaryotic cells possess neither a membrane-bound nucleus nor the organelles associated with eukaryotic cells. Bacteria (choice C) *are* prokaryotic cells. As noted in the text, there is still debate as to whether viruses (choice A) are in fact alive. They do not possess any organelles.

27.1.3.2 Fungal Reproduction

Fungi reproduce either **sexually** or **asexually**. Asexual fungal reproduction occurs through **budding**, **fission**, or **sporulation** (known also as **multiple fission**). In budding, which occurs for example among yeasts, a cell or a body of cells separates from the parent organism, grows, and becomes a new organism unto itself. In fission, a single fungal cell divides to produce two new daughter cells. In sporulation, which occurs for example in bread mold, the fungus produces spores and releases them from stem-like structures called **hyphae**. Sporulation permits a yet undeveloped organism to survive hostile environmental conditions like drought or extreme heat. A spore is metabolically inactive, encased in a thick protective wall, but under appropriate conditions it germinates and forms a new haploid fungus. Note that all forms of asexual reproduction produce progeny whose *genome is identical* to that of the parent organism.

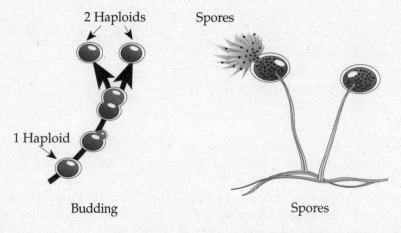

Asexual Reproduction Among Fungi Showing
Budding and Spore Formation

Figure 27.6

Sexual reproduction among fungi involves the fusion of haploid gametes from two parent fungi. The parents are usually of opposite sexual type; one type is designated (+) and the other (−). (The terms "male" and "female" are not used for the sexual reproduction of fungi.) Gametes arise from the hyphae of each parent. The haploid gametes fuse and form a diploid zygote. The zygote stage of a fungal life cycle, therefore, is diploid. The zygote undergoes meiosis (not mitosis) to produce haploid spores. These, in turn, germinate and produce new haploid organisms. Note that the newly formed organisms are normally not genetically identical to either parent, their genomes having arisen from the combination of parental genes followed by meiosis.

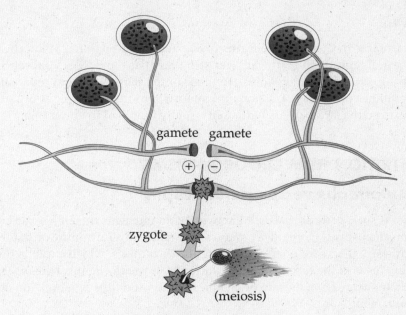

gamete gamete

(+) (−)

zygote

(meiosis)

Sexual Reproduction of Fungi

Figure 27.7

Please solve this problem:

- Which of the following are NOT associated with
  asexual reproduction among fungi?

  A. Spores
  B. Zygotes
  C. Buds
  D. Hyphae

Problem solved:

B is correct. With respect to fungal reproduction, zygotes form only in association with
sexual reproduction. They are diploid, and formed by the fusion of haploid gametes. Spores
(choice A) arise from sporulation, an asexual or sexual reproductive process. These spores are
released from hyphae (choice D). Though hyphae also produce the gametes associated with
sexual reproduction, because they are associated with asexual reproduction as well, choice D
is not correct. Buds (choice C), which arise through budding, are "pieces" of a parent
organism that separate from the parent under appropriate conditions and grow into separate
organisms.

Please solve this problem:

- Among the following processes, which one can
  give rise to progeny that are not genetically identical to the parent(s)?

  A. Sexual reproduction
  B. Asexual sporulation
  C. Budding
  D. Fission

Problem solved:

A is correct. Choices B, C, and D are forms of asexual reproduction. Although sporulation is also a form of sexual reproduction, the answer stipulates "asexual." Asexual reproduction produces offspring with identical genomes to those of the parent. Sexual reproduction in fungi, which combines processes of fusion and meiosis, produces a haploid organism whose genome derives from the two parents but is not usually identical to either one.

27.1.4 NUTRITION IN MICROORGANISMS

27.1.4.1 Autotrophs versus Heterotrophs

Microorganisms such as those discussed above obtain nutrients through a variety of processes and mechanisms. All organisms may be classified as **autotrophic** or **heterotrophic.** Autotrophs synthesize their own energy through photosynthesis, which exploits the radiant energy of the sun, or, as in the case of chemoautotrophs, through chemical means. Heterotrophs cannot obtain their energy from the sun or chemical bonds and thus must rely on other organisms for nutrition.

Heterotrophs either possess digestive systems or do not. A heterotroph that *does* digest can be further subcategorized as a **herbivore**, a **carnivore**, or an **omnivore**. Herbivores obtain their nutrition from plants only. Carnivores obtain their nutrition from animals only, and omnivores obtain nutrition from plants *and* animals.

Heterotrophic microorganisms do *not* possess digestive systems. Such microorganisms may be classified in several categories. **Parasites** obtain nutrition directly from the body of a living organism *to the detriment of that organism.* (This is not to say that all parasites lack digestive systems. Many parasites, large and small, have well-developed digestive systems.) **Saprophytes** absorb nutrients from the remains of dead organisms. Some heterotrophic microorganisms are *neither* parasitic nor saprophytic. There are those, for example, that derive nutrition from living organisms *without* harming them.

Saprophytic organisms facilitate the release and recycling of numerous substances, promoting their availability to other organisms whose survival depends on them. These subtsances include carbon and nitrogen, as well as the mineral components of a variety of organic compounds.

Please solve this problem:

- An organism that lacks a digestive system and obtains nutrients from other living organisms while harming the organism is:

  A. autotrophic.
  B. saprophytic.
  C. carnivorous.
  D. parasitic.

Problem solved:

D is correct. If an organism cannot synthesize its own nutrients it is a heterotroph. If, further, it lacks a digestive system, it is not a herbivore, carnivore, or omnivore. It is either a parasite or a saprophyte. If it feeds on the remains of deceased organisms it is a saprophyte. If it feeds on living organisms and harms them in the process, it is a parasite.

Please solve this problem:

- An organism that synthesizes its own energy is called:

  A. autotrophic.
  B. heterotrophic.
  C. saprophytic.
  D. omnivorous.

Problem solved:

A is correct. If an organism synthesizes its own energy, it is autotrophic. The term "heterotroph" (choice B) refers to those organisms that do not synthesize their own energy, and the terms "saprophytic" (choice C) and "omnivorous" (choice D) are subcategories within the classification heterotroph.

Please solve this problem:

- Which of the following is characteristic of saprophytic organisms?

  A. They obtain energy through photosynthesis.
  B. They recycle biological substances.
  C. They obtain nutrients from living organisms.
  D. They harm other living organisms.

Problem solved:

B is correct. Saprophytes are heterotrophs that (a) lack a digestive system and (b) absorb nutrients from the remains of dead organisms. Saprophytes often recycle a variety of substances that are useful to other organisms within their ecosystem.

27.1.4.2 Bacterial Metabolism

27.1.4.2.1 Aerobes vs. Anaerobes

Bacteria use many different nutritional strategies. Some bacteria are autotrophs while others are heterotrophs. Some heterotrophs are saprophytes, some are parasites, and some are neither (deriving nutrition from living organisms *without harming them*). Regardless of their status as autotrophs, heterotrophs, parasites, or saprophytes, all must convert energy into a form that is usable by the cell. The process by which that conversion occurs is **respiration**.

For some bacteria respiration requires oxygen and for others it does not. Respiration that requires oxygen is called **aerobic**. Respiration that does not require oxygen is called **anaerobic**. Anaerobic bacteria may be called **obligate anaerobes** or **facultative anaerobes**. Obligate anaerobes are unable to live in the presence of oxygen. Some facultative anaerobes will use oxygen in their respiratory process if it is available, but will conduct anaerobic respiration in its absence. Other facultative anaerobes always conduct anaerobic respiration but are indifferent to the presence of oxygen.

Please solve this problem:

- Which of the following characterizes anaerobic respiration?

    A. It is a respiratory process that cannot operate in the presence of oxygen.
    B. It is a respiratory process that can operate in the absence of oxygen.
    C. It is dependent on the remains of other organisms.
    D. It is dependent on living organisms and harm to them.

Problem solved:

B is correct. Anaerobic respiration does not require oxygen but oxygen does not, on the other hand, render it inoperative. Choice A, therefore, is incorrect. It is true that obligate anaerobic organisms cannot survive in the presence of oxygen, but that is not because anaerobic respiration itself requires an anaerobic environment. Choices C and D refer to nutritional mechanisms, not to respiratory mechanisms; neither has any direct bearing on anaerobic respiration.

Please solve this problem:

- Which of the following classes of bacteria can survive in the presence or absence of oxygen?

    A. Aerobes
    B. Obligate anaerobes
    C. Facultative anerobes
    D. Saprophytes

Problem solved:

C is correct. The term "facultative anaerobe" only specifies bacteria that can survive whether or not oxygen is present; it does not say anything definitive about the organism's respiratory processes. Choice A is wrong because aerobes must have oxygen, and choice B is wrong because obligate anaerobes die in the presence of oxygen. In choice D, the term "saprophyte" refers to nutrition, not respiration.

27.1.4.2.2 Nitrogen-Fixing Bacteria

Mutualism is a relationship between two organisms in which each confers a benefit on the other. For example, one specialized form of bacteria enters into a mutualistic relationship with the root nodules of certain legumes (such as pea plants). These **nitrogen-fixing bacteria** convert nitrogen into a form that can be used by the legume. The legume benefits from the association by being provided with nitrogen in a form it can readily utilize to synthesize protein. Meanwhile, the legume provides nutrition for the bacteria.

Please solve this problem:

- Nitrogen-fixing bacteria are classified as:

    A. saprophytes.
    B. parasites.
    C. autotrophs.
    D. heterotrophs.

Problem solved:

D is correct. Nitrogen-fixing bacteria are heterotrophs; they cannot synthesize their own food and so must obtain their nutrients from other organisms. Choice A is incorrect because saprophytes derive their nutrients from dead organisms. Choice B is also incorrect. Although parasites absorb nutrients directly from the body of their host, they harm the host in doing so. Choice C is incorrect because the autotrophs conduct photosynthesis or obtain their energy from inorganic chemical bonds. Nitrogen-fixing bacteria do not.

27.2 MASTERY APPLIED: SAMPLE PASSAGE AND QUESTIONS

Passage

Viral population growth varies depending on the nature of the virus itself and on the nature of the host it infects. Some of the viruses that infect bacteria have growth cycles that are measured in minutes, whereas some of the viruses that infect human cells have growth cycles measured in hours.

Figure 1 depicts a growth curve for an infecting virus.

At the onset of viral infection of a host cell, the virus actually disappears: The virus particle is undetectable within the infected cell. This stage of the viral growth cycle is termed the *eclipse period*. Although the viral particle vanishes during the eclipse period, its nucleic acid is present and active. After the passage of some time, new viral nucleic acid molecules accumulate within the cell to a detectable level. The *latent period* is the interval between the onset of infection and the first extracellular appearance of the virus. Viral-related changes to cell morphology and function occur near the end of the latent period, which is known as the cytopathic effect (CPE). The cytopathic effect culminates in the rupture and death of affected cells. Some viruses can replicate without producing CPE in the host cell.

Table I outlines the various stages associated with the viral growth cycle. The virus first attaches to receptor proteins located on the periphery of the host cell. It gains entrance into the host cell by one of several mechanisms. Once inside the cell, the virus may then appropriate the host cell's machinery to replicate itself

Viral gene expression begins with mRNA synthesis. mRNA is then translated by host cell ribosomes into viral proteins. These early proteins are enzymes required for viral genome replication. As the replication of the viral genome continues, the cell synthesizes late mRNA. The late mRNA is translated into structural capsid proteins to enclose new viral particles. Progeny viral particles are assembled, enclosing nucleic acid within a capsid protein. The release of new viruses is accomplished either by rupture of the cell membrane (the route taken by unenveloped viruses) or by budding out through an envagination of the cell membrane. Those that are shed by budding are enveloped viruses, they are enclosed in a lipoprotein envelope derived from the host's cell membrane.

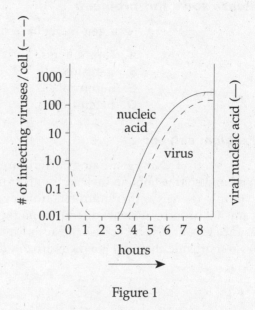

Figure 1

Early Events	Parent virus attaches and penetrates host cell
	Parent virus genome is removed from protein coat
Middle Events	Host cell synthesizes early viral proteins
	Host cell replicates viral genome
	Host cell synthesizes late viral proteins
Late Events	New viruses assembled
	New viruses emerge from host cell

Table 1

1. An important early protein that is most likely translated from mRNA is:

   A. a protease.
   B. a polymerase.
   C. an antibody.
   D. a peptidase.

2. Which of the following is (are) possible templates for the synthesis of viral mRNA?

   I. Viral DNA
   II. Viral RNA
   III. Cellular DNA

   A. I only
   B. II only
   C. III only
   D. I and II only

3. Researchers find that a test-tube mixture containing only purified viral RNA and purified protein yields correctly assembled viruses. Among the following, the LEAST reasonable conclusion is that:

   A. specificity of viral assembly lies within the RNA and protein.
   B. enzymatic activity is not required for correct viral assembly.
   C. viral particles are capable of spontaneously disassembling.
   D. energy is not required for viral particles to assemble.

4. The eclipse period for the viral growth curve represented in Figure 1 occurs during the period:

   A. 0 to 1.5 hours.
   B. 1.5 to 2.5 hours.
   C. 1.5 to 3.5 hours.
   D. 3.5 to 5.5 hours.

5. Which of the following is NOT true of the cytopathic effect?

   A. It affects all host cells within which viral replication takes place.
   B. It is associated with changes in a cell's shape and function.
   C. It culminates in cell lysis and cell death.
   D. It occurs at approximately the same time as the first extracellular appearance of the virus.

6. The latent period coincides with which of the following events listed in Table 1?

   A. Early events only
   B. Early and middle events only
   C. Middle and late events only
   D. Early, middle, and late events

7. Intact poliovirus is able to penetrate only the cells of humans and other primates. Experimentation has shown, however, that purified RNA from the virus can enter a nonprimate cell, undertake the complete viral growth cycle, and give rise to thousands of new polioviruses. The new viral particles thus produced can infect only primate cells. Among the following, the most reasonable conclusion that can be drawn from the experiment is that:

A. viral protein-cell receptor interaction, facilitated by the capsid protein, is necessary to initiate the normal viral growth cycle in poliovirus.

B. viral protein-cell receptor interaction is not necessary for infection by purified poliovirus RNA, so host range specificity no longer applies.

C. purified poliovirus RNA is infectious despite the lack of a protein capsid, proving that protein provides the genetic material for viral progeny.

D. in a nonprimate host cell, purified nucleic acid from the poliovirus is capable only of initiating replication.

27.3 MASTERY VERIFIED: ANSWERS AND EXPLANATIONS

1. *B is the correct answer.* The passage states that protein created early in the virus growth cycle is used in the replication of viral nucleic acid. Polymerases are required for nucleic acid synthesis. Choice A is incorrect because a protease degrades protein. Choice C is incorrect because an antibody, although a protein, functions in the immune system of higher organisms and plays no role in the synthesis of nucleic acid. Choice D is incorrect because peptidases hydrolyze peptide bonds and thus degrade proteins. They are not involved in nucleic acid synthesis.

2. *D is the correct answer.* Viruses contain, as their nucleic acid, either RNA or DNA. Viral reproduction requires the replication of the viral genome. An RNA virus appropriates a host cell's synthetic machinery and uses it to synthesize mRNA from *its own* RNA; a DNA virus uses host cell machinery to synthesize mRNA from *its own* viral DNA. Items I and II, therefore, are accurate statements. Item III is not.

3. *C is the correct answer.* The question asks the student to find the conclusion that is *least* justified by the data. The observation that viral particles spontaneously assemble under the circumstances described should not lead the observer to conclude that disassembly is also spontaneous. Choice A is a plausible conclusion; the viral particles assembled themselves without exogenous instruction or molecular intervention. Choice B represents a reasonable conclusion.

   Despite the absence of an energy source in the test-tube mixture, the viral particles assembled themselves properly. Choice D is a sensible inference since the experimental conditions did not provide an energy source.

4. *C is the correct answer.* During the eclipse period, the virus is not detectable within the host. Figure 1 shows no virus between 1.5 and 3.5 hours after infection.

5. *A is the correct answer.* The question requires only that the student carefully read the passage. At the end of its third paragraph, it is stated that "[s]ome viruses can replicate without producing CPE in the host cell." Choices B, C, and D are statements that, according to the passage, are true.

6. *D is the correct answer.* The passage identifies the latent period as that between the onset of infection and the appearance of extracellular viruses. According to Table 1, early, middle, and late events all occur during that period.

7. *B is the correct answer.* The question concerns host cell specificity, which is governed by the interaction between viral capsid and host membrane receptors. The experiment reveals that without its protein coat, poliovirus can infect a host cell that is otherwise inaccessible to it. New progeny, complete with protein coats, are *un*able to infect any cells other than those of primates. The absence of the protein coat, it appears, frees the virus from the limitations imposed by host cell specificity.

   Choice A contradicts the data. The experiment reveals that capsid proteins are not necessary for the complete assembly of normal poliovirus. Choice C is also erroneous; the observation that purified poliovirus RNA can cause infection in the absence of a protein coat indicates that nucleic acid, not protein, is the operative genetic material. Choice D is incorrect as well. The experiment indicates that purified nucleic acid is fully capable of directing the full cycle of viral replication, and thereby capable of producing normal progeny.

CHAPTER 28

PRINCIPAL BIOCHEMICAL PATHWAYS OF THE CELL

28.1 MASTERY ACHIEVED

28.1.1 ENZYMATIC FACILITATION OF CELLULAR REACTIONS

A cell's survival is dependent on the biochemical reactions it conducts. Most of these reactions would not proceed at a rate consistent with survival were it not for the availability of **catalysts**. In a biochemical context **enzymes** catalyze reactions; the cell's survival depends on its enzymes.

Whether a reaction is ultimately exothermic or endothermic, it requires energy at the outset. This energy is called the **activation energy**. Like all catalysts, *enzymes reduce a reaction's activation energy*. In so doing, they increase reaction rate. Like any catalyst, an enzyme itself undergoes *no net change* during the course of the reaction it catalyzes. An enzyme emerges from a chemical reaction unaltered in quantity and condition. Indeed, a single enzyme molecule will typically catalyze the same reaction over and over again.

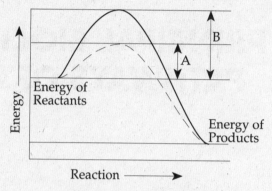

A = activation energy with enzyme

B = activation energy without enzyme

— — — catalyzed reaction

——— uncatalyzed reaction

Comparative Energies of Activation of a
Reaction, Catalyzed and Uncatalyzed

Figure 28.1

Although an enzyme increases the rate at which a given reaction occurs, it does not affect
the **equilibrium concentrations** of the reactants or products.

Please solve this problem:

- A catalyst:

    A. increases activation energy.
    B. decreases activation energy.
    C. promotes exothermicity.
    D. decreases free energy.

Problem solved:

B is the correct answer. All catalysts (including enzymes) serve to reduce activation energy.
They do not promote exothermicity or endothermicity and they have no effect on free energy.

Please solve this problem:

- After an enzyme has catalyzed a reaction several
    times, the quantity of the enzyme within that cell
    will have:

    A. decreased.
    B. increased.
    C. remained unchanged.
    D. increased, decreased, or remained unchanged,
        depending on the reaction.

Problem solved:

C is the correct answer. Enzyme concentration undergoes no net change during the course of the reaction it catalyzes. Enzymes are "recycled"; an enzyme molecule will catalyze a reaction over and over again.

28.1.1.1 Mechanism of Enzymatic Action

The first step in the functioning of an enzyme is the formation of a transient **enzyme-substrate complex**.

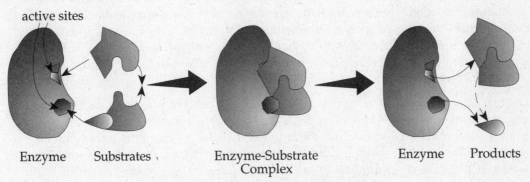

Lock and Key Theory of Enzymatic Activity

Figure 28.2

An enzyme associates with its substrate at the **active site(s)**, which are sites on the enzyme's surface shaped to accommodate the substrate molecules. The enzyme's active sites draw substrate molecules close together, allowing the substrates to interact. Substrates normally react when they are incorporated into an enzyme-substrate complex. Therefore, while an enzyme-substrate complex is formed from enzyme and substrates, its dissociation liberates enzyme and product(s).

Substrate A + Substrate B + Enzyme → Enzyme-Substrate Complex → Enzyme + Product(s).

Enzyme specificity refers to the fact that an enzyme is usually specific to one reaction. An enzyme functions because of the relationship of its physical conformation to the substrates on which it acts. Generally, the active site is structurally unreceptive to any molecules except those substrates to which the enzyme is specific, and so only reactions involving those substrates will be catalyzed. An early theory proposed to explain this specificity was called the **lock and key** hypothesis; it stated that the enzyme's shape accomodated precisely the shape of the substrate. This hypothesis has been elaborated upon in the **induced fit** hypothesis, which states that the enzyme's shape compels the substrate to take on the shape of the reaction's transition state. This hypothesis is now the prevailing model for enzyme activity.

28.1.1.2 Limitations of Enzymatic Activity

Most enzymes are proteins. Any condition that affects the stability of a protein molecule, therefore, potentially affects an enzyme's stability and its ability to function. Such conditions include pH and temperature. A given enzyme will only function *within a particular range of pH and within a particular temperature range.*

An enzyme will only function within a very small pH range. For most enzymes, this pH is between 6.5 and 8.0 (which is the normal physiological pH range), but there are enzymes whose optimum pH range falls outside this range. For example, pepsin, the proteolytic enzyme that operates in the stomach, works best in the pH range of the stomach, which is approximately 1.5 to 2.5. Similarly, most enzymes work best at physiological temperatures (around 37° C). Below this temperature, enzymatic activity slows, but the structure of the enzyme remains intact. Above this temperature, the enzymes three-dimensional structure begins to break down. Since, as we discussed, the enzyme's shape is critical to its proper function, enzymatic activity falls off dramatically at temperatures exceeding 37°C by a significant amount. This breakdown in the enzyme's shape is called **denaturation** and it occurs under conditions that disrupt hydrogen bands, which are responsible for holding the protein's tertiary structure together. Denaturation also explains the drop-off in enzymatic activity that occurs at pHs outside an enzyme's optimum range. If favorable pH and temperature conditions are restored, the enzyme will usually renature, or return to its functional conformation.

The rate of a catalyzed reaction depends on both the concentration of substrate and the concentration of enzymes. When substrate is first added to a reaction system, only a few molecules will be required to catalyze the reaction. In other words, only a few enzyme molecules are involved in enzyme-substrate caomplexes (ES); most remain as free enzymes molecules (E). As the concentration of substrate is increased, the proportion of ES will increase while the proportion of free E decreases. With continued addition of substrate, eventually all of the enzymes in the system will be involved in ES complexes; the addition of more substrate will not increase the overall rate of the reaction, since there is no more available enzyme to accomodate the additional substrate. At this point, the only way to increase the overall rate of reaction (assuming that external conditions, e.g., temperature, remain constant) is to add more enzyme to the system.

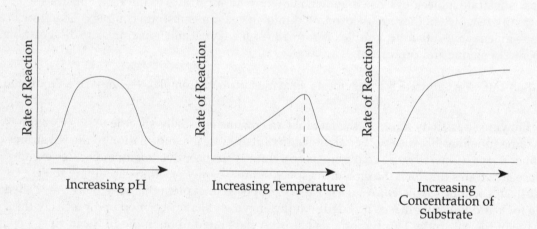

Factors That Affect Enzyme Function
Figure 28.3

Certain enzymes require for their activity the availability of **cofactors** or **coenzymes**. Cofactors are inorganic substances such as Fe^{2+} or Cu^{2+} ions. Coenzymes are organic substances, such as vitamins.

Please solve this problem:

- All of the following are true of enzymes EXCEPT:

  A. they increase the rate at which a reaction will take place.
  B. they lower the activation energy of a reaction.
  C. most are proteins.
  D. they increase the equilibrium concentration of product.

Problem solved:

D is the correct answer. Choices A, B, and C are true statements. Enzymes (like all catalysts) increase reaction rate by lowering activation energy. They do not, however, alter equilibrium concentrations of the product or reactant.

Please solve this problem:

- Among the following choices, which would most likely happen to an enzyme exposed to a temperature of 150 °C?

  A. Saturation
  B. Desaturation
  C. Denaturation
  D. Excessive activity

Problem solved:

C is the correct answer. Every enzyme operates best within a relatively narrow range of temperature. This is the principal reason that changes in human body temperature threaten health. If body temperature exceeds the upper or lower limits of various enzymes, then death or severe cell injury may result. In particular, excessively high temperatures disrupt the enzyme molecule's three-dimensional structure. This process is called denaturation.

28.1.1.3 Enzyme Inhibition

Enzymes exert control over the cell's activities by determining which reactions occur and which do not. Enzymes themselves are controlled by a process called **feedback inhibition**: an enzyme's activity may be inhibited by accumulation of product. Some reaction products are toxic in high concentrations; feedback inhibition prevents the cell from producing an excessive quantity of product. Also, accumulating too much product can be a waste of energy.

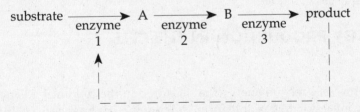

Feedback Inhibition of Enzyme Action

Figure 28.4

Competitive inhibition occurs when two molecules, one of which is the substrate and one of which us called the **inhibitor**, compete for an enzyme's binding site. The substrate, if bound to the enzyme, will participate in the reaction, but the inhibitor will not. For the time during which the inhibitor is bound to the enzyme, the enzyme is essentially nonfunctional. By effectively reducing the concentration of enzyme in a reaction system, it suppresses the rate of reaction.

Please solve this problem:

- The saturation point of an enzyme is reached when:

    A. the concentration of end products of the reaction exceeds the cell's need.
    B. all available active sites on enzyme molecules are occupied by substrate molecules.
    C. an enzyme-substrate complex is formed from reactants and enzyme.
    D. the enzyme experiences feedback inhibition.

Problem solved:

B is the correct answer. The saturation point is that point at which the concentration of substrate is sufficiently high that all available enzyme molecules are in use; the active sites are saturated and no additional substrate will increase the reaction rate.

Please solve this problem:

- If, during a particular enzymatic reaction, product concentration becomes excessively high, which of the following processes would most likely reduce enzymatic activity?

    A. Saturation
    B. Denaturation
    C. Competitive inhibition
    D. Feedback inhibition

Problem solved:

D is the correct answer. Feedback inhibition refers to a phenomenon in which the accumulation of product inhibits the activity of the enzyme. This mechanism prevents the cell from accumulating excess product.

28.1.2 ENERGY PRODUCTION IN THE CELL

28.1.2.1 ATP

Most cellular processes rely on energy that is stored in the cell until it is needed and available for conversion to a usable form. **Adenosine triphosphate (ATP)** is the form in which most cells store their energy just before use. ATP is dubbed the cell's "energy currency." In a molecule of ATP, adenine (a nitrogenous base) is linked to ribose (a sugar), which is also linked to a chain of three phosphate (PO_4) groups. The bonds that link the two phosphate groups furthest from the adenosine moiety are **high-energy bonds**. Their disruption releases more energy than does disruption of other bonds in the molecule. (Remember that no bond releases energy when broken. The energy from disruption actually comes from the subsequent formation of bonds that are more stable.)

Although removal of both the second and third phosphate groups yield about the same amount of free energy under standard conditions, it is the third phosphate group that is removed most often in psysiological systems. The liberated energy is then used to drive otherwise unfavorable processes.

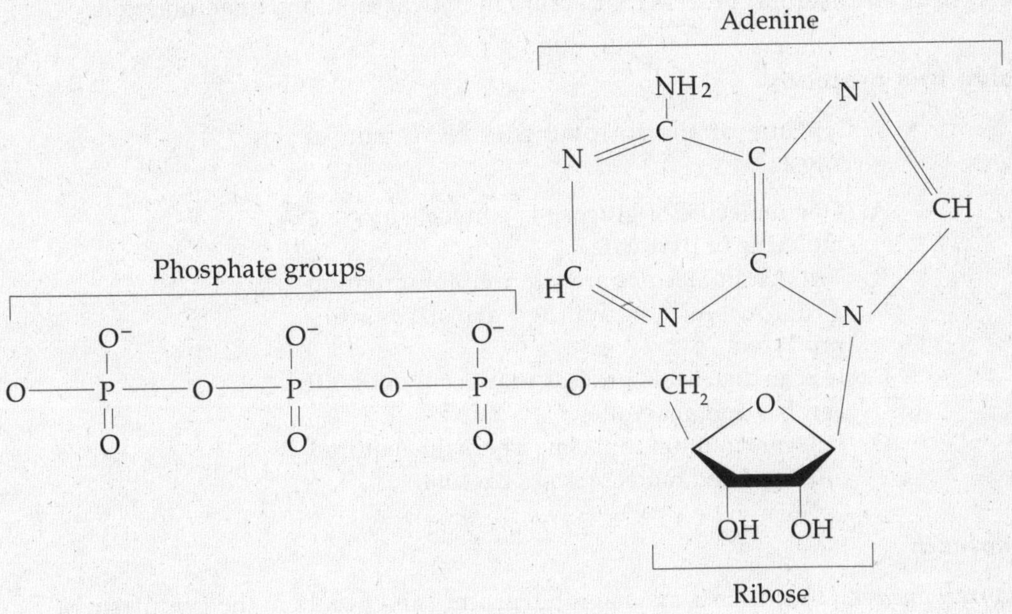

Adenosine Triphosphate (ATP)

Figure 28.5

The energy required to synthesize ATP is derived from glucose molecules stored in the cell. Glucose is a six-carbon monosaccharide. The chemical bonds within the molecule are broken by a series of reactions. The energy released by the formation of more stable bonds is an energy source for ATP production.

28.1.2.2 Anaerobic Processes

ATP can be produced both **anaerobically** and **aerobically**. **Glycolysis** and **fermentation** are anaerobic processes. The essential characteristics of each process are discussed below.

28.1.2.2.1 GLYCOLYSIS

Glycolysis is a series of enzymatic reactions that break down a glucose molecule to yield two molecules of pyruvic acid (a three-carbon molecule). This process requires an initial input of two ATP molecules but it leads to the production of four ATP molecules, for a net gain of two ATP molecules. Glycolysis also generates two molecules of NADH, which constitute the reduced form of two NAD^+ molecules. In this reduced form NADH stores energy that will ultimately generate additional ATP.

Here is the formula for glycolysis:

$$2\,ATP + 1\,Glucose + 2\,NAD^+ \rightarrow 2\,Pyruvic\,Acid + 4\,ATP + 2\,NADH$$

Note that:

- The cell experiences a net gain of two ATP molecules and two NADH molecules (from 2 molecules of NAD^+) for each molecule of glucose that undergoes glycolysis.

- Glycolysis occurs in the cell's cytoplasm, where the substrates and enzymes necessary for its several steps are available.

- Glycolysis is an anaerobic process that occurs in both aerobic and anaerobic cells.

Please solve this problem:

- Which one of the following is NOT true of glycolysis?

  A. One molecule of glucose is converted to one molecule of pyruvate.
  B. Two ATP molecules are required for initiation and four ATP molecules are ultimately produced.
  C. It is an anaerobic process that occurs in both aerobes and anaerobes.
  D. It occurs in the cytoplasm, where the required enzymes and molecules are present.

Problem solved:

A is the correct answer. Glycolysis is an anaerobic process and occurs in the cytoplasm of both aerobic and anaerobic organisms. Moreover, it requires, for its initiation, two molecules of ATP, and produces 4 ATP for a net yield of 2ATP. Choices B, C, and D, therefore, are true statements. Choice A is false because for each molecule of glucose that enters the glycolytic pathway, *two* molecules of pyruvic acid are produced.

28.1.2.2.2 FERMENTATION

If oxygen is unavailable, the pyruvic acid that is produced through glycolysis undergoes fermentation. **Fermentation** is an anaerobic process in which pyruvic acid is converted to either **lactic acid** or **ethyl alcohol**. Certain bacteria, fungi, and human muscle cells (under anaerobic conditions) conduct fermentation. During exercise human muscles may experience a lack of oxygen, called **oxygen debt**, which leads the pyruvic acid to undergo fermentation. This produces two molecules of lactic acid. It is the lactic acid that causes muscle fatigue. When yeast cells undergo fermentation they yield ethanol and carbon dioxide (a process long exploited by humans to produce wines and other alcohol-containing beverages). The process of fermentation does *not* produce any ATP molecules in addition to those derived from glycolysis.

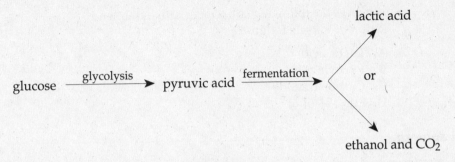

Anaerobic Pathways

Figure 28.7

Please solve this problem:

- Which of the following statements best characterizes glycolysis?

  A. It is an aerobic process that yields lactic acid.
  B. It is an aerobic process that yields ethyl alcohol.
  C. It is an anaerobic process that produces a net yield of two ATP molecules.
  D. It is an anaerobic process that produces a net yield of four ATP molecules.

Problem solved:

C is the correct answer. Glycolysis involves the degradation of a six-carbon molecule (glucose) into two three-carbon molecules (pyruvic acid). The process requires an input of two ATP molecules and produces four ATP molecules, for a net yield of two ATP molecules. Glycolysis occurs in the absence of oxygen, that is, anaerobically.

Please solve this problem:

- Which of the following best characterizes fermentation?

  A. It is an aerobic process that yields lactic acid.
  B. It is an aerobic process that yields ethyl alcohol.
  C. It is an anaerobic process that produces no ATP.
  D. It is an anaerobic process that produces four ATP molecules.

Problem solved:

C is the correct answer. Under anaerobic conditions, fermentation follows glycolysis. Through fermentation, pyruvic acid is converted to either (a) lactic acid or (b) ethyl alcohol and carbon dioxide. Fermentation does not produce ATP.

Please solve this problem:

- Which of the following substances causes the sensation of muscle fatigue?

    A. Lactic acid
    B. Pyruvic acid
    C. Carbon dioxide
    D. Ethyl alcohol

Problem solved:

A is the correct answer. A rapidly exercising muscle may require more oxygen than is delivered to it. The result is that it experiences oxygen debt and cannot carry on the aerobic processes that would otherwise follow glycolysis. The pyruvic acid produced during glycolysis instead undergoes fermentation and is converted to lactic acid, which causes muscle fatigue.

28.1.2.3 Aerobic Processes

When the necessary oxygen is available, aerobic organisms do not conduct fermentation, but rather direct pyruvic acid toward aerobic pathways, ultimately producing thirty-six molecules of ATP from each molecule of glucose. Aerobic cells use molecular oxygen as the final oxidizing agent—the final electron acceptor—in their respiratory pathways. In terms of harvesting energy from glucose, aerobic respiration is far more efficient than anaerobic respiration.

Aerobic respiration involves several phases. These are: glycolysis (which is anaerobic), and the **Krebs cycle, electron transport**, and **oxidative phosphorylation** (which require oxygen, and are aerobic). When the cell conducts aerobic respiration, the pyruvic acid molecules formed during glycolysis enter the mitochondria (where all aerobic reactions occur). In the mitochondria each pyruvic acid molecule is converted to acetyl CoA in preparation for the Krebs cycle.

28.1.2.3.1 The Krebs Cycle

The **Krebs cycle** (also known as the **citric acid cycle** or **tricarboxylic acid cycle**) is composed of eight reactions designed to harness the energy released from the stepwise oxidation of pyruvate. You are advised to know the fundamental principles of the Krebs cycle and to be able to identify the processes and molecules associated with its critical steps.

Pyruvate produced during glycolysis is channeled to the Krebs cycle via the multienzyme complex pyruvate dehydrogenase, located in the mitochondrial matrix. In a reaction known as oxidative decarboxylation, pyruvate dehydrogenase catalyzes the release of carbon dioxide from pyruvate, and the resulting molecule is oxidized (two electrons are transferred to NAD^+ to produce NADH). The acetyl group that is produced is then combined with coenzyme A to yield acetyl CoA.

$$\text{pyruvate} + \text{CoA} + NAD^+ \rightarrow \text{acetyl CoA} + CO_2 + \text{NADH}$$

Acetyl CoA, a two-carbon molecule, enters the Krebs cycle and reacts with the four-carbon oxaloacetate molecule to produce the six-carbon citrate molecule (citric acid).

$$\text{acetyl CoA} + \text{oxaloacetate} \rightarrow \text{citrate}$$

Citrate then undergoes a series of oxidation-reduction reactions that lead to the removal of two carbon groups as CO_2 and the reduction of four **electron carrier molecules.** Specifically, three molecules of NAD^+ and one FAD molecule are reduced, as shown in the following reactions:

$$NAD^+ + 2e^- + 2H^+ \rightarrow NADH + H^+$$
$$FAD + 2e^- + 2H^+ \rightarrow FADH_2$$

(Customarily, when writing NADH, the "$+H^+$" is omitted.) These reduced electron carriers store energy, and they will themselves be oxidized in a later stage of aerobic respiration, thereby releasing their energy into a process that generates ATP.

In essence, the Krebs cycle begins with a molecule of citric acid formed from the combination of a molecule of acetyl CoA and a molecule of oxaloacetate. The removal of two carbons from the six-carbon citrate regenerates the four-carbon oxaloaceteate, which can then recombine with another molecule of acetyl CoA to initiate another turn of the cycle. The energy released during the oxidation-reduction reactions is used to produce NADH and $FADH_2$ by reduction from the electron acceptors NAD^+ and FAD.

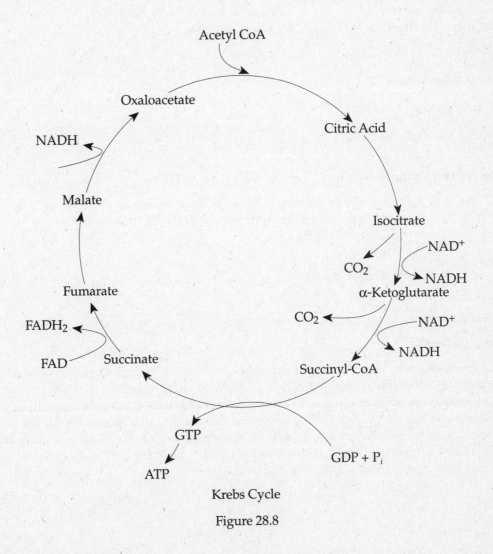

Krebs Cycle

Figure 28.8

28.1.2.3.2 Products Generated

In addition to the reduced electron carriers, one molecule of GTP (guanosine triphosphate) is produced from GDP (guanosine diphosphate) and inorganic phosphate during each turn of the Krebs cycle. GTP's phosphate bond is essentially equivalent in energy to ATP's, as evidenced by the fact that most of the GTP transfers its third phosphate group to ADP to produce ATP.

Each turn of the Krebs cycle, therefore, oxidizes citric acid in a stepwise fashion and stores the liberated energy in the following forms:

(a) three molecules of NADH;

(b) one molecule of $FADH_2$; and

(c) one molecule of GTP.

Two molecules of CO_2 are also produced, regenerating the four-carbon oxaloacetate molecule for the next turn of the cycle.

Note that glycolysis generates *two* molecules of pyruvic acid, and in the presence of sufficient oxygen each will generate a molecule of acetyl CoA. Therefore, one molecule of glucose generates two turns of the Krebs cycle, producing:

(a) four molecules of CO_2

(b) six molecules of NADH

(c) two molecules of $FADH_2$

(d) two molecules of GTP

Please solve this problem:

- Which of the following does NOT represent an energy-rich molecule from which ATP will ultimately be formed?

    A. NADH
    B. $FADH_2$
    C. CO_2
    D. GTP

Problem solved:

C is the correct answer. As evidenced by the presence of two oxygen atoms and one carbon atom, carbon dioxide (like water) represents a highly oxidized compound. Within the realm of biochemical systems, neither water nor carbon dioxide contains significant amounts of chemical energy. Indeed, H_2O and CO_2 are the end-products of physiologic oxidative processes, in which chemical energy is drawn from high-energy molecules to produce both highly oxidized compounds that are low in energy and high-energy molecules that store the energy in a form that is more readily useable by the cell.

The oxidation of glucose—beginning with glycolysis and proceeding through the aerobic processes of the Krebs cycle, electron transport, and oxidative phosphorylation—produces as end-products (1) stored energy (in molecules of ATP), and (2) the low-energy compounds carbon dioxide and water. The end of the Krebs cycle represents an intermediate point in this process; much of the energy drawn from glucose molecules resides in molecules of NADH and $FADH_2$.

During the Krebs cycle, the high-energy molecule GTP is usually converted to ATP, making choice D true.

28.1.2.3.3 ELECTRON TRANSPORT

The inner membrane of the mitochondrion contains an array of molecules known as the **electron transport chain** or the **cytochrome carrier system**, many of these molecules contain iron. The process of electron transport begins with the NADH and $FADH_2$ molecules produced by the Krebs cycle. These reduced coenzymes pass electrons to flavomononucleotide (FMN) and then to coenzyme Q (CoQ); the coenzymes NAD^+ and FAD are thus regenerated. The electrons are then passed from CoQ along the electron transport chain. With each transfer from one carrier molecule to the next, the electrons are passed to molecules whose centers of positive charge have a progressively increased tendency to attract them. That means that each transfer involves the processes of oxidation and reduction; the donor molecule is oxidized (loses electrons) and the recipient molecule is reduced (gains electrons). With each transfer, energy is released. The process of oxidative phosphorylation ultimately uses this energy to produce ATP (**28.1.2.3.4**).

Once the electrons have been passed down the electron transport chain, they are passed to protons and oxygen atoms, forming H_2O.

Please solve this problem:

- The role of oxygen in the electron transport chain is to:

    A. generate CO_2 from carbon derived from cytochrome carrier molecules.
    B. serve as the ultimate reducing agent for the storage of energy.
    C. mediate the movement of electrons from NADH and $FADH_2$ to the cytochrome carrier molecules.
    D. accept electrons donated by NADH and $FADH_2$.

Problem solved:

D is the correct answer. The cytochrome carrier system "passes electrons" from one oxidizing agent to the next, releasing energy with each pass. The ultimate oxidizing agent (electron acceptor) is oxygen, which, when combined with the electrons (and free-floating protons) forms water.

Please solve this problem:

- The cytochrome carrier system serves to:

    A. oxidize water and carbon dioxide so that the energy they contain can be released for use by the cell.

    B. liberate energy through a series of oxidation-reduction reactions.

    C. move energy from glucose to NADH and $FADH_2$.

    D. move energy from GTP to ATP.

Problem solved:

B is the correct answer. The cytochrome carrier system (electron transport chain) is composed of a series of molecules that pass electrons from one to the other, the donor being oxidized and the recipient being reduced. Energy is liberated through this process.

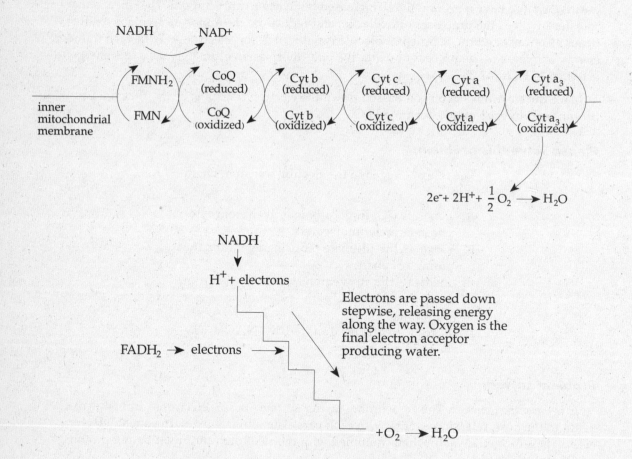

The Cytochrome Carrier System

Figure 28.9

28.1.2.3.4 OXIDATIVE PHOSPHORYLATION

The electron transport process releases energy. Certain complexes in the electron transport chain use it to *pump hydrogen ions (H+) outward from the mitochondrial matrix into the space between the outer and inner membranes*. This creates an electrochemical gradient; the concentration of positive charge and of hydrogen ions in the intermembrane space exceeds that within the matrix. A gradient like this stores potential energy. This potential energy once resided in the glucose molecule with which the respiratory process began.

Protons move back across the inner membrane in an attempt to eliminate the gradient. In order to do so, however, they must pass through channels that are composed of the enzyme **ATP synthetase**. When protons pass through these channels, the potential energy is used to drive synthesis of ATP from ADP and inorganic phosphate, a process called **oxidative phosphorylation**.

Electron transport and oxidative phosphorylation are said to be coupled. Although each process can be described separately, one occurring before the other, this is not strictly accurate. Electron transport and oxidative phosphorylation occur together, like the release of a watch spring and the movement of its hands. Electron transport provides energy for the movement of hydrogen ions from the matrix to intermembrane space. Oxidative phosphorylation occurs as the hydrogen ions move back from intermembrane space into the matrix. Processes that are linked in this way are said to be **coupled**.

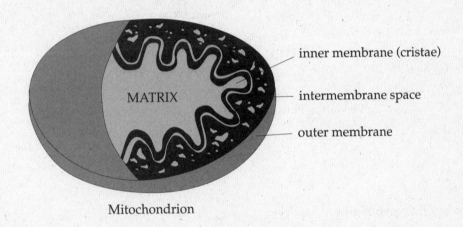

Mitochondrion

Structure of the Mitochondrion

Figure 28.10

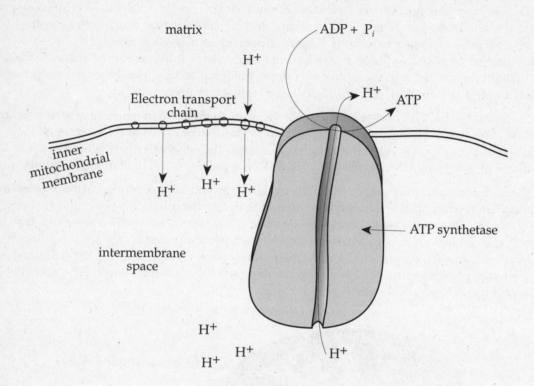

matrix

ADP + P_i

H^+

Electron transport chain

H^+ ATP

inner mitochondrial membrane

H^+ H^+ H^+

ATP synthetase

intermembrane space

H^+

H^+

H^+ H^+

Oxidative Phosphorylation via ATP Synthetase

Figure 28.11

Please solve this problem:

- The movement of hydrogen ions from the mitochondrial matrix to the intermembrane space serves to:

  A. provide the energy gradient necessary to initiate and perpetuate the sequential delivery of electrons from one cytochrome carrier to the next.

  B. establish an electrochemical gradient that promotes the passive diffusion of protons and a concomitant conversion of potential energy to chemical energy.

  C. provide an environment in which electrons may be accepted by oxygen and free-floating protons and thereby regenerate water molecules disrupted during the Krebs cycle.

  D. promote the synthesis of enzymes necessary to generate ATP molecules from ADP and inorganic phosphate.

Problem solved:

B is the correct answer. The electron transport chain uses some of the energy liberated through oxidation-reduction reactions to pump protons from the matrix into the intermembrane space. This gradient stores potential energy. The protons flow down their gradient, through ATP synthetase complexes, back into the matrix. ATP synthetase converts the potential energy of the gradient into chemical energy when it catalyzes the synthesis of ATP from ADP and inorganic phosphate.

Please solve this problem:

- Oxidative phosphorylation occurs:

   A. in the mitochondrial cytoplasm before electron transport.
   B. on the nuclear membrane before electron transport.
   C. on the inner mitochondrial membrane contemporaneous with electron transport.
   D. in the cytoplasm, after electron transport.

Problem solved:

C is the correct answer. As noted in the text, the process of oxidative phosphorylation refers to the formation of ATP from ADP and inorganic phosphate. It is driven by the release of potential energy, which is stored in the electrochemical gradient created by the movement of hydrogen ions from the mitochondrial matrix into the intermembrane space. That movement of hydrogen ions is fueled by energy released into electron transport. Oxidative phosphorylation is coupled with electron transport, and it occurs on the inner mitochondrial membrane, through the action of ATP synthetase. Choices A, B, and D inaccurately describe the site at which oxidative phosphorylation occurs and do not reflect the concept that electron transport and oxidative phosphorylation are coupled.

28.1.2.4 Quantitative Comparison of ATP Production: Aerobic and Anaerobic Respiration

Glycolysis yields a net production of two ATP molecules per molecule of glucose degraded. The full process of aerobic respiration, including glycolysis (which is an anaerobic step), yields a total of 36 ATP molecules per glucose molecule degraded in eukaryotes.

Please solve this problem:

- With regard to cellular respiration, which of the following statements is true?

   A. Glycolysis requires two ATP molecules and produces two ATP molecules, yielding a net production of zero ATP molecules.
   B. The Krebs cycle produces three molecules of NADH for each molecule of glucose that is degraded.
   C. Carbon dioxide is formed during the Krebs cycle.
   D. Electrons and hydrogens are passed along a chain of electron transport molecules in a process that requires the input of energy.

Problem solved:

C is the correct answer. During the Krebs cycle, two carbon dioxide molecules are released. Choice A is false because glycolysis offers a net yield of two ATP molecules, requiring two at initiation and generating four by completion. Choice B is similarly false. The Krebs cycle produces three molecules of NADH per molecule of acetyl CoA that enters the cycle. However, two molecules of acetyl CoA enter the cycle per molecule of glucose degraded (each arising from a molecule of pyruvic acid). Choice D is false because it describes electron transport as a process that requires the input of energy. The process liberates energy; it is an oxidative process, with oxygen serving as the electron acceptor.

Please solve this problem:

- In comparison to anaerobic respiration, aerobic respiration yields:

  A. greater quantities of ATP because the presence of oxygen, a strong oxidizing agent, facilitates greater oxidation of the glucose molecule.
  B. greater quantities of ATP because aerobic processes avoid the accumulation of lactic acid.
  C. lesser quantities of ATP because oxygen has such a strong affinity for electrons that it obstructs the electron transport system.
  D. lesser quantities of ATP because iron within the cytochrome carrier system competes for active sites on the ATP synthetase molecule.

Problem solved:

A is the correct answer. As noted in the text, aerobic respiration makes more efficient use of the glucose molecule than anaerobic resipiration. At the end of the glycolysis, NADH is reoxidized to NAD^+ during fermentation, a process that does not produce ATP. In aerobic respiration, however, NADH and $FADH_2$ donate their electrons into the electron transport system, which converts some of the stored energy into a gradient that is used to produce more ATP. In order to do this, however, there must be a final electron acceptor, or else the electrons would accumulate. Oxygen fulfills this role.

Please solve this problem:

- Which of the following statements most likely represents the reason that oxidative phosphorylation occurs on the inner mitochondrial membrane?

    A. ATP synthetase is located on the membrane.
    B. The membrane serves as the barrier that maintains the electrochemical gradient.
    C. The membrane permits active transport of protons.
    D. The membrane permits passive diffusion of protons.

Problem solved:

A is the correct answer. The inner mitochondrial membrane where ATP synthetase is located. Even were that information not provided in the text, you might infer it, since such an enzyme is necessary for the synthesis of ATP. Choices B, C, and D make inaccurate statements.

28.2 MASTERY APPLIED: SAMPLE PASSAGES AND QUESTIONS

28.2.1 Passage I

The smooth endoplasmic reticulum of the cells of the liver and other tissues is the site of numerous enzymes that metabolize drugs. Forming a significant class of such enzymes are the mixed function oxidases (MFO), also called monooxygenases. To function effectively, MFO enzymes require a reducing agent and molecular oxygen. A typical reaction involving a monooxygenase results in the consumption of one molecule of oxygen per substrate molecule. One of the oxygen atoms is incorporated into the product while the other is incorporated into water.

Homogenization and fractionation of the cell yield microsomes. Microsomes are vesicles that retain the morphological and functional traits of the intact endoplasmic reticulum. Two important microsomal enzymes that catalyze the oxidation-reduction reaction mentioned above are the flavoprotein, NADPH-cytochrome P-450 reductase and the hemoprotein, cytochrome P-450. Cytochrome P-450 serves as the terminal oxidase in the reaction. An overview of the oxidative cycle involved in microsomal drug oxidation is presented in Figure 1.

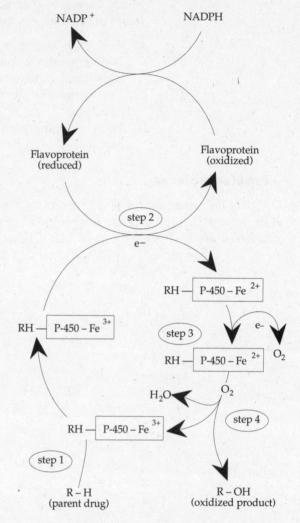

Cytochrome P-450 Cycle in Drug Oxidations

Figure 1

1. Drugs are metabolized largely in the:
   A. peroxisomes of all cells.
   B. cell membrane of liver cells.
   C. endoplasmic reticulum of liver cells.
   D. mitochondria of most cells.

2. Cytochrome P-450 reduction constitutes the rate-limiting step in hepatic drug oxidations. If the concentration of cytochrome P-450 reductase is higher than that of the other enzymes involved in the reaction, what is a possible explanation for cytochrome P-450 reduction being the rate-limiting step?

A. Cytochrome P-450 reductase is a poor reducing agent.
B. Cytochrome P-450 reductase is a poor oxidizing agent.
C. The reduction of cytochrome P-450 has a higher energy of activation than the other steps in the reaction.
D. The reduction of cytochrome P-450 has a lower energy of activation than the other steps in the reaction.

3. Which of the following choices is a cellular process with a biochemical reaction similiar to the cytochrome P-450 cycle?

A. Oxidative phosphorylation/electron transport
B. Glycolysis
C. Conversion of glucose to pyruvic acid
D. Anaerobic respiration

4. Which of the following choices is a reducing agent employed in the cytochrome P-450 cycle (Figure 1)?

A. Water
B. Molecular oxygen
C. NADPH
D. NADP

5. Which of the following statements accurately describes the orientation of phospholipids found in the lipophilic membranes of the endoplasmic reticulum?

A. The hydrophilic tail faces the interior of the bilayer sheet while the hydrophobic head is positioned facing the cytoplasm.
B. The hydrophilic tail faces the cytoplasm while the hydrophobic head is positioned toward the interior of the bilayer sheet.
C. The hydrophobic tail faces the cytoplasm while the hydrophilic head is positioned toward the interior of the bilayer sheet.
D. The hydrophobic tail faces the interior of the bilayer sheet while the hydrophilic head is positioned facing the cytoplasm.

6. Among many of the drugs and substrates processed by the cytochrome P-450 cycle, high lipid-solubility constitutes the only common property. The best explanation for this phenomenon is that:

A. substrate specificity is high for this enzyme complex.
B. substrate specificity is low for this enzyme complex.
C. the energy of activation is decreased for this reaction.
D. the energy of activation is increased for this reaction.

7. Which of the following statements is NOT an accurate description of the reaction steps featured in Figure 1?

A. Oxidized (Fe^{3+}) cytochrome P-450 combines with a drug substrate in Step 1.

B. NADPH gains an electron from flavoprotein reductase, which in turn further oxidizes the oxidized cytochrome P-450 drug complex.

C. NADPH loses electrons to flavoprotein reductase.

D. The cytochrome P-450–substrate complex with reduced oxygen transfers the oxygen to the drug substrate to form oxidized product.

8. The site of mixed function oxidases is associated with which other distinguishing feature(s)?

   I. It bears smooth segments of membrane not associated with protein synthesis.

   II. It bears rough segments of membrane associated with protein synthesis.

   III. Portions of it are attached to ribosomes.

A. I only

B. I and III only

C. II and III only

D. I, II, and III

28.2.2 Passage II

Cholesterol is a sterol, which is a kind of lipid. Located primarily in eukaryotic cell membranes, it regulates membrane fluidity. An amphipathic molecule, cholesterol's hydrophobic moiety is a fatty acid chain and hydrocarbon chain of sphingosine; its hydrophilic moiety consists of a hydroxyl group. Cholesterol is also a precursor to steroid hormones, such as progesterone, testosterone, estradiol, and cortisol. It is synthesized from acetyl CoA. Its metabolism must be carefully regulated, however. High serum levels of cholesterol can result in disease and death, particularly by contributing to the deposition of plaques in arteries throughout the body.

A lack of LDL (low density lipoprotein) receptors leads to hypercholesterolemia and atherosclerosis. Low density lipoproteins comprise the major carriers of cholesterol in the blood. In familial hyper–cholesterolemia, cholesterol is deposited in various tissues as a result of high plasma concentrations of LDL-cholesterol. The molecular defect associated with familial hypercholesterolemia is the lack of, or defect in, functional receptors for LDL. Affected individuals who are homozygous for the condition are virtually devoid of receptors for LDL, while heterozygous individuals possess approximately one-half the normal number of receptors. Both conditions impair entry of LDL into the liver and other cells, leading to increased plasma levels of LDL.

A precursor of cholesterol is 3-hydroxy-3-methylglutarate (HMG). Two preparations are used to treat hypercholesterolemia: Drug A and Drug B (Figure 2). Both drugs contain molecular groups that are structural analogs of HMG, and both act by inhibiting HMG-CoA reductase, which is a rate-limiting enzyme in the production of cholesterol. The enzyme is synthesized in greater quantities when cholesterol supplies are low and in lesser quantities when cholesterol supply is high. Inhibition of *de novo* cholesterol synthesis leads to a reduction of intracellular supply of cholesterol (Figure 1).

As a result, the cell increases production of cell-surface LDL receptors that can bind and internalize circulating LDL particles. Increased catabolism of LDL and reduced cholesterol synthesis result in a decrease in plasma cholesterol level.

Both therapeutic preparations are most effective in individuals who are heterozygous for familial hypercholesterolemia (see Figure 2). Patients who are homozygous for the condition lack the LDL receptors entirely, limiting the benefit they can derive from these agents.

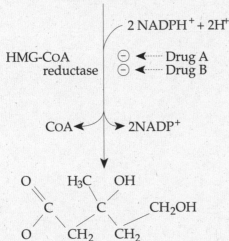

HMG-CoA

$2 NADPH^+ + 2H^+$

HMG-CoA
reductase $\ominus$ ◄------ Drug A
$\ominus$ ◄------ Drug B

CoA ◄ ► $2NADP^+$

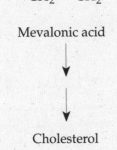

Mevalonic acid

Cholesterol

Figure 1

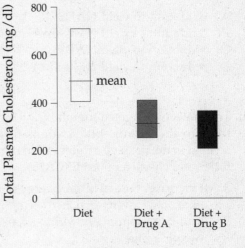

Figure 2

1. High LDL levels are likely to accumulate in the blood plasma when:

   A. receptors for LDL are sparse or nonfunctional.
   B. catabolism of LDL is increased.
   C. HMG-CoA reductase activity is enhanced.
   D. Drugs A and B are administered.

2. Bile salt constitutes a principal breakdown product of cholesterol. Synthesized in the liver and stored in the gall bladder, it is:

   A. an enzyme that is released into the small intestine.
   B. an emulsifier that is released into the stomach.
   C. an enzyme that promotes hydrolysis by lipases.
   D. an emulsifier that aids in food absorption.

3. Figure 1 indicates that during conversion of HMG-CoA to mevalonic acid, NADPH molecules undergo:

    A. oxidation to yield NADP⁺.
    B. oxidation to yield HMG-CoA.
    C. reduction to yield NADP⁺.
    D. reduction to yield HMG-CoA.

4. The molecule targeted for inhibition by the two therapeutic preparations described in the passage exhibits all of the following characteristics EXCEPT:

    A. it increases the activation energy required for a given reaction to occur.
    B. it functions optimally within a narrow pH range.
    C. it is subject to denaturation at high temperatures.
    D. it is not consumed in a reaction.

5. According to Figure 2, which experimental treatment(s) is (are) associated with the widest range of values for total blood plasma cholesterol?

    A. Diet
    B. Diet plus Drug A
    C. Diet plus Drug B
    D. No variation in range of values among the variables is apparent.

6. An increase in dietary cholesterol would most likely have which of the following effects?

    A. LDL particles would cease to carry cholesterol in the blood.
    B. Synthesis of HMG-CoA reductase in the liver would be increased.
    C. Synthesis of HMG-CoA reductase in the liver would be reduced.
    D. Synthesis of steroid hormones would be decreased.

7. The initial precursor for cholesterol synthesis is also a direct participant in which of the following processes?

    A. Glycolysis
    B. Fermentation
    C. The Krebs cycle
    D. Oxidative phosphorylation

28.3 MASTERY VERIFIED: ANSWERS AND EXPLANATIONS

28.3.1 PASSAGE I

1. *C is the correct answer.* The passage states that drugs are metabolized primarily in the smooth endoplasmic reticulum of liver cells, among others: "The smooth endoplasmic reticulum of the cells of the liver and other tissues is the site of numerous enzymes that metabolize drugs." Choice A is not correct because peroxisomes, which contain the enzyme catalase, serve in the metabolism of hydrogen peroxide. Choice B, too, is wrong. The cell membrane regulates the flow of material into and out of the cell. It is not associated with drug metabolism. Choice D is false. The mitochondria function in cellular respiration and the passage does not indicate otherwise.

2. *C is the correct answer.* By definition, the rate-limiting step of a reaction is the one with the highest energy of activation. Choices A and B are nonsensical because an enzyme is never an oxidizing or reducing agent.

3. *A is the correct answer.* Both pathways rely on oxidation-reduction reactions. The cytochrome P-450 cycle serves in drug metabolism, whereas oxidative phosphorylation (coupled with the electron transport chain) promotes ATP production.

   Choices B, C, and D refer to a single process: anaerobic respiration. None describes a process that closely resembles the cytochrome P-450 cycle.

4. *C is the correct answer.* Regardless of the seeming complexity of Figure 1, a quick examination reveals that flavoprotein is reduced as NADPH is converted to NADP. NADPH, therefore, serves as the reducing agent.

5. *D is the correct answer.* The phospholipid molecule of the membrane contains a hydrophobic moiety, the tail, and a hydrophilic moiety, the head. The hydrophobic tail faces the interior of the bilayer sheet, and the hydrophilic head faces the cytoplasm.

6. *B is the correct answer.* Enzymes are ordinarily highly specific with respect to substrate. This trait explains why, in most cases, a given enzyme will catalyze only a very specific reaction. In this case, however, the same enzyme system will act on a variety of substrates, which suggests that enzyme specificity is low. Enzymes always serve to reduce (not increase) activation energy, but that fact is not relevant to the question. Choices C and D, therefore, are incorrect.

7. *B is the correct answer.* The question does not require a comprehensive understanding of Figure 1 nor of the process it depicts. The student is not expected to have previously heard of cytochrome P-450. Rather, the answer can be determined by examining the diagram.

   According to the figure, Step 2 causes NADPH to lose (not gain) electrons to the flavoprotein reductase, which in turn *reduces* the oxidized cytochrome P-450 drug complex. (That is why Fe^{3+} went to Fe^{2+} in Step 2.) Choice B makes a *false* statement and is therefore *correct*.

8. *A is the correct answer.* The passage states that the site of MFOs is the smooth endoplasmic reticulum. Only Item I properly describes smooth ER.

28.3.2 PASSAGE II

1. *A is the correct answer.* The passage states that deficiencies in LDL receptors impair the movement of LDL into tissue cells and out of the bloodstream. Choice B is contrary to information provided in the third paragraph: catabolism of LDL inside cells is dependent on removing the LDL from the blood and internalizing it in the cell. Increased catabolism would *reduce* the quantity of circulating LDL in the blood, not increase it.

   Choice C is incorrect because HMG-CoA reductase is involved in the production of cholesterol from precursors within the cell. Enhancing its activity would likely result in greater manufacture of cholesterol, while blood-borne LDL-cholesterol molecules are not taken up by the cells.

   Choice D is likewise incorrect. The passage states that both therapeutic preparations increase production of LDL receptors which then bind to LDL particles, removing them from the blood.

2. *D is the correct answer.* The answer draws on the student's knowledge of bile and its function. It has little connection to the passage. On the basis of the question itself, you can be reasonably sure that bile is not an enzyme because it is not a *protein*. Bile is an emulsifier but is not released into the stomach. It is released into the small intestine.

3. *A is the correct answer.* Oxidation-reduction reactions always occur together. The NADPH is serving as an electron donor, which results in the reduction of HMG-CoA. As a result of losing those electrons to HMG-CoA, NADPH is oxidized to $NADP^+$.

4. *A is the correct answer.* According to the passage, the molecule inhibited by both preparations is HMG-CoA reductase. The suffix "ase" ordinarily signifies an enzyme. All properties associated with an enzyme therefore apply. Since the question turns on the word "except," any false statement is correct. Enzymes *reduce* the activation energy; they do not increase it. Choices B, C, and D make statements that accurately describe enzyme properties.

5. *A is the correct answer.* The total plasma cholesterol values for diet range from 400 mg/dl to approximately 700 mg/dl, compared to a range of roughly (a) 250 mg/dl to 400 mg/dl for diet plus Drug A, (b) 200 mg/dl to 350 mg/dl for diet plus Drug B. The widest range, then, is associated with diet alone.

6. *C is the correct answer.* The availability of increased amounts of dietary cholesterol would tend to increase levels of cholesterol in the plasma and in the cells that normally take it in *from* the plasma. The pathways and mechanisms normally responsible for cholesterol synthesis would thus tend to be less active. HMG-CoA reductase catalyzes a reaction necessary for the synthesis of cholesterol. As stated in the passage it is normally a rate-limiting enzyme. When plasma and cells have an increased supply of cholesterol, synthesis of the enzyme is reduced.

7. *C is the correct answer.* The passage states that the initial precursor for cholesterol synthesis is acetyl CoA. Acetyl CoA also participates in the Krebs cycle: it combines with oxaloacetate to form citrate.

CHAPTER 29

HUMAN PHYSIOLOGY I: GAS EXCHANGE, CIRCULATION, DIGESTION, AND MUSCULOSKELETAL FUNCTION

29.1 MASTERY ACHIEVED

29.1.1 GAS EXCHANGE AND THE RESPIRATORY SYSTEM

The term **respiration** has two distinct but related meanings. It refers to (a) the *oxidation of nutrients* to liberate energy and (b) the process of *gas exchange* in the organism as a whole. In human beings, gas exchange involves the intake of oxygen and its delivery to the cells, and the removal of carbon dioxide from the cells and its delivery to the environment.

29.1.1.1 Inspiration

29.1.1.1.1 REGULATION OF BREATHING

Although respiration is under some voluntary control, it is *normally an involuntary behavior*. In higher organisms respiration is controlled by the **medulla oblongata**, a relatively primitive component of the brain. Signals that initiate each cycle of breathing arise from that part of the medulla oblongata known as the **respiratory center**.

The **diaphragm** is the major muscle of respiration. The **phrenic nerve** carries signals from the medulla oblongata to the diaphragm and the diaphragm is thus stimulated to contract. Contraction of the diaphragm initiates **inspiration**, the process of breathing in.

29.1.1.1.2 NEGATIVE PRESSURE

The diaphragm is a large, dome-shaped muscle located between the **thorax** and **abdomen**. When it is relaxed its dome arches upward. When it contracts it flattens with its center drawn downward. Contraction causes the space between the lungs and diaphragm to increase, creating a *negative pressure differential* between the lungs and the diaphragm. The lungs respond to this by expanding, creating a negative pressure differential between the interior of the lungs and the outside air. This negative pressure differential is equilibrated by the inflow of air, which we experience as "drawing a breath." As the diaphragm contracts, so do the **intercostal muscles**, which are accessory muscles of respiration. Contraction of the intercostal muscles further expands the chest cavity, augmenting the pressure differential created by the contracting diaphragm.

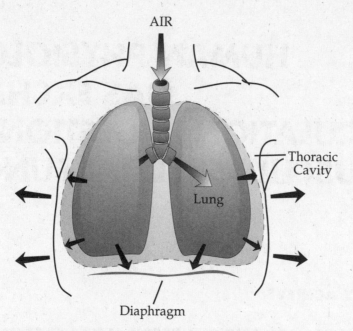

Expansion of Thoracic Cavity and the Creation
of Negative Pressure

Figure 29.1

The **elasticity** of the lung causes it to resist expansion. The negative pressure created by contraction of the diaphragm and accessory muscles must be sufficient to overcome the lung's natural tendency to collapse (as can be seen when a lung is punctured). With the lungs expanded and filled with air, inspiration is complete.

29.1.1.2 Expiration

Expiration occurs when the respiratory center *ceases* to send its signal to the diaphragm. The diaphragm relaxes and the lungs shrink, much like an emptying balloon. Air is forced from the lungs through the respiratory tract and out into the environment. Because expiration occurs when the diaphragm relaxes, it is normally a *passive process*.

Please solve this problem:

- The phrenic nerve carries its signal:

    A. from the cerebral cortex to the lungs.
    B. from the lungs to the cerebral cortex.
    C. from the medulla oblongata to the diaphragm.
    D. from the diaphragm to the lungs.

Problem solved:

C is the correct answer. The signal that initiates inspiration originates in the respiratory center of the medulla oblongata and is sent to the diaphragm via the phrenic nerve.

Please solve this problem:

- Expansion of the lungs occurs in response to:

  A. elimination of elasticity within the lungs.
  B. relaxation of the diaphragm.
  C. negative pressure within the esophagus.
  D. negative pressure between the diaphragm and
     the lungs.

Problem solved:

D is the correct answer. Contraction of the diaphragm increases the space between the lungs and the diaphragm, thus creating a negative pressure in the pleural cavity around the lungs. This negative pressure causes the lungs to expand and consequently produces a negative pressure within the lungs themselves. That negative pressure is equilibrated by air flowing inward through the respiratory tract.

29.1.1.3 Structural Features of the Respiratory Tract

29.1.1.3.1 Trachea, Bronchi, Bronchioles, and Alveoli

Air travels to the lungs through the **respiratory tract**. Air enters the respiratory tract through the nose and mouth, both of which serve to *warm and moisten* air as it enters the body. Mucus and the hairs lining the **nares** (nostrils) trap large particles that might be present in incoming air. After air enters through the nose it passes through the **nasopharynx**, then the **oropharynx**.

Air travels through the oropharynx and the **larynx** and into the **trachea**. The trachea is a mucous-membrane-lined tubular structure whose lumen (i.e., the airway) is kept open by the **cartilaginous rings** that are embedded in its wall.

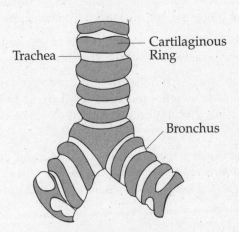

Section of Respiratory Tract

Figure 29.2

The trachea branches into a **left** and a **right bronchus**, which, like the trachea, are tubular structures kept open by a set of cartilaginous rings. The left and right bronchi themselves branch, giving rise to bronchi of progressively smaller size. Ultimately, the passages are called **bronchioles**. At the end of the bronchioles are minute air sacs called **alveoli**.

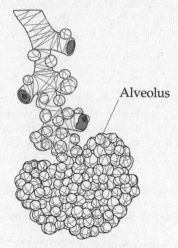

Alveolus

Terminal Bronchioles with
Alveoli

Figure 29.3

Very small foreign particles that reach the respiratory tract may be trapped by mucus. From there they are removed by the perpetual beating of **cilia**—the hair-like structures on the cells that coat the airway. Small particles sometimes escape this defense and enter the alveoli, where they are **phagocytized** (ingested and digested) by **macrophages** (phagocytic cells).

The respiratory tract's most important function is to convey air to the alveoli, *delivering oxygen to* the blood and *removing carbon dioxide from* the blood (for expulsion from the body).

Each alveolus is surrounded by a rich network of **pulmonary capillaries**. The blood that enters these capillaries contains somewhat more carbon dioxide than oxygen, because this blood has returned from systemic circulation, where it took carbon dioxide from the cells and delivered oxygen to the cells.

Ordinary air contains about twenty percent oxygen; its carbon dioxide content is less than one percent. Alveolar air contains relatively less oxygen and more carbon dioxide due to the mixing of atmospheric oxygen with residual air remaining in the alveoli and respiratory tract after each episode of expiration.

Please solve this problem:

- The cartilaginous rings that surround the trachea and bronchi serve to:

  A. keep the airway open.
  B. create the negative pressure generated by contraction of the diaphragm.
  C. maintain the movement of cilia within the airway.
  D. facilitate the transmission of respiratory signals from the medulla oblongata.

Problem solved:

A is the correct answer. The horseshoe-shaped cartilaginous rings that surround the trachea and bronchi hold the airway open (patent). You might think of a vacuum cleaner hose, which maintains its patency through the rigidity of stiff rings that support its otherwise collapsible walls.

Both the **pulmonary capillary wall** and the **alveolar wall** are permeable to carbon dioxide and oxygen. Like any substances in solution separated by a permeable membrane, carbon dioxide and oxygen move by passive diffusion down their respective concentration gradients until the concentrations are equalized. Oxygen passes from the alveolus, where its concentration is relatively higher, to the surrounding capillary blood, where its concentration is relatively lower. Carbon dioxide moves from the capillary blood, where its concentration is relatively higher, to the alveolus, where its concentration is relatively lower.

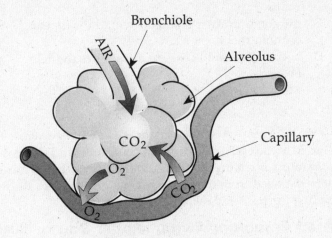

Gas Exchange at the
Alveolar-Capillary Interface

Figure 29.4

This kind of ongoing gas exchange requires continual maintenance of the concentration gradients that drive it. This is achieved by (a) the inspiratory and expiratory processes and (b) the systemic and pulmonary circulations. Inspiration and expiration draw carbon dioxide out of the alveoli while replenishing them with oxygen. Blood circulates continuously throughout the body, delivering oxygen to the cells and removing carbon dioxide from them.

Please solve this problem:

- Outgoing air from the body follows which one of the following pathways?

  A. Bronchi, bronchioles, trachea, alveoli
  B. Bronchioles, bronchi, trachea, alveoli
  C. Alveoli, bronchioles, bronchi, trachea
  D. Trachea, bronchi, bronchioles, alveoli

Problem solved:

C is the correct answer. Incoming air travels through, in order, the trachea, the bronchi, the bronchioles, and the alveoli; outgoing air follows the reverse pathway out of the body.

Please solve this problem:

- Inspiration and expiration are necessary for the maintenance of gas exchange between an alveolus and a pulmonary capillary because:

    A. the phrenic nerve sends signals directly to the alveoli.
    B. gas exchange is dependent on the equality of gas concentrations across the alveolar membrane.
    C. the concentration gradients would disappear without them.
    D. body cells would cease to metabolize in their absence.

Problem solved:

C is the correct answer. With respect to alveolar air, gas exchange across the alveolar membrane tends to increase the carbon dioxide concentration and decrease oxygen concentration. In order to maintain the concentration gradient that drives the gas exchange, carbon dioxide must be expelled from the lungs and oxygen must be drawn inward. Expiration serves the first purpose and inspiration the second.

29.1.1.3.2 SURFACE TENSION OF ALVEOLI AND THE ROLE OF SURFACTANT

Surface tension results from the force of attraction among molecules in a liquid. If this liquid comes in contact with a substance with which it cannot establish intermolecular bonds, surface tenstion results, compelling both substances to minimize contact with each other. The polar water molecules that line the alveoli are in contact with air, a nonpolar substance. The resulting surface tension would normally cause the water to coalesce into a drop (because the shape with the smallest surface-to-volume ratio is a sphere), collapsing the alveoli in the process, if there were no means to alleviate the surface tension.

In humans and other higher organisms, surface tension is relieved through the use of a **surfactant**. A surfactant has a polar end and a nonpolar end; a good example of one is a phospholipid. In the alveoli, the polar end of the surfactant dissolves into the water and the nonpolar end dissolves into the air, thereby separating the two from each other and eliminating the surface tension. Surfactant may be absent from newborns, in which case the alveoli remain collapsed. This is called **respiratory distress syndrome**.

Please solve this problem:

- A decreased concentration of surfactant leads to:

    A. a decrease in surface area for alveolar gas exchange.
    B. an inability to inspire air.
    C. a decrease in pulmonary elastic recoil.
    D. an inability of the phrenic nerve to transmit signals to the diaphragm.

Problem solved:

A is the correct answer. If alveoli collapse, then the surface area for gas exchange decreases. Alveoli are more likely to collapse when surfactant is not present in sufficient quantities.

29.1.1.4 Gas Exchange at the Alveolar Surface

29.1.1.4.1 THE BIOCHEMISTRY OF THE BLOOD GASES

When carbon dioxide produced by metabolizing cells enters the blood stream, it readily combines with water to form **carbonic acid** (H_2CO_3) in the presence of carbonic anhydrase, found in red blood cells:

$$CO_2 + H_2O \rightleftharpoons H_2CO_3$$

While still in the red blood cell, carbonic acid dissociates into hydrogen ions and bicarbonate ions (HCO_3^-):

$$H_2CO_3 \rightleftharpoons H^+ + HCO_3^-$$

Some carbon dioxide also combines directly with hemoglobin (HbO_2), producing **carboxyhemoglobin** ($HBCO_2$) and oxygen:

$$CO_2 + HbO_2 \rightleftharpoons HbCO_2 + O_2$$

When blood reaches the alveolar capillary bed, the chemical processes just described tend to move in the *reverse direction* in accordance with Le Châtelier's principle. *Molecular carbon dioxide* is regenerated and passively diffuses across the capillary wall into the alveolar space.

Please solve this problem:

- Vigorous exercise would tend to:

    A. reduce blood pH.
    B. increase blood pH.
    C. decrease blood carbon dioxide concentration.
    D. increase blood oxygen concentration.

Problem solved:

A is the correct answer. Increased metabolic activity of any tissue or organ produces increased quantities of carbon dioxide, which is carried away from the tissues by the blood. The gas combines with water to form carbonic acid, which then dissociates into protons and bicarbonate ions. An increase in proton concentration is the same as a decrease in pH.

29.1.1.4.2 REGULATORY CONTROL OF BLOOD GAS LEVELS

The respiratory center in the medulla oblongata monitors blood concentrations of several molecules and regulates respiratory rate accordingly in order to maintain homeostasis. Specifically, it is sensitive to blood oxygen, carbon dioxide, and hydrogen ion levels. When blood oxygen is low, blood carbon dioxide is high, and/or blood pH is low, the respiratory center signals the lungs to increase respiratory rate. In general, these three conditions will all occur at the same time, for example when the organism is exercising vigorously. When blood oxygen is high, blood carbon dioxide is low, and/or pH is low, the lungs are signaled to decrease respiratory rate. Of these factors, respiratory rate is most sensitive to carbon dioxide concentration. **Hyperventilation** may accompany extreme anxiety and may lead to increased blood pH.

To review:

- Respiratory rate *increases* in response to *decreased oxygen* concentration in the blood; *increased carbon dioxide* concentration in the blood; and *decreased blood pH*.

- Of these factors respiratory rate is most sensitive to the *carbon dioxide* concentration.

The homeostatic mechanisms just described also operate in the inverse. Respiratory rate decreases in response to increased concentration of oxygen in the blood, decreased concentration of carbon dioxide in the blood, and increased blood pH. **Hyperventilation**, which may accompany a state of extreme anxiety, produces low carbon dioxide concentration in the blood, and can lead to high blood pH.

Please solve this problem:

- Decreased blood pH will:

    A. increase respiratory rate, and it accompanies an increased delivery of oxygen to the alveoli.
    B. increase respiratory rate, and it accompanies an increased level of carbon dioxide in the blood.
    C. decrease respiratory rate, and it accompanies reduced synthesis of carbonic acid.
    D. decrease respiratory rate, and it accompanies increased synthesis of hemoglobin.

Problem solved:

B is the correct answer. Decreased blood pH may arise from an increased level of carbon dioxide in the blood. High carbon dioxide concentration promotes formation of carbonic acid, which dissociates into hydrogen ions and bicarbonate ions, reducing blood pH. The respiratory center of the medulla oblongata responds by increasing respiratory rate. The respiratory center is most sensitive, however, to blood carbon dioxide levels. An increased carbon dioxide concentration raises respiratory rate, and decreased carbon dioxide concentration reduces respiratory rate.

29.1.2 BLOOD FLOW

29.1.2.1 The Heart and Circulation in Overview

The heart is responsible for pumping blood throughout the body. Its muscular tissue is called **myocardium**. In humans the heart is four-chambered, with two chambers on the left and two on the right. The two upper chambers, left and right, are the **atria**, and the lower chambers, left and right, are the **ventricles**. Hence, the heart has a left atrium and a left ventricle, and a right atrium and a right ventricle. Each atrium/ventricle pair is connected by a valve through which blood flows.

29.1.2.2 Systemic Circulation

29.1.2.2.1 ARTERIAL CIRCULATION

All components of the **arterial circulation** carry blood *away* from the heart. Blood first exits the left ventricle and enters the large **artery** called the aorta.

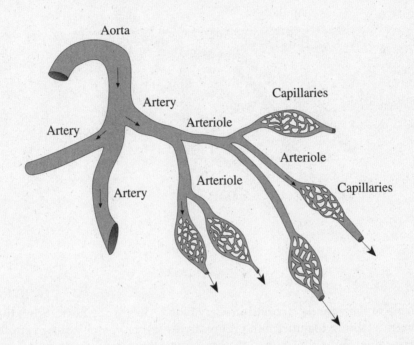

The aorta branches into arteries of progressively smaller size. These arteries continue to branch as they spread out to reach the body's tissues, becoming the very small **arterioles**. Arterioles continue branching to become millions of microscopic **capillaries**.

29.1.2.2.2 CAPILLARY BED EXCHANGE

Capillaries are found in every living part of the body, where they serve many functions. The most important is that of bringing *oxygen and nutrients* to all the cells of the body, simultaneously removing waste and the end products of respiration. The capillaries serve also as **thermoregulators**. Skin capillaries alter their diameter in response to changes in body temperature. In cold weather, when the body must conserve heat, capillaries constrict to reduce blood flow, thus reducing loss of heat into the environment. When the body becomes too warm, skin capillaries dilate, allowing blood to reach the body surface, and so facilitating the radiative loss of heat.

29.1.2.2.3 VENOUS CIRCULATION

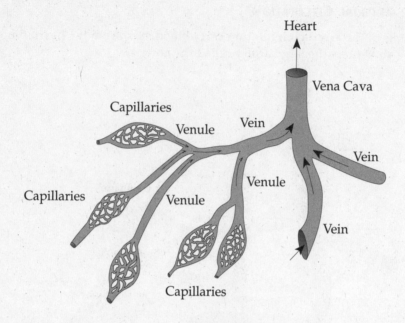

Venous Circulation

Figure 29.6

All components of the **venous circulation** carry blood toward the heart. From the **capillary bed** vessels *converge*, joining together into progressively larger vessels called **venules**, which converge to form **veins**. Veins continue to converge until they form two large veins called the **superior vena cava** and the **inferior vena cava**, each of which delivers blood directly to the heart's *right atrium*.

Please solve this problem:

- Outline the route of blood through the circulation, beginning with a capillary. Refer to the size of the operative vessels and the direction of flow.

Problem solved:

From any capillary, blood flows toward the heart in vessels of increasing size. It enters venules, then veins, and finally one of the two venae cavae, which empty blood into the heart's right atrium. Blood leaves the heart from the left ventricle via the aorta which, by branching, forms arteries, arterioles, and capillaries.

29.1.2.3 The Heart Valves

Like many pumps, the heart has **valves** which are essential to its function. The valves are situated *between the atrium and ventricle on each side* of the heart. Valves are also located at the *outlets of the right and left ventricles*, where the right ventricle delivers blood to the **pulmonary artery** and the left ventricle delivers blood into the aorta. The heart has four valves:

- **tricuspid valve,** located between the right atrium and right ventricle

- **pulmonary valve**, located between the right ventricle and pulmonary artery

- **mitral (bicuspid) valve**, located between the left atrium and left ventricle

- **aortic valve**, located between the left ventricle and aorta

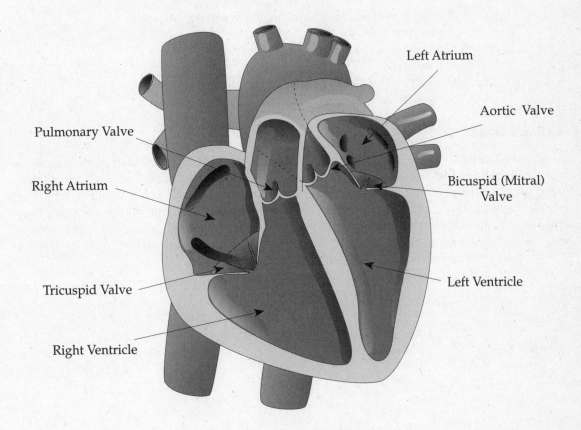

The Valves of the Heart

Figure 29.7

Heart valves operate via flexible **leaflets**, or **cusps**, which open when pressure is applied in the forward direction, and close when pressure is applied in the backward direction. Healthy heart valves are *unidirectional*. When pressure in forward and backward directions is equal, the valve assumes its **native position**, closed.

The terms "tricuspid" and "bicuspid" are used both as names of particular valves and descriptively. The tricuspid, pulmonary, and aortic valves are *tricuspid*. The mitral, or bicuspid, valve is the only *bicuspid* valve in the human heart.

The heart valves serve two functions. First, by preventing backflow they assure that *blood travels only in the forward direction*. Second, they facilitate the generation of the pressure necessary to propel blood through the circulation.

Please solve this problem:

- Which of the following correctly describes the order in which blood travels through the chambers of the heart?

  A. Right ventricle, left ventricle, right atrium, left atrium
  B. Right ventricle, right atrium, left ventricle, left atrium
  C. Left atrium, right atrium, left ventricle, right ventricle
  D. Left atrium, left ventricle, right atrium, right ventricle

Problem solved:

D is the correct answer. You might answer by naming any of the cardiac chambers first, so long as you then list the remaining three chambers in appropriate order. Choice D selects the left atrium as starting point and then correctly orders the remaining three chambers; left ventricle, right atrium, right ventricle. Choices A, B, and C are incorrect, *not* for the point they name as the beginning, but for the order they describe. If, for example, the right ventricle is named as the beginning of the circulatory system it must be followed with left atrium, left ventricle, and right atrium.

29.1.2.4 Pulmonary Circulation

Blood moves from the right to the left side of the heart by traveling first through the right and left **pulmonary arteries**, through the **pulmonary circulation**, and then to the left ventricle via the **pulmonary veins**.

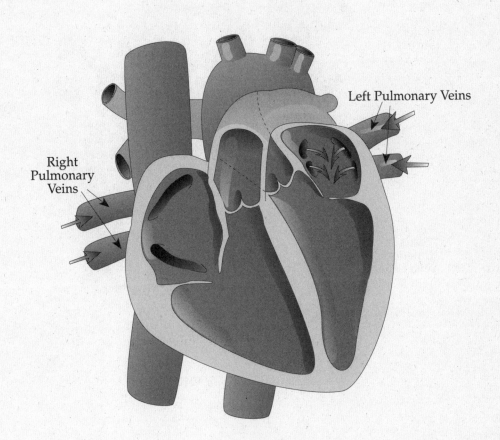

Right Pulmonary Veins

Left Pulmonary Veins

The Pulmonary Veins

Figure 29.8

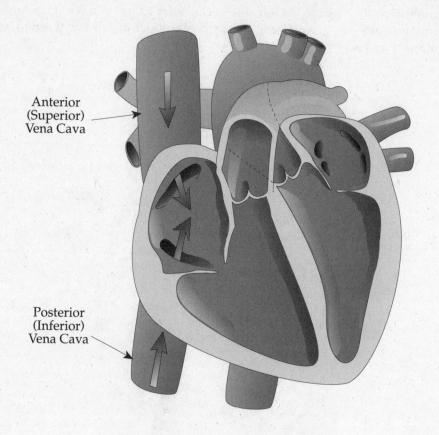

Anterior and Posterior Vena Cava

Figure 29.9

Blood entering the right side of the heart via the superior and inferior venae cavae arrives at the right atrium. The right atrium delivers this blood to the right ventricle through the tricuspid valve, which closes when the ventricle contracts. Ventricular contraction propels blood through the pulmonary valve into the **pulmonary trunk**, which almost immediately divides into the left and right pulmonary arteries. These bring blood to the left and right lungs, respectively. Blood traveling toward the lungs is relatively deoxygenated and is relatively rich in carbon dioxide.

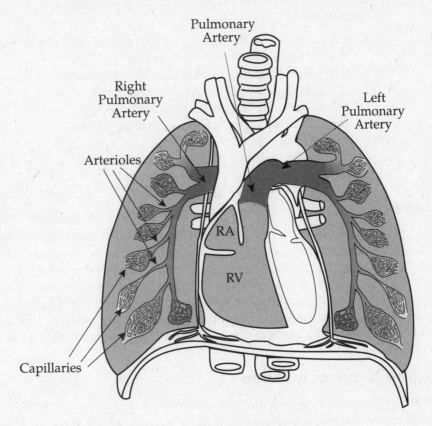

Pulmonary Circulation

Figure 29.10

At each lung the pulmonary artery branches repeatedly, leading into capillary beds which flood the tissues surrounding the alveoli with blood. The blood arriving in the capillary beds has low oxygen and high carbon dioxide concentrations relative to the alveolar air. At the alveoli, carbon dioxide is removed from capillary blood in exchange for oxygen. From the capillaries the vessels come together, forming venules, small veins, larger veins, and ultimately two left pulmonary veins and two right pulmonary veins. These veins return oxygenated blood to the left atrium. After passing through the mitral valve into the left ventricle, blood is moved into the systemic circulation.

Please solve this problem:

- Which of the following is true regarding human circulation?

    A. Pulmonary and systemic circulations comprise one continuous circulation.
    B. The systemic circulation delivers blood to the entire body with the exception of the lungs.
    C. Pulmonary circulation branches off the systemic circulation in the right side of the heart, where it then travels to the lungs.
    D. The pulmonary and systemic circulations are parallel, but separate and nonintersecting.

Problem solved:

A is the correct answer. Pulmonary and systemic circulations constitute two components of a continuous loop. Choice B confuses the fact that the pulmonary circulation travels to the lungs with the fact that systemic circulation eventually feeds capillary beds throughout the body. Although not explicitly stated, the student can infer that the lungs have two separate capillary beds. In the pulmonary circulation, capillaries bring deoxygenated blood to the alveoli for gas exchange, and in the systemic circulation capillary beds bring oxygenated blood to the alveoli to provide the lung tissues with oxygen. Choices C and D contradict the notion of a continuous circulation.

29.1.2.5 The Heart as a Pump

Contraction is the means by which the heart serves its function as pump. The myocardium, like any muscle, is **contractile**; it undergoes continuous cycles of precisely coordinated phases of contraction and relaxation.

In Stage 1A (Figure 29.11), all four cardiac chambers are relaxed. This creates relatively low pressure within each chamber, allowing the blood from the systemic circulation to rush into the right atrium via the superior and inferior venae cava, and into the left atrium from the four pulmonary veins returning from the lungs. Most of this blood flows directly into the ventricles through the open atrioventricular valves. In the next stage (1B), the two atria simultaneously contract, forcing blood into both ventricles. In Stage 2 the two atria are relaxed and the two ventricles, now filled with blood, contract. **Ventricular contraction** opens the aortic and pulmonary valves. From the left, blood rushes into the systemic circulation. On the right it enters the pulmonary circulation, moving toward the lungs for oxygenation.

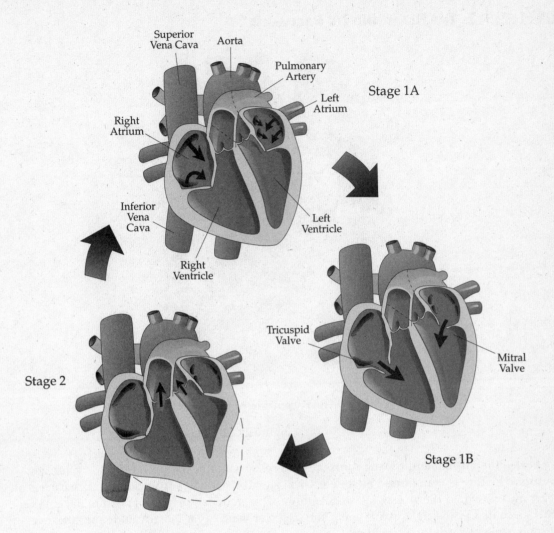

Blood Flow During Stages of Heart Contraction

Figure 29.11

Stages 1A and 1B together are called **diastole**, while stage 2 is called **systole**. In diastole the atria are first relaxed, and then contracted. The ventricles remain relaxed throughout diastole. In systole, the two ventricles contract.

29.1.2.5.1 THE PULSE

The force of propulsion of the blood as it enters the aorta from the left ventricle is transmitted throughout the body and can be felt in the periphery as the arterial **pulse**. The **radial pulse** is commonly measured by a clinician to obtain the heart rate, although numerous other pulses can be found in arteries throughout the body.

29.1.2.5.2 THE HEART AND ITS PACEMAKER

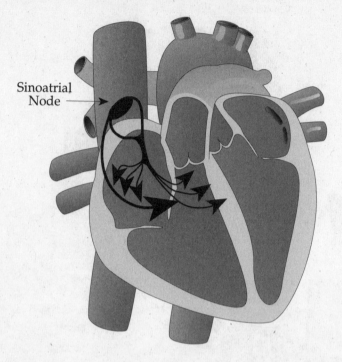

Sinoatrial
Node

The Pacemaker of the Heart

Figure 29.12

At rest the normal adult heart contracts and relaxes at an average rate of 70 cycles per minute. The rate is maintained by an electrical signal that comes from a specialized mass of heart muscle called the **sinoatrial**, or **SA**, **node**. This node is the heart's normal **pacemaker** and is situated in the right atrium near the superior vena cava. The SA node initiates every normal cycle of cardiac contraction.

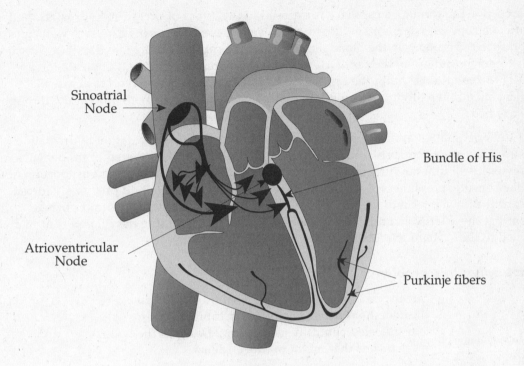

Sinoatrial Node

Atrioventricular Node

Bundle of His

Purkinje fibers

Electrical Conduction of the Heart

Figure 29.13

The pacemaker signal from the SA node is conducted electrically through the walls of the atria to the **atrioventricular node** (**AV node**), located near the intersection of the four heart chambers. From the AV node the signal passes along the **septum** between the ventricles, by way of another specialized set of myocardial fibers called the **bundle of His**. From the bundle of His, the signal moves through the **Purkinje fibers** and spreads throughout the ventricular walls.

29.1.2.6 Composition of the Blood

Blood cells are broadly divided into two types: **red cells** and **white cells**. Blood also contains **platelets**, which are cell fragments of a white cell type called **megakaryocyte**. Blood is also composed of a host of ions, and proteins such as **albumin** and **immunoglobulins**.

Red cells, or **erythrocytes**, carry oxygen and carbon dioxide. White blood cells, or **leukocytes**, mediate the cellular immune system. Included among leukocytes are the **lymphocytes**. Platelets are essential in helping the blood to clot when a vessel has been injured. All blood cells arise from precursor cells within the **bone marrow**.

Several terms are commonly used in discussion of blood composition. **Hematocrit** represents the percentage of whole blood volume occupied by red cells, and is typically measured by **centrifugation** of a blood sample. **Plasma** refers to the blood stripped of its cells. **Serum** refers to blood stripped of the proteins that precipitate when clotting occurs; it is **defibrinated** plasma.

29.1.2.7 Capillary Exchange

Blood flowing through a capillary is exposed to two types of pressure: **hydrostatic** and **oncotic**. Oncotic pressure is a specific form of osmotic pressure across capillary walls due to the presence of proteins in the blood. From within the capillary lumen, hydrostatic pressure tends to push fluid out of the capillary, while oncotic pressure exerts an opposite force, tending to keep fluids within the capillary. The interaction of the two forces across the capillary membrane produces a number of phenomena associated with blood flow through the capillary bed.

At the proximal, or arterial, end of a capillary in the systemic circulation hydrostatic pressure exceeds oncotic pressure within the lumen, and fluids are therefore propelled across the vessel's wall into the surrounding interstitial fluid. At the distal, or venous, portion of the capillary oncotic pressure prevails, and ninety-nine percent of the fluid previously forced outward is drawn back into the capillary. The remaining 1 percent of the fluid pushed outward at the arterial end remains in the interstitium (surrounding tissue) and is ultimately returned to the systemic circulation via the lymphatic system.

Please solve this problem:

- Edema, an abnormal increase in fluid content in the interstitial spaces surrounding capillary beds, is manifested clinically as swelling. Describe the mechanisms that might produce edema.

Problem solved:

Edema is caused by disruption of the hydrostatic/oncotic pressure dynamics and/or compromise of the vessel membrane integrity. Either condition can arise in both capillaries and lymph vessels. When lymph vessels are affected, normal drainage of tissue fluid is disturbed. An increase in hydrostatic pressure forces fluid out of capillaries; the capillaries then fail to reabsorb the fluid in adequate amounts. Increased hydrostatic pressure within lymph vessels, as might be caused by a distal blockage, exerts a similar effect, and prevents normal lymphatic drainage. Backward-directed increases in venous pressure (seen in right-sided heart failure), venous blockage (in thrombophlebitis, for example), or valvular insufficiency (as in varicose veins) all increase capillary hydrostatic pressure. Excessive renal retention of salt and water can also increase fluid volume and thus capillary hydrostatic pressure, producing edema.

Diminished capillary oncotic pressure reduces the blood's tendency to draw fluid back from the interstitium into the capillary. Insufficient plasma concentrations of albumin (called hypoalbuminemia) reduces the blood's ability to draw water inward across the capillary membrane, and edema results. Hypoalbuminemia might be caused, for example, by liver failure or malnutrition. Finally, disruption of capillary wall integrity, precipitating loss of plasma proteins, reduces the ability of the vessels to hold and resorb fluid, causing edema. Such breakdown is seen, for example, in allergy and burns.

29.1.3 THE LYMPHATIC SYSTEM

The **lymph vessels**, mentioned above, comprise another body-wide vessel system: the lymph system. Unlike blood vessels, the lymph vessels do not form a complete circuit, but begin as thin, blind-ending vessels in the interstitium. These coalesce and ultimately converge to form two large **lymphatic ducts** that return lymph fluid to the venous circulation by emptying into the large veins of the neck and upper chest.

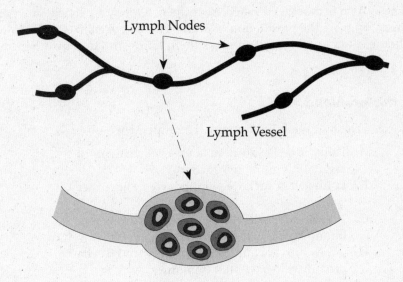

Figure 29.14

29.1.3.1 Lymph Nodes

Numerous **lymph nodes** are found along each lymph vessel. These nodes contain a concentration of *lymphocytes*, which fight infection. Lymphocytes also circulate freely in the blood stream. Infection in one part of the body causes swelling of regional lymph nodes as lymphocytes in the nodes multiply to combat the infection.

29.1.3.2 Other Lymphatic Organs

The **spleen** and **thymus** are also components of the lymphatic system. The spleen, located under the stomach, functions much like a large lymph node, except that the spleen acts as a lymphatic filter for blood while lymph nodes filter the lymph fluid. In addition, the spleen destroys senescent (aged) erythrocytes.

Found in the middle of the upper chest, the thymus is a small lymphoid organ that is especially active between birth and puberty. **T-lymphocytes** mature in the thymus, which degenerates during adolescence and adulthood, becoming largely nonfunctional.

29.1.3.3 Lymphocytes

Lymphocytes are a class of white blood cell (leukocyte). They are broadly divided into two classes: **T lymphocytes (T cells)** and **B lymphocytes (B cells)**. T cells are the basis of **cell-mediated immunity**. They have their origins in the bone marrow, but mature in the thymus. Several subtypes of T cells have been identified, including **helper**, **suppresser**, and **killer T cells**. B cells also originate in the bone marrow. They participate in humoral immunity by producing antibodies, which belong to a class of proteins called immunoglobulins. The humoral immune system is mobilized when an antigen, a foreign particle or a portion of an invading organism, triggers the production of antibodies by specialized cells called plasma cells. The antibodies bind to antigens and mark them for destruction by other immune cells.

Please solve this problem:

- Which of the following is a true statement?

  A. Killer T cells kill B cells as a mechanism of regulating immune function.
  B. Leukocytes include lymphocytes and other cell types.
  C. T cells and B cells reside in the marrow, where immunoglobulins proliferate.
  D. T cells provide humoral immunity, and B cells provide cell-mediated immunity.

Problem solved:

B is the correct answer. Lymphocytes are a subclass of leukocyte. Choice A is incorrect because the normal function of killer T cells is directed against foreign substances, not against other immune cells. Both T cells and B cells have their origins in the bone marrow, but once mature they do not normally reside there, as choice C incorrectly suggests. (T cells mature in the thymus.) The reverse of choice D is true—correctly stated, B cells provide humoral immunity and T cells are the source of cell-mediated immunity.

29.1.4 THE DIGESTIVE SYSTEM

Macronutrients (which are found in both liquid and solid foods) can be grouped into three types: **carbohydrate**, **protein**, and **fat**. In order to be of use to the body, these foods must be broken down into smaller particles that can be absorbed from the lumen of the digestive tract into the blood stream. Digestion is of two types: **mechanical** and **chemical**. Mechanical digestion begins with the shredding and grinding of food into small pieces by chewing (mastication). It continues with vigorous churning in the stomach. Chemical digestion occurs by means of enzymes produced by several different organs associated with the alimentary canal. Enzymes break food down into absorbable molecules.

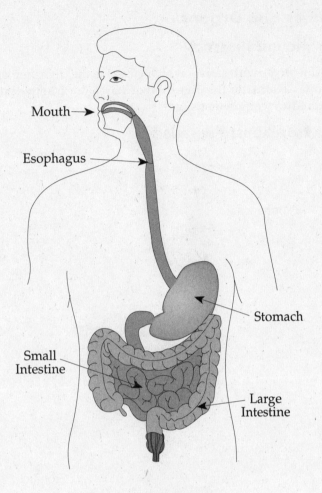

The Gastrointestinal Tract

Figure 29.15

Figure 29.15 identifies the basic organs of the human digestive tract. Food enters through the mouth, goes down the **esophagus** into the **stomach**, and then passes through the **small intestine** and the **large intestine**.

29.1.4.1 Enzymes and Organs

29.1.4.1.1 THE MOUTH: INGESTION

As food is chewed it mixes with saliva, which contains the digestive enzyme **salivary amylase**. Salivary amylase initiates the digestion of starch (a carbohydrate), hydrolyzing glycosidic bonds to produce component sugars.

29.1.4.1.2 THE ESOPHAGUS: PERISTALSIS

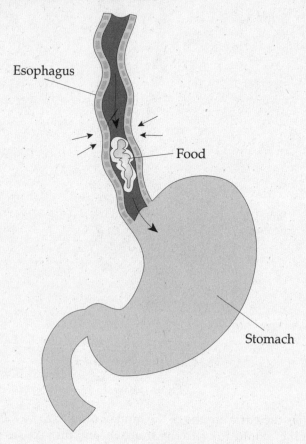

Peristalsis

Figure 29.16

The esophagus has no enzymatic function but serves as a conduit for food from the mouth to the stomach. It is a muscular structure with separate sets of muscle fibers arranged circumferentially and longitudinally. Transit through the esophagus results from a highly coordinated series of contractions, involving both circular and longitudinal muscles, known as **peristalsis**. This process squeezes a bolus of chewed food downward to the stomach. Peristalsis continues throughout the gastrointestinal tract.

29.1.4.1.3 The Stomach: Acidification

Among the stomach's most striking features is its relatively *low pH*. Specialized cells in the lining of the stomach called **parietal cells** secrete **hydrochloric acid (HCl)** into the stomach's lumen. The **vagus nerve** stimulates the production and secretion of HCl. The acidity of the stomach is essential to the functioning of the gastric enzyme **pepsin**. Secreted by **chief cells** in the stomach wall, pepsin initiates the chemical breakdown of proteins. Once food has been churned and digested by pepsin, it passes through the **pyloric sphincter** into the first section of the small intestine, the **duodenum**.

Please solve this problem:

- What are the primary digestive functions of the mouth, esophagus, and stomach? What enzymes, if any, are associated with each?

Problem solved:

The mouth performs the function of mastication—the mechanical breakdown of food with the teeth. Further, it secretes amylase-containing saliva, which begins the digestion of starch. The esophagus transports food from the mouth to the stomach through the synchronized muscular contractions called *peristalsis*. The stomach initiates protein digestion (and performs some mechanical digestion as well). The parietal cells within the walls of the stomach secrete hydrochloric acid, rendering the lumen highly acidic (the pH is normally between 1.5 and 2.5). The stomach also secretes pepsin, which works only in an acidic environment. Pepsin breaks down proteins.

29.1.4.1.4 The Small Intestine: Pancreatic Enzymes

In the small intestine the liquid food mixture, or **chyme**, is processed by enzymes that act on protein, carbohydrate, and fat. Unlike pepsin, which is produced by the organ into which it is released, the enzymes of the small intestine are synthesized in a separate organ—the **pancreas**. **Pancreatic enzymes** are delivered directly to the duodenum via the **pancreatic duct**.

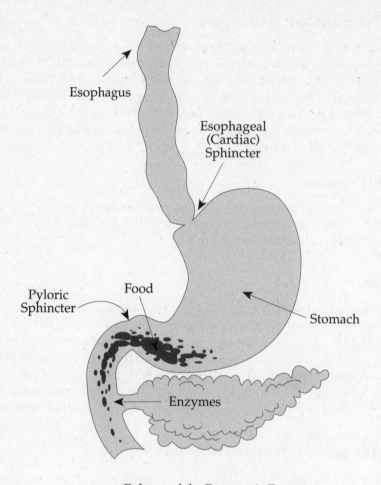

Release of the Pancreatic Enzymes

Figure 29.17

Some pancreatic enzymes are secreted into the small intestine in an inactive form. These inactive precursors are called **zymogens**. To be *activated*, zymogens must be cleaved by yet another enzyme. For example, among the zymogens released into the intestine is **trypsinogen**. The pancreatic enzyme trypsinogen is activated by an enzyme in the duodenum called **enterokinase**, also called **enteropeptidase**. The activation process produces **trypsin**, an active protein-degrading enzyme. Trypsin, moreover, cleaves a number of other protein-degrading enzyme precursors into their active forms.

You should be familiar with the names and targets of a number of digestive enzymes. **Pancreatic amylase**, chemically identical to salivary amylase, continues the digestion of carbohydrates, which was initiated in the mouth. **Pancreatic lipase**, as its name suggests, serves in the enzymatic breakdown of fats (lipids). Trypsin and **chymotrypsin** are the two most important proteolytic, or protein-digesting, enzymes in the gastrointestinal tract. These two enzymes break peptide bonds, reducing large proteins into small chains composed of only a few amino acids.

Food particles are broken down by digestive enzymes into smaller subunits; these enter the blood stream by being absorbed across the wall of the small intestine into regional capillaries. From the small intestine, blood travels directly to the liver, where further processing occurs.

Please solve this problem:

- Characterize a zymogen.

Problem solved:

A zymogen is a digestive enzyme's inactive precursor. It prevents the exposure of non-target material to the digestive process of an active enzyme. Cleavage by another enzyme activates a zymogen. The pancreatic enzyme trypsinogen, for example, is a zymogen; its active form is trypsin.

Please solve this problem:

- Pancreatic enzymes are secreted into the:

    A. pancreas.
    B. liver.
    C. stomach.
    D. small intestine.

Problem solved:

D is the correct answer. The question asks you to distinguish the origin of the pancreatic enzymes from their site of action. Pancreatic enzymes are produced in the pancreas and secreted through the pancreatic duct into the duodenum of the small intestine.

29.1.4.1.5 THE LIVER AND BILE

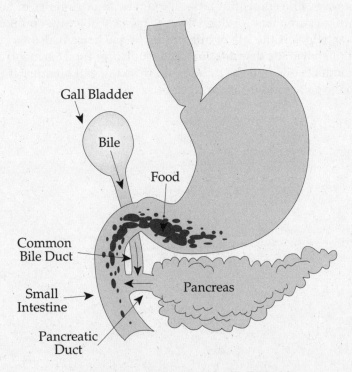

Release of Bile from the Gall Bladder

Figure 29.18

Also active in the duodenum is **bile**, which is produced in the **liver** and stored in the **gall bladder**. Bile is a complex mixture of water, electrolytes, cholesterol, bilirubin, steroid hormones and several other substances. Unlike pancreatic secretions, bile contains no enzymes, but instead acts as an **emulsifier** helping to separate large globules of *fat molecules* into smaller globules in order to increase the surface area available for the action of **lipase**. Bile enters the midsection of the duodenum via the **common bile duct**.

Bile production is only one of the important functions of the liver. The liver also plays a significant role in carbohydrate metabolism (for example, converting glucose to a storage form, **glycogen**), converts amino acids to **keto acids** and **urea**, and processes toxins. Another of its functions is the degradation of senescent erythrocytes.

Please solve this problem:

- Which one of the following statements is true regarding the gall bladder?

    A. The gall bladder produces bile, which emulsifies fats.
    B. The gall bladder produces bile, which enzymatically degrades fats.
    C. Bile has no enzymatic activity in the digestive system.
    D. Bile enters the gall bladder for storage via the common bile duct.

Problem solved:

C is the correct answer. Bile emulsifies fats—it reduces large globules of fats into smaller globules in order to prepare them for digestion by lipase. Choices A and B mistake the gall bladder for the liver, which is the site of bile production. Choice B also wrongly describes the role of bile as that of enzymatic degradation. Bile emulsifies fat. D is incorrect because the *common bile duct* conducts bile into the duodenum from the gall bladder; it is the *cystic duct* that carries bile to the gall bladder for storage.

29.1.4.1.6 THE LARGE INTESTINE: RESORPTION

The soft, watery mixture of indigestible and nonabsorbable food remnants reaching the end of the small intestine finally arrives at the **large intestine**, or **colon**. The most important function of the large intestine is the *resorption of large amounts of water* from its lumen.

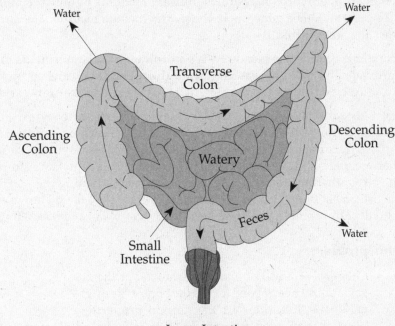

Large Intestine

Figure 29.19

Several liters of water per day are delivered to the upper digestive tract. The water comes from what the individual has imbibed and also from the fluid that carried enzymes from the pancreas (and other secretory organs) into the gastrointestinal tract. Failure to resorb adequate quantities of this water would lead to **dehydration** through water loss, as occurs when one has diarrhea. Normal feces consists of undigested food particles, other body waste products, and only a small amount of water.

29.1.5 THE MUSCULOSKELETAL SYSTEM

The musculoskeletal system, as its name implies, is comprised of the skeleton and the muscles of the body. While the skeleton includes the cartilage and teeth, its main constituent is bone.

29.1.5.1 Bone

Bone serves several important functions. As the major component of the skeleton, bone provides an *anchor for muscular contraction*. Bones also provide structural support and protection for organs and nerves. Red blood cells and platelets are formed in the **marrow** of bone. In addition, bone serves as a storage depot for calcium, phosphate, and other ions of biological significance. Bone takes up and releases such substances in response to changing needs and conditions. It serves to maintain a variety of ion concentrations within acceptable limits.

29.1.5.1.1 Basic Composition of Bone

Bone is a *dynamic connective tissue* composed principally of **matrix** and cells.

Bone matrix is composed of *organic* and *inorganic* substances in approximately a 1:1 ratio. The principal *inorganic constituents of bone are calcium and phosphorous,* which together form a crystalline compound called **hydroxyapatite**. Significant amounts of noncrystalline calcium phosphate are also present. Other minerals in the matrix include bicarbonate, citrate, magnesium, potassium, and sodium.

The organic component of matrix is mostly **Type I collagen** and amorphous **ground substance**. The ground substance consists largely of **glycosaminoglycans** and **proteins**. Hydroxyapatite and collagen create the characteristic hardness and resistance of bone.

Bone is a living tissue with three different cell types: **osteoblasts**, **osteocytes**, and **osteoclasts**. Osteoblasts are located on the inner surfaces of bone tissue, while osteocytes occupy minute spaces (**lacunae**) within the bony matrix. Osteoblasts synthesize Type I collagen and other organic components of the matrix. Osteocytes, which are simple osteoblasts with greatly reduced synthetic capacity, are responsible for maintaining the matrix. While the osteocyte and the osteoblast build and nourish bone, the osteoclast (also known as a **multinucleated giant cell**) promotes ongoing *breakdown, resorption, and remodeling* of bone.

Please solve this problem:

- Chemical removal of either the mineral or the organic substance of bone leaves the bone in its original shape, but alters its mechanical properties. What changes would be produced by removal of the mineral component? The organic component?

Problem solved:

The mineral composition of bone is largely a crystalline substance, hydroxyapatite. Dissolution of the mineral component would make the bone softer and more flexible. Collagen, composed of protein chains, can be correctly presumed to impart some flexibility to bone. The removal of the organic component of the bone matrix results in an inflexible, hard, brittle substance, subject to ready destruction under force.

29.1.5.1.2 Gross Morphology of Bone: Compact and Spongy

Gross examination of cut bone reveals two distinct bone morphologies. The outer, dense portion is called **compact bone**. The inner spongy-looking area is called **spongy bone**, due to its many small, *marrow-filled cavities*.

Bone marrow is of two types: **red** and **yellow**. In addition to the bone cell types described above, other cell species inhabit the marrow. Red marrow is the site of red blood cell and platelet production and some immune cell development and maturation. Yellow marrow is filled with **adipocytes** (fat cells).

In the newborn, all marrow is red. In the mature adult, red marrow is confined primarily to flat bones such as ribs, clavicles, pelvic bones, and skull bones. Under stress of blood loss or poor oxygen supply, however, yellow marrow may be transformed into red marrow to increase red blood cell production.

Despite differences in their gross appearances, compact and spongy bone are similarly constituted. Each consists of matrix and cells.

29.1.5.1.3 HISTOLOGY OF BONE: HAVERSIAN SYSTEMS

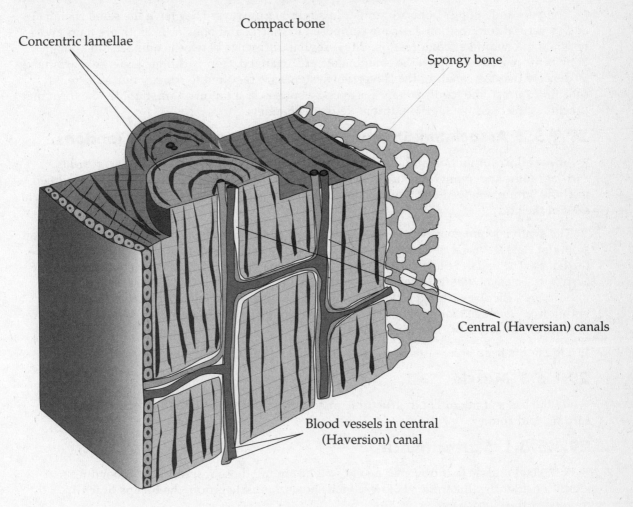

On microscopic examination, a cross section of compact bone shows several sets of concentric **lamellae** rings. Each set of concentric lamellae, running parallel to the bone's long axis, is an **Haversian system**. Haversian systems exist to distribute nutrients throughout compact bone. Many Haversian systems together give compact bone its strength.

At the center of each Haversian system is a canal known as an **Haversian canal**. An Haversian canal runs the length of an Haversian system. This canal carries blood vessels and nerves, and is filled with loose connective tissue. Shallow indentations mark the surfaces of the lamellae.

In spongy bone, thin segments of bone, known as **spicules**, surround the many small marrow spaces. Because of their thinness, the spicules within spongy bone are able to absorb nutrients directly from the marrow contained within their cavities, and so do not require Haversian systems for nutrient delivery.

Please solve this problem:

- In what ways are compact and spongy bone similar? Dissimilar?

Problem solved:

Compact and spongy bone are similar in a number of ways. They have the same chemical and structural composition. Both are composed of matrix and bone cells. Both are hard and resistant to bending or compression. The essential difference between compact and spongy bone is the manner in which the components are arranged. Compact bone is densely arranged, so densely that the canals of the Haversian systems are required to convey nutrients to its cells. In contrast, the hard substance of spongy bone is laid out in a thin, bubble-like form that precludes the need for special nutrient delivery channels.

29.1.5.2 Associated Structures: Joints, Ligaments, and Tendons

Joints allow for motion and flexibility and may be grouped into three classes: **fibrous**, **cartilaginous**, and **synovial**. Fibrous joints are composed of collagen fibers and are designed to allow minimal movement. Synovial joints allow for the great range and extent of movement seen in the body.

The synovial joint consists of the approximated ends of two bones, covered with a common **synovial capsule** made of fibrous tissue. This capsule encloses a sac of **synovial fluid** between the bones. The ends of the bones, nearly in contact, are covered with smooth, tough **articular cartilage**. The synovial fluid contained in the joint space acts as a lubricant, which, with the underlying articular cartilage, allows smooth movement of the joint, protecting the bones within from damage that might otherwise result from friction. Examples of synovial joints are those of the knees, hips, shoulders, and fingers.

Ligaments keep bones attached across joints. **Tendons** attach muscles to bones.

29.1.5.3 Muscle

On the basis of microscopic structure, muscle may be divided into three types: **skeletal**, **cardiac**, and **smooth**.

29.1.5.3.1 SKELETAL MUSCLE

A skeletal muscle that traverses a joint will be among those responsible for bending that joint. Consider the illustration below, which shows a muscle group, the **biceps brachii**, traversing the elbow joint.

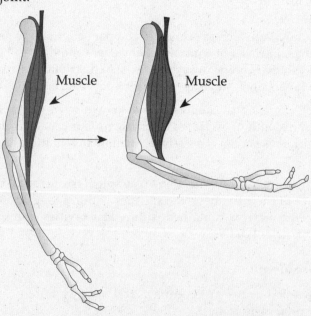

Biceps Brachii Flexes Elbow Joint

Figure 29.21

The biceps brachii attaches to the upper end of the forearm and the shoulder, crossing the elbow joint. Contraction of this muscle causes the elbow joint to bend. If the biceps muscle existed alone, as shown in the schematic diagram, the individual would be able to flex (bend) the elbow joint, but he would have no ability to straighten it (without application of some external force).

The two illustrations below demonstrate the manner in which the elbow joint is straightened.

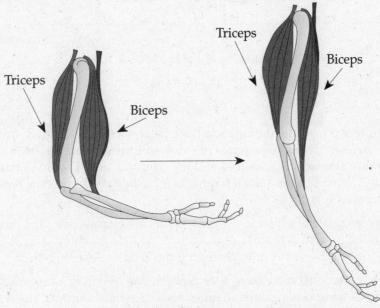

Flexion and Extension at the Elbow Joint

Figure 29.22

Active straightening of the elbow joint is possible, however, because of the action of the triceps, shown in Figure 29.22. When muscles such as the biceps and triceps pull in opposite directions across a joint, they are said to be **antagonistic** to one another.

29.1.5.3.2 MUSCLE FIBER

A skeletal muscle cell is a long, multinucleated cell, in which many striations are visible. Because of their length, skeletal muscle cells are commonly referred to as muscle "fibers." A group or bundle of skeletal muscle fibers (cells) is referred to as a **fascicle**.

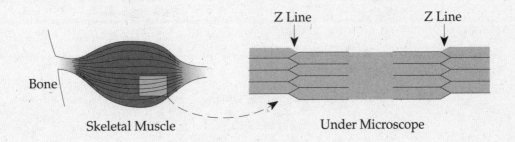

Skeletal Muscle

Figure 29.23

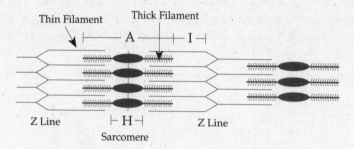

Functional Unit of the Muscle Fiber

Figure 29.24

A single **sarcomere** is a segment of muscle fiber between two Z lines, as shown in Figure 29.24. A sarcomere is composed of a series of **thick and thin filaments** arranged parallel to each other. Each **thin filament** is anchored at one end to a Z line. The **thick filaments** have no connection to the Z lines. Thin and thick filaments interdigitate in the very regular manner depicted in the figure.

Filaments are composed of proteins. Thin filaments are composed of the protein **actin** and thick filaments of the protein **myosin**. Contraction of muscle is achieved by the *sliding of actin and myosin filaments*, each over the other, bringing the Z lines closer together.

Various sectors of the sarcomere have been named. The length of a myosin (thick) filament corresponds to the **A band**. Because the filament itself does not contract, the A band has a fixed length, equal to that of the myosin strands. The space between the end of a group of thick filaments and the Z line is referrred to as the **I band**. In the middle of the sarcomere, containing only myosin filaments with no overlapping actin filaments, is the **H band**.

29.1.5.3.3 INTERACTION OF ACTIN AND MYOSIN

In order for thin and thick filaments to interact and cause muscle contraction, they must somehow link. Regularly spaced **crossbridges** extend from the myosin filaments to the actin filaments to provide the needed link.

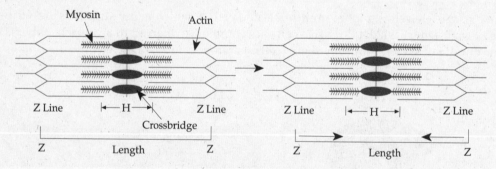

Shortening of Sarcomere During Contraction

Figure 29.25

At regular intervals (corresponding to the frequency of myosin crossbridges), actin filaments have sites containing **troponin**, a 3-subunit molecule with a binding site for calcium ions. Associated with each troponin complex is a long thin **tropomyosin** molecule that wraps in a long helix around the actin filament. In the absence of calcium ion, the actin site for myosin's crossbridges is blocked by the tropomyosin strand, and thus unavailable for binding. The *binding of calcium to troponin leads to a conformational change* in the tropomyosin that makes the myosin crosslink binding site available. Calcium, then, makes possible the crosslinking of myosin filaments to actin filaments and, therefore, the contraction of the sarcomere.

29.1.5.3.4 DEPOLARIZATION

Muscle contraction begins with the arrival of a **depolarizing nerve signal** at the neuromuscular junction. The signal, which crosses the neuromuscular junction via the diffusion of the neurotransmitter **acetylcholine**, depolarizes the **sarcoplasmic reticulum**, a specialized and widely branching endoplasmic reticulum that contains a high concentration of calcium ions. Depolarization of the sarcoplasmic reticulum leads to movement of calcium ions into the space surrounding actin and myosin, making calcium available for binding to troponin. In order for synchronized depolarization and crosslinking to occur, the action potential is carried deep into the muscle cells by a series of invaginations of the *sarcolemma* (muscle cell membrane) called the **T tubules**.

Please solve this problem:

- List in simple terms the order of events in muscle contraction, beginning with a nerve impulse to the muscle.

Problem solved:

A nerve impulse arrives at the neuromuscular junction, causing the release of acetylcholine, the neurotransmitter involved in muscle contraction. Depolarization of muscle cell membranes is carried throughout the fiber by the T tubules. The depolarization causes a release of calcium ions, which bind to troponin on the actin filaments. This causes a conformational change that uncovers myosin binding sites on the actin filaments. Myosin crossbridges are then able to attach to the actin and flex, pulling the actin fiber along the myosin fiber. This causes the simultaneous shortening of sarcomeres all along the muscle cell.

29.1.5.3.5 ENERGY REQUIREMENTS

In their natural condition, actin and myosin are bound together in a state of contraction (this partially explains the phenomenon of rigor mortis). **Relaxation** requires energy. ATP sits at an ATPase site on the crossbridge head. Hydrolysis of this ATP is normally slow, but when interacting with actin as its cofactor, myosin quickly cleaves the ATP molecule into phosphate and ADP with a concomitant release of energy. The energy enables the release of actin from myosin, and a new ATP molecule quickly replaces the hydrolyzed one. This sequence— calcium release, contraction, ATP hydrolysis, muscle relaxation—occurs over and over whenever visible muscle contraction occurs.

Muscle's energy requirement during strenuous activity is great. The increased oxygen demand of very active muscle is met by arterial dilation, which increases the delivery of oxygenated blood to the muscle. When vigorous, sustained exercise requires more oxygen than is supplied, an "oxygen debt" arises. To compensate, pyruvate is anaerobically converted to lactic acid, which causes muscle cramps and pain.

29.1.5.3.6 CARDIAC MUSCLE

Cardiac muscle is **striated**, much like skeletal muscle. Unlike skeletal muscle, however, its cells branch and bind to adjacent cells, giving it an interwoven appearance. Another distinguishing feature of cardiac muscle is that of transverse lines called **intercalated discs**. The structure and function of cardiac muscle is similar to that of skeletal muscle.

29.1.5.3.7 SMOOTH MUSCLE

Smooth muscle is under **involuntary control**. It is the operative muscle of such diverse organs and systems as blood vessels, stomach, intestines, skin, glands, and ducts. Its cells are **mononucleated**, **elongated**, and **nonstriated**. Although the arrangement of actin and myosin filaments is less regular in smooth muscle than in skeletal or cardiac muscle, the mechanism of contraction is thought to be similar. In smooth muscle, calcium interacts with a binding protein called **calmodulin**. **Cyclic AMP** is involved in regulating contraction.

Please solve this problem:

- Identify the muscle type of each of the following organs or structures: wall of the right ventricle; wall of the gall bladder; wall of a large artery in the quadriceps; the quadriceps; the diaphragm; the iris of the eye.

Problem solved:

The wall of the right ventricle and the other cardiac chambers are the only sites at which cardiac muscle is found. The walls of the gallbladder, of arteries throughout the body, and in the iris are all composed of smooth muscle fibers. The quadriceps and the diaphragm are both composed of skeletal muscle.

29.2 MASTERY APPLIED: SAMPLE PASSAGE AND QUESTIONS

Passage

Bone is a dynamic organ composed of cells, matrix, and minerals. Osteoclasts, osteoblasts, and osteocytes, together with the matrix, comprise healthy bone. Bone continuously remodels itself along lines of stress (areas that bear weight). Normal bone repair in humans begins when osteoclasts resorb old bone in order to provide space for new bone. Osteoblasts, meanwhile, lay down new bone in the area. Under normal conditions, these two processes occur at the same rate, maintaining the strength of bone.

As the result of aging, however, bone remodeling can be disrupted. Dissolved bone can be diverted to the serum, causing more bone to be lost during remodeling than is replaced. The new, incompletely remodeled bone is then vulnerable to fracture. Osteoporosis results from reduced bone mass (osteopenia) while the bone matrix remains normally mineralized.

Adequate serum levels of calcium are crucial to maintaining healthy bone. Underabsorption of calcium by the GI tract threatens normal bone metabolism and leads to reduced bone mass. Low levels of serum calcium activate a biofeedback system involving calcium, vitamin D, and parathyroid hormone. The activated system causes bone destruction in order to release calcium into the blood stream. Figure 1 depicts the regulatory activity of parathyroid hormone.

Other conditions that adversely affect bone include hyperparathyroidism, renal failure, and vitamin D deficiency. Drugs implicated in the development of osteoporosis include steroids, which reduce bone mass, and phenytoin, which alters the metabolism of vitamin D in the liver.

Another structural defect arising from an abnormality of bone turnover is Paget's disease. Affected bones become softened and enlarged, and those bearing weight become curved. In pagetic bone there is a pronounced increase in bone resorption, compounded by a secondary burst of new bone formation. Both processes are accelerated, producing bone that is both very dense and structurally inferior. Viewed through a microscope, pagetic bone shows a chaotic architecture that bears little structural resemblance to the honeycombed appearance of healthy bone. Furthermore, osteoclasts typically contain fifty to one hundred nucleii per cell in pagetic bone compared to four or five in osteoclasts from normal bone. These pagetic osteoclasts are also oversized and more numerous compared to those in healthy bone.

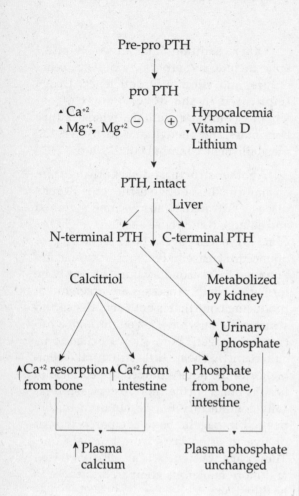

Figure 1

2. Hydroxyapatite and collagen are the principal components of:

   A. hard bone matrix.
   B. Haversian canals.
   C. cartilage matrix.
   D. lacunae.

3. The most appropriate pharmaceutical to administer to a patient with osteoporosis would be one that:

   A. inhibits the effects of osteoblasts.
   B. increases the production of osteoclasts.
   C. decreases both bone resorption and bone formation.
   D. decreases bone resorption without affecting bone formation.

4. In Paget's disease, affected bone undergoes increased vascularization. All of the following could be possible effects on the body EXCEPT:

   A. pagetic bone can pose a risk of serious bleeding if it breaks.
   B. pagetic bone can exert an extra strain on cardiac tissue.
   C. increased warmth can be detected directly over the site of pagetic bone.
   D. decreased hemoglobin concentrations can occur in areas of nonpagetic bone.

5. Which of the following is a pathophysiological process associated with osteopenia?

   A. Decreased rate of bone resorption
   B. Decreased gastrointestinal absorption of calcium
   C. Increased production of osteoblasts
   D. Increased rate of bone formation

1. Which of the following applies to osteoclasts?

   I. They are multinucleated cells.
   II. They are a type of bone cell.
   III. They deposit new bone during bone remodeling.

   A. II only
   B. I and II only
   C. II and III only
   D. I, II, and III

6. Parathyroid hormone has which of the following effects?

   A. It increases the body's metabolic rate.
   B. It decreases glucose levels in the blood stream.
   C. It increases the blood's concentration of calcium.
   D. It increases heart rate and blood pressure.

7. The serum calcium regulation pathway involving calcium, vitamin D, and parathyroid hormone could best be described as:

   A. a negative feedback loop.
   B. a positive feedback loop.
   C. allosteric regulation.
   D. competitive binding.

8. Based on Figure 1, when parathyroid hormone reaches the liver:

   A. it is metabolized into four moieties that are then metabolized by the kidney.
   B. it is metabolized into two moieties that then enter different biochemical pathways.
   C. it is metabolized into a molecule called proparathyroid.
   D. it is not metabolized.

29.3 MASTERY VERIFIED: ANSWERS AND EXPLANATIONS

1. *B is the correct answer.* The fifth paragraph states that osteoclasts contain more than one nucleus per cell. Statement I is accurate. The first paragraph states that bone cells include osteoblasts, osteocytes, and osteoclasts, so statement II is accurate as well. The first paragraph also states that osteoclasts resorb old bone, making statement III inaccurate.

2. *A is the correct answer.* Osteoblasts secrete bone matrix, containing mostly collagen. The bone matrix then becomes hardened when hydroxyapatite is deposited at the site. Choice B is incorrect because Haversian canals are found at the center of Haversian systems within compact bone. Blood vessels and nerves run through the Haversian canal. Choice C is incorrect as well: cartilage matrix is composed of collagen and proteoglycans. Choice D is incorrect because lacunae are small cavities or wells. Cartilage cells (chondrocytes) and bone cells (osteocytes) reside in the lacunae.

3. *D is the correct answer.* An agent that decreases bone resorption without affecting bone formation would constitute the ideal drug. The imbalance of bone remodeling processes would be compensated by such a pharmacological approach. Choice A is incorrect because osteoblasts build bone. Inhibiting their effects would worsen the condition rather than remedy it. Choice B too, is incorrect. Osteoclasts degrade bone. Increasing their numbers would likewise worsen the condition. Choice C is wrong because although a drug that decreases bone resorption would improve the osteoporotic condition, decreasing bone formation as well would worsen osteoporosis.

4. *D is the correct answer.* The hemoglobin content of red blood cells remains the same throughout the body. Blood supply may increase at sites of pagetic bone, but it is not possible for a variation in blood supply to affect hemoglobin content of blood. Choice A is correct because it is possible that increased blood vessels in the pagetic bone are supplying the site with blood. Therefore, it is reasonable to predict that a break at this site poses the risk of excessive bleeding. Choice B is also correct: It is possible that the increased need for blood by pagetic bone makes the heart work harder to supply blood to the site. This might exacerbate cardiac pathology. Choice C is correct because it is possible for the large volume of blood that supplies pagetic bone to cause an increase of heat at the diseased site.

5. *B is the correct answer.* The passage states that absorption of calcium is critical to proper bone formation. If calcium is inadequately absorbed, bone formation (and mass) will be adversely affected. Choice A is incorrect because decreased rate of bone resorption would not deplete bone mass (an increased rate would, however). Choice C is incorrect as well: increased osteoblast production means increased bone formation. Choice D is incorrect because an increased rate of bone formation would *build* bone; it would have an effect opposite of that associated with osteopenia.

6. *C is the correct answer.* Parathyroid hormone, secreted by the parathyroid gland, is responsible for increasing concentrations of calcium in the blood stream. Choice A is not correct. Thyroid hormone (not parathyroid hormone), secreted by the thyroid gland, increases the body's metabolic rate. Choice B is incorrect because insulin, secreted by the pancreas, causes glucose levels in the blood to decrease. Choice D is wrong because epinephrine and norepinephrine, secreted by the adrenal medulla, increase heart rate and blood pressure.

7. *A is the correct answer.* Low levels of calcium trigger an increase in the secretion of parathyroid hormone (PTH), and higher calcium levels reduce PTH release (Figure 1). This is an instance of negative feedback control on PTH. Choice B is incorrect: in a positive feedback loop the end product promotes the creation of additional product. Choice C, too, is wrong. Allosteric regulation occurs in the governing of enzyme activity, not hormone levels. Choice D is incorrect because competitive binding involves competition between substrates for an enzyme's active site. It does not relate to hormonal regulation.

8. *B is the correct answer.* Figure 1 indicates that upon reaching the liver, intact PTH is broken down into two separate molecules, called N-terminal PTH (on the left) and C-terminal PTH (on the right). One is then metabolized by the kidney (to the right) and the other enters an alternate pathway (to the left). Therefore the correct answer choice must describe two moieties which then enter separate pathways.

HUMAN PHYSIOLOGY II: THE RENAL, ENDOCRINE, AND NERVOUS SYSTEMS, AND THE SENSORY ORGANS AND SKIN

30.1 MASTERY ACHIEVED

30.1.1 THE RENAL SYSTEM

In humans the **kidneys** are the main organs of excretion. Together with the **ureters**, **bladder**, and **urethra** they form the urinary system.

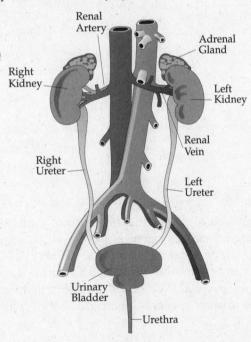

Gross Structure of the Human Urinary Tract

Figure 30.1

30.1.1.1 Gross and Microscopic Structure of the Kidney

On gross examination, the kidney consists of two portions: an outer portion, called the **renal cortex**, and an inner portion, called the **renal medulla**. The medulla is composed of wedge-shaped tissue structures called the **renal pyramids**. A hollow **renal pelvis** makes up the innermost portion of the kidney, around which the medulla and cortex are wrapped. The pelvis, located in the kidney's hilus, is actually an extension and expansion of the ureter, which leads to the **urinary bladder**.

The basic structural and functional unit of the kidney is the **nephron**. Each nephron consists of a **renal corpuscle**, continuous with a long "urinary pipeline," or **renal tubule**. Each kidney consists of more than a million nephrons. This discussion of renal function will focus on a single, representative nephron.

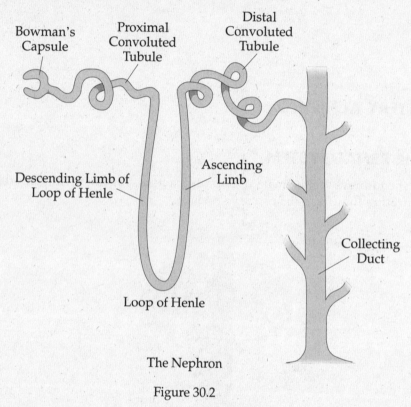

The Nephron

Figure 30.2

The renal corpuscle is comprised of two elements: a tuft of capillaries, called the **glomerulus**, and a surrounding **Bowman's capsule**. The Bowman's capsule is a double-walled cup formed as an enlargement of the **proximal** end of the renal tubule. The capsule's inner wall (**visceral layer**) is porous and permeable to plasma and other small blood constituents. The exterior wall of the capsule (**parietal layer**) is neither porous nor permeable. The space enclosed by the two walls, the **urinary space**, is the origin of the renal tubule.

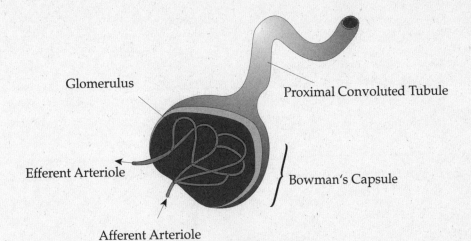

Glomerulus

Proximal Convoluted Tubule

Efferent Arteriole

Bowman's Capsule

Afferent Arteriole

A Renal Corpuscle

Figure 30.3

Fluid filtered from blood through the glomerular capillary tuft enters the renal tubule at the Bowman's capsule.

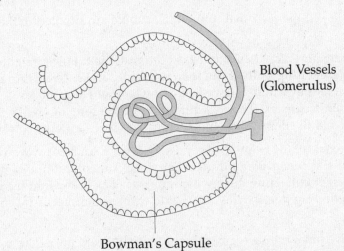

Blood Vessels (Glomerulus)

Bowman's Capsule

Filtration of Blood at the Glomerulus

Figure 30.4

Starting at the capsule, the renal tubule follows a twisting course, conventionally partitioned into five major segments. The first segment of the tubule, situated immediately beyond the Bowman's capsule, is called the **proximal convoluted tubule**, because it is most proximal (closest) to the beginning, or glomerular, tip of the nephron.

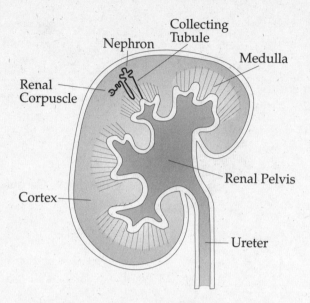

The Kidney Showing Position of a Nephron

Figure 30.5

The renal corpuscle and the proximal convoluted tubule are situated in the cortex of the kidney.

After making a characteristic series of twists and turns, the tubule straightens out in the second segment, or **descending limb of the loop of Henle**, and extends into the pyramids of the renal medulla, the kidney's midsection. There, the loop of Henle makes a 180° hairpin turn and passes into the third segment, the **ascending limb of the loop of Henle**, which, running approximately parallel to the descending limb, courses back up into the cortex.

In the cortex, the renal tubule begins a second set of twists and turns, which constitute its fourth segment, the **distal convoluted tubule**. Each distal convoluted tubule then empties into the fifth segment, a larger **collecting duct**, which courses back down into the medullary pyramids. A single collecting duct carries away fluid from numerous distal convoluted tubules.

In summary, the five renal tubule segments, sequentially from proximal to distal, are: (1) the proximal **convoluted tubule;** (2) the descending limb of the loop of Henle; (3) the ascending limb of the loop of Henle; (4) the distal convoluted tubule; and (5) the collecting duct.

Many nearby collecting ducts merge to form one **papillary duct**. Papillary ducts then empty into the funnel-shaped sections of the **renal pelvis** called the **calyces** (singular: calyx). From the renal pelvis, the **ureter** carries the urine away from the kidney to the **urinary bladder** where it is stored until it passes from the body in **micturition** (urination).

Please solve this problem:

- Urine passes directly to the outside of the body through which of the following structures?

    A. The urethra
    B. The ureter
    C. The collecting duct
    D. The renal tubule

Problem solved:

A is the correct answer. The urethra passes from the bladder to the outside of the body; it is from here that urine is excreted. A ureter passes from each kidney to the bladder. Collecting ducts channel urine to the renal pyramids, which are still far from the point of excretion from the body. The renal tubule refers to the portion of the nephron beginning immediately distal to the renal corpuscle.

Please solve this problem:

- Which of the following is an INCORRECT statement?

    A. Glomeruli are continuous with the proximal convoluted tubule.
    B. The proximal convoluted tubule is continuous with the distal convoluted tubule.
    C. The ureter empties into the bladder.
    D. Distal portions of each nephron coalesce to form, ultimately, a structure that is continuous with the ureter.

Problem solved:

A is the correct answer. As noted in the text, the glomerulus is a tuft of capillaries which, together with Bowman's capsule, constitutes the renal corpuscle. The glomerulus is not *continuous* with Bowman's capsule. Rather, certain blood constituents pass *through the walls* of the glomerular capillaries to reach Bowman's capsule. Bowman's capsule *is* continuous with the proximal convoluted tubule, which is continuous with the descending limb of the loop of Henle, which is continuous with the ascending limb of the loop of Henle, which is continuous with the distal convoluted tubule, which is continuous with the collecting duct. The collecting ducts coalesce to form papillary ducts, which, in turn, ultimately join to form the renal pelvis. The renal pelvis is continuous with the ureter, and the ureter empties into the bladder.

Please solve this problem:

- Which of the following choices correctly characterizes the glomerulus?

    A. It is closely associated with the distal convoluted tubule.
    B. It is composed primarily of blood vessels.
    C. There is one per kidney.
    D. It is situated distal to Bowman's capsule.

Problem solved:

B is the correct answer. The glomerulus is a tuft of capillaries, and capillaries are blood vessels. Blood is filtered through the glomerulus into Bowman's capsule, which means that the glomerulus is *proximal* (not distal) to Bowman's capsule. Therefore, it is not closely associated with the distal convoluted tubule. There is one glomerulus associated with each nephron, which means that there are an enormous number of glomeruli (not one) associated with each kidney.

30.1.1.2 Filtrate Transit Through the Nephron

30.1.1.2.1 FILTRATION AT THE GLOMERULUS

The blood to be filtered by the kidney is delivered via the **renal artery**. The artery branches into **afferent** ("approaching") **arterioles**, which travel to individual renal corpuscles, where they branch profusely to form the **glomerular capillaries** inside a Bowman's capsule. Leaving plasma and other small blood constituents in the Bowman's capsule for renal tubular processing, the branched glomerular capillaries join together again to form the **efferent** ("exiting") **arterioles**.

Filtration occurs across the glomerular capillary walls into Bowman's capsule. Because the efferent arterioles are narrower than the afferent ones, and because the efferent arterioles can constrict, a high blood pressure (about 60 mm Hg) can be created in the capillaries of the glomerulus. This pressure forces fluid to leave the capillaries, and the low pressure and permeable inner wall of the Bowman's capsule provides an outlet. The cell membranes of the capillaries allow all but cells, platelets, and macromolecules (such as large proteins) to pass through into the capsular space. Thus, the blood reaching the glomerular capillaries via the afferent arterioles has the same composition of sugars, amino acids, ions, and water as the fluid that filters out of the capillaries into the capsule. Once fluid exits the capillary into the urinary space of Bowman's capsule, it is referred to as **glomerular filtrate**.

Please solve this problem:

- Which of the following laboratory findings would most likely indicate disease?

    A. The absence of large proteins in the urine
    B. The absence of white blood cells in the urine
    C. The presence of red blood cells in the urine
    D. The presence of hydroxide ions in the urine

Problem solved:

C is the correct answer. Blood coursing through the glomerular capillaries is filtered through the capillary walls into Bowman's capsule. As noted in the text, the filtrate contains a great many constituents of blood, but it does not contain blood cells. The presence of red blood cells in the urine (**hematuria**) is abnormal and a possible indication of disease. The urine does not normally contain large proteins or white blood cells; it does contain hydroxide ions.

30.1.1.2.2 THE DESCENDING LOOP OF HENLE

A greater volume of blood is filtered at the kidney each minute than a person excretes as urine in a day. Therefore, the kidney *reabsorbs* water, ions, and other substances from the glomerular filtrate. This reabsorption occurs to some degree along the entire length of a nephron, but most reabsorption occurs at the proximal convoluted tubule, where seventy-five percent of the filtrate is reabsorbed.

Filtrate within the tubule is affected by the fluid environment through which the tubule passes. The salt concentration of the interstitial fluid in the kidney is precisely regulated, so there is a concentration gradient between the cortical and medullary regions of the kidney. The salt concentration of the cortical interstitial fluid—around the renal corpuscles, proximal convoluted tubules, and upper portion of the loop of Henle—is relatively low. The interstitial salt concentration increases at deeper levels within the medulla.

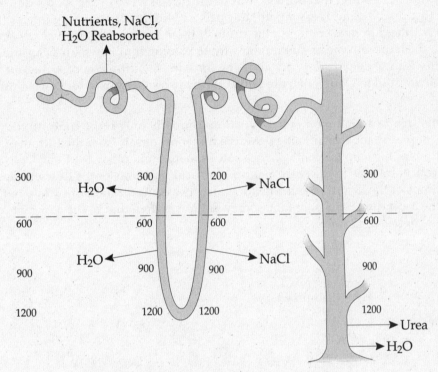

Fluid Transport Through the Loop of Henle

Figure 30.6

As filtrate travels through the descending loop of Henle, it encounters increasingly higher salt concentrations in the surrounding interstitial environment. To maintain osmotic equilibrium across a membrane, fluid and/or solutes must cross the membrane. Because the wall of the descending limb of the loop of Henle is permeable to water but nearly impermeable to solutes, water must pass out of the loop to equalize concentrations inside the renal tubule with those outside the tubule.

30.1.1.2.3 THE ASCENDING LOOP OF HENLE

Like the descending loop of Henle, the ascending loop also traverses the concentration gradient of the surrounding interstitial fluid; the dynamics are reversed, however. The concentration gradient decreases as the tubule extends into the relatively dilute interstitial environment of the cortex. As in the descending loop, the osmotic differential across the cells of the tubule walls will equalize the intratubal pressure with the pressure of the interstitial environment. Unlike the descending limb, however, the ascending limb is impermeable to water, but becomes permeable to sodium. As the filtrate travels through the ascending tubule, it becomes dilute once again, extruding sodium first by passive diffusion and then by active transport across tubule walls into the interstitial environment. Passage through the loop of Henle has restored the filtrate's solute concentration at the cortical portion of the ascending limb to levels nearly equal to those of the pre-loop filtrate at the cortical portion of the descending limb.

On first examination, the loop of Henle may appear to have no function, as it seems to produce no change in solute concentration. However, the ascending limb contains a *reduced volume* of filtrate. The water that diffused out of the tubule walls of the loop's descending limb has been reabsorbed by, and is essentially trapped within, the surrounding interstitial space, and is thus withheld from excretion in the urine. If there were no *tubular reabsorption* mechanism, the large volume of glomerular filtrate passing into Bowman's capsule each day would swiftly lead to dehydration. By allowing for one-way diffusion of water out of the nephron, the limbs of the loop of Henle afford the body a mechanism for conservation of water.

The tubular reabsorption mechanism functions properly only if the concentration gradient around the loop of Henle is maintained. **Active transport** of salt from the filtrate of the ascending limb of the loop of Henle plays a role in maintaining that gradient. Consequently, the filtrate concentrations in the corresponding cortical segments of the descending and ascending limbs of the loop of Henle are not equal. The concentration of filtrate in the cortical portion of the ascending limb is, in fact, somewhat lower than that in the adjacent cortical portion of the descending limb.

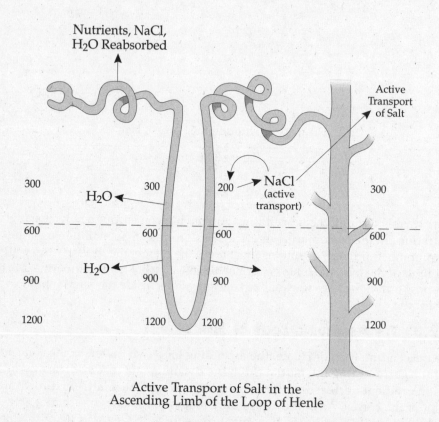

Active Transport of Salt in the
Ascending Limb of the Loop of Henle

Figure 30.7

Please solve this problem:

- The kidney maintains a concentration gradient in its interstitial fluid, with the concentration of sodium and other ions increasing several fold from the cortex to the medulla. Discuss this gradient in relation to the composition of filtrate in the descending loop of Henle.

Problem solved:

Water will diffuse across a membrane to equalize ionic concentrations on both sides of the membrane. In the descending limb of the loop of Henle, the filtrate encounters a progressively increasing concentration of solute across the tubular membrane as it travels toward the medulla. Thus, water from the filtrate diffuses across the loop membrane into this surrounding interstitial fluid, which increases the concentration of tubular ions and dilutes the interstitial fluid. Despite this diluting effect of reabsorbed filtrate water, other mechanisms work to maintain the interstitial concentration gradient. Hence, the process of tubular filtrate concentration continues as it passes through the increasingly concentrated environment of the medulla near the hairpin loop.

Please solve this problem:

- Which of the following choices properly characterizes fluid in the distal convoluted tubule?

  A. Its concentration of protein is markedly higher than that of the proximal convoluted tubule.
  B. Its chlorine concentration is markedly lower than that of the proximal convoluted tubule.
  C. Its sodium concentration is markedly lower than that of the proximal convoluted tubule.
  D. Its volume is markedly less than that of the proximal convoluted tubule.

Problem solved:

D is the correct answer. As described in the text, the passage of filtrate through the loop of Henle and its limbs allows for the conservation of water. That is, a net movement of water occurs *from* the tubule outward into the interstitium. Although the tubular fluid experiences little change in its concentrations of solutes as it passes from descending to ascending limbs, it undergoes a pronounced diminution in volume. Protein molecules are not normally filtered through the glomerulus into the tubular fluid. Protein concentration within the tubular fluid should be very nearly zero at all portions of the nephron. The presence of protein in the urine (**proteinuria**) is a classic sign of kidney disease.

30.1.1.3 Hormonal Regulation of Water Retention

From the cortical end of the ascending limb of the loop of Henle (also called the distal end, because it is farthest from the glomerulus), filtrate passes into the distal convoluted tubule, and from there into a collecting duct. A significant amount of water reabsorption can occur in each of these latter segments. As filtrate flows from the proximal (cortical) end of the collecting duct down toward a papillary duct of the renal pelvis, it encounters the same increasing interstitial salt concentration as it did in the descending limb of the loop of Henle. Again, a concentration gradient exists across the tubule walls, but because the collecting duct is impermeable to salt, the filtrate does not receive any solutes from the surrounding environment.

The permeability of the collecting tubule to water, however, can be regulated depending on the body's need to conserve or eliminate water. This regulation is accomplished by the hypothalamic hormone antidiuretic hormone (ADH). When dehydration stimulates release of ADH from the posterior pituitary, where it is stored, it increases the collecting duct's permeability to water; water moves outward from duct to interstitium and is conserved. When the body is adequately hydrated ADH secretion is diminished, reducing the permeability of the collecting duct, thereby trapping the water within the tubule and producing an increased volume of more dilute urine.

Please solve this problem:

- A woman preparing to undergo a sonogram drinks six 8-ounce glasses of water before the procedure. What will likely be the effect of her water intake on blood levels of ADH, a hormone released by her posterior pituitary?

Problem solved:

ADH increases the collecting duct's permeability to water, promoting water conservation. In this case, the patient is overhydrated. In order to reestablish homeostasis, she must excrete a relatively large volume of urine, so the posterior pituitary reduces its secretion of ADH.

Please solve this problem:

- Which of the following choices does NOT accompany increased secretion of ADH?

    A. Decreased urine volume
    B. A more dilute urine
    C. Increased movement of water from collecting ducts to interstitium
    D. Water conservation

Problem solved:

B is the correct answer. ADH increases the collecting duct's permeability to water, causing (a) movement of water from the collecting duct to the interstitium, (b) the production of a concentrated urine, relatively low in volume, and (c) the concomitant conservation of water. ADH concentrates the urine; it does not dilute it.

Please solve this problem:

- In the condition known as diabetes insipidus, ADH secretion is impaired. Among the following, which symptom will the patient most likely experience?

  A. Increased thirst
  B. Decreased thirst
  C. Low urine output
  D. High content of protein in the urine

Problem solved:

A is the correct answer. The absence of ADH will decrease the permeability of the collecting duct to water. Water will not move from the collecting duct to the interstitium, even in the face of relative dehydration. The patient will excrete relatively high volumes of dilute urine. She will thus experience a tendency toward high salt concentrations and low volume of her body fluids. If the patient's thirst mechanism is intact (as it ordinarily is in diabetes insipidus), she will experience increased thirst and will compensate by drinking. In the absence of kidney disease the urine will not contain protein; that is, in the healthy kidney, protein is not filtered out of the glomerulus.

30.1.2 THE ENDOCRINE SYSTEM

Some of the body's most important homeostatic mechanisms are found in the **endocrine system**, which promotes communication among various tissues and organs through the secretion of **hormones**. Hormones are secreted by **endocrine organs**, more commonly called **endocrine glands**. Hormones usually act at considerable distances from the sites of their release. They are released from an endocrine gland into the **bloodstream**, by which they are carried to their **target cells**. Exocrine organs, by contrast, are not components of the endocrine system. They secrete **enzymes** into ducts that carry them directly to their sites of action.

The **pancreas** is both an endocrine gland and an exocrine gland. Its secretion of **insulin** is an *endocrine* function; its secretion of **digestive enzymes** is an *exocrine* function. Insulin is secreted into the blood and carried through the bloodstream to its site of action. Digestive enzymes are secreted into the **pancreatic duct**, which carries them to the **small intestine** where they act.

Most endocrine hormones act slowly and for longer periods (i.e., minutes to years) to maintain the body in relative homeostasis. Their secretion is modulated by changes in bodily needs and conditions.

Because they are secreted directly into the blood stream, endocrine hormones come into contact with nearly every cell of the body. Despite that fact, a given hormone may not have any effect on a given cell type. Many hormones affect a cell only if the cell has, on its surface membrane, a **receptor** that binds them. Other hormones encounter their receptors inside the cell. A hormone's target cells, then, are those cells that have receptors for it. A given cell type might be the target of one hormone, many hormones, or no hormones, depending on the number and kind of receptors it possesses.

602 ■ FLOWERS & SILVER MCAT

Please solve this problem:

- Which one of the following choices is NOT characteristic of an endocrine gland?

  A. It secretes enzymes that act on distant organs
  or cells.
  B. It helps to maintain homeostasis.
  C. It secretes hormones that exert their effects at
  a distant site.
  D. It secretes hormones that are transported
  through the blood stream to reach their sites
  of action.

Problem solved:

A is the correct answer. Endocrine glands secrete *hormones*, not enzymes. (Exocrine glands
secrete enzymes.) Endocrine glands do function in the maintenance of homeostasis—their
hormones affect target cells and organs, which compensates in response to changes in internal
and external bodily environments. Generally, hormones act at sites remote from the points at
which they are released, and they reach their sites of action via the bloodstream.

Please solve this problem:

- Which of the following findings would justify an
  investigator in classifying the kidney as an endocrine organ?

  A. It passes urine to the bladder via a duct system.
  B. It receives a large blood supply.
  C. It modulates the excretion of fluid in order to
  maintain fluid balance.
  D. It secretes a substance that travels through the
  blood and affects the degree of muscle tone
  in small arteries and arterioles in order to
  modulate blood pressure in response to variable conditions.

Problem solved:

D is the correct answer. An endocrine organ is one that secretes hormones. Hormones travel
in the blood, reach their target sites, and act to promote homeostasis. If the kidney secretes a
substance that travels through the blood to modulate blood pressure, it secretes a hormone
and is an endocrine organ. In fact, the afferent arterioles leading to the glomerulus secrete a
substance called **renin**. Renin converts a blood protein to angiotensin I, and then angiotensin I
is converted to angiotensin II. Angiotensin II increases smooth muscle tone in small arteries
and arterioles, thus increasing blood pressure.

30.1.2.1 Principal Endocrine Organs

The higher regulatory organs of the endocrine system are the **hypothalamus** and the **anterior** and **posterior pituitary glands**. These regulatory organs affect target organs—either directly or through other, intermediate endocrine glands.

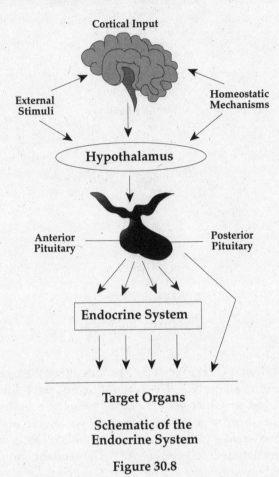

Cortical Input

External Stimuli

Homeostatic Mechanisms

Hypothalamus

Anterior Pituitary

Posterior Pituitary

Endocrine System

Target Organs

Schematic of the Endocrine System

Figure 30.8

30.1.2.1.1 THE PANCREAS

As already noted, the **pancreas** is both an exocrine and an endocrine organ; it is an exocrine organ because it secretes digestive enzymes (see Chapter 29). It is as an endocrine organ because it secrets hormones, two of which are **insulin** and **glucagon**. These two hormones regulate **glucose** transport, storage, and metabolism. They are secreted by pancreatic **islet cells** located in the **islets of Langerhans**.

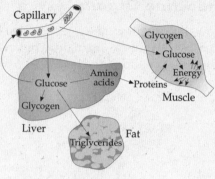

Insulin effects

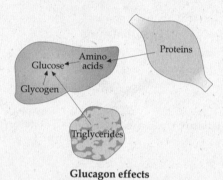

Glucagon effects

Pancreatic Enzymes

Figure 30.9

Glucose reaches the blood when it is ingested or produced by the liver and released to the blood. In the absence of insulin, all body cells—except those of the brain and liver—are relatively impermeable to glucose. Glucose in the blood tends to remain in the blood when insulin secretion is low. When insulin secretion is high, however, circulating glucose is taken up by the body cells, and the blood's glucose level is decreased. The cells that receive the glucose either store it or metabolize it to produce ATP. The student should note, once again, that *the brain takes up glucose from the blood whether or not insulin is secreted.* When the liver takes up glucose, it converts large quantities of it to **glycogen**, a long carbohydrate molecule that serves to store glucose.

The student should recall that insulin secretion: (1) increases cellular uptake of glucose; (2) promotes formation of glycogen from glucose in the liver; and (3) reduces glucose concentration in the blood.

Glucagon has effects that are opposite to the second and third of the effects just listed: it promotes the **breakdown** of glycogen in the liver, through a process termed **glycogenolysis**. The breakdown of glycogen produces glucose, which is, in turn, released into the blood. Glucagon also promotes the manufacture of glucose in the liver through a process termed **gluconeogenesis**. Gluconeogenesis involves the synthesis of glucose—not from glycogen, but from lactate, amino acids, and triglycerides. This newly formed glucose is also released into the blood. The most easily detectable effect of glucagon, therefore, is to increase the blood's glucose levels. You should note, however, that glucagon does not have effects opposite to the first of those listed above: it does *not decrease* cellular uptake of glucose.

In the service of homeostasis, a high blood glucose level normally stimulates the secretion of insulin. The insulin causes the body cells to take up glucose and thus lowers the blood glucose level. A low blood glucose level tends to decrease insulin secretion and to raise glucagon secretion. The increased glucagon secretion causes the release of glucose from the liver and raises the blood glucose level.

Hyperglycemia refers to excessively high levels of glucose in the blood and is typically due to diminished insulin secretion or activity. **Hypoglycemia** refers to excessively low levels of glucose in the blood and may result from elevated levels of insulin or insufficient glucagon levels in the body.

Please solve this problem:

- Which of the following is a pair of hormones secreted by the pancreas?

  A. Glycogen and glucose
  B. Insulin and glycogen
  C. Insulin and glucagon
  D. Amylase and lipase

Problem solved:

C is the correct answer. Insulin and glucagon are two of the endocrine hormones secreted by the "endocrine" pancreas into the blood; the "exocrine" pancreas, in contrast, secretes digestive enzymes, including amylase and lipase, directly into the digestive tract via ducts.

Please solve this problem:

- If a patient were to lose consciousness because his blood levels of glucose were low and his brain was receiving an inadequate supply of fuel, which of the following would be the best treatment?

  A. Administration of insulin
  B. Administration of glucagon
  C. Administration of glycogen
  D. Administration of oxygen

Problem solved:

B is the correct answer. The patient has fallen unconscious because his brain has no source of glucose, which it needs to produce ATP, its energy "currency." In order to supply the brain with glucose, the physician must raise the glucose levels of the blood. Administration of glucagon will cause the liver to release glucose into the blood and thus make it available to the brain. The physician should not administer insulin, which would worsen the patient's condition. Insulin tends to promote the uptake of glucose by all bodily cells, lowering blood glucose levels even further. (The condition described in the question often arises in diabetics who have received too much exogenous insulin.)

Please solve this problem:

- Among the following choices, which is most likely to produce hyperglycemia ?

    A. A hepatic condition in which gluconeogenesis is impaired

    B. A hepatic condition in which glucagon fails to exert its effects

    C. A pancreatic condition in which glucagon is not secreted

    D. A pancreatic condition in which insulin is not secreted

Problem solved:

D is the correct answer. Hyperglycemia refers to excessive quantities of glucose in the blood. It is caused by either excessive secretion of glucagon or impaired secretion of insulin. In most cases, it is produced by impaired secretion of insulin, as in diabetes mellitus Type I. If gluconeogenesis were impaired, as is suggested in Choice A, one potential source for blood glucose would be eliminated and blood glucose levels would, if anything, be reduced. The same is true for Choices B and C; suppression of glucagon function, by whatever means, would inhibit gluconeogenesis and glycogenolysis, thereby reducing blood glucose levels, if anything.

30.1.2.1.2 THE ADRENAL GLAND

An **adrenal gland** sits on each kidney; that is, humans have both a left and a right adrenal gland. Each gland has two distinct regions that are developmentally and functionally distinct. The two regions are related more in name than in function, and are termed the **adrenal cortex** and the **adrenal medulla**.

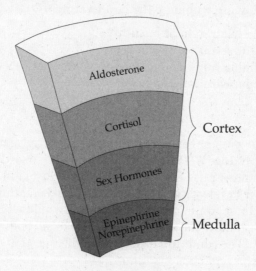

The Adrenal Gland

Figure 30.10

30.1.2.1.3 The Adrenal Cortex

The **adrenal cortex** comprises the outer portion of the adrenal gland. It produces a class of endocrine hormones called **corticosteroids**, subdivided into four groups: the **mineral corticoids**, the **glucocorticoids**, the **anabolic hormones**, and the **sex hormones**.

The mineral corticoids include **aldosterone**, which acts primarily at the distal convoluted tubule of the kidney to promote sodium-potassium exchange. Aldosterone increases the activity of sodium-potassium pumps, which remove three sodium ions from the renal filtrate for every two potassium ions it transports into the filtrate. In promoting an uneven exchange of sodium and potassium at the distal tubule, aldosterone increases the interstitial concentration of solutes, and so tends to promote the movement of water from tubule to interstitium. The ultimate effects of aldosterone are: (1) to increase urinary excretion of potassium; (2) to increase interstitial sodium concentration; and (3) to increase water conservation (as an effect secondary to the increase of insterstitial sodium concentration). As a result, it is not surprising that aldosterone secretion is stimulated by high levels of extracellular potassium, low levels of extracellular sodium, and low fluid levels (blood volume).

The glucocorticoids have a wide range of effects on many organ systems. One such effect is similar to that of glucagon: they increase blood glucose levels, especially in response to environmental stressors. The glucocorticoids also strengthen cardiac muscle contractions, increase water retention, and have anti-inflammatory and antiallergic activities.

30.1.2.1.4 The Adrenal Medulla

The adrenal medulla secretes two hormones: **epinephrine** and **norepinephrine**, together referred to as **catecholamines**. Epinephrine is known also as **adrenaline**, and norepinephrine as **noradrenaline**. Receptors for norepinephrine and epinephrine are widely distributed throughout the body. The hormones are normally released in very small quantities, and are largely reserved for stressful situations in which the body prepares for the so-called "fight or flight" response. Nerve impulses arriving at the adrenal medulla stimulate catecholamine release. There are several types of catecholamine receptors; each type differs in the nature of its response to catecholamine binding. In general, epinephrine and norepinephrine increase heart rate, raise blood pressure, and increase alertness.

30.1.2.1.5 The Thyroid and Parathyroid Glands

The **thyroid** is a flat gland located in the neck, in front of the larynx. Most cells of the body have receptors for **thyroxine** (thyroid hormone, T_4), or for its analog, **triiodothyronine** (thyroid hormone, T_3), both of which are synthesized in the follicles of the thyroid gland. (Thyroxine contains four molecules of iodine, while triiodothyronine contains three molecules of iodine.) Thyroid hormone produces a generalized increase in metabolism throughout the body. More specifically, thyroid hormone stimulates increased oxygen demand and heat production, as well as growth and development.

Hypothyroidism refers to an inadequate production of thyroid hormone. The hypothyroid patient tends to be overweight and slowed down in physical (and sometimes mental) activities. Although rare in areas where modern medicine is available, **cretinism** arises from a deficiency of thyroid hormone in the first six months of life.

Thyroid hormone requires iodine. Insufficient dietary iodine intake produces a decrease in thyroid hormone production. A feedback mechanism stimulates the thyroid to increase its function and, as a result, the thyroid undergoes excessive growth (hypertrophy), producing the condition known as **goiter**. Goiter manifests as a large prominence in the anterior aspect of the neck. The prominence is the overgrown thyroid itself.

Calcitonin is produced in the **parafollicular cells** of the thyroid. Although its importance in the body is not fully understood, calcitonin administered therapeutically reduces blood calcium concentration and inhibits the normal process of bone resorption.

The **parathyroids** are a set of four small glands located on the posterior aspect of the thyroid gland. **Parathyroid hormone**, or **parathormone**, exerts effects opposite to those of calcitonin. Through actions on various organs, parathyroid hormone increases levels of blood calcium. It acts to (1) increase bone resorption and consequent calcium release; (2) increase intestinal calcium uptake; and (3) promote calcium reuptake at the kidney. It is secreted in response to low blood levels of calcium.

30.1.2.1.6 THE ANTERIOR PITUITARY

Central control of the individual endocrine glands described above is provided by neural input from both the hypothalamus and the anterior pituitary, which are also endocrine organs. The hypothalamus serves as a high-level coordinating and regulating center for both the endocrine system and the autonomic nervous system. It integrates a variety of information from the **cerebral cortex** and **limbic systems**, and regulates output from the **pituitary glands**.

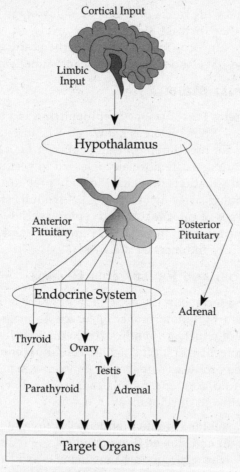

Position of the Pituitary Glands
in the Endocrine Pathway

Figure 30.11

The **pituitary gland** is a small structure on the underside of the brain. The anterior pituitary secretes a number of regulating hormones that act as "chemical switches," stimulating or inhibiting other endocrine glands. One such regulatory hormone released by the anterior pituitary is **thyroid-stimulating hormone (TSH)**. TSH stimulates the thyroid gland to secrete thyroid hormone. Release of TSH is, in turn, governed by the hypothalamus through its secretion of **thyrotropin-releasing hormone (TRH)**. TRH acts on the anterior pituitary to stimulate TSH secretion.

The anterior pituitary also controls secretion of glucocorticoids by the adrenal cortex through the action of **adrenocorticotropic hormone (ACTH)**. Released into the circulation by the pituitary, ACTH stimulates adrenocortical secretion of cortisol. The hypothalamus plays a role in the secretion of ACTH through secretion of **corticotropin-releasing hormone (CRH)**, which stimulates the pituitary to secrete ACTH.

In addition to hormones that regulate the release of other hormones at a distant gland, the anterior pituitary secrets other hormones that interact directly with certain target organs. Two such hormones are **growth hormone** (or **somatotropin**, **STH**), and **prolactin**. Growth hormone influences the development of skeletal muscle, bone, and organs in infants and children. Without growth hormone, children fail to develop normally. Prolactin directly targets the female breasts, where it stimulates breast development and milk production. The anterior pituitary also secretes hormones involved in the menstrual cycle.

Please solve this problem:

- Which of the following would most likely be observed in a patient who secretes excessive quantities of thyroid hormone?

  A. Decreased cellular uptake of oxygen
  B. Decreased cellular uptake of glucose
  C. Increased cellular production of carbon dioxide and water
  D. Increased blood pH

Problem solved:

C is the correct answer. Thyroid hormone acts to increase metabolic rate—to increase the rate at which cells burn fuel. The patient who secretes excessive quantities of thyroid hormone is hypermetabolic: he burns fuel at a greater rate than normal. The burning of fuel produces carbon dioxide and water, since in aerobic respiration oxygen serves as the ultimate oxidizing agent (electron acceptor). The increased metabolic rate would likely be associated with an increase—not a decrease—in uptake of oxygen and glucose. Hyperthyroidism does not ordinarily affect blood pH. Any tendency it might have to do so, however, would bring about a decrease, not an increase, in pH. The increased production of carbon dioxide would promote increased formation of carbonic acid, which, on dissociation, reduces pH (increases hydrogen ion concentration).

Please solve this problem:

- A tumor that secretes aldosterone would most likely lead to:

    A. an increased concentration of potassium in the urine.
    B. an increased concentration of potassium in the blood.
    C. an increased urinary output.
    D. a decreased metabolic rate.

Problem solved:

A is the correct answer. Tumors commonly secrete hormones—often in an unpredictable and uncontrollable fashion. These hormones produce effects normally associated with the particular hormones. Aldosterone promotes an exchange of sodium and potassium ions between the distal tubular filtrate and the surrounding interstitium: potassium moves into the tubular filtrate, to be excreted in the urine; and sodium moves out of the tubule, producing increased sodium concentration in the interstitium and a relative increase in the amount of water reabsorbed from the tubules. Aldosterone (a) increases urinary potassium concentration, (b) decreases extracellular potassium concentration, (c) decreases urinary sodium concentration, (d) increases extracellular sodium concentration, (e) decreases the volume of urine, and (f) increases bodily blood and bodily fluid volume.

Please solve this problem:

- An impairment of parathyroid hormone secretion will lead to:

    A. depletion of bone.
    B. an increased sodium concentration in the blood.
    C. a decreased calcium concentration in the blood.
    D. a decreased metabolic rate.

Problem solved:

C is the correct answer. Parathyroid hormone increases calcium concentration in the blood by promoting (a) resorption of bone (which releases calcium into the blood), (b) calcium absorption in the digestive tract, and (c) calcium reabsorption in the kidney. A deficiency of parathyroid hormone will lead to a decreased calcium concentration in the blood.

Please solve this problem:

- The hypothalamus affects secretion of corticosteroids by releasing:

    A. enzymes that catalyze secretory reactions in the adrenal cortex.
    B. catecholamines.
    C. thyroid releasing hormone.
    D. corticotropin releasing hormone (CRH).

Problem solved:

D is the correct answer. Corticosteroids are released from the adrenal cortex, which is stimulated by adrenocorticotropic hormone (ACTH) released from the anterior pituitary. The anterior pituitary releases ACTH in response to the release of CRH from the hypothalamus.

Please solve this problem:

- The adrenal medulla releases:

    A. insulin and glucagon.
    B. epinephrine and norepinephrine.
    C. glucocorticoids, mineral corticoids, anabolic hormones, and sex hormones.
    D. aldosterone.

Problem solved:

B is the correct answer. Functionally, the adrenal medulla and the adrenal cortex are two separate endocrine glands; anatomically they are adjoined. The cortex (not the medulla) secretes corticosteroids, which include: the mineralocorticoids (aldosterone, for example); the glucocorticoids (cortisol, for example); the anabolic hormones; and the sex hormones. The adrenal medulla releases epinephrine (adrenaline) and norepinephrine (noradrenaline). Insulin and glucagon are secreted by the pancreas, not the adrenal gland.

30.1.2.1.7 THE POSTERIOR PITUITARY

The two hormones secreted by the posterior pituitary are **antidiuretic hormone** (**ADH**, or **vasopressin**), whose function has been discussed in connection with the kidney, and **oxytocin**, which is released at childbirth (parturition), causing the uterus to contract and push the fetus through the birth canal. Both ADH and oxytocin are *synthesized* in the hypothalamus and *stored* in the posterior pituitary, from which they are released directly into the bloodstream as needed.

30.1.2.2 Hormonal Regulation of the Menstrual Cycle

The **menstrual cycle** is a series of hormonally-induced events that prepare the woman's body for pregnancy. Typically, the cycle takes 28 days to complete, with the first day of menstrual bleeding conventionally recognized as Day 1 of the cycle.

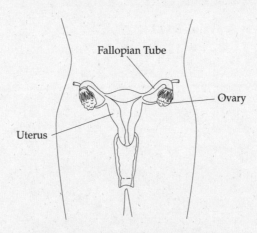

The Female Reproductive Organs

Figure 30.12

30.1.2.2.1 THE FOLLICULAR PHASE

The first phase of the menstrual cycle begins around day 5, after the onset of menstrual bleeding, and is known as the **follicular phase**, or **proliferative phase**, owing its name to the rapid growth of the **ovarian follicle**. During this phase, the anterior pituitary gland secretes two hormones which stimulate the growth of one follicle containing several ova, only one of which fully matures. The two follicular hormones are **follicle stimulating hormone (FSH)** and **luteinizing hormone (LH)**. The follicle itself is secretory, releasing **estrogen** as it develops. The follicular phase ranges from seven to twenty-one days. Increased ovarian **estrogen** release prevents maturation of more than one follicle at a time.

30.1.2.2.2 THE LUTEAL SURGE AND OVULATION

At the end of the follicular stage (which occurs on or about day 14), there is a surge in LH secretion from the anterior pituitary. This surge causes the release of the ovum from the enlarged follicle into the fallopian tube. The release of the ovum from the follicle is known as **ovulation**.

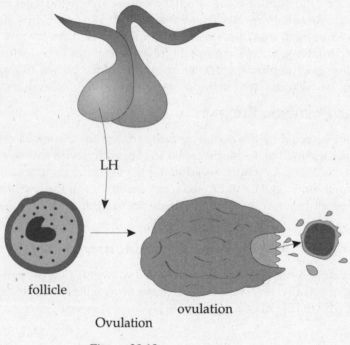

LH

follicle

ovulation

Ovulation

Figure 30.13

30.1.2.2.3 THE ROLE OF ESTROGEN AND PROGESTERONE

After ovulation, the ruptured follicle—which remains in the ovary—is referred to as the **corpus luteum**. The corpus luteum secretes estrogen and progesterone. Progesterone promotes the rapid thickening and vascularization of the uterine lining in preparation for the implantation of a fertilized ovum.

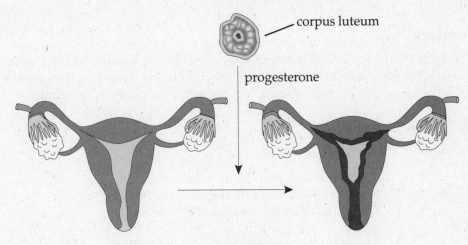

corpus luteum

progesterone

Luteal Phase

Figure 30.14

30.1.2.2.4 UTERINE SHEDDING

If the mature ovum is not fertilized, it will not implant into the uterine lining. At approximately thirteen days after ovulation (day 27 of the cycle), the corpus luteum degenerates and ceases to secrete estrogen and progesterone. With progesterone no longer available to maintain the thickened uterine lining, the lining begins to slough off the uterine wall. This causes severing of the newly formed vasculature and the bleeding that is characteristic of human menstruation. After an average of five days, the shedding of the uterine lining is complete, and a new proliferative phase begins.

If the ovum is fertilized (which would occur on or about day 14), the developing placenta begins to secrete human chorionic gonadotropin (HCG). HCG prevents the corpus luteum from degenerating, allowing it to continue secreting progesterone. This maintains the integrity of the uterine lining and allows the pregnancy to continue. Before the end of the first month of pregnancy, the placenta begins to secrete estrogen and progesterone and the corpus luteum degenerates. These hormones are secreted at continuously increasing levels throughout pregnancy.

Please solve this problem:

- Follicle stimulating hormone (FSH) is secreted by:

    A. the hypothalamus.
    B. the follicular cells.
    C. the ovaries.
    D. the anterior pituitary gland.

Problem solved:

D is the correct answer. Follicle stimulating hormone (FSH) is secreted by the anterior pituitary gland. Together with luteinizing hormone (LH), also secreted by the anterior pituitary, FSH stimulates one follicle to develop, ultimately to produce an ovum.

Please solve this problem:

- The luteal surge causes:

    A. sudden shedding of the uterine lining.
    B. release of the ovum into the oviduct.
    C. implantation of a fertilized ovum in the uterus.
    D. the second meiotic division of a secondary oocyte.

Problem solved:

B is the correct answer. The phrase "luteal surge" refers to a sudden increase in the secretion of luteinizing hormone (LH) from the anterior pituitary; this event is associated with the release of an ovum (a haploid cell produced by the first meiotic division of the primary oocyte) into the oviduct (the fallopian tube). If the ovum encounters a sperm in the oviduct, it will undergo fertilization. If it does not undergo fertilization, then after approximately fourteen days, the corpus luteum (the remains of the follicle from which the ovum was released) ceases to produce estrogen and progesterone, and the uterine lining is shed. If the ovum is fertilized, it implants in the uterus.

Please solve this problem:

- Which of the following correctly characterizes the corpus luteum?

    A. It secretes estrogen and progesterone.
    B. It undergoes meiosis.
    C. It is located in the uterine lining.
    D. It is non-secretory.

Problem solved:

A is the correct answer. The corpus luteum is the remnant of the ruptured follicle after ovulation occurs. Its cells secrete estrogen and progesterone. The secretion of progesterone promotes growth of the uterus and prepares it for implantation. If implantation does not occur, the corpus luteum ceases to secrete estrogen and progesterone. The uterine lining then begins to deteriorate and menstrual bleeding begins.

Please solve this problem:

- Name the hormones that control the female menstrual cycle and describe their functions.

Problem solved:

FSH, LH, and estrogen are secreted during the follicular phase; estrogen and progesterone are secreted from the corpus luteum for approximately two weeks following ovulation. Upon fertilization and implantation, human chorionic gonadotropin (HCG) is secreted from the developing placenta, and stimulates the corpus luteum to continue progesterone and estrogen secretion. In the absence of implantation and the consequent absence of placental HCG, the corpus luteum degenerates, and its hormonal secretion terminates. Without progesterone, the endometrial lining deteriorates. Menstrual bleeding follows. Also, in response to the post-luteal fall in circulating levels of estrogen and progesterone, FSH production rises, initiating a new proliferative phase.

30.1.2.3 The Testes

30.1.2.3.1 STRUCTURAL FEATURES

Each **testis** contains the specialized reproductive organs, called **seminiferous tubules**, which contain **spermatogonia**, the precursors of spermatozoa formation. The interstitial cells, situated among the twisted seminiferous tubules, secrete **testosterone** under the stimulus of pituitary LH (also called **interstitial cell stimulating hormone**, **ICSH**, in mature males). This predominantly male sex hormone does not become plentiful until puberty. Like the other endocrine hormones, testosterone is secreted into the bloodstream and comes into contact with all parts of the body.

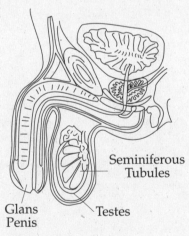

Seminiferous Tubules

Glans Penis

Testes

Male Reproductive System

Figure 30.15

30.1.2.3.2 ROLE OF TESTOSTERONE

Testosterone serves diverse functions. In the testes, its principal role is to promote **spermatogenesis**, the division of spermatogonia cells within the seminiferous tubules to produce haploid spermatozoa (see Chapter 25). Testosterone also promotes the development of secondary sex characteristics, which in adolescent males include: deepening of the voice; growth of facial, axillary, and pubic hair; and enlargement of the penis and scrotum.

Please solve this problem:

- Which of the following would most likely result from impaired secretion of testosterone in the mature male?

  A. degeneration of the testes
  B. sudden and pronounced feminization
  C. absence of gamete production
  D. increased metabolic rate

Problem solved:

C is the correct answer. Testosterone promotes spermatogenesis in the seminiferous tubules, leading to production of spermatozoa, or the male gametes. If testosterone secretion is impaired, the gametes will not be produced. Sudden and pronounced feminization does not accompany impaired testosterone secretion in a mature male. (A degree of feminization may be achieved in the mature male by exogenous administration of female sex hormones.) The testes do not degenerate in the absence of testosterone. The metabolic rate bears no direct connection to testosterone secretion.

30.1.3 THE NERVOUS SYSTEM

30.1.3.1 The Anatomy of the Nervous System

The human nervous system is comprised of two principal divisions: the **central nervous system (CNS)** and the **peripheral nervous system (PNS)**.

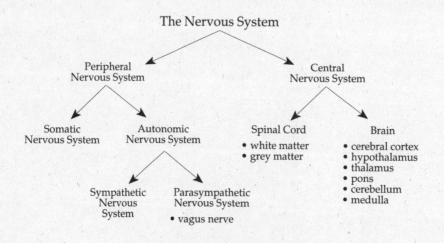

The Divisions and Subdivisions
of the Nervous System

Figure 30.16

The central nervous system consists of all neurons and neuronal connections within, among, and between the brain and spinal cord. The peripheral nervous system consists of all neurons and neuronal connections lying outside the brain and spinal cord. You should understand, however, that the dichotomy between the central and peripheral nervous systems is somewhat artificial. In fact, the two systems are fully adjoined.

30.1.3.2 The Central Nervous System

30.1.3.2.1 THE BRAIN

During embryonic development the anterior section of the **neural tube** gives rise to the brain, and the posterior portion forms the spinal cord. The brain and spinal cord are connected and in communication with one another. Together, they form the central nervous system. Both components of the CNS—brain and spinal cord—are protected by layers of connective tissue (the **meninges**), bone, and circulating **cerebrospinal fluid (CSF)** that acts as a liquid shock absorber.

The embryonic precursors of adult brain structures are the **forebrain**, the **midbrain**, and the **hindbrain**. From the forebrain arise the **cerebral cortex**, the **thalamus**, and the **hypothalamus**. The midbrain gives rise to structures which govern visual and auditory reflexes and coordinate information on posture and muscle tone. The hindbrain becomes the **cerebellum**, the **pons**, and the **medulla**.

The **cerebrum** (not to be confused with the cerebellum) is composed of **two hemispheres** divided by a **longitudinal fissure**; it is the largest portion of the human brain. The cerebral cortex is readily observable as an outer layer of **gray matter** overlying the cerebrum. The gray matter of the cerebral cortex contains neuronal cell bodies which conduct the highest of intellectual functions. It integrates and interprets sensory signals of all kinds. The size of the cerebral cortex in humans is unparalleled by that of any other species. This quantity of cortical material correlates with the highly developed functions of language and cognition that distinguish humans from other species. The student should note that the cerebral cortex also governs voluntary motor activity.

Situated on the underside of the brain is the hypothalamus, which maintains homeostasis through hormonal regulation. Posterior to the hypothalamus is the thalamus, which relays information between the spinal cord and the cerebral cortex. The pons serves to connect the spinal cord and medulla with upper regions of the brain. The cerebellum is responsible for posture, muscle tone, and spatial equilibrium. Connected to the pons above and to the spinal cord below, the medulla exerts regulatory control over involuntary processes such as heart rate, respiration, blood pressure, and reflex reactions like coughing.

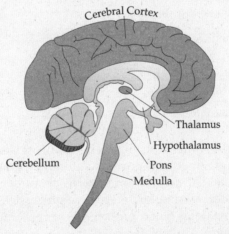

Basic Structures of Brain (Midline View)

Figure 30.17

Please solve this problem:

- A patient who shows loss of balance and inability to perform tasks that call for rapid and refined coordination of musculature most likely suffers from dysfunction at which of the following sites?

    A. Cerebellum
    B. Corpus callosum
    C. Medulla
    D. Hypothalamus

Problem solved:

A is the correct answer. The cerebellum controls such functions as balance and the ability to perform tasks that call for rapid and refined coordination of musculature. (Sewing and piano playing are examples of such activity.)

Please solve this problem:

- A patient who shows loss of ability to think abstractly most likely has a lesion affecting the:

    A. cerebral cortex.
    B. hypothalamus.
    C. thalamus.
    D. spinal cord.

Problem solved:

A is the correct answer. The processes of abstract thought are most closely associated with the cerebral cortex. A grossly observable loss in that regard is almost certainly associated with a lesion of the cerebral cortex.

Please solve this problem:

- In humans, appetite and body temperature are under the control of the:

    A. cerebellum.
    B. cerebrum.
    C. medulla.
    D. hypothalamus.

Problem solved:

D is the correct answer. The hypothalamus maintains homeostasis, adjusting body temperature, fluid balance, and appetite. It governs autonomic functions and links the endocrine and nervous systems. The cerebellum governs posture, muscle tone, and equilibrium. The cerebrum controls complex integrative processes, such as learning, memory, and reasoning. The medulla regulates blood pressure, heart beat, and respiration, and controls reflex activity, such as sneezing.

30.1.3.2.2 THE SPINAL CORD

The spinal cord governs simple motor reflexes. It relays information from other sites of the body to the brain, and from the brain to other sites of the body. The interior of the spinal cord contains **gray matter**, which is composed of cell bodies of spinal cord neurons. The exterior is composed of **white matter**, or **myelinated** spinal cord axons. White matter derives its name from the pale appearance of **myelin**, which insulates the axons.

Please solve this problem:

- The phrase "gray matter" refers to:

    A. the substance of the cerebral cortex.
    B. the substance of the spinal cord.
    C. neuronal axons within the central nervous system.
    D. neuronal cell bodies within the central nervous system.

Problem solved:

D is the correct answer. As it happens, the cell bodies of most neurons within the central nervous system have a grayish appearance on gross inspection. Within brain and spinal cord alike, the gray matter refers, generally, to the cell bodies of the enormous numbers of neurons that are situated there. White matter refers to the myelinated axons of these neurons.

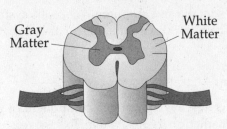

Cross Section of a Spinal Cord
Showing White and Gray Matter

Figure 30.18

30.1.3.2.3 THE PERIPHERAL NERVOUS SYSTEM

The peripheral nervous system (PNS) is divided into the **somatic nervous system** and the **autonomic nervous system**. The somatic nervous system governs voluntary activities, sending motor fibers to skeletal muscle. The autonomic nervous system controls involuntary actions, such as those of the digestive, respiratory, circulatory, and excretory systems. Its constituent neuronal components are the **sensory receptors** and the **cranial** and **spinal nerves**.

30.1.3.2.4 THE AUTONOMIC NERVOUS SYSTEM: SYMPATHETIC AND PARASYMPATHETIC SUBDIVISIONS

The autonomic nervous system has two subdivisions: the **parasympathetic nervous system** and the **sympathetic nervous system**. Many organs are innervated by both of these systems, which exert opposing effects. Cardiac muscle, smooth muscle, and the endocrine glands are innervated by the autonomic nervous system.

The sympathetic nervous system prepares the body for the "fight or flight" response, for example, in times of crisis. When activated, it increases heart rate and blood pressure, and *inhibits*, temporarily, the **vegetative functions**, like gastrointestinal motility and digestive secretion. In contrast, the parasympathetic nervous system decreases the heart rate and increases digestive activity. Note that the **vagus nerve** sends parasympathetic innervation to the thoracic and abdominal regions.

Please solve this problem:

- Which of the following statements is false?

    A. The parasympathetic and sympathetic nervous systems are subdivisions of the autonomic nervous system.
    B. The somatic and the autonomic nervous systems are subdivisions of the sympathetic nervous system.
    C. The spinal cord and the brain are constituents of the central nervous system.
    D. The peripheral and the central nervous systems constitute the two broad divisions of the nervous system.

Problem solved:

B is the correct answer. The somatic and autonomic nervous systems are subdivisions of the peripheral nervous system. The other three statements characterizing the subdivisions of the nervous system are accurate.

Please solve this problem:

- The vagus nerve is a principal component of the parasympathetic nervous system. Excessive activity of the vagus nerve would most likely produce:

    A. high heart rate and blood pressure.
    B. an impaired cough and gag reflex.
    C. failure of the stomach to secrete hydrochloric acid.
    D. abdominal cramping and diarrhea.

Problem solved:

D is the correct answer. The parasympathetic and sympathetic nervous systems are components of the autonomic nervous system. The sympathetic system mediates the so-called "fight or flight" response, tending to increase heart rate and blood pressure. The parasympathetic system controls such functions as coughing, gagging, digestion, and parturition. Hyperactivity of the vagus nerve would be expected to enhance motility of the digestive tract, producing abdominal cramping and diarrhea. Choices B and C describe what would be expected with *deficient* activity of the vagus nerve.

30.1.3.3 The Neuron

Nerves, **ganglia**, and the brain are composed of clusters of nerve cells. **Afferent nerves** transmit nerve impulses to the CNS, and **efferent nerves** conduct impulses from the CNS to the muscles or glands.

30.1.3.3.1 ASSOCIATED STRUCTURES AND FUNCTIONS

The **neuron**, or nerve cell, is the fundamental cellular unit of the nervous system. In addition to the organelles normally found in eukaryotic cells, the neuron contains a number of unique organelles specialized for the transmission of electrical impulses. Cytoplasmic extensions of the cell, called **dendrites**, act like antennae, or sensors: they receive stimuli. A single, elongated cytoplasmic extension, known as the **axon** (or nerve fiber), is specialized to transmit signals. The distal end of the axon bears small extensions called **synaptic knobs**, which contain **synaptic vesicles**. The synaptic vesicles store **neurotransmitters**, the molecules that transmit chemical signals from one neuron to the next. In some situations, a neurotransmitter will exert an excitatory effect on a neuron, while in others it will have have an inhibitory effect.

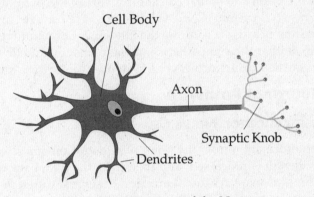

Specialized Features of the Neuron

Figure 30.19

Please solve this problem:

- If two neurons communicate in series, then the signal from one neuron reaches the other neuron via:

    A. direct contact between synaptic knobs.

    B. direct contact between axons of the first neuron and dendrites of the second neuron.

    C. release of a chemical by the first neuron and its receipt by the second neuron.

    D. direct contact between each neuron and an interneuron.

Problem solved:

C is the correct answer. One neuron relays its message to the next by releasing a chemical messenger, called a neurotransmitter, from synaptic vesicles. Direct contact is *not* a means of communication between two neurons. Rather, the neurotransmitter is released from the axon's synaptic knob into the synaptic space, and is taken up by receptors on the second neuron's surface.

Please solve this problem:

- A given neuron emanates from the spinal cord and synapses directly with a skeletal muscle cell. Which of the following correctly characterizes the neuron?

  A. It is an efferent neuron.
  B. It is an afferent neuron.
  C. It belongs to the sympathetic nervous system.
  D. It belongs to the parasympathetic nervous system.

Problem solved:

A is the correct answer. If a neuron conducts its impulse from the central nervous system to the periphery (a skeletal muscle, for example) it is an efferent, or effector, neuron. (An afferent neuron conducts its impulse toward the central nervous system.) Because the neuron lies, for the most part, outside the brain and spinal cord, it is a part of the peripheral nervous system (PNS), not the central nervous system (CNS). It belongs to the somatic, and not to the autonomic, nervous system because it controls the movement of voluntary (skeletal) muscle. Therefore, it belongs to neither the sympathetic nor the parasympathetic system, both of which are components of the autonomic nervous system.

30.1.3.4 The Neuronal Pathway

30.1.3.4.1 CLASSIFICATION OF NERVE CELL TYPES

The transmission of information from the point of registration of a stimulus at one site of the body to the CNS, where it is processed, and then from the CNS back to the site of the body that responds to the stimulus, requires the interaction of several different types of neurons. **Sensory receptor cells** register a given stimulus, such as a smell or a sound. **Sensory neurons** (also called afferent neurons) receive information from the sensory receptors and send it to the central nervous system, where one or more **interneurons** receive and process the information. In some cases, such as olfactory transduction, the receptor is a modified part of the sensory neuron itself. **Motor neurons** (also called **effector** or **efferent** neurons) convey signals from the central nervous system to the target muscle or gland. Interneurons (also called **associative neurons**) relay signals from neuron to neuron.

30.1.3.4.2 THE SIMPLE REFLEX ARC

A **simple reflex arc**—like the Achilles reflex or a patellar reflex (knee-jerk response)—requires two neurons. In the course of either one of the simple reflex arcs mentioned, a tap on the tendon stretches the attached muscle fibers. Specialized endings of affector (or sensory) neurons, called **stretch receptors**, are wrapped around individual muscle fibers, and register the tap-induced fiber stretch. The sensory neuron synapses with the dendrites of a motor neuron, which then sends an axonal impulse to the muscle fiber bundle. The motor neuron's impulse causes the release of the neurotransmitter **acetylcholine** at the site where the neuron synapses with the muscle (the **neuromuscular junction**). The acetylcholine release begins the series of steps culminating in muscle fiber contraction.

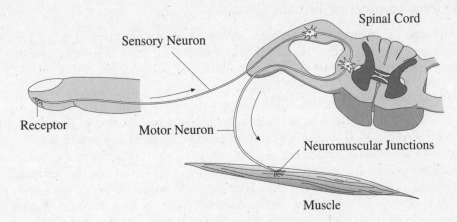

Anatomical Basis of Simple Reflex Arc

Figure 30.20

Please solve this problem:

- Cite the components involved in the Achilles reflex and describe their respective functions.

Problem solved:

A simple reflex arc is a monosynaptic reflex requiring sensory receptors, a sensory neuron, and a motor neuron. Tapping on a muscle's tendon with a mallet will cause its fibers to stretch. The stretch of the fibers is registered by sensory neuron stretch receptors located on the muscle. The neuron transmits the stretch signal to the central nervous system (spinal cord), where it synapses with a motor neuron. The motor neuron then transmits its signal back to the muscle, releasing acetylcholine at the neuromuscular junction and causing the muscle to contract.

Please solve this problem:

- Which of the following is not normally a component of a simple reflex arc?

  A. An efferent neuron
  B. An afferent neuron
  C. An interneuron
  D. The peripheral nervous system

Problem solved:

C is the correct answer. As noted in the text, a simple reflex arc (like the patellar response or the Achilles response) involves one afferent (affector) neuron, with specialized receptors at its dendritic end, and one efferent neuron, which synapses with the afferent neuron in the spinal cord. It does not involve any interneurons (associative neurons). Since the important parts of this pathway lie outside the brain and spinal cord, the simple reflex arc is said to belong to the peripheral nervous system.

30.1.3.5 PROPAGATION OF NEURAL IMPULSES

If a neuron receives a stimulus of sufficient strength, an action potential is created in the neuron. An action potential is the "signal" that is transmitted from neuron to neuron, carrying information from one part of the body to another.

30.1.3.5.1 THE RESTING POTENTIAL

Across the cell membrane of an axon, there is an uneven distribution of ions, created and maintained by the ATP-fueled sodium-potassium pump. Through the action of this pump, three sodium ions are pumped out of the cell for every two potassium ions that are pumped in. This creates several gradients: the excess of positive charges outside the cell relative to the inside gives rise to a charge gradient of approximately –70 millivolts (mV); the excess of sodium ions outside the cell relative to the inside gives rise to a concentration gradient, as does the excess of potassium ions inside the cell relative to the outside. In addition, the cell membrane is slightly permeable to potassium, allowing some ions to leak out of the cell and further contributing to the charge gradient. The membrane is impermeable to sodium.

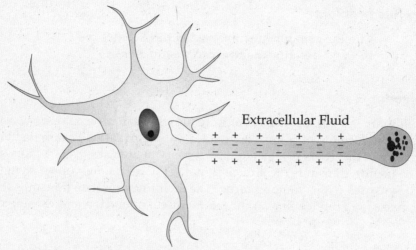

Extracellular Fluid

The Interior of a Resting Neuron is Negative Relative to its Exterior

Figure 30.21

Please solve this problem:

- A resting neuron may have which of the following eletrical potentials across its membrane?

    A.   0 mV
    B. +50 mV
    C. +20 mV
    D. –70 mV

Problem solved:

D is the correct answer. The relative excess of positive charges outside the cell compared to the inside (as a result of the action of the sodium-potassium pump) gives rise to a negative electrical potential across the membrane (as measured from the inside of the cell).

Please solve this problem:

- Which of the following correctly characterizes a neuron's resting potential?

  A. It is maintained by passive diffusion.
  B. It is maintained by an ATP-dependent mechanism.
  C. It creates a relative negative charge outside the neuronal membrane.
  D. It is attributable to a transmembrane calcium imbalance.

Problem solved:

B is the correct answer. The neuron's resting potential is maintained by an uneven distribution of cations across the membrane. The uneven distribution is not a stable situation, since passive diffusion tends to eliminate electrical and chemical gradients. Rather, the cell must expend energy to maintain it, which requires ATP.

30.1.3.5.2 THRESHOLD

The signal received at the dendrites slightly decreases the electrical polarity of the neural membrane. This small voltage change causes a few **voltage-gated sodium channels** to open. Sodium enters the cell, further reducing the membrane potential. However, in order to initiate a neuronal response—i.e., to achieve an **action potential**—the signal must be sufficiently intense. The neuronal response is termed "all-or-none": while the stimulus can be incremental, the neuron either responds with an action potential or does not fire at all. The stimulus intensity required to set off an action potential is called the **threshold** level.

30.1.3.5.3 DEPOLARIZATION

Once the threshold level of stimulation is exceeded, a series of events is triggered that are together called an **action potential**. The first event of the series is the opening of **voltage-gated channels** that are specific for sodium. As their name implies, they open in response to the change in voltage, or potential difference, across the cell membrane. Once these open, sodium rushes into the cell, down its concentration gradient. This causes the inside of the cell to become more positive; whereas the resting cell membrane potential is around –70 mV, the influx of sodium ions increases the potential to approximately +50 mV. The influx of sodium ions and the concomitant change in membrane potential is referred to as **depolarization.**

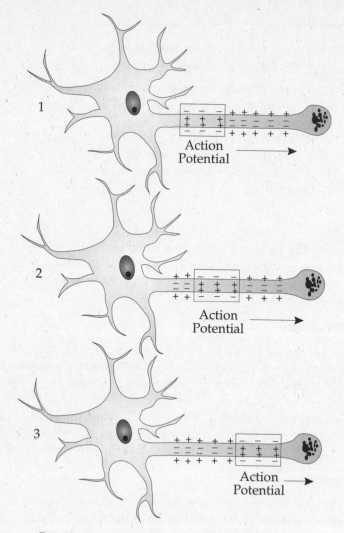

Propagation of a Nerve Impulse Along the Axon

Figure 30.22

30.1.3.5.4 REPOLARIZATION

When the cell membrane potential reaches its peak, at around +50 mV, the sodium voltage-gated channels close and other channels, also voltage-gated but specific for potassium, open, allowing potassium to rush out of the cell, down its concentration gradient. The loss of positive charge from the interior of the cell causes the membrane potential to become more negative. This part of the action potential is called **repolarization**.

Potassium efflux does not stop when the membrane potential reaches –70 mV, however. The potassium voltage-gated channels do not close until the cell potential is somewhat more negative than -70 mV. This phase of the action potential is called **hyperpolarization**. Once the potassium channels close, the action of the sodium-potassium pump, combined with the continued slight efflux of potassium, reestablishes the resting potential of –70 mV.

During and for a short time after an action potential, it is impossible to elicit a new action potential, no matter how strong the stimulus. This period is called the **absolute refractory period**. For a few milliseconds after the absolute refractory period, a period called the **relative refractory period**, an action potential will be initiated only if the stimulus is exceedingly strong.

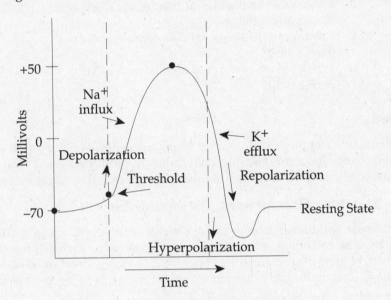

Principal Stages and Ion Flows
Associated with an Action Potential

Figure 30.23

Please solve this problem:

- Depolarization of the neuron starts with:

    A. active pumping of sodium inward across the neuronal cell membrane.
    B. a change in the neuronal membrane's potassium permeability.
    C. a change in the neuronal membrane's sodium permeability.
    D. a change in the neuronal membrane's calcium permeability.

Problem solved:

C is the correct answer. Depolarization begins when voltage-gated channels for sodium open, allowing sodium to rush into the cell down its concentration gradient.

Please solve this problem:

- Repolarization of the neuron is caused by:

    A. active pumping of sodium inward across the neuronal cell membrane.

    B. a change in the neuronal membrane's potassium permeability.

    C. a change in the neuronal membrane's sodium permeability.

    D. a change in the neuronal membrane's calcium permeability.

Problem solved:

B is the correct answer. Repolarization occurs when potassium voltage-gated channels open in response to the change in membrane potential caused by sodium influx. The loss of positive charge from the interior of the cell reestablishes the relative negative charge there.

30.1.3.5.5 SALTATORY CONDUCTION: THE MYELIN SHEATH

Certain neurons can conduct an impulse faster and more efficiently due to the **myelination** of their axons. **Schwann cells** encase long, discrete sections of the axons of neurons in the PNS by wrapping layers of their plasma membranes around the axon, creating **myelin sheaths**. Small areas of the axon remain unmyelinated at regular intervals along the axon's length. These unsheathed areas are called the **nodes of Ranvier**. The highly insulating properties of the Schwann cells serve to block transmission of the depolarizing nerve impulse where myelin sheaths cover the axon, leaving the exposed nodes of Ranvier as the only sites available for electrical propagation along the axon. It is not necessary, then, for depolarization to occur along the entire membrane, a process that would consume a relatively long period of time. Myelin insulation significantly accelerates the transmission of the impulse as depolarization jumps from one node of Ranvier to the next (**saltatory conduction**), effectively skipping across the long, insulated portions of the axon.

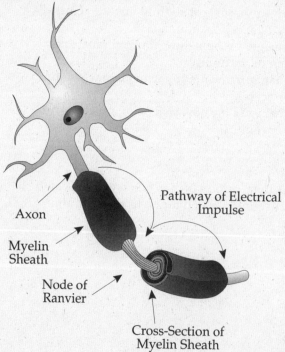

Myelinated Axon Showing Cross-Section of Schwann Cell Layers

Figure 30.24

Please solve this problem:

- Nodes of Ranvier are:

    A. exposed areas of axon that permit saltatory conduction.
    B. segments of axon that are encased in Schwann cells.
    C. insulated regions of a myelinated axon.
    D. sections of axon that contain a double membrane.

Problem solved:

A is the correct answer. The insulating properties of the myelin sheaths allow the nerve impulse to jump from one exposed node of Ranvier to the next, permitting more efficient and rapid propagation of the impulse.

Please solve this problem:

- The myelin sheath is composed of:

    A. a low molecular weight salt.
    B. a high molecular weight salt.
    C. the plasma membranes of Schwann cells.
    D. interneurons.

Problem solved:

C is the correct answer. The myelin sheath of the neurons in the PNS is composed of multiple wrapped layers of Schwann cells. It facilitates saltatory conduction, wherein an impulse jumps from one node of Ranvier to the next. The propagation along a myelinated neuron is much faster than that along an unmyelinated neuron.

30.1.3.5.6 IMPULSE TRANSMISSION AT THE SYNAPSE

Once the neural impulse arrives at the end of the axon, it triggers fusion of the synaptic vesicles with the terminal end of the axonal membrane, called the **presynaptic membrane**. This fusion causes release of neurotransmitters from the synaptic vesicles into the **synaptic cleft**—the space between the presynaptic membrane and the **postsynaptic membrane**. At the **synapse** the distance between the two neurons is minute enough to permit rapid diffusion of neurotransmitter from the first to the second neuron. Synaptic transmission transpires during a minimum interval of 0.5 ms (the **synaptic delay**), and ensures efficient communication of the neural signal across the synaptic cleft.

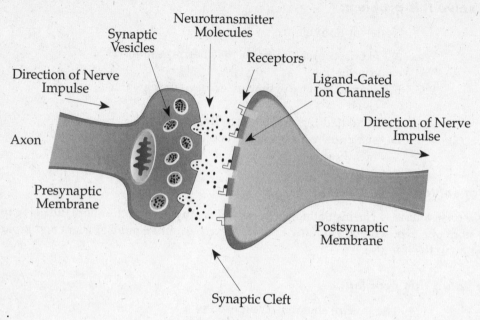

Figure 30.25

After neurotransmitters diffuse across the synaptic cleft, they bind to receptor molecules on the postsynaptic membrane. The membrane receptor molecules and neurotransmitters are specific for one another. Most postsynaptic receptors are **ligand-gated**, with specific neurotransmitters serving as ligands. Binding of the neurotransmitter to receptors at the postsynaptic membrane induces a conformational change in the receptors that opens ion channels within the membrane. The resulting influx of ions produces the electrical change that acts as a signal to the neuron. Relatively weak stimuli produce relatively weak signals: those signals that are below threshold level produce only small, localized depolarizations in the postsynaptic neuron (the "none" of the all-or-none reaction). A signal of sufficient strength to reach threshold level will initiate an action potential (the "all" of the all-or-none reaction).

The nervous system contains more than thirty different chemicals that act as neurotransmitters. One of these neurotransmitters, acetylcholine, triggers muscle contractions and is degraded by the enzyme **cholinesterase**. **Epinephrine** (adrenaline) increases heart rate and blood pressure and decreases metabolic activity, such as that of the smooth muscle of the digestive system. Epinephrine is oxidized and methylated to inactive metabolites by **monoamine oxidase** (**MAO**) and **catechol-O-methyl transferase** (**COMT**), respectively.

Please solve this problem:

- Which of the following statements does NOT accurately describe events associated with the neural impulse?

  A. Ligand-gated channels open upon binding of postsynaptic receptors with the appropriate neurotransmitter.
  B. Voltage-gated channels for sodium open in the course of an action potential, permitting efflux of sodium from the neuron.
  C. Voltage-gated channels for potassium open during repolarization, permitting efflux of potassium from the neuron.
  D. Both ligand-gated channels and voltage-gated channels are required for successful transmission of a nerve impulse from one neuron to the next.

Problem solved:

B is the correct answer. Voltage-gated sodium channels open during an action potential to allow influx of sodium ions down their concentration gradient. Each of the remaining options is an accurate statement of events occurring during neural transmission.

Please solve this problem:

- Acetylcholine serves as neurotransmitter at autonomic ganglia. What is the effect of acetylcholine on the postsynaptic membrane?

  A. It induces a change that ultimately renders the postsynaptic neuron more permeable to sodium.
  B. It renders the neuron more permeable to epinephrine and norepinephrine.
  C. It induces the production of synaptic knobs.
  D. It induces the production of synaptic vesicles.

Problem solved:

A is the correct answer. When a neurotransmitter (like acetylcholine) crosses the synaptic cleft and reaches the postsynaptic neuron, it initiates depolarization of the postsynaptic neuron (unless its stimulus is subthreshold). As a result, the postsynaptic neuron increases its permeability to sodium.

Please solve this problem:

- Which of the following would explain the failure of neurotransmitter to elicit an action potential in a postsynaptic neuron?

  A. The postsynaptic neuron has receptors specific to the neurotransmitter.
  B. The neurotransmitter produces a subthreshold response.
  C. The postsynaptic neuron has been facilitated.
  D. The postsynaptic neuron is an interneuron.

Problem solved:

B is the correct answer. Neuronal response to a stimulous is all-or-none. If a stimulus fails to reach a threshold, the neuron will not fire. Inadequate quantities of neurotransmitter or the prior inhibition of the neuron may prevent neurotransmitter from initiating depolarization. (Facilitation of the neuron would tend to reduce the stimulus necessary to bring about depolarization.) That the postsynaptic neuron should be an interneuron does not affect the dynamics just described. Interneurons, like other types of neurons, respond to stimuli in an all-or-none fashion.

30.1.4 THE SENSORY ORGANS

Humans can respond to five types of stimuli: **tactile (touch), olfactory (smell), gustatory (taste), auditory (hearing),** and **visual.** Sensory receptors provide the organism with crucial information about its environment. The sensory receptors convey information to the organism in the form of action potentials that carry the information to the central nervous system.

Mechanoreceptors include **stretch receptors, tactile receptors, proprioceptors** (which provide cues to changes in pressure or tension in muscles), and **auditory receptors.**

Chemoreceptors register taste and smell.

Thermoreceptors, electroreceptors, and **photoreceptors** respond to heat, electrical energy, and light energy, respectively.

Sensory receptors located in the olfactory epithelium of the nasal cavity detect odors.

The hair-like projections of the **taste receptors,** located in the taste buds, are sensitive to molecules in the mouth. The four basic types of gustatory receptors register **sourness, sweetness, saltiness,** and **bitterness.**

30.1.4.1 The Vestibular and Auditory Systems

The ear serves two distinct functions: (1) maintenance of postural equilibrium, and (2) reception of sound. There are three basic divisions of the ear—external, middle, and inner. The **inner ear** is the location of the **vestibular apparatus,** which interprets positional information required for maintaining equilibrium. The vestibular apparatus consists of a membranous **labyrinth** situated within the three **semicircular canals.** The semicircular canals are oriented perpendicularly to one another. Movement of the head causes movement of fluid within the labyrinths and displacement of specialized hair cells (the **crista**) located in the **ampulla** at the base of the semicircular canals. The direction and degree of head movement determine the angle and extent of fluid-mediated hair cell displacement, in turn initiating sensory impulses conveyed via the **vestibular nerve** to centers in the cerebellum, midbrain, and cerebrum, where directional movement and position are interpreted.

The auditory system involves all three divisions of the ear. The external (or outer) ear is composed of the **pinna**, which funnels sound waves into the **ear canal**. At the middle ear, sound waves cause vibrations in the **tympanic membrane**, setting into motion the three auditory bones, the **malleus**, **incus**, and **stapes**. The arrangement of these bones is like that of levers, so that movement of the malleus is amplified by the incus, and movement of the incus is amplified by the stapes. Movement of the stapes is transmitted across the **oval window** into the inner ear, setting up vibrations in the fluid of the **cochlea**, which causes bending of **auditory hair cells** in the **organ of Corti**. The **cochlear nerve** and the vestibular nerve form the two branches of the **acoustic nerve** (8th cranial nerve).

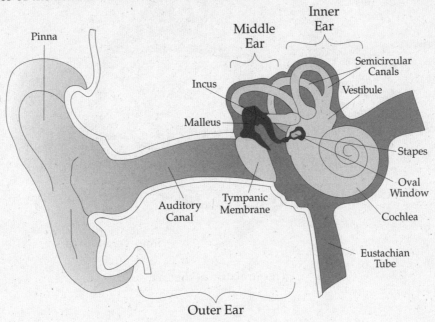

The Structure of the Ear

Figure 30.26

30.1.4.2 The Visual System

The transmission of light through the human eye follows the following pathway: light enters the **cornea**, traverses the **aqueous humor**, passes through the **pupil**, and proceeds through the **lens** and the **vitreous humor** until it reaches the light receptors of the **retina**. Electrical signals are then transmitted via the **optic nerve** to visual centers in the brain.

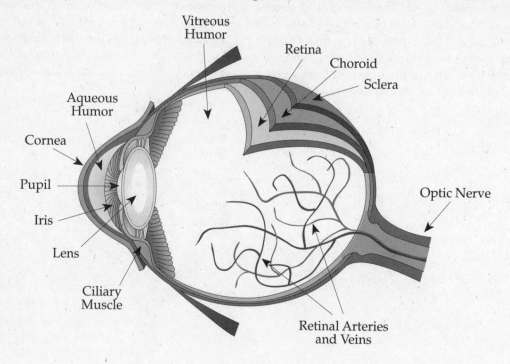

The Structure of the Eye

Figure 30.27

The lens is a transparent structure that focuses light rays on the retina. **Myopia** (nearsightedness) occurs when the lens focuses light from a distant object in front of the retina. **Hyperopia** (farsightedness) occurs when light from a nearby object is focused behind the retina.

The retina senses light rays with two types of photoreceptors located in its outer layer: (1) **rods**, which are specialized to register dim light; and (2) **cones**, which are specialized to register bright light as well as color. Both rods and cones contain pigments allowing them to absorb energy from light rays.

The pigment that mediates rod reception is **rhodopsin**.

Cones are subdivided into three types: red-absorbing, blue-absorbing, and green-absorbing. Light reception in cones is mediated by **opsin**, which is similar to rhodopsin.

The **iris**, the colored part of the eye, contains muscles that dilate and constrict it to regulate the amount of light that reaches the **retina**. The **ciliary muscle** changes the shape of the lens as the eye shifts its focus from distant to nearby objects.

30.1.5 THE SKIN

Constituting the largest organ in the body, the skin functions to: (1) maintain body temperature; (2) register information from the environment; and (3) provide a barrier against infection. The skin is composed of three layers: the **epidermis**, the **dermis**, and the **subcutaneous** tissue.

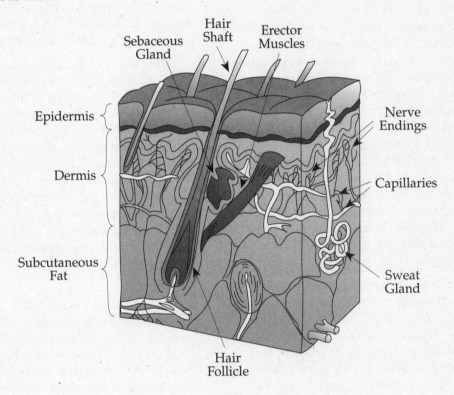

Diagram of Human Skin Showing
Three Dermal Layers

Figure 30.28

The epidermis is composed of stratified squamous epithelium and has a layered, flat cell structure. The external layer of the epidermis is the **stratum corneum**, composed of many layers of dead cells containing the protein **keratin**. The stratum corneum is waterproof and provides resistance to invasion of the body by microorganisms. The stratum corneum continuously renews itself by sloughing off cells, which are replaced by keratinized epithelial cells from deeper layers. Below the stratum corneum, the **stratum germinativum** is where skin cells replicate through mitosis, and where keratin is produced. Cells from the germinativum layer migrate upward to the surface, away from the capillary beds that nourish the skin. As they lose contact with capillaries, the cells die and form the layers of the corneum.

The dermis directly underlies the stratum germinativum of the epidermis, and contains the blood vessels, nerve endings, sebaceous glands (which secrete oils), and sweat glands. The sweat glands secrete water and ions in response to high temperatures and sympathetic stimulation, serving to maintain a stable body temperature and optimal balance of sodium and chloride ions in the body. Subcutaneous tissue contains primarily **adipose** (or fat) tissue.

30.2 MASTERY APPLIED: SAMPLE PASSAGE AND QUESTIONS

Passage

Schizophrenia refers to a group of mental disorders characterized by a disturbance of the thinking processes. The traditional animal model for schizophrenia has been a simple rodent model of amphetamine-induced excitation. When dopamine antagonists such as haloperidol and chlorpromazide (agents that counter the actions of the neurotransmitter dopamine by blocking dopamine receptors) are administered, symptoms of amphetamine-induced excitation in the rodents diminish according to a dose-response relationship. This appears to support the dopamine theory of schizophrenia, which postulates that excessive amounts of dopamine cause the disorder.

While excess dopamine plays a part in the expression of schizophrenia, it does not cause the disorder. Schizophrenia involves numerous neurotransmitter systems. In fact, the frontal cortex systems of schizophrenics are actually hypoactive for dopamine—not hyperactive, as originally proposed. The underactive cortex exerts a reduced modulating influence on the limbic system, producing an increase in dopamine activity in the midbrain.

The N-methyl-D-aspartate (NMDA) subgroup of glutamate receptors is emerging as an important component in the etiology of schizophrenia. The receptor complex modulates calcium channels and contains recognition sites for glutamate, spermidine, and zinc, which act as agonists (exerting excitatory effects) or antagonists (blocking excitatory effects). Glutamate has excitatory effects; in excess, it is toxic and destroys brain tissue.

Glutamate, dopamine, norepinephrine, and serotonin all play a role in the normal function of the brain's frontal cortex. The frontal cortex governs proper functioning of the glutamate pathways descending to the limbic system. The glutamate system, in turn, influences release of dopamine through *tonic leak,* a process in which neurons constantly release a low level of dopamine. Tonic leak maintains dopamine receptors at a normal sensitivity level.

Research with the glutamate antagonist phencyclidine (PCP) (see Figure 1) shows that phencyclidine leads to hypoactivity of the frontal cortex. This causes reduced outflow of glutamate, less NMDA receptor stimulation, decreased tonic signal, and reduced tonic leak. The net result is hypersensitivity to action potentials at the receptor level. Because dopamine is simultaneously associated with hypoactivity at the frontal cortex and hyperactivity at the receptor level, this phenomenon is explained by the *simultaneous dopamine activity/underactivity model.*

A drug that blocks only dopamine would block hyperactivity at the receptor level but would not address the frontal cortex dopamine deficit seen in the phencyclidine model. Serotonin antagonist drugs, such as risperidone and clozapine, correct this problem by blocking serotonin receptors. This has the effect of increasing dopamine activity in the frontal cortex: the dopamine increase restores glutamate levels, allowing a rise in tonic level and producing a reduction in receptor sensitivity. By this mechanism, schizophrenia can be treated with a pure serotonin blocker.

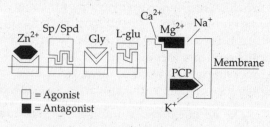

Key:

Sp/Spd = Spermidine
Gly = glycine
L-glu = glutamate

Figure 1

1. Which one of the following does NOT occur during an action potential?

   A. Sodium flows into the interior of the neuron.
   B. The neuron becomes depolarized.
   C. The interior of the neuron becomes positive relative to its exterior.
   D. Calcium flows out of the neuron.

2. A physician whose treatment strategy is based on the simultaneous overactivity/underactivity model of schizophrenia would be most likely to prescribe which of the following therapeutics for her patients?

   A. A dopamine antagonist
   B. A serotonin blocker
   C. Haloperidol
   D. Chlorpromazine

3. A researcher testing the dopamine hypothesis of schizophrenia constructs a graph of his data points comparing symptoms of amphetamine-induced excitation with dosage of dopamine antagonists administered to the rats. Which of the following graphs would most nearly match his results?

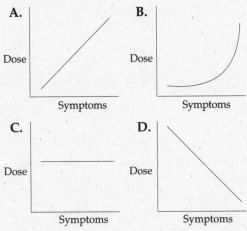

4. The glutamate antagonist phencyclidine has the effect of:

   A. impeding the release of neurotransmitter from synaptic vesicles of neurons.
   B. overstimulating the dendrites of neurons.
   C. blocking the neurotransmitter pathway across the synapse.
   D. accelerating saltatory conduction along the axon of neurons.

5. As a result of tonic leak:

   A. dopamine levels fluctuate from zero to very high across a 24-hour period.
   B. normal neuron sensitivity to neurotransmitter is maintained.
   C. dopamine has toxic effects and destroys tissue.
   D. the glutamate system is maintained at normal functioning.

6. Traditional antipsychotics often produce side effects that require additional medicine that is anticholinergic in nature. The therapeutics given to counter the side effects target which of the following neurotransmitters?

   A. Acetylcholine
   B. Serotonin
   C. Thyroid hormone
   D. Norepinephrine

7. Based on Figure 1, the hallucinogen phencyclidine exerts its effect by:

   A. blocking the outer portion of the NMDA receptor channel.
   B. producing a conformational change in the exterior portion of the receptor channel.
   C. entering and then blocking the open NMDA receptor channel.
   D. competing with the binding of zinc at the zinc receptor site.

8. Which of the following has an excitatory effect on the NMDA receptor complex?

   A. Zinc
   B. Spermidine
   C. Phencyclidine
   D. Calcium

30.3 MASTERY VERIFIED: ANSWERS AND EXPLANATIONS

1. *D is the correct answer.* The relevant ion flows associated with an action potential are the influx of sodium and the efflux of potassium, not calcium efflux. Choices A, B, and C are all true statements: during an action potential, a neuron's membrane becomes permeable to the influx of sodium down its concentration gradient and undergoes a depolarization. (The cell's interior undergoes a change in potential relative to the exterior from approximately –70 mV to approximately +50 mV.)

2. *B is the correct answer.* A serotonin blocker increases dopamine activity in the frontal cortex, as outlined in the simultaneous overactivity/underactivity theory described in the passage. Choice A is not correct: a dopamine antagonist would be the therapy of choice according to the dopamine theory of schizophrenia; it does not address the problem of frontal cortex dopamine underactivity, however. Both Choices C and D are dopamine antagonists, the therapy of choice for the dopamine theory.

3. *D is the correct answer.* The passage states that a dose-dependent relationship exists between a dopamine antagonist and the amphetamine-induced symptoms observed in rodents. Thus, the answer choice can be narrowed down to one that shows a set of data points that rise or fall in uniform increments. The passage also states that the symptoms diminish according to a dose-response relationship. The correct answer must therefore depict an inverse relationship. The graph in choice D shows a uniform inverse relationship between symptom level and dose level. As dose increases, symptoms decrease. Choice A correctly depicts a dose-dependent relationship. However, it does not show an *inverse* relationship. According to this graph, as dose increases, so do symptoms. Therefore, choice A is incorrect. Neither choice B nor C shows an inverse relationship. Both are incorrect.

4. *B is the correct answer.* Phencyclidine causes hypersensitivity to action potentials at the receptor level. As such, the dendrites will be more readily stimulated to undergo an action potential. Choice A is incorrect. Phencyclidine causes hypersensitivity of neurons to action potentials; choice A implies the opposite. Choice C is wrong as well. Phencyclidine causes hypersensitivity of neurons to action potentials, and Choice C indicates the opposite. Choice D, too, is wrong. The passage states that hypersensitivity of neurons to action potentials is due to increased sensitivity of receptors to dopamine. Neurotransmitter receptors are located on the dendrites of the neuron, not along the axon.

5. *B is the correct answer.* Tonic leak preserves normal sensitivity of neurons to neurotransmitters. Choice A is incorrect: tonic leak produces a constant low level of dopamine. Choice C is also incorrect: the passage states that high levels of glutamate have toxic effects and damage tissue, while tonic leak refers to low levels of dopamine release. According to the passage, the glutamate system governs the rate of tonic leak, and choice D indicates the opposite.

6. *A is the correct answer.* Anticholinergic drugs oppose the effects of the neurotransmitter acetylcholine. Choice B is incorrect: although serotonin is a neurotransmitter, it is not affected by anticholinergics. Choice C is incorrect because thyroid hormone is not a neurotransmitter and anticholinergics do not act upon thyroid hormone. Choice D is wrong as well, since norepinephrine is not acted upon by an anticholinergic.

7. *C is the correct answer.* Figure 1 shows that PCP is able to enter the NMDA receptor channel and then block the channel inside the passageway. Choice A is incorrect: Figure 1 indicates that PCP blocks the inner portion of the NMDA receptor channel, not the outer portion, where magnesium binds. Choice B is incorrect as well. Figure 1 does not indicate that a conformational change occurs at the NMDA receptor channel. Choice D, too, is wrong. According to Figure 1, zinc does not compete with PCP at the zinc receptor site: PCP acts on the receptor channel.

8. *B is the correct answer.* According to Figure 1, spermidine is an agonist: it has excitatory effects. Choice A is incorrect: Figure 1 indicates that zinc acts as an antagonist, with inhibitory effects. Choice C, too, is incorrect, as Figure 1 shows that phencyclidine is an antagonist: it has inhibitory effects. Choice D is wrong as well. The NMDA receptor channel is permeable to calcium, sodium, and potassium, according to Figure 1. While these ions have important effects on the neuron, they are labeled as neither agonists nor antagonists.

CHAPTER 31

MECHANISMS OF HEREDITY

31.1 MASTERY ACHIEVED

31.1.1 GENES, LOCI, AND ALLELES

A **gene** is a specific sequence of nucleotides (A-adenine, T-thymine, C-cytosine, or G-guanine; see Chapter 24) that is capable of directing the production of a particular protein. Because some nucleotide sequences found on DNA serve as chemical "switches" to start or stop protein production, and others simply act as spacers between genes and do not contain directions for protein production, not all nucleotide series constitute genes.

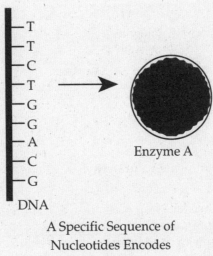

A Specific Sequence of
Nucleotides Encodes
Enzyme A

Figure 31.1

A gene is a hereditary unit, passed from parents to offspring, coding for a specific protein that expresses itself as some specific physical or metabolic trait. Hair color, for example, is a physical trait, while lactose intolerance is a metabolic trait. Lactose-intolerant individuals lack the gene responsible for the synthesis of the enzyme essential for the proper digestion of lactose, a component sugar of dairy products.

Both a gene and its related trait are passed on to the offspring, although in cases where an individual's parents have passed on contrasting genes—say, one for white skin color, and one for brown skin color—one of the parental genes may dominate over the other, or alternatively, an expression reflecting a mixture of the two may result. Occurring at trait-specific sites on chromosomes, a gene is reproduced and transmitted to an offspring through the combined processes of **meiosis** and **mitosis**. The place on a chromosome at which a gene is located is called the **locus** (plural: loci). For two homologous chromosomes, a gene found at a particular locus on one chromosome will code for the same trait as the gene at that locus on the other. While the aligned genes (**alleles**) code for the same specific trait, the maternal and paternal trait frequently differ, so that each allele might code either for the same expression of a specific trait, or for differing expressions of it.

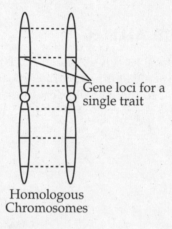

Gene loci for a single trait

Homologous
Chromosomes

Figure 31.2

Please solve this problem:

- All of the following accurately characterize a gene EXCEPT:

    A. It is inherited.
    B. It codes for a protein or enzyme.
    C. It occupies a fixed position on a chromosome.
    D. Each segment of a DNA strand comprises a gene.

Problem solved:

D is correct. Many segments of a DNA strand do not contain a gene. Choices A through C can be eliminated because they accurately describe the characteristics of a gene. A gene is a particular sequence of nucleotides that codes for an enzyme or other protein. A gene occupies a fixed position on a chromosome and can be passed on to successive generations.

Please solve this problem:

- Trace the molecular pathways that produce a given trait in an organism.

Problem solved:

A DNA molecule contains sequences of nucleotides that comprise genes. A gene codes for a specific enzyme or other protein. The proteins catalyze reactions or participate in physiological processes that are associated with the appearance of particular traits in the organism. Traits range from readily apparent characteristics, such as eye color or height, to subtle traits, such as a heightened (or diminished) ability to process alcohol or higher (or lower) resistance to environmental hazards such as pollution or ultraviolet radiation.

Please solve this problem:

- Each of the thousands of genes found on a diploid chromosome occupies a site on the chromosome called a:

   A. allele.
   B. locus.
   C. gene.
   D. nucleotide.

Problem solved:

B is correct. The locus of a gene is the physical site that the gene occupies on the chromosome. Alleles are at loci that are aligned on homologous chromosomes.

31.1.2 GENOTYPE VS. PHENOTYPE

The alleles for a given trait represent an organism's **genotype** for the trait; together, through the related cellular processes of DNA transcription and RNA translation, the two alleles produce the organism's **phenotypic** expression of the trait. With regard to genotype, a given individual may be termed **homozygous** or **heterozygous** for a given trait, the former indicating that both alleles code for identical expressions of the trait, and the latter signifying that the alleles code for differing expressions. A brief discussion of eye color should prove illustrative. For purposes of the discussion, we assume that there are only two alleles, B and b, and two eye colors, blue and brown.

Alleles of an Individual Homozygous for Eye Color

Figure 31.3

The genotype of an individual with blue eyes consists of two alleles that code for blue eye color, designated (*bb*). This individual is homozygous with regard to eye color because both alleles for the trait are identical. The individual's associated phenotype (the trait that is expressed and discernible in the individual) is "blue-eyed." Alternatively, an individual possessing brown eyes (phenotype: "brown-eyed") may possess one of two alternate genotypes: two alleles, each coding for brown color, designated (*BB*), which is a homozygous genotype; or one allele for brown eye color and one allele for blue eye color, designated (*Bb*), and heterozygous for eye color. An organism heterozygous for a given trait possesses different alleles for the trait, each coding for different protein products.

Alleles of an Individual Heterozygous for Eye Color

Figure 31.4

Please solve this problem:

- Distinguish between genotype and phenotype.

Problem solved:

Genotype refers to the genetic makeup of an individual. Phenotype refers to the outward appearance of an individual, or the manifestation of an individual's genotype.

Please solve this problem:

- Define the terms *allele*, *homozygous*, and *heterozygous*.

Problem solved:

Genes that code for the same trait in an individual are called alleles. Alleles code for a specific characteristic of an individual (e.g., hair texture or eye color), but do not always code for the same expression of that trait (i.e., straight vs. curly, or blue vs. brown).

Heterozygous refers to a genotype in which paired alleles code for different versions of a trait (e.g., in a guinea pig, one allele codes for a short-haired coat and one allele codes for a long-haired coat).

Homozygous refers to a condition in which two alleles encode for the same expression of a trait (e.g., in a fruit fly, both alleles code for normal wings).

31.1.3 DOMINANT VS. RECESSIVE GENES

An organism that is heterozygous for a given trait normally expresses only one of the contributing alleles for the trait, as one allele of the pair is **dominant** over the other allele. The dominant allele is expressed, while the **recessive** allele—remaining a component of the genotype, and therefore heritable by offspring—lies dormant. By convention, a capital letter symbolizes the dominant allele (such as *B* for brown eye color), and a lower-case letter designates the recessive allele (such as *b* for blue eye color).

It should be understood that an organism that is heterozygous for a given trait will be indistinguishable from an individual that is homozygous dominant for that trait, so if the dominant phenotype is observed, we can know nothing definitive about that organism's genotype. On the other hand, an organism that possesses the recessive phenotype can have only one genotype: homozygous recessive.

Please solve this problem:

- If straight hair (*HH*) is a dominant trait and curly hair (*hh*) is recessive, which of the following genotypes would NOT be expressed as straight hair?

  A. (*HH*)
  B. (*Hh*)
  C. (*hH*)
  D. (*hh*)

Problem solved:

D is correct. Only Choice D, which shows two alleles for the recessive gene (*hh*), offers a genotype that will be expressed as curly hair. Choice A shows a genotype which is homozygous for the dominant trait, straight hair (*HH*). Both Choices B and C present heterozygous genotypes, which will express themselves as the straight hair phenotype.

31.1.4 THE PUNNETT SQUARE

The **Punnett square** is a tool used to determine the statistical probability of the outcome of a mating (**cross**) between two individuals. The outcome ratio of the offspring genotype derived from the Punnett square describes the average, or expected, outcome of the cross. It does not, however, predict the *actual* outcome of a single parental pairing. The Punnett square shown below depicts the pattern of transmission of eye color trait from parents to offspring. The paternal alleles are (*bb*), which indicate a homozygous blue-eyed male. The maternal alleles are (*Bb*), indicating a heterozygous brown-eyed female. The Punnett square predicts that half of the offspring of these parents will be heterozygous and brown-eyed, like the mother, while the other half will be homozygous and blue-eyed, like the father.

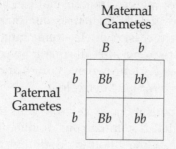

Maternal
Gametes

2 Bb : 2 bb
B = brown eye color allele
b = blue eye color allele

Outcome of Cross between
Heterozygous Brown-eyed Female and
Homozygous Blue-eyed Male

Figure 31.5

Thus, the Punnett square predicts the *probability* that each of the possible genotypes and phenotypes will appear in the offspring.

31.1.5 MENDEL'S LAWS: THE LAW OF SEGREGATION AND THE LAW OF INDEPENDENT ASSORTMENT

By studying the behavior of gene transmission for single-locus traits, the Austrian geneticist Gregor Mendel established that parental genes are conveyed to offspring according to the **law of segregation** and the **law of independent assortment**. The law of segregation holds that, in the process of meiosis, the homologous chromosomes of a diploid cell become separated into different gametes, ensuring that each gamete contains one allele for a given trait. Hence, a heterozygous pointy-eared individual whose genotype is (*Pp*) produces gametes in which half contain the allele for pointy ears (*P*) and the other half contain the gene for round ears (*p*). There will be no gametes that contain both the *P* and the *p* alleles.

The law of independent assortment states that genes for different traits that are carried on different chromosomes are distributed independently of each other when the gametes are formed through meiotic division. According to this law, the trait for eye color, for example, sorts independently from the trait for hair color, or from any other heritable trait. The law of independent assortment does not apply to **linked genes**, which are carried on the same chromosome, and therefore are usually inherited together.

Please solve this problem:

- According to Mendelian genetics, what would be the likely genotypes in the F1 generation (the first generation) after a cross between a plant that produces yellow, smooth seeds [*YYSS*] and a plant producing green, wrinkled seeds [*yyss*]?

  A. 100% (*YYSS*)
  B. 100% (*YySs*)
  C. 50% (*YySs*), 50% (*YYSS*)
  D. 75% (*YySs*), 25% (*YYSS*)

Problem solved:

B is correct. A cross between the homozygous parent plants described above would yield F1 generation plants with only one genotype—that of (*YySs*)—and one phenotype—yellow, smooth seeds.

Please solve this problem:

- According to Mendelian genetics, which of the following would be the most likely ratio of phenotypes in the offspring of a cross between two plants from the F1 generation described immediately above, each plant having genotype (*YySs*)?

  A. 1:3:3:9 for yellow, smooth; yellow, wrinkled; green smooth; and green wrinkled
  B. 3:1:3:9 for yellow, smooth; yellow, wrinkled; green, smooth; and green, wrinkled
  C. 9:3:3:1 for yellow, smooth; yellow, wrinkled; green, smooth; and green, wrinkled
  D. The phenotypic outcome of such a cross cannot be determined using the Punnett square.

Problem solved:

C is correct. A cross of the heterozygous F1 plants (*YySs*) x (*YySs*) would yield F2 generation plants bearing sixteen genotypes. The phenotypic ratio of the F2 plants is 9:3:3:1 for yellow, smooth; yellow, wrinkled; green, smooth; and green, wrinkled.

31.1.6 GENETIC VARIABILITY

31.1.6.1 Genetic Recombination: Crossing Over During Synapsis

When linked genes are sufficiently far apart on a chromosome, the process of **crossing over** may occur, in which equal sections of chromatid between a pair of homologous chromosomes are exchanged. Crossing over occurs during the first prophase of meiosis, when homologous chromosomes align side by side during **synapsis**, forming a **tetrad**. Crossing over leads to **genetic recombination**. While the two chromosomes possess the same genes, they may carry different alleles for those genes. A chromosome that carried the dominant allele for a given trait may, after crossing over, carry the recessive trait. Such reassortment of genes increases **genetic variability**, expanding the total number of gene combinations that can result from a given cross.

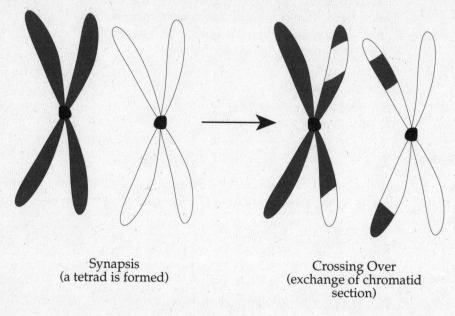

Synapsis
(a tetrad is formed)

Crossing Over
(exchange of chromatid
section)

Figure 31.6

Please solve this problem:

- Explain why crossing over leads to genetic recombination.

Problem solved:

The process of crossing over involves the mutual exchange of sections of DNA between chromatids of a homologous chromosome pair. Instead of producing an exact replica of the parent chromosomes, crossing over results in chromatids whose allelic combinations differ from those of the parent chromatids. The exchanged DNA sections contain blocks of genes which have changed the offspring gametes' chromatid composition, and this alteration constitutes genetic recombination.

Please solve this problem:

- What feature of the meiotic reduction division allows for the phenomenon of crossing over?

    A. Replication
    B. Migration
    C. Equatorial division
    D. Synapsis

Problem solved:

D is correct. Crossing over occurs during the first prophase of meiosis. Homologous chromosomes align themselves in what is termed *synapsis*. The pair of homologous chromosomes that forms during synapsis is called a *tetrad*. The physical juxtaposition of the homologous chromosomes at this stage makes crossing over possible.

31.1.6.2 Genetic Recombination: Mutation

Mutation contributes to genetic recombination (and, therefore, to increased variability) by producing new genes. The deletion, addition, or substitution of one or more nucleotides can alter the product of that gene. In some cases, the mutation will produce effects deleterious to the organism's survival; in other cases, the mutation will lead to an improvement in the organism's adaptability. Still other mutations may not result in any significant advantage or disadvantage to the organism.

Mutations can arise spontaneously within a cell, or can result from external environmental factors, such as exposure to sunlight (or other sources of ultraviolet radiation) or to mutagenic chemicals. Once a cell has mutated, the alteration is inherited by the cell's progeny.

Please solve this problem:

- All of the following are possible sources of genetic variability EXCEPT:

    A. mitosis.
    B. crossing over.
    C. ultraviolet exposure.
    D. spontaneous mutation.

Problem solved:

A is correct. Genetic variability can result from crossing over (Choice B), from exposure to a mutagen or sunlight (Choice C), or from spontaneous mutation. Mitosis (Choice A) does not produce genetic recombination.

Please solve this problem:

- Of the following, which is NOT a possible effect of mutation on the function of a gene?

    A. Termination of enzyme production
    B. Alteration of protein structure
    C. Saturation of enzyme
    D. No effect

Problem solved:

C is correct. A mutation may halt the production of an enzyme (Choice A) or it may lead to the production of a protein different from the one originally produced by the affected gene (Choice B). Alternatively, the mutation may have no effect on gene activity or protein synthesis (Choice D). Saturation (Choice C) is dependent on the relative amounts of substrate and enzyme available for a reaction.

Please solve this problem:

- Which of the following is NOT true regarding mutation?

    A. It may enhance fitness.
    B. It may reduce fitness.
    C. It is always inherited.
    D. It may be produced by ultraviolet light.

Problem solved:

C is the correct answer. Not all mutations are inherited. A mutation must occur in the gametes in order to be passed on to an organism's offspring. In addition, it must occur in a gamete that eventually *becomes* a new offspring in order to be inherited. Any other mutation will be lost when the parent organism dies.

31.1.6.3 Sex-linked Traits

Most traits are **autosomal**, meaning that they are carried on one of the twenty-two pairs of autosomal chromosomes in humans. Some traits, however, are **sex-linked**: they are carried on the X chromosome. (Traits that are carried on the Y chromosome are called **holandric**.) Two examples of sex-linked traits are color blindness and hemophilia.

Individuals with one X and one Y chromosome are male; individuals with two X chromosomes are female. Only males possess the Y chromosome, and thus only fathers can pass it on to offspring. The main function of the Y chromosome is to direct protein synthesis that (1) causes the embryo to develop as a male, and (2) produces male secondary sexual characteristics; it appears to have little other function. Because each of an individual's parents donates one sex chromosome to the individual, a male's X chromosome must come from the maternal parent. While the paternal contribution can be an X or Y chromosome, the maternal contribution is always an X chromosome. A female offspring, then, receives her father's X chromosome and one of her mother's X chromosomes.

As is typically the case for somatic traits, the female who is homozygous for a recessive, abnormal sex-linked trait (the female in whom both X chromosomes bear the trait's gene) will display the trait, and will pass the gene to her offspring; the female who is heterozygous for the trait (the female in whom only one X chromosome carries the abnormal gene) will be a genotypic **carrier** for the trait: she will not express the gene phenotypically herself, but she can pass it on to the next generation through her gametes. Because females possess two X chromosomes, the heterozygous female's X chromosome that lacks the abnormal gene can compensate for the fact that the other X carries it. However, if a male's X chromosome bears an abnormal gene, it will be expressed, since he lacks another X to compensate.

Figure 31.7 presents a cross between a color-blind female and a male who is not color-blind. The Punnett square predicts that female offspring will be carriers of the abnormal gene but will show normal phenotype for color-blindness; and male offspring will carry both the genotype and the phenotype for color-blindness.

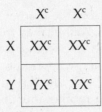

Punnett Square Showing
Transmission of Sex-Linked
Trait for Color-Blindness

Figure 31.7

Please solve this problem:

- Explain why a male with a sex-linked gene always expresses the trait, while a female carrier of the same trait does not necessarily express the phenotype.

Problem solved:

Males have one X and one Y chromosome, and females have two X chromosomes. Sex-linked traits are carried on the X chromosome. If a male receives an X chromosome that bears a particular sex-linked gene, the male must express the trait it codes for. On the other hand, a female receives one X chromosome each from both her mother and her father. If one of those X chromosomes bears an abnormal gene, her other X chromosome can mask it.

Please solve this problem:

- Arthur's paternal grandmother had three brothers, all of whom developed male pattern baldness (MPB) in their thirties. His paternal great-grandfather, grandfather, and father also had the trait. Arthur's maternal grandfather did not develop MPB, but his maternal great-grandfather, and all five brothers of his maternal grandmother, had the trait. Arthur's brother also has the trait. Given the family background, and the fact that MPB is an X-linked trait, which of the following statements is most likely to be correct?

  A. Arthur has a 25% chance of developing MPB.
  B. Arthur has a 50% chance of developing MPB.
  C. MPB affects only one generation and is not inherited.
  D. MPB may be produced by ultraviolet light.

Problem solved:

B is correct. Males receive one X gene from the mother and one Y gene from the father. If male pattern baldness is an X-linked trait, Arthur may inherit the trait on his X gene, i.e., from his mother. Therefore, the information about his father's family is irrelevant. Arthur's mother inherited one of her X genes from her father, who did not display the trait, and one from her mother, whose five brothers were all bald. Because Arthur's brother displays the trait, and so had to inherit it from his mother, Arthur's mother must be heterozygous for X-linked MPB. Arthur has a 50% chance of inheriting his maternal grandfather's X gene, which does not carry the MPB gene, and the same chance of inheriting his maternal grandmother's X gene, which carries the trait.

31.2 MASTERY APPLIED: SAMPLE PASSAGE AND QUESTIONS

Passage

Autosomal dominant (AD) inheritance is one of four basic patterns of Mendelian inheritance reflecting the types and combinations of alleles, or alternative forms of a gene, at a given site on a chromosome. A Mendelian disease is one in which a single mutant gene has a large phenotypic effect, and is transmitted in a vertical pattern, being passed from one generation to the next vertically on a pedigree.

Of the 4000 traits delineated by scientists as following Mendelian inheritance, 54% are autosomal dominant, 36% are autosomal recessive, and 10% are X-linked dominant or recessive. Of these traits, approximately 3000 have been linked to human disease. The Punnett square below illustrates the classical pattern of transmission of an autosomal dominant mutant trait from parents to offspring, where one heterozygous parent expresses the trait, while one homozygous recessive parent does not express it.

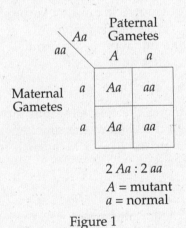

$$2\ Aa : 2\ aa$$
$$A = \text{mutant}$$
$$a = \text{normal}$$

Figure 1

1. The Punnett square presented in the passage indicates that:

   A. the parents produced four offspring.

   B. on average, mating of heterozygous parents yields a 50-50 ratio of heterozygous and homozygous offspring.

   C. on average, mating of a heterozygous and a homozygous parent yields equal numbers of heterozygous and homozygous recessive offspring.

   D. the probable outcome of heterozygous-homozygous matings is determined by the paternal chromosomal make-up.

2. Which of the following is true regarding the pedigree shown in Figure 2?

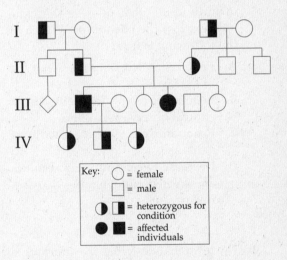

Key:
○ = female
□ = male
◐ = heterozygous for condition
● = affected individuals

Pedigree of an Autosomal Recessive Trait

Figure 2

A. The trait illustrated in the pedigree is autosomal and sex-linked because both affected offspring and heterozygotes have affected or heterozygous fathers, and only generation III involves a carrier mother.

B. The pedigree is incorrect, because genotype for the trait should skip generations in autosomal recessive inheritance.

C. Phenotypic expression of autosomal recessive traits in offspring requires that both parents be heterozygous, or that one parent is a heterozygous and the other is homozygous recessive.

D. Phenotypic expression of autosomal recessive traits in parents must result in affected offspring.

3. *Penetrance* refers to the clinical expression of a genotype. Penetrance is described quantitatively as the percentage of individuals that possess the gene who express the phenotype. Which of the following is true?

A. Penetrance describes the genotype of a disease.

B. Penetrance can be determined from clinical observation alone.

C. Penetrance describes the severity of a disease.

D. Decreased penetrance can result in an affected child having disease-free parents.

4. The term that describes the alternative forms of a given gene is:

A. *locus.*
B. *allele.*
C. *chromatid.*
D. *autosome.*

5. According to the law of independent assortment:

A. homologous chromosomes enter the same gamete during meiosis.

B. homologous chromosomes become separated into different gametes during meiosis.

C. the gene for each trait in an organism will segregate independent of those for other traits in the organism during meiosis.

D. alternative alleles for a trait enter the same gamete during meiosis.

6. Achondroplasia, a common cause of dwarfism, is an example of an autosomal dominant condition, which arises through mutation 80% of the time. The disorder is characterized by decreased cartilage production at the bone growth plates. Increased paternal age may increase the rate of this mutation. All of the following are true statements with regard to mutations EXCEPT:

A. a mutation can arise spontaneously.

B. a mutation involves a change in the nucleotide sequence of DNA.

C. a mutation can alter the production of a specific protein.

D. a mutation is always inherited by offspring.

7. Among the following phenotypes, a trait included in the subcategory that comprises 10% of Mendelian inheritance is:

A. eye color.
B. height.
C. color-blindness.
D. sickle cell anemia.

31.3 MASTERY VERIFIED: ANSWERS AND EXPLANATIONS

1. *C is the correct answer.* A Punnett square is used to determine the average or expected outcome of matings. They do not predict *actual* outcomes of individual pairings, which are subject to random variability of pairing of individual gametes. Choice A is not correct. A Punnett square describes the statistical probability of the outcome of a mating between two individuals. It does not predict the number of offspring. Choice B is incorrect as well. The Punnett square in Figure 1 indicates nothing about the mating of heterozygous parents. Choice D, too, is wrong. Although the offspring ratio (50% [*Aa*], 50% [*aa*]) looks like the paternal gametes (*Aa*), the maternal gametes (*aa*) play an equal part in determining the genotypes of the offspring.

2. *C is the correct answer.* Phenotypic expression of a recessive trait requires contribution of a recessive gene from each parent. Choice A is not correct. A gene can by definition be autosomal or sex-linked, but by definition cannot be both. Choice B is incorrect. Expression of an autosomal recessive trait does not have to skip generations. Choice D is wrong as well. Heterozygous parents contribute either one or zero recessive genes each to a zygote. Using probability, one-quarter of offspring of such parents will be affected (homozygous for the abnormal gene) and one-quarter will be homozygous for the normal gene.

3. *D is the correct answer.* An autosomal dominant parent may lack expression of the phenotype of the disease (decreased penetrance), but his or her offspring may have full penetrance of the disease genotype. Choices A and B are incorrect because penetrance is a function of phenotype, which in turn depends on genotype. Choice C is incorrect as well. Penetrance is only concerned with whether a trait is clinically observable or not.

4. *B is the correct answer.* The passage states that alleles are alternative forms of a gene. Genes, chromatids, and autosomes all refer to the genome, but not specifically to alleles.

5. *C is the correct answer.* This is an accurate statement of this law. D is not true, as described in the preceding chapter.

6. *D is the correct answer.* Choices A, B, and C accurately characterize mutations.

7. *C is the correct answer.* According to the passage, 10% of traits that follow Mendelian inheritance are X-linked (sex-linked). Therefore, the correct answer must describe a sex-linked trait. Color-blindness is a sex-linked trait. Choices A , B, and D are incorrect since none lists a sex-linked trait.

CHAPTER 32

POPULATIONS, EVOLUTION, AND ECOLOGY

32.1 MASTERY ACHIEVED

32.1.1 GENE POOL, MUTATION, AND GENETIC VARIABILITY

A **gene pool** constitutes the total possible assortment of genes found in the population of a species. Each member of a population possesses an overall genotype (and therefore phenotype) that differs in some aspect from the other members of a population. The differences among the members' genotypes is an expression of the genetic variability present in the population. Genetic variability is predominantly the result of random **mutation**—the spontaneous addition, transfer, rearrangement, or deletion of one or several nucleotides in a section of DNA. The mutation may confer an advantage or disadvantage on the organism with regard to its survival and ability to reproduce. If the mutation is heritable, the organism's progeny may also possess the advantageous or disadvantageous trait.

32.1.2 THE DYNAMICS OF EVOLUTION

Evolution is a change in the genetic makeup of a given population. The term applies to **populations**: a single individual is not capable of evolving. Evolution acts upon the population's gene pool. Advantageous mutations become incorporated into the gene pool, while those that confer serious disadvantage generally do not remain in the gene pool. Organisms placed at a serious disadvantage will usually not survive long enough to reproduce. Mutations producing deleterious effects of a subtler nature, however, tend to persist in the gene pool over time. At some future time, a change in circumstances may then cause the gene to provide some advantage, after which the gene will become more prevalent in the population.

32.1.2.1 Environment and Alteration of a Gene Pool

A new environment usually poses new challenges to the survival of an organism. Consequently, those organisms whose genes confer traits advantageous to their survival and reproduction in the new environment tend to proliferate at the expense of other organisms in the population. Over time, the gene pool of the population will shift, with the frequency of advantageous genes increasing and that of deleterious genes decreasing.

A case in point is the mutant sickle cell allele, which produces an altered form of hemoglobin designated HbS. The aberrant hemoglobin has the tendency to cause the red blood cell in which they are housed to sickle. The sickled cells will often clump and clog smaller blood vessels. Homozygous individuals for HbS normally do not survive to adulthood. Heterozygous individuals, whose genotype for hemoglobin consists of one allele for HbS and one allele for HbA (normal hemoglobin), are disadvantaged by the sickling of those red blood cells harboring HbS, but are also able to produce normal hemoglobin and a certain percentage of normal-shaped red blood cells.

Significantly, the allele for HbS also confers increased resistance to a virulent form of malaria caused by the protozoon *Plasmodium*. In environments where the likelihood of infection with the virulent form of malaria is high—such as in areas of Africa, Southern Asia, and India—the frequency of the HbS allele in the gene pool can rise as high as 40% in the population. Alternatively, in environments that do not pose the risk of malarial infection (where possession of the allele conferring malarial resistance does not confer an advantage)—such as in North America—the frequency of the HbS allele is reduced in the population to as low as 4%.

32.1.2.2 Darwinian Fitness

Fitness, according to Charles Darwin, refers to the ability of an organism's genotype to persevere in subsequent generations. There is competition among organisms in a population; therefore not all previously existing and newly mutated alleles can be perpetuated in the finite gene pool of a population. Those alleles that persist in the gene pool (those that have been "selected for" by the environment) will supplant alternative forms of the gene. An organism that is able to survive to reproductive age is able to pass on to its progeny whatever trait or traits that assisted in its survival. A given organism's fitness depends on the interplay between its environment and its phenotype, and is judged ultimately by its ability to survive to reproductive age.

Please solve this problem:

- Describe fitness as it applies to the Darwinian concept of evolution.

Problem solved:

Fitness, as it applies to Darwinian evolution, is the ability of a gene to persist in the gene pool through successive generations. An organism that can survive and reproduce, passing on its genotype to its offspring, embodies Darwin's concept of fitness. Differential reproduction rates dictate that all available alleles for a gene will not be inherited at equal rates from generation to generation. The factor that determines which genes persevere is natural selection. An organism possessing alleles for a trait that confers an advantage will more likely survive and, therefore, may reproduce more often than an organism that possesses an alternate form of the gene which does not confer advantage.

Please solve this problem:

- Which one of the following is essential to the process of evolution?

    A. Mutation
    B. Death of some mutant offspring before reproductive age
    C. Unchanging gene pool
    D. Physical separation of two populations of the same species

Problem solved:

A is correct. The process of evolution depends on ongoing random mutation within a population. Those mutations that favor survival are promoted simply because the individuals that possess them are more likely to survive to reproductive age and to pass them on. The process of mutation does not require that some mutant offspring die before reproductive age (although this is a common event). Evolution is the alteration in gene pool composition in a given population of a species. It may proceed in the absence of any physical separation between two populations of the species.

Please solve this problem:

- Environmental changes might produce evolution by:
    A. inducing rapid and direct genetic change in response to the stresses imposed on the environment.
    B. revealing the selective advantage conferred by a particular gene that is possessed by some but not all members of a population.
    C. halting the process of random mutation.
    D. producing mutations unfavorable to the altered environment.

Problem solved:

B is correct. Within the gene pool of a population, some genes have neither an advantageous nor a disadvantageous effect on the individual. Under some environmental change, however, such a gene might prove to be advantageous, and so confer a selective advantage on those individuals who possess it. Such individuals will be more likely to survive to reproductive age; and so, over some generations, the composition of the gene pool will change.

Please solve this problem:

- Jean Baptiste de Lamarck posited that an individual could pass a trait acquired in its lifetime on to its offspring. How does Lamarck's theory of evolution compare to the theory of evolution according to Darwin?

Problem solved:

Lamarck incorrectly theorized that an acquired trait, developed at some point during the organism's lifetime, was heritable in the same manner that a gene arising through mutation would be heritable. Additionally, Lamarck's theory of evolution embraced a direction of evolution that entailed a continual quest (and reward) for self-improvement by the organism that is absent in evolution. According to Darwin's theory of evolution (since borne out, of course), only traits that are coded for by the genes in the gametes can be transferred to offspring. Furthermore, the advantage that a trait confers to an organism depends primarily on the environment in which the organism finds itself.

32.1.2.3 Speciation

32.1.2.3.1 REPRODUCTIVE ISOLATION

Speciation—one type of **divergent evolution**—refers to the evolution of a new species of plant or animal from a preexisting, or parent, species. The two populations evolve separately over time until what had originally been a common gene pool has evolved into two distinct gene pools. **Reproductive isolation** is insularity of a gene pool from genetic mixing. Reproductive isolation occurs when two species capable of interbreeding are prevented from doing so. Their reproductive isolation can take the form of temporal isolation (e.g., breeding that is confined to a specific time of day, season, or year), ecological isolation (e.g., different habitat requirements for two species within the same geographical area), or behavioral isolation (e.g., courtship behavior that is species-specific), among others. Often more than one form of reproductive isolation exists as a barrier to the mixing of genes between species.

Please solve this problem:

- Which of the following describes an instance of reproductive isolation?

    A. A rattlesnake becomes separated from other rattlesnakes and therefore cannot mate.
    B. Two distinct populations of the same species show subtle differences in traits and genotypes.
    C. Two populations of frogs share a common ancestor but will no longer interbreed because their mating seasons do not overlap.
    D. Each species of flycatcher, a bird, is associated with its own characteristic song.

Problem solved:

C is the correct answer. Reproductive isolation requires two things: (1) that two populations once interbred; and (2) that they no longer do. Only choice C provides evidence that both of these criteria are met.

32.1.2.3.2 ADAPTIVE RADIATION

When a given population of a species has undergone a sufficient change in genotype to render it reproductively isolated from other populations of its parent species, it has evolved into a new species. The term applied to this form of speciation is **adaptive radiation**. Adaptive radiation is associated with reduced competition and an alteration of the organism's original **niche**. An organism's niche represents the organism's "environment" in its broadest sense, encompassing an organism's habitat, food sources, territory, range, and mating behavior.

One method by which adaptive radiation arises is through geographical separation, such as through the migration of glaciers, or the development of a land bridge or a mountain range. A population that migrates to and colonizes new territory will be subject to a different set of criteria for selection of its genotype—criteria that are based on the conditions of the new environment. Ultimately, those organisms able to survive and procreate in the new environment will belong to a gene pool that is reproductively isolated from the gene pool to which they originally belonged before of their migration. This form of adaptive radiation is called **allopatric speciation**.

The other form of adaptive radiation that can occur is **sympatric speciation**. Sympatric speciation occurs in the absence of geographical isolation: it occurs in a geographical area shared by the parent and the new species. Two closely related populations of one species can diverge, such that their differences allow them to exploit different niches within the same environment. Because adaptive radiation involves the creation of one or more species from a parent species, it acts to increase biological diversity.

Please solve this problem:

- Define the term *adaptive radiation*. Describe two mechanisms that give rise to this form of evolution. Does adaptive radiation increase or decrease biological diversity?

Problem solved:

Adaptive radiation is a form of evolution characterized by the creation of one or more new species that arise from a preexisting ancestral species. A key requirement for adaptive radiation is the reproductive isolation of a population of a species. One mechanism giving rise to adaptive radiation is geographical separation, such as occurs with the development of a land bridge, the movement of a glacier, or the appearance of a mountain range. Another mechanism leading to adaptive radiation is the divergence of two gene pools of populations inhabiting the same geographical region. Speciation can occur in this case when two populations are able to exploit different niches in the same environment. Either mechanism of adaptive radiation increases biological diversity by increasing the number of species that exist.

Please solve this problem:

- Adaptive radiation results in all of the following EXCEPT:

  A. reduced competition.
  B. overall increase in the number of species.
  C. change of an organism's original niche.
  D. convergence of species.

Problem solved:

D is correct. Choice D is the only one of the choices that fails to describe an effect of adaptive radiation. Adaptive radiation entails a divergence of species, ultimately increasing biological diversity.

Please solve this problem:

- Which of the following is associated with both allopatric and sympatric speciation?

    A. Gross geographic separation
    B. Occupation of a new niche
    C. Increased competition among original and newly developed species
    D. Decreased exploitation of resources

Problem solved:

B is the correct answer. Both allopatric and sympatric speciation involve the occupation of a new niche by one or several populations, which in time gives rise to new species. Choice A describes allopatric speciation only. Choices C and D are false for both allopatric and sympatric speciation; both will decrease competition among species and will increase the efficiency of exploitation of resources.

32.1.3 PREDICTION OF GENE FREQUENCY IN A POPULATION

32.1.3.1 The Hardy-Weinberg Law

The frequency with which a given trait occurs in a population remains steady, according to the **Hardy-Weinberg law.** The Hardy-Weinberg law only applies, however, to an ideal population that adheres to the following criteria: (a) a large population; (b) absence of mutations; (c) absence of immigration or emigration; (d) random reproduction; and (e) no geneotypes are favored, with respect to reproductive success. When these criteria are satisfied, the frequency with which an allele occurs in a population will remain constant. For example, if a gene has only two possible alleles, B and b, where B occurs 60% of the time and b occurs 40% of the time, those percentages will remain the same if the five Hardy-Weinberg criteria are met. The numerical forms of the Hardy-Weinberg law are:

$$p^2 + 2pq + q^2 = 1,$$
$$\text{and}$$
$$p + q = 1$$

where p and q represent the frequencies of specific alleles in a population.

32.1.3.2 Genetic Drift

When a population is small in number, the Hardy-Weinberg law does not apply; instead a pattern of gene transmission known as **genetic drift** takes effect. A change in the initial frequency of alleles due to chance matings becomes more likely in a small population. As a result, within the population, certain genes disappear while other genes become more prevalent in the population. The variation in gene frequency arises by chance, *not* by selection processes that emphasize the survival of the fittest.

Please solve this problem:

- The **founder effect** is a form of genetic drift that results when a small population colonizes a new area. All of the following would apply in the founder effect EXCEPT:

  A. The gene frequencies of an isolated colony may differ substantially from those of the larger population from which the colony broke off.

  B. The population of the colony is sufficiently small for genetic drift to alter the gene pool.

  C. Any differences in the colony's gene frequency from its original population are more likely to be adaptive than random.

  D. Members of the colony may possess only a small portion of the available alleles of the gene pool of the population they left behind.

Problem solved:

C is correct. Genetic drift, of which the founder effect is one form, entails random changes in the allelic frequencies of populations. Choice A lists a common effect of genetic drift on a population, while choices B and D list conditions under which genetic drift may alter the gene pool.

Please solve this problem:

- Among the following, which will NOT alter the gene frequencies of a population?

  A. Genetic drift
  B. Natural selection
  C. Hardy-Weinberg equilibrium
  D. Mutation

Problem solved:

C is correct. The Hardy-Weinberg law establishes the stability of gene frequencies. When the the Hardy-Weinberg law applies, the frequency with which a trait occurs in a population remains steady. A series of conditions must be met, however, in order for the Hardy-Weinberg law to take effect: large population, absence of mutations, absence of immigration or emigration, random reproduction, and the condition that any one gene has the same chance of reproducing as any other gene. Choices A, B, and D—genetic drift, natural selection, and mutation—are incorrect, because all can alter the gene frequencies of a population. Genetic drift produces random evolutionary changes in allele frequency; natural selection selects favorable alleles over unfavorable ones, leading to changes in the gene pool; and mutation entails direct changes in the nucleotide sequence of DNA, potentially producing new alleles.

32.1.4 TAXONOMIC ORGANIZATION

Taxonomy—the classification of organisms—is based upon the binomial system proposed by Carolus Linnaeus in the mid-eighteenth century. An organism is classified according to a hierarchical scheme and is given a two-part name based on its assumed evolutionary relationship to other organisms based on available data. The order of classification, from most comprehensive to most specific, is: kingdom, phylum, class, order, family, genus, and species.

The most exclusive unit of classification is the species. Closely related species comprise a **genus**; related genera comprise a **family**; related families comprise an **order**; related orders comprise a **class**; related classes make up a **phylum**; and related phyla comprise a **kingdom**. Among phyla, the chordates are identifiable by the presence at some point during development of: (1) a dorsal nerve cord, (2) gill slits, and (3) a notochord. Of the chordates, vertebrates are recognized by possession of: (a) a vertebral column, (b) a closed circulatory system, (c) a developed nervous system, and (d) a developed sensory apparatus.

Please solve this problem:

- Order the following groupings of *Homo sapiens* (humans) according to the binomial system of classification: Mammalia (Class), Hominidae (Family), Chordata (Phylum), Vertebrata (Subphylum), *Homo* (Genus), Primata (Order), *sapiens* (species), Animalia (Kingdom).

Problem solved:

Kingdom	Animalia
Phylum	Chordata
Subphylum	Vertebrata
Class	Mammalia
Order	Primates
Family	Hominidae
Genus	*Homo*
Species	*sapiens*

32.1.5 COEXISTENCE, ECOLOGICAL NICHE, AND ECOSYSTEM

Another form of classification pertains to the nature of the relationship a given member of one species may have with a member of another species. A prolonged intimate association between a member of one species and a member of another species is referred to as **symbiosis**. Symbiotic relationships are classified into three types: **mutualism, commensalism**, and **parasitism**. Each partner of a mutualistic relationship derives benefit from the association; in fact, two such individuals are frequently unable to survive independently of one another. Nitrogen-fixing bacteria and the legume root nodules they colonize constitute a mutualistic partnership: the plants receive nitrogen in a form that they can use, and the bacteria derive nutrition and shelter from the plant host.

Commensalism involves one partner that benefits from the symbiotic association, and one partner that neither benefits nor is harmed by the association. Epiphytes, small "air plants" that use trees to anchor themselves, are the partner that derives benefit. The tree to which the epiphyte attaches represents the partner that is unaffected by the association. Parasitism is a symbiotic relationship in which one organism benefits and the other is harmed. An example of parasitism is the association between tapeworm and humans. The tapeworm derives food from its human host to the detriment of the human.

The behaviors described all allow a given organism or organisms to fill a particular niche within their ecosystem. As described above, the term *niche* encompasses all parameters of the "environment" of an organism; numerous niches are utilized by similar and different species in any given ecosystem. The term **ecosystem** is an equally complex concept: it characterizes a self-sustaining natural system, composed of both living and nonliving components, as well as all of the interactions between them that help to mold it into a stable system.

Please solve this problem:

- Elucidate the benefits or costs to organisms belonging to the following symbiotic relationships: mutualism, parasitism, and commensalism.

Problem solved:

In mutualism, both organisms benefit from their intimate relationship; in parasitism, one organism benefits, while the other organism is harmed; in commensalism, one organism benefits, while the other organism neither benefits nor is harmed. All three relationships constitute forms of symbiosis, an intimate living arrangement between two organisms of different species.

32.2 MASTERY APPLIED: SAMPLE PASSAGE AND QUESTIONS

Passage

According to the principle of competitive exclusion, one species will always predominate over another if both are in competition for the same resource within the same community. The competition, states the theory, will cause the elimination of one of the two species from the community. To test the validity of the theory, two experiments were performed.

Experiment 1

At step 1, two species of bacteria, Species A and Species B, were cultured in separate flasks containing identical media. As shown in Figure 1, it was noted that the population of Species A showed a growth rate greater than that of Species B. At step 2, organisms belonging to both species were grown together in a single flask under the same conditions used in step 1. As shown in Figure 1, Species A survived and Species B died out.

Experiment 2

At step 1, two species of algae, Species C and Species D, were grown in separate flasks containing identical media. As measured by dry weight (Figure 2), the population of Species C grew more rapidly than did that of Species D. At step 2, Species C and D were grown together in a single flask under the same conditions used in step 1. The resulting data indicated that the population of Species D grew more rapidly than did that of Species C, the latter species eventually dying out (see Figure 2).

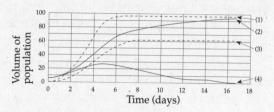

Key: (1) Species A (alone)
        (2) Species A (with Species B)
        (3) Species B (alone)
        (4) Species B (with Species A)

Figure 1

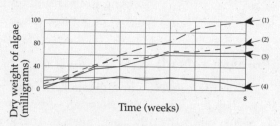

Key: (1) Species C (alone)
        (2) Species D (alone)
        (3) Species D (with Species C)
        (4) Species C (with Species D)

Figure 2

1. Organisms belonging to Species X are in competition for resource R. One organism belonging to the species acquires by mutation the ability to use resource S as a substitute for resource R. Which of the following choices best describes the situation?

   A. Competitive inhibition
   B. Hardy-Weinberg law
   C. Adaptive radiation
   D. Genetic drift

2. Among the following choices, which best describes the meaning of "fitness" in Darwinian terms?

   A. Ability to undergo random mutation
   B. Ability to escape predators
   C. Ability to adjust to changing environmental conditions
   D. Ability to reproduce

3. Among the following choices, which is best supported by the data derived from Experiment 1?

   A. Species A is more fit than Species B under the experimental conditions.
   B. Species A is more fit than Species B under all conditions.
   C. The period of Species A's presence on the earth is longer than that of Species B.
   D. If Species A and Species B lived in separate communities, Species B would become extinct before Species A.

4. Which of the following conclusions is contradicted by the data obtained in Experiments 1 and 2?

   A. Species A has an adverse effect on the reproductive capacity of Species B when they are cultured together.
   B. Species D has an adverse effect on the reproductive capacity of Species C when they are cultured together.
   C. If two species compete for the same resource, one will always outcompete the other.
   D. A species will better compete with another species if, when living in the absence of the other species, it shows greater population growth than does the other species.

5. With respect to Figure 1, which of the following choices most likely explains the apparent elimination, over time, of the gap between Curves 1 and 2?

   A. Adaptation of Species A
   B. Evolution of Species A
   C. Mutation within Species A
   D. Elimination of Species B

6. Taken together, do the two experiments support the theory of competitive exclusion?

   A. Yes, because in each case the two competing species show different rates of population growth.
   B. Yes, because in each case one of the two competing species fails to survive.
   C. No, because the two experiments involve different species.
   D. No, because the two experiments do not necessarily involve the same growth medium or environments.

7. With reference to the first experiment, what was the difference after 10 days between the size of the population of Species B when grown alone and the population of Species B when grown together with Species A?

   A. 10 units
   B. 20 units
   C. 50 units
   D. 60 units

32.3 MASTERY VERIFIED: ANSWERS AND EXPLANATIONS

1. *C is the correct answer*. Adaptive radiation refers, generally, to the situation in which a subpopulation of a species is able to occupy a new ecological niche. Through additional evolution, its progeny adapt themselves to the new niche and may, ultimately, generate a separate species. Competitive inhibition (choice A) refers to an enzyme-related phenomenon. The Hardy-Weinberg law accounts for the stability of gene frequencies in a large population that meets specific criteria (choice B); and genetic drift (choice D) refers to changes in a small population's gene pool through random processes.

2. *D is the correct answer*. The measure of "fitness" in Darwinian terms is the organism's ability to survive for as long as is necessary to reproduce.

3. *A is the correct answer*. Choice A is directly supported by data. Choice B is not refuted, but we have almost no evidence regarding this statement. We only know that Species A is more fit under one set of conditions; we have no evidence regarding any other possible set of circumstances. We have no evidence at all for either C or D.

4. *D is the correct answer*. Choices A, B, and C are consistent with the data. While the data does not directly address reproductive capacity, it does not contradict the conclusions stated in choices A and B. It is also logically possible that the greater population growth of Species A in the first experiment and of Species D in the second experiment is attributable to such adverse influences. In Choice C, it is true that in each experiment performed, one of the two species survived. The data does contradict the statement made in Choice D, however, since in the second experiment, Species C showed greater population growth when grown alone, but died out when grown together with Species D.

5. *D is the correct answer*. Examination of Figure 1 shows that the growth of Species A in the presence of Species B (Curve 2) increases as the population of Species B decreases (Curve 4). This logic suggests that the elimination of Species B gives Species A greater access to the resources for which Species B was competing.

6. *B is the correct answer*. According to the passage, the theory of competitive exclusion provides that if two species compete for the same resource, one must ultimately be eliminated. In both cases, one of the species did die out. In the first case, Species B died out; and in the second case, Species C died out. The statements that are made in Choices A, C, and D are not relevant to the question.

7. *C is the correct answer*. Curve 3 represents Species B's population growth when grown alone, and Curve 4 represents Species B's population growth when Species B is grown together with Species A. At 10 days, the population of Species B is 60 units when grown alone, and 10 units when grown with Species A; 60 – 10 = 50 units.

CHAPTER 33

CARBON BONDING

33.1 MASTERY ACHIEVED

33.1.1 ORBITAL HYBRIDIZATION

As we mentioned in Chapter 13, the location of an atom's electrons is conventionally described in terms of atomic orbitals that represent spatial probabilities, and are labeled s, p, d, and f. This model, called the **atomic orbital theory**, describes the way in which electrons are arranged to build up atoms. Now let's look at how complex bonds are formed between atoms.

Consider the formation of beryllium chloride ($BeCl_2$):

$$Be + Cl_2 \rightarrow BeCl_2$$

Chlorine's atomic number is 17, and the configuration of its outer shell is $3s^2 3p^5$; it features one unpaired electron in the third p orbital of the third shell. Beryllium's atomic number is 4, and its electron configuration is $1s^2 2s^2$; it has no unpaired electrons. How does the beryllium atom form two bonds with an atom of chlorine?

The beryllium atom redistributes its electrons in the following manner: (1) one electron is "promoted" from a $2s$ orbital into an empty $2p$ orbital, leaving two unpaired electrons—one in the $2s$ orbital and one in the $2p$ orbital; (2) the $2s$ orbital and the $2p$ orbital then "hybridize" to form two sp orbitals that both contain an unpaired electron; (3) each of these two hybridized sp orbitals is able to donate an electron to a covalent bond.

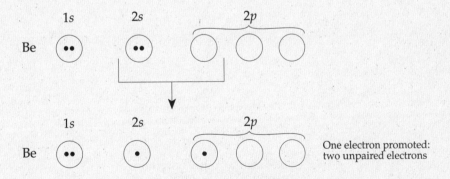

Promotion of electron from s orbital to p orbital

This process is known as **orbital hybridization**. The hybridization just described is termed *sp* **hybridization** because it involves the combination of one *s* orbital and one *p* orbital.

Please solve this problem:

- The process of orbital hybridization facilitates:

    A. the breaking of stable covalent bonds.
    B. the conversion of ionic bonds to covalent bonds.
    C. the generation of an increased number of unpaired electrons.
    D. the pairing of otherwise unpaired electrons within a single atom.

Problem solved:

C is the correct answer. As you now know, the process of orbital hybridization involves the movement of an electron from a subshell of relatively lower energy into a vacant orbital of relatively higher energy. This process leaves an unpaired electron in the lower energy orbital and creates an unpaired electron in a higher energy orbital, increasing the number of unpaired electrons that are capable of forming bonds.

sp^2 **hybridization** involves hybridization among one *s* orbital and two *p* orbitals. The formation of boron trifluoride (BF_3) illustrates this process.

Fluorine's atomic number is 9, and its electron configuration is $1s^2 2s^2 2p^5$; it has one unpaired electron in the third *p* orbital of its second shell, and shares it to form a covalent bond. Boron's atomic number is 5, so its electron configuration is $1s^2 2s^2 2p^1$; it carries one unpaired electron in its 2*p* orbital. To form three bonds, boron must reconfigure its electron distribution to create three unpaired electrons. In this way, one of the two 2*s* electrons is moved to an empty *p* orbital to generate three *sp*^{2} hybrid orbitals, each with one unpaired electron.

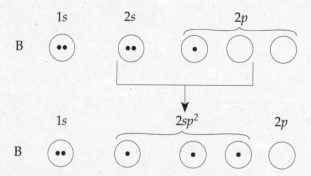

sp^2 hybridization: one 2*s* orbital
merges with two 2*p* orbitals

Orbital hybridization is most relevant to medicine in the context of carbon bond formation. With an atomic number of 6, carbon has the electron configuration of $1s^2 2s^2 2p^2$; it carries two unpaired electrons in the *p* subshell.

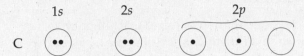

The electron configuration of carbon

Based on its configuration, a carbon atom appears to share only two electrons and should therefore only be able to form two covalent bonds, but carbon can form *four* covalent bonds! How is this possible?

The carbon atom undergoes *sp^3* **hybridization**: it forms four hybridized orbitals from one *s* orbital and three *p* orbitals. The atom promotes one of its paired 2*s* electrons into the vacant, third *p* orbital, leaving an unpaired electron in the *s* orbital and an unpaired electron in each of the three *p* orbitals. The *s* and the three *p* orbitals hybridize to form four equivalent *sp^3* hybrid orbitals, each of which is capable of donating an electron to a covalent bond.

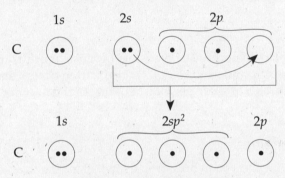

Formation of three 2sp^2 orbitals
and a lone 2*p* orbital in a *sp^2*-
hybridized carbon atom

Please solve this problem:

- If an atom undergoes *sp^3* hybridization, it will form:

    A. three orbitals equivalent in energy and in bonding properties.

    B. four orbitals equivalent in energy and in bonding properties.

    C. three orbitals that differ in energy and in bonding properties.

    D. three orbitals that differ in energy, but not in bonding properties.

Problem solved:

B is the correct answer. *sp^3* hybridization means hybridization among one *s* orbital and three *p* orbitals, and the hybrid orbitals that are created are equivalent in *all* respects.

Please solve this problem:

- An investigator hypothesizes that although sp, sp^2 and sp^3 hybridizations are observed, sp^4 and sp^5 hybridizations are not possible. Is this hypothesis correct?

    A. Yes, because no subshell carries more than three p orbitals.
    B. Yes, because such a predominance of p subshells would contravene the equivalence of hybrid orbitals.
    C. No, because a p subshell may house as many as six electrons.
    D. No, because hybrid orbitals do not conform to any rules or laws that govern unhybridized orbitals.

Problem solved:

A is the correct answer. The hypothesis is plausible because hybridization occurs among the orbitals that belong to the s, p, and d subshells. Hybridization occurs among *orbitals*, and since there are not more than three p orbitals per subshell, that is the number of p orbitals available for hybridization.

Please solve this problem:

- With respect to hybrid orbitals, which of the following is FALSE?

    A. Hybrid oribitals increase the number of bonds in which an atom might participate.
    B. Hybrid orbitals are equivalent in their energy characteristics and bonding properties.
    C. Hybrid orbitals always promote double or triple bonding.
    D. Hybrid orbitals may or may not promote double or triple bonding, depending on the atoms involved.

Problem solved:

C is the correct answer. Hybridization does not only occur in the case of double and triple bonds. As you can see, we've just gone over several instances in which hybridization promoted single bonds. For example, the molecules BF_3 and $BeCl_2$ involve hybridization, but all bonds are single.

33.1.1.1 Carbon-Carbon Double and Triple Bonding; Sigma and Pi Bonding

As we just explained, the carbon atom may undergo sp^3 hybridization. Alternatively, it may undergo a hybridization process in which one electron from an s orbital is moved to a p orbital, and instead of forming four equivalent sp^3 orbitals, three equivalent sp^2 orbitals and one p orbital are formed, each holding one unpaired electron.

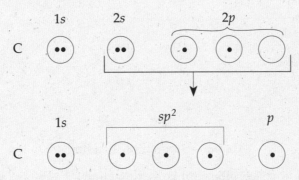

Formation of three sp^2 orbitals and
a lone p orbital in carbon atom

Each of the sp^2 orbitals and the p orbital are capable of donating an electron to a covalent bond to produce a **carbon-carbon double bond**, usually with each carbon atom also singly bonded to two other constituents.

R   R

sp^2 C $\underset{sp^2}{\overset{p}{——}}\underset{sp^2}{\overset{p}{——}}$ C sp^2

sp^2 sp^2

R   R

Carbon-carbon double bonding

Carbon may also undergo **triple bonding**, in which the initial hybridization involves the formation of one sp hybrid orbital (from the combination of one s orbital and one p obital) and two p orbitals.

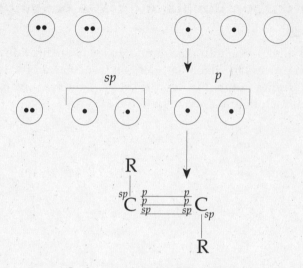

Carbon–carbon triple bonding

Any bond between (a) two *s* orbitals, (b) an *s* orbital and a *p* orbital, (c) single lobes of a *p* orbital, (d) two *sp* hybrid orbitals, or (e) two hybrid *sp²* orbitals is called a σ **bond**. A bond in which both lobes of a *p* orbital from one atom overlap with both lobes of a *p* orbital from another is called a π **bond**. In a the carbon-carbon double bond, one bond is a σ bond that arose from the overlap of two *sp²* orbitals and the other is a π bond that arose from the overlap of two *p* orbitals. Within the carbon-carbon triple bond, one bond is a σ bond that arose from the overlap of two *sp* orbitals and the remaining two are π bonds that arose from the bilobar overlap of two *p* orbitals.

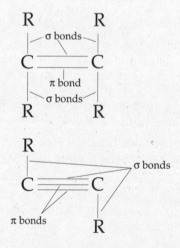

π bonds and σ bonds of carbon-carbon
double and triple bonds

Please solve this problem:

- The carbon-carbon triple bond involves the overlap of:

  A. two hybrid sp^2 orbitals and one lobe of each of two p orbitals.
  B. two hybrid sp orbitals and both lobes of each of two p orbitals.
  C. two hybrid sp orbitals and one lobe of each of two p orbitals.
  D. three p orbitals.

Problem solved:

B is the correct answer. The carbon-carbon triple bond involves hybridization that creates one sp hybrid orbital and two p orbitals. The sp orbital of one carbon atom overlaps with the sp orbital of another to form a σ bond, and both lobes of the two p orbitals of one carbon atom overlap with two lobes of two p orbitals of the other to form two π bonds.

33.1.2 POLAR BONDING AND DIPOLE MOMENT

As we mentioned in Chapter 14, the terms "polarity" and "polar bonds" generally refer to covalent bonds in which electrons are not shared equally. One of the atoms, the more electronegative, takes on a partial negative charge while the other takes on a partial positive charge. A **dipole** is a *molecule* (not a bond) whose polar bonds provide it with both a positive and negative end. If a molecule is a dipole, it has a **dipole moment** equal to:

$$\mu = e\,d$$

where:

μ = dipole moment, measured in the unit Debye (D)

e = charge, measured in electrostatic units (esu)

d = distance between the centers of the positive and negative charge, measured in centimeters (cm)

The following is a table of dipole moments.

H_2	0	HF	1.75	CH_4	0
O_2	0	H_2O	1.84	CH_3Cl	1.86
N_2	0	NH_3	1.46	CCl_4	0
Cl_2	0	NF_3	0.24	CO_2	0
Br_2	0	BF_3	0		

Dipole Moments, D

Generally, the elements with the greatest electronegativity are located in the upper right region of the periodic table, and those with the least electronegativity are in the lower left region. It is helpful to know that in terms of electronegativity:

$$F > O > N > Cl > Br > C > H$$

An organic molecule may contain polar bonds but have no dipole moment, meaning that the *molecule* itself is not then a dipole. Determining whether a particular molecule is a dipole requires an examination of its bonds, the relative electronegativities of its atoms and the spatial relationships of each bond to every other.

A molecule that is symmetrical and composed of a central carbon atom and two or more identical substituents will not form a dipole, even if the bonds between carbon and its substituents are polar. Consider, for example, the molecules carbon dioxide (CO_2) and carbon tetrachloride (CCl_4). Both are composed of polar covalent bonds, but because each is symmetrical and carries equivalent bonds on each aspect of its central carbon atom(s), it shows no net dipole moment.

Look at the structure of carbon dioxide:

$$O = C = O$$

Oxygen is more electronegative than carbon, and each oxygen atom tends to carry a negative charge, leaving the central carbon atom with a slightly positive charge. Because, however, the two negatively charged entities are equally distant from the carbon and arranged symmetrically around it, they "cancel" each other. The molecule is not a dipole, despite its polar bonds.

Carbon tetrachloride is tetrahedrally arranged: a central carbon atom is attached to four chlorine atoms.

Carbon tetrachloride:
tetrahedral, dipole moment = 0

Chlorine is more electronegative than carbon, and so each bond is polar. But because the molecule is symmetrical and the polarity of all the bonds are equal, the negative charges have a center that coincides with the positive carbon atom, and the molecule is not a dipole; it has no dipole moment.

If a molecule is not symmetrical, or if the central carbon is bound to atoms of differing electronegativities, centers of positive and negative charge will not coincide and the molecule will show a dipole moment. Methyl chloride (CH_3Cl), for example, is tetrahedrally shaped and so fulfills the criterion of symmetry. But chlorine is more electronegative than carbon and carbon is more electronegative than hydrogen. The center of positive charge lies below the central carbon atom in the diagram, but the center of negative charge lies somewhere *between* the central carbon atom and the chlorine atom:

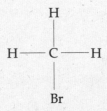

CH₃Cl dipole moment = 1.86 D

The molecule is therefore a dipole and shows a dipole moment.

Please solve this problem:

- An organic molecule will always show a dipole moment if

    A. some or all of its bonds are polar.
    B. some or all of its bonds are ionic.
    C. it is symmetrically oriented.
    D. its centers of positive and negative charge fail to coincide.

Problem solved:

D is the correct answer. Remember, a molecule that contains polar bonds may or may not be a dipole, depending on whether its centers of negative and positive charge coincide. Even if a molecule is composed of polar bonds, it will not show a dipole moment if it is symmetrically arranged and all of its bonds are equivalent. Such is the case, for example, in the molecules CO_2, which is linearly arranged, and CCl_4, which is tetrahedrally arranged.

Please solve this problem:

H
|
H — C — H
|
Br

- The bromomethane molecule pictured above is most likely:

    A. a dipole, because bromine is more electronegative than carbon and hydrogen.
    B. a dipole, because the molecule contains four covalent bonds.
    C. not a dipole, because the molecule lacks double and triple bonds.
    D. not a dipole, because it involves no hybridized orbitals.

Problem solved:

A is the correct answer. Bromine is more electronegative than carbon and carbon is more electronegative than hydrogen. Although the molecule is somewhat symmetrically shaped, the centers of positive and negative charge do not coincide. The center of positive charge is near the carbon atom, and the center of negative charge is somewhere between the carbon and bromine atoms.

Please solve this problem:

• The molecule pictured above is most likely:

A. a dipole, because carbon is more electronegative than nitrogen.

B. a dipole, because nitrogen is more electronegative than carbon.

C. not a dipole, because the centers of positive and negative charge do not coincide.

D. not a dipole, because the molecule is linear and symmetrical in shape and composition.

Problem solved:

D is the correct answer. Nitrogen is more electronegative than carbon. For each carbon-nitrogen triple bond, carbon carries a relative positive charge, and nitrogen carries a relative negative charge. However, the molecule is symmetrical in terms of shape and composition. The negative charges on the nitrogen atoms produce a center of negative charge midway between them. That, in turn, coincides with the center of positive charge that occurs midway between the two carbon atoms. The molecule, therefore, is not a dipole, even though it carries polar bonds.

Please solve this problem:

• The water molecule pictured above is most likely:

A. a dipole, because the molecule is not symmetrically shaped.

B. a dipole, because hydrogen is more electronegative than oxygen.

C. not a dipole, because the centers of positive and negative charge coincide.

D. not a dipole, because the oxygen atom is bound to two other atoms, not four.

Problem solved:

A is the correct answer. Although the water molecule's oxygen atom is bound to two hydrogen atoms, the molecule is *bent*, not symmetrical. Centers of positive and negative charge fail to coincide. Note that choice D is incorrect because a central atom does not need to be bound to four atoms to eliminate a dipole moment. One example of this is carbon dioxide, which lacks a dipole moment although carbon is bonded only to two oxygens, because the molecule is linear.

33.1.3 HYDROGEN BONDING

Hydrogen has a relatively low electronegativity, and if it is bound to an atom of relatively high electronegativity (like oxygen, nitrogen, or fluorine), the molecule has a considerable dipole moment. In a solution of any such molecules, the positive end of one molecule is drawn to the negative end of another; the molecules experience what is called **dipole-dipole attraction**. Although the molecules neither exchange nor share electrons, they experience a binding attraction called a **hydrogen bond**. The strength of a hydrogen bond is about 5%-10% of that of a true covalent bond.

Hydrogen bonding is observed between water molecules:

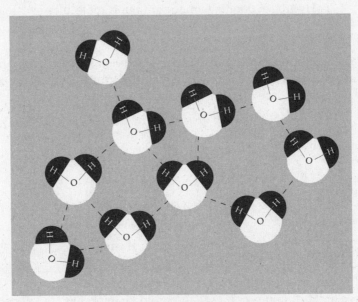

Hydrogen bonding in water
Figure 33.1

Hydrogen bonding also occurs between ammonia (NH_3) molecules in solution:

Hydrogen bonding among ammonia molecules

...and between a variety of other molecules that are discussed in other chapters. Hydrogen bonding may also arise in aqueous solutions in which the solute carries an OH group, as in an alcohol or a carboxylic acid.

Hydrogen bonding in alcohols

The existence of hydrogen bonds increases a substance's boiling point, in fact, carboxylic acids and water have higher boiling points than would be expected, calculated from their molar mass. In fact, in the absence of hydrogen bonding, water would be a gas at room temperature. Also, solid water (ice) takes the form of a crystalline structure because of hydrogen bonding—this structure imposes much empty space between molecules. The empty space markedly reduces the density of water as it freezes, and makes water one of the few substances whose solid form is less dense than its liquid form.

Please solve this problem:

- With respect to hydrogen bonding, which of the following statements is FALSE?

  A. It does not arise among a sample of hydrogen molecules.
  B. It is partially caused by the relatively low electronegativity of the hydrogen atom.
  C. It constitutes weak covalent bonding.
  D. It arises from dipole-dipole interactions.

Problem solved:

C is the correct answer. Hydrogen bonding is a form of dipole-dipole interaction. Specifically, it refers to interactions among dipolar molecules in which hydrogen, which has relatively low electronegativity, is bound to an atom with high electronegativity. The hydrogen of one molecule associates with another molecule's negative region. The name "hydrogen bonding" arose because hydrogen appears so frequently in organic chemistry and has such low electronegativity that it frequently gives rise to dipolar molecules. The essential nature of the hydrogen bond, however, is similar to that of any other dipole-dipole interaction. Note that choice A does make a true statement: A sample of hydrogen (H_2) molecules will not exhibit hydrogen bonding because the hydrogen molecule is not a dipole. The bond between the two hydrogens is obviously not polar.

Please solve this problem:

- Hydrogen bonding increases boiling point because it:

  A. promotes adherence among molecules in the liquid state.
  B. mimics the presence of an ionic solute.
  C. causes molecules to disperse more readily.
  D. increases vapor pressure.

Problem solved:

A is the correct answer. Hydrogen bonding is a form of dipole-dipole interaction and it promotes adherence among the molecules within a given sample. For such molecules, escape from the liquid to the gas phase requires sufficient energy not only to produce a phase change but also to initially separate the adherent molecules. For this reason, hydrogen bonding increases boiling point. Note that choices C and D are clearly incorrect; the conditions they reflect would indicate a *decrease* in boiling point.

33.1.4 ELECTRON DELOCALIZATION AND RESONANCE STRUCTURES

33.1.4.1 Electron Delocalization

The **delocalization of electrons** increases a structure's stability. For example, the H_2 molecule is more stable than the H atom, partially because the covalent bond that joins two H atoms allows each of two electrons to move around *two* hydrogen nuclei instead of being confined to one. The O_2 molecule is more stable than the oxygen atom for the same reason; the covalent bond allows the valence electrons to move around two nuclei instead of one.

33.1.4.2 Resonance

The term **resonance** refers to a molecule or ion that has a configuration that cannot be accurately represented by a conventional diagram because one or more of its electrons is **delocalized**. Consider, for example, the carboxylate ion. It is formed by deprotonation of COOH, which is the sidechain of carboxylic acids (Chapter 38).

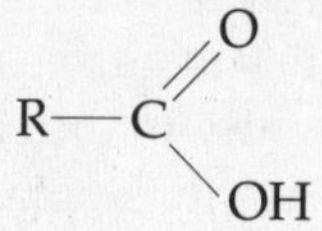

After losing a hydrogen ion, the carboxylate ion bears a negative charge and can be thought of as either this:

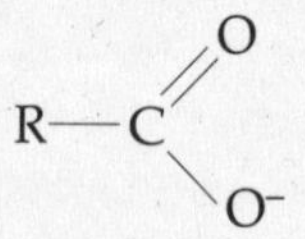

or this:

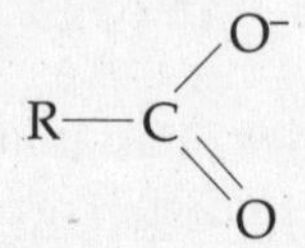

Although the carboxylate ion is sometimes said to resonate between the two forms shown, no such resonance truly occurs. Instead, the carboxylate ion represents a **resonance hybrid** between the two structures, each of which is said to contribute to the true structure. The "extra" electron—which imparts the negative charge—is delocalized; it is not affiliated with either of the terminal oxygen atoms alone, but is dispersed between the two oxygen atoms. It can be represented in the following way:

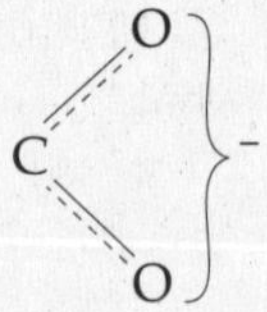

Nitrogen dioxide (NO_2) is a resonance structure and is said to "resonate" between these two configurations:

$$N \underset{O}{\overset{O}{\Big|}}$$

But in fact, neither of the N-O bonds is a true double bond. Instead, each has a partial double-bond character, and the structure is better represented as:

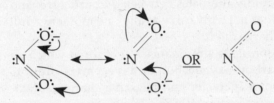

Here, as always, resonance denotes the delocalization of electrons. In the case of NO_2, the delocalized electrons are those in the double bond. They are not truly localized between the nitrogen atom and one of the oxygen atoms alone; they are "spread out" between the nitrogen atom and both oxygen atoms.

33.1.4.3 The Significance of Resonance: Stability

The term "resonance" does not really describe a *process* of resonance; it describes the delocalization of electrons, which enhances stability. If one or more of the electrons associated with a molecule or an ion have relatively greater freedom to "roam" among separate nuclei, the entire species is stabilized.

Consider again a prototypical carboxylic acid. Its acidity—or its willingness to part with a hydrogen ion—depends partially on the stability of the anion that would be created by depronation.

$$R - C \underset{OH}{\overset{O}{\Big|}} \longrightarrow R - C \Big\}^{-} + H^{+}$$

The carboxylate ion is particularly stable because it is a resonance structure. Now consider a prototypical alcohol:

$$R - C - OH$$

Alchohols are less acidic than carboxylic acids because their anions are not stabilized by resonance.

$$R - C - OH \longrightarrow R - C - O^{-} + H^{+}$$

Please solve this problem:

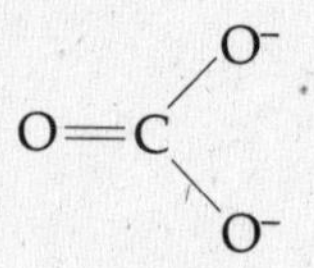

- The carbonate ion is often depicted as shown above. It has been discovered, however, that the ion's three carbon-oxygen bonds are of equal length and character. The most likely explanation is that the ion:

    A. represents a resonance structure in which positive charge is delocalized, and there is partial triple bond character between the central carbon atom and one of the oxygen atoms.

    B. rapidly alternates between two structures and does not truly carry at any one moment a full charge of −2.

    C. represents a resonance structure in which all carbon-oxygen bonds have partial double bond character and negative charge is delocalized among three oxygen atoms.

    D. does not represent a resonance structure.

Problem solved:

C is the correct answer. A resonance structure depicts the delocalization of electrons, which may include electrons that participate in a bond. Although a resonance structure may be depicted as "resonating" between two or more forms, no resonance truly occurs. Instead, the structure constitutes a hybrid of possible resonance forms. If the resonance involves delocalization of charge, the charge is at all times evenly distributed among those atoms where it is said to resonate. If the resonance involves delocalization of bonding electrons, the relevant bonds are of equal character. In the case of the carbonate ion, the equivalence of the three carbon-oxygen bonds is explained by resonance; each has partial double bond character. The charge of −2 is delocalized and is "shared" among the three oxygen atoms. The three resonance structures are:

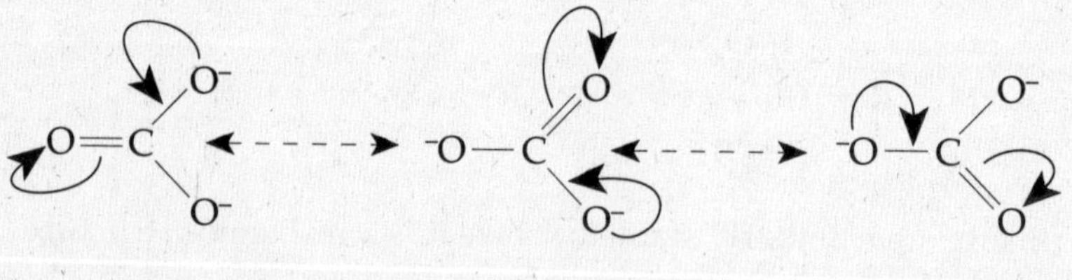

and another representation is:

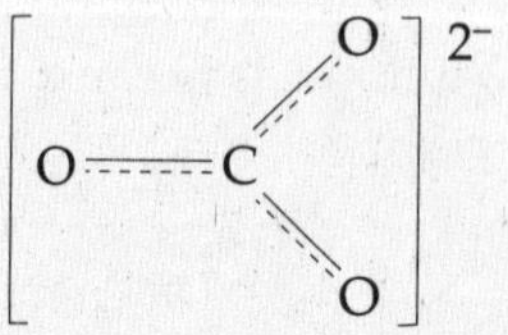

Please solve this problem:

$$CH_2 = CH - CH_2 \cdot \qquad \cdot CH_2 - CH = CH_2$$

$$1 \qquad\qquad\qquad\qquad 2$$

- The allyl radical is a hybrid of the two structures shown above. Which of the following is true?

   A. Neither structure actually exists.
   B. Both structures exist but differ in stability.
   C. Both structures exist and are identical in their stability.
   D. A sample of allyl radical is composed 50% of one structure and 50% of the other.

Problem solved:

A is the correct answer. As stated in the text, resonance hybrids are not really composed of two molecules. Instead, the resonance structure represents a hybrid molecule that has, in part, the character of each of its contributing structures. A resonance hybrid is analogous to the hybrid created by the mating of a horse and donkey. The resulting mule is not a horse at one moment and a donkey at another. Rather, it is an entity unto itself, resembling a horse in some respects and a donkey in others.

33.2 MASTERY APPLIED: SAMPLE PASSAGE AND QUESTIONS

Passage

In order to perform their metabolic functions, organisms require a supply of free energy. In most biological systems, the immediate donor of free energy is adenosine triphosphate (ATP) which, when hydrolyzed, yields free energy, adenosine diphosphate (ADP), and inorganic phosphate, P_i.

The standard free energy of hydrolysis of ATP to form ADP and inorganic phosphate is –7.3 kcal/mole. This is low compared with the –2.2 kcal/mole yielded in the hydrolysis of glycerol-3-phosphate.

$$ATP + H_2O \rightleftharpoons ADP + P_i$$

$$\Delta G^\circ = -7.3 \text{ kcal/mol}$$

$$\text{glycerol-3-phosphate} + H_2O \rightleftharpoons \text{glycerol} + P_i$$

$$\Delta G^\circ = -2.2 \text{ kcal/mol}$$

The relatively low standard free energy associated with ATP hydrolysis means that for the ATP molecule, phosphate group transfer potential is higher than it is for glycerol-3-phosphate. The relatively large phosphate group transfer potential for ATP reflects the difference between the standard free energy of the reactants (ATP and H_2O) and that of the products (ADP and inorganic phosphate). In part, the relative stability of the products is traceable to the resonance stabilization of inorganic phosphateshown in Figure 1 to the right.

For the molecules phosphoenolpyruvate, acetyl phosphate, and phosphocreatinine (Figure 2), phosphate group transfer potential is higher than it is for ATP. Among the significant phosphorylated compounds in biological systems, ATP is associated with an intermediate phosphate group transfer potential. It is for that reason that ATP is well-suited to serve as a phosphate carrier

and, therefore, as an immediate donor of free energy in metabolic processes. If phosphate group transfer potential were extremely high, ADP would not take on phosphate to form ATP. If it were extremely low, the ATP molecule would resist hydrolysis and would be unable to serve as a ready source of free energy.

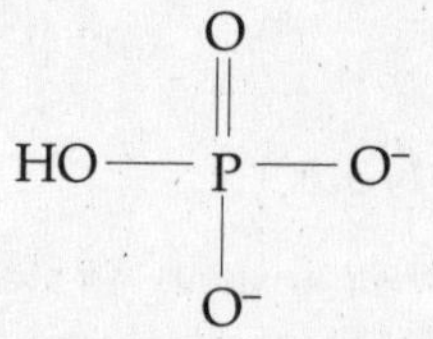

Figure 1

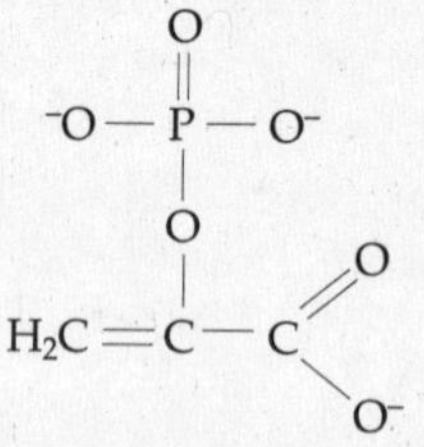

Phosphoenolpyruvate

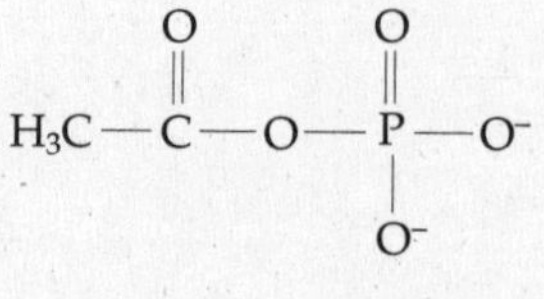

Acetyl phosphate

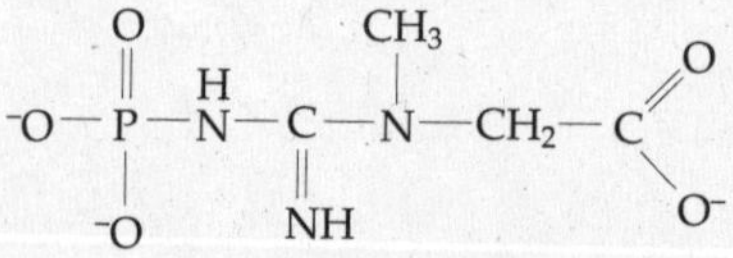

Phosphocreatine

Figure 2

Compound	$\Delta G°$ (kcal/mol)
Phosphoenolpyruvate	–14.8
Carbamoyl phosphate	–12.3
Acetyl phosphate	–10.3
Creatine phosphate	–10.3
Pyrophosphate	–8.0
ATP (to ADP)	–7.3
Glucose-1-phosphate	–5.0
Glucose-6-phosphate	–3.3
Glucose-3-phosphate	–2.2

Table 1
Free energies of hydrolysis for some
biologically significant phosphorylated molecules

1. In the molecule of acetyl phosphate shown in Figure 2, the carbon atom that is double bonded to oxygen:

   A. has undergone sp^2 hybridization.
   B. has undergone sp^3 hybridization.
   C. has formed no σ bonds.
   D. is in a higher energy state than unbound atomic carbon.

2. Among the following choices, which most likely contributes to the stability of the dehydrogenated phosphocreatine molecule shown in Figure 2?

   A. Repulsion between negative charge and positive charge
   B. Repulsion between negative charge and negative charge
   C. Low acidity of the carboxyl (COOH) group
   D. Electron delocalization within the carboxylate (COO⁻) moiety

3. Which among the following choices is LEAST likely to represent a structure that contributes to the inorganic phosphate resonance structure?

   A.

   B.

   C.

   D.

4. Within the molecule acetyl phosphate, shown in Figure 2, the single carbon-carbon bond is:

   A. dipolar ionic.
   B. nonpolar ionic.
   C. nonpolar covalent.
   D. polar covalent.

5. Which of the following molecules would show the greatest difference between its own standard free energy and that of the products that result from its hydrolysis into inorganic phosphate and the corresponding dephosphorylated molecule?

A. Glucose-3-phosphate
B. Creatinine phosphate
C. Carbamoyl phosphate
D. Adenosine triphosphate

6. At physiologic pH, the ATP molecule is sufficiently deprotonated as to carry four negative charges. Which of the following choices, if added to the surrounding medium, would most likely DECREASE the molecule's phosphate group transfer potential?

A. An inorganic base
B. An inorganic acid
C. An inorganic salt
D. An organic nonpolar solute

7. A chemist considers the ramifications of hypothetical evolutionary trends in which organisms had not developed the capacity to synthesize ATP. Among the following compounds, which would be most thermodynamically suited to assume its role as immediate donor of phosphate?

A. Glucose-6-phosphate
B. Carbamoyl phosphate
C. Phosphoenolpyruvate
D. Pyrophosphate

33.3 MASTERY VERIFIED: ANSWERS AND EXPLANATIONS

1. *A is the correct answer.* Although an unbound carbon atom has only two unpaired electrons in its outer shell, it can form up to four sigma bonds by hybridizing its orbitals. In this case three sigma bonds and one pi bondare formed from sp^2 hybridized orbitals.

2. *D is the correct answer.* The carboxylate (COO^-) moiety is a resonance structure; it represents a hybrid between between two structures: each carbon-oxygen bond has a partial double bond character. The electrons that form the bond are highly delocalized; they move about the positively charged nuclei of two oxygen atoms and a carbon atom. The negative charge carried by the COO^- moiety is delocalized, being accommodated by the two oxygen atoms.

3. *A is the correct answer.* Figure 1 shows one of the structures that contributes to the orthophosphate resonance structure. The other structures show delocalization of electrons by the movement of the double bond about the molecule and the dispersal of the molecule's two negative charges. Choice A shows the addition of a proton (hydrogen ion) to one of the oxygen molecules, which changes the molecule's constitution. The structure shown in choice A is not molecularly equivalent to the structure shown in Figure 1 or to those shown in choices B, C, and D.

4. *D is the correct answer.* Ionic bonds arise only between atoms of markedly different electro-negativities; they result in a true exchange of electrons. A polar covalent bond arises between atoms whose electronegativities are significantly different, but not so different as to produce an ionic bond. In a polar covalent bond, electrons are *shared unequally*: one atom carries a partial negative charge, and the other a partial positive charge. However, the MCAT test-taker must be aware that a carbonyl carbon carries a partial positive charge due to the high electronegativity of oxygen. This partial positive charge makes the bond between these two carbons a polar covalent bond.

5. *C is the correct answer.* The substance that has the lowest standard free energy of hydrolysis will be the one for which the difference between the standard free energy of products and reactants is greatest. Among the molecules listed in choices A–D, carbamoyl phosphate shows the lowest standard free energy of hydrolysis: –12.3 kcal/mol.

6. *B is the correct answer.* The four negative charges associated with the ATP molecule at physiologic pH are attributable to deprotonation—loss of hydrogen ions. Addition of an inorganic or organic base would decrease the ambient concentration of hydrogen ions and (a) promote deprotonation, and (b) increase the degree of negative charge. Addition of an inorganic acid would have the opposite effect. It would (a) increase ambient hydrogen ion concentration, and (b) *re*protonate the ATP molecule.

The ATP molecule's four negative charges repel one another and impair its stability, favoring its hydrolysis. Addition of an acid and the resulting reprotonation of the ATP molecule will reduce its number of negative charges and therefore stabilize it. If the ATP molecule's stability is increased, its tendency to be hydrolyzed and hence to transfer a phosphate group will be decreased.

The addition of a base would have the opposite effect: by promoting deprotonation of the molecule, it would increase the degree of negative charge, destabilize the molecule, increase its tendency to undergo hydrolysis, and increase its phosphate group transfer potential. The addition of inorganic salt would depend on the K_a for that salt and thus is not the best answer. A nonpolar solute would not affect the ATP molecule's stability.

7. *D is the correct answer.* According to the passage's last paragraph, ATP is well-suited to its role as immediate donor of phosphate because it shows an intermediate value for standard free energy of hydrolysis. Among the biologically significant phosphorylated compounds, the best replacement would be another molecule that has a free energy of hydrolysis in the mid-range. Choices A, B, and C are molecules whose standard free energies of hydrolysis are either extremely high or extremely low. Pyrophosphate, on the other hand, has the value of –8.0, which is relatively close to that of ATP and is in the mid-range.

CHAPTER 34

STEREOCHEMISTRY

34.1 MASTERY ACHIEVED

Two molecules are said to be **isomers** if they have the same atomic content and the same molecular formula, but differ in the way their atoms are arranged. **Structural isomers** are compounds that have the same molecular formulas but different atom to atom connectivity. Structural isomers have different chemical and physical properties.

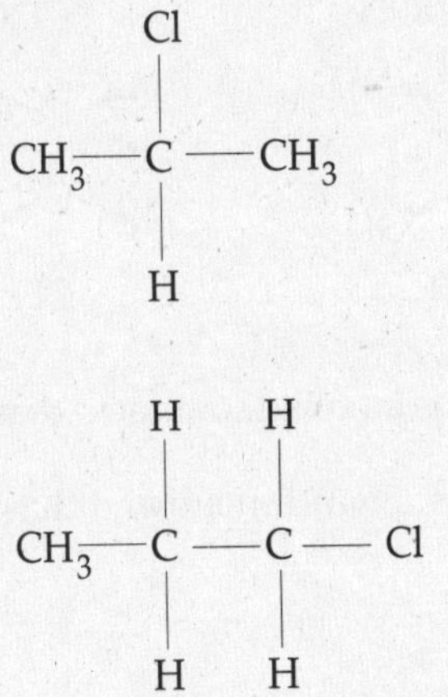

$$CH_3 - \underset{\underset{H}{|}}{\overset{\overset{Cl}{|}}{C}} - CH_3$$

$$CH_3 - \underset{\underset{H}{|}}{\overset{\overset{H}{|}}{C}} - \underset{\underset{H}{|}}{\overset{\overset{H}{|}}{C}} - Cl$$

Structural isomers

Stereoisomers are isomers in which atoms are bonded similarly but have different spatial arrangements. There are two types of stereoisomers; geometric and optical. The class of **geometric isomers** gives rise to what are called **cis** and **trans** configurations.

Cis-2-butene and *trans*-2-butene, for example, are geometric isomers.

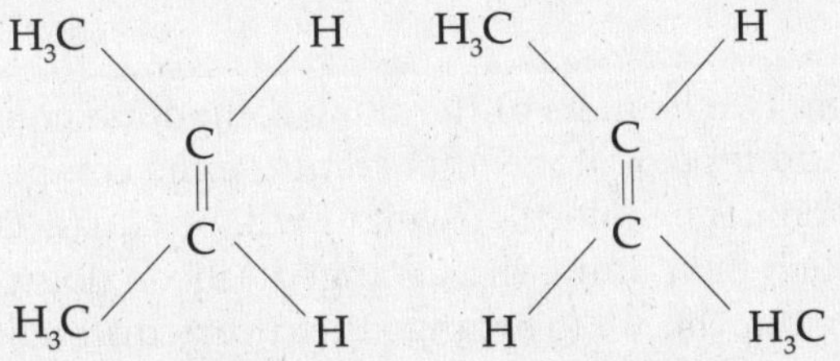

cis–2–Butene   trans–2–Butene

Geometric isomers

As you can see in the cis configuration, the two CH_3 ligands are located on the same side of the carbon-carbon double bond. In the trans configuration, the two CH_3 ligands are located on opposite sides of the molecule's carbon-carbon double bond.

Optical isomers are stereoisomers; they are also non-superimposable mirror image molecules. Optical isomers may be further divided into the subtypes **enantiomers** and **diastereomers**. Enantiomers are nonsuperimposable mirror-image stereoisomers, and diastereomers are nonsuperimposable *non*-mirror-image stereoisomers.

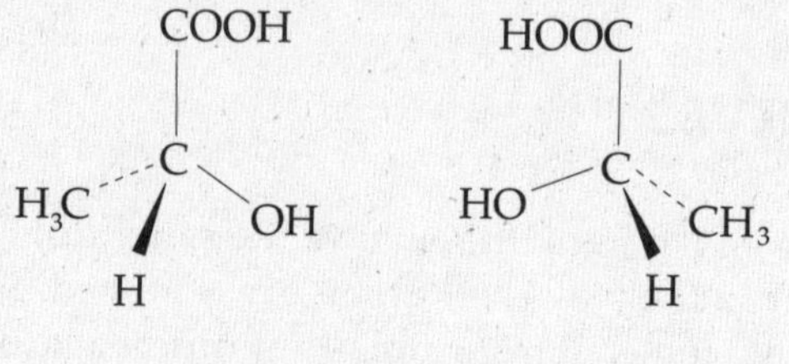

Lactic acid enantiomers

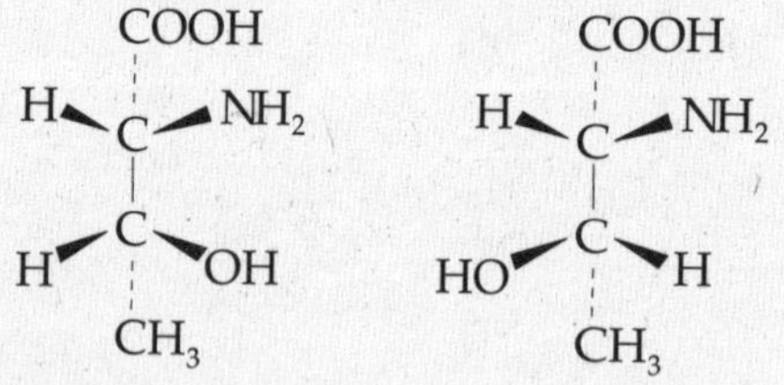

2-Amino-3-hydroxybutanoic acid diastereomers

Stereoisomers: Enantiomers and diastereomers

Please solve this problem:

- For two isomers, which of the following might be different?

  A. Molecular weight
  B. Molecular structure
  C. Both A and B
  D. Neither A nor B

Problem solved:

B is correct. By definition, two isomers of the same compound contain the same atomic constituents: the number and type of atoms that compose the compounds are identical. Therefore, for any pair of isomers, molecular weight will be equal. Two isomers differ, however, in the way in which their atoms are arranged. (By analogy, two persons might own identical items of furniture but choose to arrange them very differently. The weight of each set of furniture is equal; the arrangement of each set is different.)

Please solve this problem:

- The terms cis and trans represent alternate configurations of:

    A. all structural isomers.
    B. all stereoisomers.
    C. all geometric isomers.
    D. all optical isomers.

Problem solved:

C is correct. As noted in the text, cis and trans always refer to a pair of geometric isomers. Cis refers to isomers for which identical constituents are situated on one side of the molecule; trans refers to a pair of isomers for which identical constituents are situated on opposite sides of the molecule.

Please solve this problem:

- Two substances are analyzed and are found to have identical molecular formulas but different physical properties. An investigator postulates that the two substances represent a pair of structural isomers. Is the hypothesis plausible?

    A. Yes, because structural isomers have different molecular weights and, thus, different chemical properties.
    B. Yes, because structural isomers can represent very different substances with different chemical properties.
    C. No, because a pair of structural isomers has different molecular formulas.
    D. No, because structural isomers would most likely show similar behaviors and properties.

Problem solved:

B is correct. Two molecules may have the same atomic content and the same molecular formula but *differ* significantly in the way its constituent atoms are bonded and arranged. Such molecules are structural isomers and can possess very different physical properties.

34.1.1 CHIRALITY AND ENANTIOMERISM

A molecule is **chiral** if it cannot be superimposed on the molecule that represents its mirror image. A chiral molecule and its mirror image, in turn, are a pair of **enantiomers**. Consider the two enantiomers of the lactic acid molecule shown below:

$$\begin{array}{cc}
\text{COOH} & \text{COOH} \\
\text{H} - \text{C} - \text{OH} \quad & \quad \text{HO} - \text{C} - \text{H} \\
\text{CH}_3 & \text{CH}_3
\end{array}$$

Lactic acid

Observe that if we attempt to superimpose one molecule on the other, we fail. If the OH and H groups are superimposed on one another, the COOH and CH₃ groups will not coincide. If the COOH and CH₃ groups are superimposed on one another, the OH and H groups will not coincide. These two mirror image molecules cannot be superimposed on one another.

The two nonsuperimposable mirror image molecules that follow from chirality are, of course, isomers. More specifically, they are stereoisomers and more specifically still, they are enantiomers. A pair of enantiomers, then, is made up of two molecules that represent mirror images of each other, but cannot be superimposed on one another. Chirality gives rise to enantiomers, and enantiomers arise *only* from chirality. Therefore:

- If a molecule is chiral, its mirror image is its enantiomer, and its enantiomer is its mirror image.

- Any molecule for which there is an enantiomer is chiral.

- A molecule that is not chiral is sometimes called *a*chiral.

34.1.1.1 Chirality and the Chiral Center

Within any molecule, a **chiral center** refers to any central atom bonded to four **different** atoms or groups. Oftentimes, chiral centers are labeled as such by an asterix. The prototypical chiral center conforms to the model:

$$\begin{array}{c}
\text{Z} \\
\text{Y} - \text{C*} - \text{W} \\
\text{X}
\end{array}$$

Most chiral molecules important to organic chemistry have carbon as their chiral center. The letters W, X, Y, and Z refer to the four atoms or groups to which the chiral center (carbon) is bound. In the lactic acid molecule shown earlier, W, X, Y, and Z would correspond to OH, CH₃, H, and COOH, respectively. OH, CH₃, H, and COOH represent four different atoms or groups.

Consider a molecule of bromochloromethane:

$$
\begin{array}{c}
\text{Cl} \\
| \\
\text{H} - \text{C} - \text{H} \\
| \\
\text{Br}
\end{array}
$$

Bromochloromethane

The central carbon in bromochloromethane is bound to four atoms; however, two of the bonded atoms are H atoms, each of these *identical* to the other. The bromochloromethane molecule does not conform to the orientation:

$$
\begin{array}{c}
\text{Z} \\
| \\
\text{Y} - \text{C*} - \text{W} \\
| \\
\text{X}
\end{array}
$$

Rather, it conforms to this model:

$$
\begin{array}{c}
\text{Z} \\
| \\
\text{W} - \text{C} - \text{W} \\
| \\
\text{X}
\end{array}
$$

Therefore, it is not chiral.

The presence in any molecule of *one and only one* chiral center means that the molecule is chiral. As will be discussed in **34.1.2,** however, some molecules have *more than one* chiral center, and these molecules are not chiral. Moreover, some molecules are chiral even though they have no chiral centers. (The MCAT will seldom introduce a chiral molecule that has no chiral centers.)

Please solve this problem:

- An investigator discovers a molecule that has one and only one chiral center. Is he justified in concluding that the molecule is not superimposable on its mirror image?

    A. Yes, because the presence of one or more chiral centers always indicates chirality.

    B. Yes, because the presence of one and only one chiral center always indicates chirality.

    C. No, because some chiral molecules are superimposable on their mirror image molecules.

    D. No, because some enantiomeric pairs are superimposable on one another.

Problem solved:

B is correct. If a molecule has one and only one chiral center, it is chiral. Chirality refers to the condition in which a molecule is not superimposable on its mirror image molecule.

Please solve this problem:

- An investigator discovers a molecule that has no chiral centers. Is she justified in concluding that such a molecule may have an enantiomer?

    A. Yes, because a molecule may have no chiral centers and still be chiral.
    B. Yes, because a molecule that is achiral may nonetheless have an enantiomer.
    C. No, because a molecule without a single chiral center cannot be chiral.
    D. No, because enantiomers arise only when a molecule has a single chiral center.

Problem solved:

A is correct. A molecule with no chiral centers *may* be chiral, although it usually isn't. The molecule that represents the mirror image of any chiral molecule is, by definition, its enantiomer. Choice B is incorrect because an achiral molecule cannot have an enantiomer. Choices C and D are also wrong. A molecule may have no chiral centers and yet be chiral; a molecule with more than one chiral center may also be chiral.

Please solve this problem:

- Which of the following is true?

    A. Chirality requires at least one chiral center.
    B. The presence of one or more chiral centers always produces chirality.
    C. Both A and B
    D. Neither A nor B

Problem solved:

D is correct. It is possible for a molecule to have no chiral centers and yet be chiral; it is also possible for a molecule to have more than one chiral center and yet be achiral.

Please solve this problem:

- Which of the following is true?

    A. If a molecule has exactly one chiral center, it is nonsuperimposable on its mirror image molecule.
    B. If a molecule is nonsuperimposable on its mirror image molecule, it has exactly one chiral center.
    C. Both A and B
    D. Neither A nor B

Problem solved:

A is correct. Again, if a molecule has one and only one chiral center, it is chiral and is not superimposable on the molecule that represents its mirror image.

34.1.1.2 Classification of Enantiomers: R and S

Every chiral center and its four bonded entities may have either R or S configuration. R and S refer to a chiral center's **absolute configuration.** This is how to assign R or S:

(1) First, examine the chiral center and assign to each of its bonded groups or atoms a priority number of 1, 2, 3, or 4.

$$
\begin{array}{c}
Z \\
| \\
Y - C^* - W \\
| \\
X
\end{array}
$$

The constituent with the highest atomic number is assigned priority 1, and the constituent with the lowest atomic number is assigned priority 4.

(2) Draw the chiral center according to this model, positioning the atom with the lowest priority (4) in the back (represented by the straight dotted line):

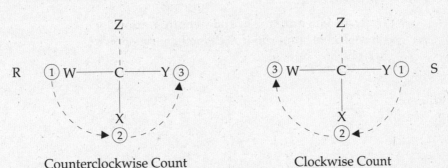

Counterclockwise Count   Clockwise Count

(3) Ignore the atom with priority number 4, and draw an arrow from the constituent with the highest priority to the one with the lowest priority. Does the arrow point in a clockwise or counterclockwise direction? If it proceeds clockwise, you have drawn the R configuration. If it proceeds counterclockwise, the chiral center has S configuration.

For the hypothetical chiral center shown above, the figure on the right represents the R configuration, and the one on the left represents the S configuration.

Consider a molecule of chloroiodomethanesulfonic acid, which has a single chiral center:

$$
\begin{array}{c}
H \\
| \\
I - C^* - Cl \\
| \\
SO_3H
\end{array}
$$

Of the atoms attached to the chiral carbon, hydrogen has the lowest atomic number, so the chiral center is drawn according to the model shown above, with hydrogen in the back position. Priority numbers are assigned to the remaining three atoms. Iodine has the highest atomic number, chlorine the next highest, and sulfur the lowest of the three. Thus, iodine is given priority number 1, chlorine number 2, and sulfur number 3. If we count 1-2-3 on the left molecule below, we move clockwise: the molecule on the left represents the R-configuration. If we count 1-2-3 on the right molecule, we move in the counterclockwise direction: the molecule on the right represents the S-configuration.

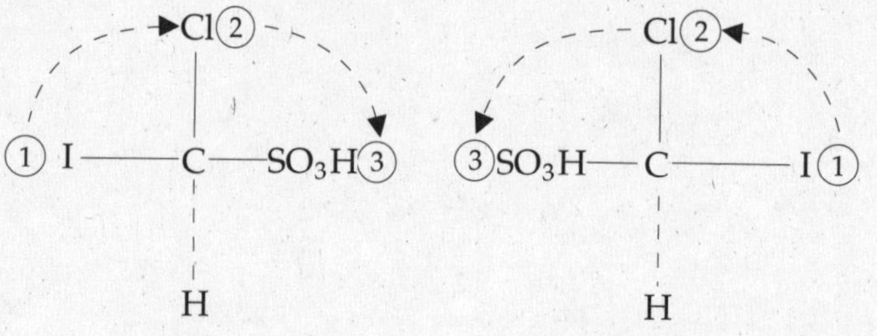

Clockwise Count
R-Configuration

Counterclockwise Count
S-Configuration

Please solve this problem:

- Draw and identify the R- and S-configurations of the molecule bromochloroiodomethane, as shown below:

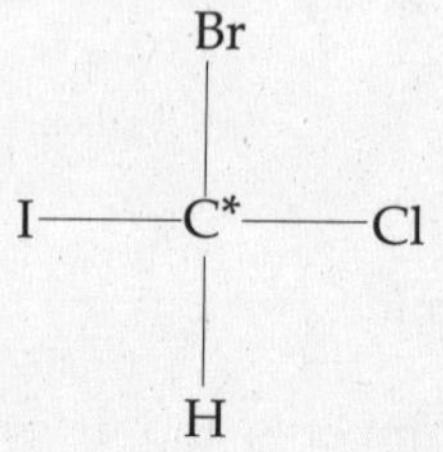

Problem solved:

To identify the R- and S-configurations, we examine the flat projection and assign priority numbers. Each of the bonded entities is a single atom, and the order of priorities is easily ascertained from the periodic table. Iodine has a higher atomic number than bromine, which has a higher atomic number than chlorine, which has a higher atomic number than hydrogen. Priority numbers are assigned as follows:

iodine, 1; bromine, 2; chlorine, 3; hydrogen, 4

The chiral center (which, in this case, embodies the entire molecule) is drawn according to the model shown above, with hydrogen pointed backward:

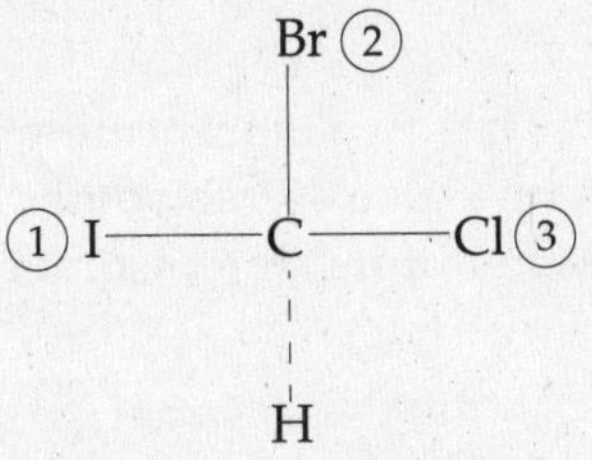

R-bromochloroiodomethane 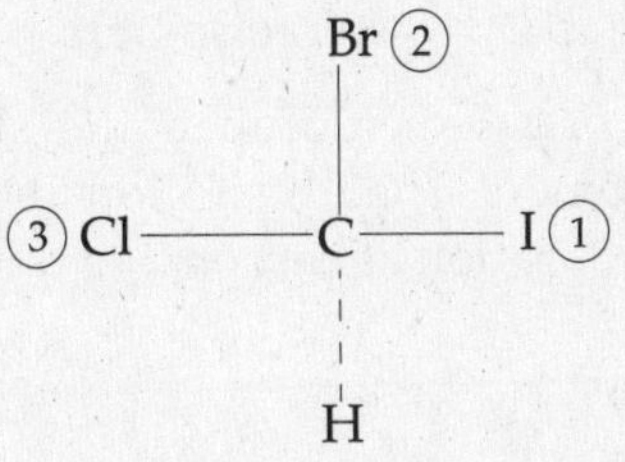   s-bromochloroiodomethane

For each of the resulting structures, we count 1-2-3 and note whether our progress is clockwise or counterclockwise. For the structure on the left, progress is clockwise. For the structure on the right, progress is counterclockwise. As such, the structure on the left is the R configuration, and the structure on the right is the s configuration.

34.1.2 DIASTEREOMERS

Some molecules have more than one chiral center. Consider this illustration of 2, 3-dichloropentane:

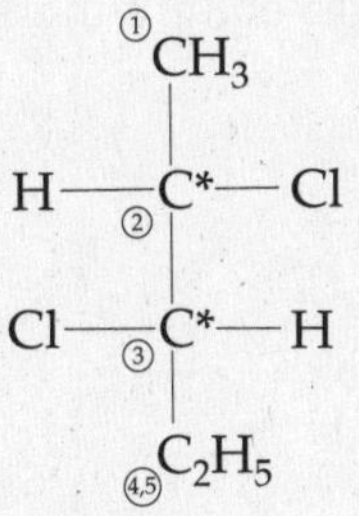

2, 3-dichloropentane

Two of the carbon atoms are chiral. The chiral center at carbon 2 conforms to the model:

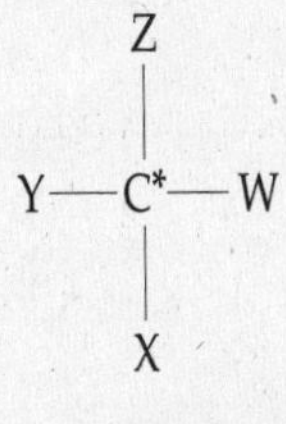

and the lettered variables in this case correspond to the following constituents:

Cl, **W**; C_3H_6Cl, **X**; H, **Y**; and CH_3 **Z**.

The X component corresponds to the entire group that is bonded to carbon 2. It consists, then, of carbon 3, and everything that's bonded to it.

Carbon 3 is also chiral, the lettered variables correspond to the following constituents:

H, **W**; C_2H_5, **X**; Cl, **Y**; C_2H_4Cl, **Z**

For carbon 3, the Z component corresponds to carbon 2 and everything bonded to it.

For any molecule with the number of chiral centers, n, the potential number of its stereoisomers is 2^n. For example, a molecule with one chiral center yields $2^1 = 2$ stereoisomers. A molecule with 2 chiral centers yields up to $2^2 = 4$ stereoisomers. A molecule with 3 chiral centers yields up to $2^3 = 8$ stereoisomers.

The molecule of 2, 3-dichloropentane, shown above, has two chiral centers, and gives rise to $2^2 = 4$ stereoisomers. The illustration above depicts one such stereoisomer. Let us now reverse the configuration at carbon 2 and identify another of its stereoisomers:

$$①CH_3$$
$$H—②C^*—Cl$$
$$H—③C^*—Cl$$
$$④,⑤C_2H_5$$

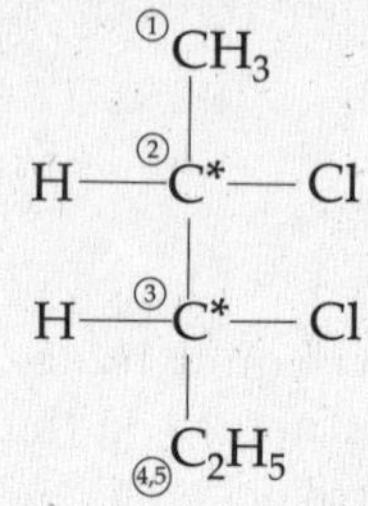

The drawing just shown does *not* represent the mirror image of the previous drawing. By definition, therefore, it is not the enantiomer of the molecule originally drawn. It is, however, a stereoisomer of that molecule. More specifically, it is its **diastereomer**. Diastereomerism arises when a molecule has more than one chiral center and produces more than one stereoisomer—only one of which, naturally, can be its mirror image. The other two stereoisomers are its diastereomers and are enantiomers of each other.

1.
$$CH_3$$
$$H—C—Cl$$
$$Cl—C—H$$
$$C_2H_5$$

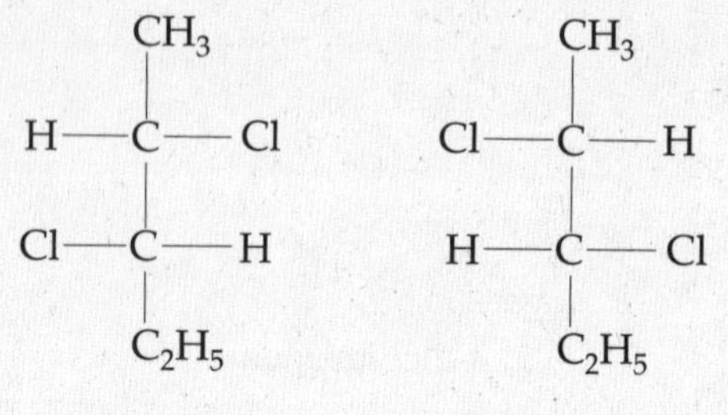

$$CH_3$$
$$Cl—C—H$$
$$H—C—Cl$$
$$C_2H_5$$
2.

$$CH_3$$
$$H—C—Cl$$
$$H—C—Cl$$
$$C_2H_5$$
3.

$$CH_3$$
$$Cl—C—H$$
$$Cl—C—H$$
$$C_2H_5$$
4.

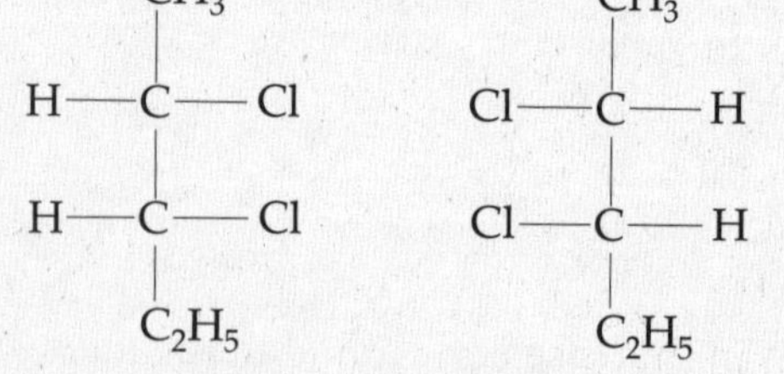

Stereoisomers of 2,3-Dichloropentane

Examine the molecules immediately above and note that 2,3-dichloropentane exists as four stereoisomers. These four stereoisomers embody two pairs of enantiomers. Either member of such a pair constitutes the diastereomer of a member of the other pair. In the illustration above, molecules 1 and 2 are a pair of enantiomers. Molecules 3 and 4 are a pair of enantiomers. Molecules 1 and 3 are a pair of diastereomers and molecules 2 and 4 are a pair of diastereomers. *All four molecules are stereoisomers of 2,3-dichloropentane.*

Please solve this problem:

- A molecule with 5 chiral centers may have a maximum of how many stereoisomers?

    A. 5
    B. 10
    C. 16
    D. 32

Problem solved:

D is correct. If a molecule has n chiral centers, then it has 2^n potential stereoisomers. If a molecule has 5 chiral centers, it has up to $2^5 = 32$ stereoisomers.

Please solve this problem:

- A molecule with 5 chiral centers may have a maximum of how many pairs of enantiomers?

    A. 5
    B. 10
    C. 16
    D. 32

Problem solved:

C is correct. As just noted, a molecule with 5 chiral centers has up to 32 stereoisomers. Each stereoisomer has one enantiomer, and so the total of 32 stereoisomers represents 16 pairs of enantiomers. Any member of one such pair is a diastereomer of any member of *another* such pair.

Please solve this problem:

- An investigator creates a substance that has 3 chiral centers. She isolates one of its stereoisomers, which she calls "stereoisomer W." Stereoisomer W may have a maximum of how many diastereomers?

    A. 4
    B. 6
    C. 8
    D. 12

Problem solved:

B is correct. The substance has 3 chiral centers and has, therefore, $2^3 = 8$ potential stereoisomers. Stereoisomer W is one of them, and like any of the eight stereoisomers, it has one enantiomer. The remaining six stereoisomers are its diastereomers.

Please solve this problem:

- An investigator discovers a substance containing 4 chiral centers. She isolates one of its stereoisomers, which she calls "stereoisomer X." How many diastereomers might stereoisomer X have?

   A. 14
   B. 16
   C. 24
   D. 32

Problem solved:

A is correct. The substance has 4 chiral centers and up to $2^4 = 16$ stereoisomers. Stereoisomer X is one of them; and, like any of the sixteen stereoisomers, it has one enantiomer. The remaining fourteen stereoisomers are its diastereomers.

34.1.3 OPTICAL ACTIVITY AND RACEMIZATION

Chiral compounds are **optically active**. *A compound that is optically active rotates the plane of polarized light.* For any enantiomeric pair, one enantiomer rotates the plane of polarized light to the right and is called the **dextrorotatory** or **d-enantiomer**. The other rotates the plane of polarized light to the left and is called the **levorotatory** or **l-enantiomer**. Rotation to the right is also associated with a positive (+) sign, and rotation to the left, with a negative (–) sign. For any given pair of enantiomers, therefore, the d-enantiomer is called the **(+)-enantiomer** and the l-enantiomer, the **(–)-enantiomer**.

Consider again, the compound bromochloroiodomethane, as shown below:

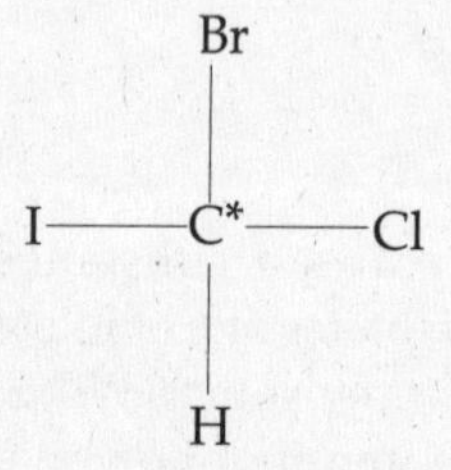

$$
\begin{array}{c}
Br \\
| \\
I - C^* - Cl \\
| \\
H
\end{array}
$$

One of this molecule's enantiomers is the d-enantiomer, meaning that it rotates the plane of polarized light to the right, and the other is the l-enantiomer, meaning that it rotates the plane of polarized light to the left.

To determine which enantiomer is dextrorotatory and which is levorotatory, one must use a **polarimeter**. The polarimeter consists of an eyepiece and two lenses, with a chamber between the two lenses in which a substance is placed. The instrument will indicate in which direction the plane of light is rotated. If the plane of light is rotated to the right, then the substance is the d-enantiomer; the other enantiomer is the l-enantiomer.

Other than evaluation via polarimetry, the chemist has no means of distinguishing between l-enantiomers and d-enantiomers. There is no analysis or examination of a chiral molecule's structure that reveals the direction in which it rotates polarized light.

Moreover, dextrorotatory and levorotatory are not equivalent to R and S. As described in **34.1.1.2**, R and S are achieved by convention, not by test for properties or behavior. For one chiral molecule, the R-enantiomer might be dextrorotatory, and the s-enantiomer, levorotatory, while for another chiral molecule, the s-enantiomer might be dextrorotatory, and the r-enantiomer, levorotatory. One must not equate r with d, or s with l.

On the other hand, the designations r and s do refer to a pair of enantiomers. If, for some chiral molecule, you learn, via polarimetry, that the r-enantiomer is levorotatory, then you should conclude that the s-enantiomer is dextrorotatory. If for some other substance you learn that the s-enantiomer is levorotatory, you can conclude that the r-enantiomer is dextrorotatory.

Please solve this problem:

- An investigator identifies the r-enantiomer of a particular enantiomeric pair. With no additional testing, which of the following may she justifiably conclude?

    A. The r-enantiomer rotates the plane of polarized light to the right.
    B. The r-enantiomer rotates the plane of polarized light to the left.
    C. Both A and B
    D. Neither A nor B

Problem solved:

D is correct. By convention, each member of an enantiomeric pair is assigned an r or s, which does not necessarily correspond to the direction in which it rotates polarized light. Because the investigator is dealing with a chiral molecule, she *can* conclude that it rotates the plane of polarized light, but she *cannot* know in which direction the rotation occurs (unless she or someone else has tested the molecule via polarimetry).

Please solve this problem:

- An investigator identifies the s-enantiomer of a particular enantiomeric pair. With no additional testing, which of the following may she justifiably conclude?

    A. The s-enantiomer rotates the plane of polarized light.
    B. The s-enantiomer rotates the plane of polarized light in a direction opposite to that in which the r-enantiomer rotates it.
    C. Both A and B
    D. Neither A nor B

Problem solved:

C is correct. Optical activity is a property of chirality. Both members of any enantiomeric pair rotate the plane of polarized light—one to the left, and one to the right. In the absence of polarimetry, one cannot determine which enantiomer—r or s—rotates the light in which direction. One does know, however, that (a) each enantiomer rotates the plane of polarized light either to the right or to the left, and (b) the other enantiomer rotates it in the opposite direction.

Please solve this problem:

- An investigator identifies a chiral compound having 2 chiral centers and isolates three of its stereoisomers. Assuming this compound has four stereoisomers, which of the following may she justifiably conclude?

    A. All three stereoisomers rotate the plane of polarized light in the same direction.
    B. Two of the three stereoisomers rotate the plane of polarized light in one direction, and the third rotates it in the other direction.
    C. Both A and B.
    D. Neither A nor B.

Problem solved:

B is correct. The four stereoisomers embody two pairs of enantiomers. Among the four stereoisomers, two are dextrorotatory and two are levorotatory. The investigator has isolated three of the four stereoisomers. That means that two of the three stereoisomers rotate polarized light in one direction (both to the right, or both to the left), and the third rotates it in the other direction.

34.1.3.1 Racemic Mixtures

A **racemic mixture** is any mixture of enantiomers in which dextrorotatory and levorotatory structures are of equal concentration. If, for one chiral molecule with one chiral center, a 50%-50% mixture of its two enantiomers is placed in a polarimeter, the polarimeter will show no rotation of polarized light, because the tendency of one enantiomer to rotate light to the right will equal the tendency of the other to rotate it to the left. A racemic mixture does not rotate the plane of polarized light, because the tendency of the d-enantiomer(s) to rotate rightward "cancels" the tendency of the l-enantiomer(s) to rotate leftward.

If a chiral molecule has more than one chiral center, it may yield more than one pair of enantiomers. If, for example, a chiral molecule features three chiral centers, it may give rise to $2^3 = 8$ stereoisomers, which are made up of four pairs of enantiomers. If you prepared a mixture so that all enantiomers are represented in equal proportions, the mixture would be racemic and would not be optically active.

Please solve this problem:

- A sample of x, a substance known to have a single chiral center, is subjected to polarimetry and causes no rotation of polarized light. Which of the following would explain the finding?

    A. The sample is a racemic mixture.
    B. The substance is not chiral.
    C. Both A and B
    D. Neither A nor B

Problem solved:

A is correct. The molecule has a single chiral center. It *must*, therefore, be chiral. (See **34.1.1.1.**) As explained in the text, a racemic mixture of a chiral substance will produce no net rotation of polarized light.

Please solve this problem:

- An experimenter identifies a chiral molecule with three chiral centers. He mixes two of its stereoisomers in equal concentrations and subjects the mixture to polarimetry. He notes a pronounced rotation to the left. Which of the following explains the finding?

  A. The sample is a racemic mixture.
  B. The two stereoisomers are diastereomers.
  C. Both A and B
  D. Neither A nor B

Problem solved:

B is correct. The substance has three chiral centers and gives rise, therefore, to as many as $2^3 = 8$ stereoisomers. These eight stereoisomers embody four pairs of enantiomers. Each pair, in turn, features a dextrorotatory enantiomer and a levorotatory enantiomer. The experimenter gathers a 50%-50% mixture of two stereoisomers, and on performing polarimetry notes leftward rotation. He cannot have produced a racemic mixture—a mixture of two enantiomers. If he had, he would observe no rotation. Instead, he has mixed two *diastereomers*, which are either both levorotatory, or one is more levorotatory than the other is dextrorotatory.

34.1.4 MESO COMPOUNDS

In **34.1.1.1** it was noted that a molecule with two or more chiral centers may or may not be chiral. That is because such a molecule might or might not represent a meso compound. A **meso compound** is one that is not chiral, even though it does have chiral centers.

Consider the molecule of 2, 3-dichlorobutane:

2, 3-Dichlorobutane

Note that the compound has two chiral centers, carbon 2 and carbon 3. Each carbon conforms to the model:

$$Z$$
$$|$$
$$Y—C^*—W$$
$$|$$
$$X$$

For carbon 2,

W is Cl; **X** is carbon 3 and all its bonded entities; **Y** is H; and **Z** is CH_3

For carbon 3,

W is Cl; **X** is CH_3; **Y** is H; and **Z** is carbon 2 and all its bonded entities

Consider now the mirror image of the entire molecule:

$$CH_3 \qquad\qquad CH_3$$
$$| \qquad\qquad\qquad |$$
$$H—C^*—Cl \qquad Cl—C^*—H$$
$$| \qquad\qquad\qquad |$$
$$H—C^*—Cl \qquad Cl—C^*—H$$
$$| \qquad\qquad\qquad |$$
$$CH_3 \qquad\qquad CH_3$$

2,3-Dichlorobutane and its Mirror Image

Note that the two mirror image molecules are in fact superimposable on one another. If we take the molecule on the left and, without removing it from the page, turn it upside-down in a counter-clockwise way, it is fully superimposable on the molecule to the right. These two molecules are in fact identical; they are not enantiomers. Each has a mirror image molecule superimposable on itself, and so the molecule as a whole is not chiral, even though it does feature two chiral centers.

The molecule below, 2,3-dichlorobutane, is a meso compound: it has chiral centers but is not chiral. Note the **plane of symmetry** of the meso compound. The molecule contains two chiral halves, each of which is the mirror image of the other.

$$CH_3$$
$$|$$
$$H—C^*—Cl$$
$$- - - - - - - - - -|- - - - - - - - -\text{ Plane of symmetry}$$
$$H—C^*—Cl$$
$$|$$
$$CH_3$$

A meso compound is, in a sense, two enantiomers bound within one molecule.

A molecule with more than one chiral center is not necessarily a meso compound: It is a meso compound only if it has a plane of symmetry, and hence is superimposable on its mirror image. If a molecule with more than one chiral center lacks a plane of symmetry, (1) it is not a meso compound, (2) it is chiral, (3) it is not superimposable on its mirror image, and (4) it *is* optically active.

Please solve this problem:

- Which of the following is true of a meso compound?

    A. It features a plane of symmetry.
    B. It is optically inactive.
    C. Both A and B
    D. Neither A nor B

Problem solved:

C is correct. A meso compound shows a plane of symmetry. One-half of a meso compound is the mirror image of the other half. A meso compound is optically inactive.

Please solve this problem:

- An experimenter identifies a molecule with two chiral centers. She subjects a sample of the substance to polarimetry and finds no rotation. Which of the following may she justifiably conclude?

    A. The molecule is a meso compound.
    B. She has prepared a racemic mixture.
    C. Either A or B
    D. Neither A nor B

Problem solved:

C is correct. The molecule has two chiral centers; it might be chiral, or it might be a meso compound. If it's chiral, however, its enantiomers might exist in equal proportions so as to produce a racemic mixture. It is possible that this investigator has gathered a racemic mixture. On the other hand, the molecule might be a meso compound. That is why choice C is correct.

34.2 MASTERY APPLIED: SAMPLE PASSAGE AND QUESTIONS

Passage

A neurological researcher is attempting to develop a pharmacologic agent effective in treating a degenerative disease of the cerebellum, called CDS. The disease impairs coordination of musculoskeletal movement. The researcher has isolated a substance that she calls X-TS and hypothesizes that it is effective in treating CDS. Dose-controlled studies suggest to her, however, that some samples of the substance are more effective than others. She then hypothesizes that the samples may produce different responses because they differ in their stereochemistry. Seeking to further assess and understand the matter, she conducts an experiment.

Experiment 1

A group of six normal individuals are subjected to a neurologic performance test involving a variety of tasks that assess musculoskeletal coordination. For each patient, a score is noted and recorded on a scale of 1-100. A group of six patients afflicted with CDS are subjected to the same neurologic performance test, and their scores also are noted and recorded on a scale of 1-100. Results are shown below.

Normal

Patient	Score
1	88
2	84
3	71
4	80
5	79
6	80

Afflicted

Patient	Score
1	21
2	26
3	18
4	30
5	20
6	22

Table 1

Experiment 2

Six samples of X-TS, labeled 1-6, each equal in mass, are subjected to polarimetry. The degree to which each sample rotates the plane of polarized light is noted and recorded. A group of forty-two patients is divided into six groups of seven members each, and each patient is treated daily with 50 mg of chemical derived from one of the samples 1-6. All members in one group are treated with a chemical derived from the same sample. Group 1 patients are treated with substance from sample 1, group 2 patients with substance from sample 2, and so forth.

After administration of the agent for one week, all patients are subjected to the neurologic performance test applied in Experiment 1. For each of the six patient groups, average scores are recorded and noted. Results are shown in Table 2.

Group/Sample	Rotation*	Score
1	+6.2°	29
2	+4.1°	33
3	+0.1°	43
4	−2.2°	50
5	−4.8°	65
6	−8.1°	65

*(+): rightward rotation
(−): leftward rotation

Table 2

1. Among the following, polarimetry would best determine whether a chiral molecule is:

   I. the R-versus the S-isomer.
   II. the d-versus the l-isomer.
   III. the (+)-versus the (−)-isomer.

A. I only
B. I and II only
C. II and III only
D. I, II and III

2. If an investigator subjects a sample of substance to polarimetry and finds no rotation of the plane of polarized light, is he justified in concluding that the substance is not chiral?

A. Yes, because any molecule that rotates the plane of polarized light is chiral.
B. Yes, because all chiral molecules rotate the plane of polarized light.
C. No, because some chiral molecules do not rotate the plane of polarized light.
D. No, because the sample may represent a racemic mixture.

3. The researcher described in the passage most likely performed polarimetry to determine if differences in therapeutic efficacy were due to differences in:

A. cis versus trans configuration.
B. stereoisomerism.
C. molecular formula.
D. molecular structure.

4. Among the following, the experimental data most strongly justify the conclusion that sample 6 is composed of:

A. a nonracemic mixture.
B. a levorotatory isomer only.
C. a racemic mixture.
D. achiral molecules.

5. In Experiment 2, which of the following served as a control?

A. Averaging of neurologic performance scores
B. Performance of Experiment 1
C. Notation of both the degree of rotation and the neurologic test scores
D. Use of unequal masses of sample X-TS

6. Among the following choices, which conclusion is most justified by the data derived from Experiments 1 and 2?

A. X-TS is chemically analogous to an endogenously produced substance which, when absent, produces CDS.
B. X-TS would be an ineffective treatment for CDS if the substance administered to the patient constituted a racemic mixture of (+)- and (−)-isomers.
C. X-TS is ineffective for treating CDS unless composed of a purely levorotatory form of the isomer.
D. A levorotatory form of X-TS effectively treats CDS, but benefit levels off after a certain percentage of l−isomer is attained in the compound.

7. Which of the following, if true, would most seriously question the conclusion that X-TS may be useful in treating CDS?

   A. All patients studied in Experiment 2 also had been diagnosed with an unrelated neurologic condition which produces symptoms of musculoskeletal incoordination.

   B. All of the patients studied in Experiment 2 were aware that the experiment was designed to test the efficacy of X-TS in the treatment of CDS.

   C. Patients in the early stages of CDS are frequently unaware of their disease and the dysfunction it produces, and consequently do not to seek treatment for it.

   D. Other investigators who have attempted to devise treatments for CDS have uniformly failed in their efforts.

8. The investigator concludes that X-TS is a chiral molecule consisting of one levorotatory enantiomer and one dextrorotatory enantiomer. Among the following, her conclusion would be most challenged if it were shown that:

   A. X-TS contains no carbon.
   B. X-TS is optically inactive in racemic mixtures.
   C. X-TS has more than one chiral center and is not a meso compound.
   D. X-TS has one and only one chiral center.

34.3 MASTERY VERIFIED: ANSWERS AND EXPLANATIONS

1. *C is correct.* Polarimetry allows the investigator to determine whether a particular sample of chiral substance rotates polarized light to the right or to the left. The dextrorotatory isomer—d-isomer—rotates light to the right, and the levorotatory—l-isomer—rotates it to the left. In this respect, the designations (+) and (–) are synonomous with "right" and "left," respectively. Choices II and III are accurate. Choice I is not. R and S refer to chiral *centers* (not chiral molecules) and are assigned according to a convention.

2. *D is correct.* If a substance is subjected to polarimetry and does not rotate the plane of polarized light, then either its molecules are not chiral, or they are chiral, but the sample is a racemic mixture of its dextrorotatory and levorotatory enantiomers.

3. *B is correct.* The polarimeter reveals optical activity. Optical activity refers to a substance's tendency to rotate the plane of polarized light, which closely relates to stereoisomerism. If two substances differ in the direction in which they rotate the plane of polarized light, they are stereoisomers.

4. *A is correct.* The substance in sample 6 rotates the plane of polarized light to the left. Hence it is composed of chiral molecules, since achiral molecules are not optically active. Choice D, therefore, is incorrect. Choice C is similarly incorrect; a racemic mixture has equal concentrations of opposing enantiomers and is therefore optically inactive.

   The investigator would not be justified, however, in concluding that sample 6 is composed *only* of levorotatory molecules (choice B). The sample might rotate the plane of polarized light to the left and still contain some dextrorotatory molecules, so long as the levorotatory influence is predominant. The investigator can conclude that the mixture is nonracemic since a racemic mixture is optically inactive.

5. *B is correct.* Data from Experiment 2 shows a tendency for a group's neurologic test score to increase with increasing levorotation of the administered substance. It does not show, however, what test score an afflicted patient might achieve in the absence of medication. A scientist might also question whether the medication has a harmful rather than a beneficial effect. In order to account for that possibility, the investigator would use a *control*. This would be accomplished in Experiment 2 by selecting one group of patients, providing them with no medication at all, and then subjecting them to the neurologic performance test. In Experiment 1, afflicted patients underwent neurologic testing without having received medication. Their scores of 21, 26, 18, 30, 20, and 22, yield an average of approximately 23, indicating that the patients of Experiment 2 would not have achieved better scores in the absence of any medication.

6. *D is correct.* The data show a correlation between extent of levorotation and neurologic performance that strongly suggests that a levorotatory form of X-TS constitutes an effective treatment for CDS. Furthermore, the substance that produced levorotation of –4.8° and that which produced levorotation of –8.1° yielded equal neurologic test performance. Since all samples were equal in mass when subjected to polarimetry, and all patients received 50 mg of medication per day, the results suggest that above some maximum dose the medication produces no improvement in performance.

   The passage does not provide evidence to justify choice A as more than a hypothesis. The experiments indicate that a levorotatory form of X-TS is useful, but they don't tell us how X-TS works. Choice B is incorrect as well: the data indicates that the levorotatory form of X-TS is effective in treating CDS. Moreover, there is indication that the medication will be effective without leftward rotation. If the D- and L-isomers are actually enantiomers, a racemic mixture would contain 50% L-enantiomer and 50% D-enantiomer. The data indicate that the presence of the L-enantiomer in the mixture might well bring benefit. They do not indicate that the presence of the D-enantiomer will prevent the L-enantiomer from acting.

Choice C is wrong for the same reason that choice B is wrong. The data suggest that levorotatory X-TS produces benefit, even when mixed with the dextrorotatory form. Samples 3, 4, and 5, for example, seem to contain some amount of D-isomer, since sample 6 shows even greater levorotation than they do. Yet, samples 3, 4, and 5 are associated with progressively increasing neurologic performance scores.

7. *A is correct.* If all patients studied in Experiment 2 were afflicted not only with CDS but also with another disease that produces uncoordination, the evidence may well indicate that X-TS is effective against the other disease and not against CDS. That is not to suggest that the experiment is without value. It provides a reason to believe that X-TS is effective against either disease.

Choice B is a weaker response than choice A. It is arguable that the patients could experience a "placebo effect" if they knew the purpose of the experiment. It is unlikely, however, that the placebo effect would be so pronounced; furthermore, the question asks which situation would "most seriously" question the conclusion.

Choices C and D are not relevant to the question. The fact that a patient is unaware of his or her disease has little to do with the testing of X-TS as a treatment for it. Similarly, the failure of a researcher's predecessors to achieve success does not have bearing on the outcome of her results.

8. *C is correct.* If a compound has more than one chiral center and is not a meso compound, then it gives rise to more than one pair of enantiomers. It gives rise to 2^n stereoisomers and $\dfrac{2^n}{2}$ pairs of enantioners. Each pair of enantiomers, in turn, embodies one levorotatory molecule and one dextrorotatory molecule. The investigator's conclusion as described by the question would be proven false if the conditions described in choice C were shown to be true.

Choice A is incorrect. Chirality does not depend on the presence of carbon. Although it is true that in the study of premedical organic chemistry the chiral compounds of most significance do contain carbon, some chiral compounds do not. Choice B is incorrect because racemic mixtures are optically inactive. Such a finding neither supports nor weakens the investigator's conclusion. Choice D is wrong because its statement would confirm the investigator's conclusion. If a molecule has one and only one chiral center it (a) is chiral, and (b) exists as two enantiomers—one dextrorotatory and the other levorotatory.

CHAPTER 35

THE HYDROCARBONS

35.1 MASTERY ACHIEVED

35.1.1 STRUCTURE OF HYDROCARBONS

Hydrocarbons are the simplest organic molecules; they are made up of only hydrogen and carbon. Hydrocarbons may be either **branched** or **unbranched** and either **saturated** or **unsaturated**.

Unbranched hydrocarbons consist of a straight chain of carbon atoms, while branched hydrocarbons contain branches of carbon chains.

Saturated hydrocarbons contain only C—C and C—H single bonds, while unsaturated hydrocarbons contain at least one site of unsaturation, which may be either a carbon-carbon double bond or a ring structure within the molecule. (A carbon-carbon triple bond represents two sites of unsaturation.) A hydrocarbon that possesses one or more of these features is said to be unsaturated. A saturated hydrocarbon has the general formula C_nH_{2n+2}, and an unsaturated hydrocarbon has the general formula $C_nH_{2(n-u+1)}$, where u is the number of sites of unsaturation in the molecule.

Please solve this problem:

- A chemical with the formula $C_{14}H_{18}$ has:

  A. one double bond, one triple bond, and one ring.
  B. two double bonds, one triple bond, and one ring.
  C. four double bonds and two rings.
  D. five double bonds and one triple bond.

Problem solved:

The correct answer is C. To solve this problem, we must first determine the number of sites of unsaturation (u) in this compound. Using the general formula $C_nH_{2(n-u+1)}$, we see that $n = 14$ and $18 = 2(14 - u + 1)$. Therefore, $u = 6$. Choice C is the only answer choice that contains six unsaturation sites.

35.1.2 NOMENCLATURE OF HYDROCARBONS

35.1.2.1 Unbranched Molecules

Hydrocarbons are named using a system of prefixes, each of which denotes the number of carbons in the molecule. These prefixes are:

Number of carbons	Prefix
1	meth-
2	eth-
3	prop-
4	but-
5	pent-
6	hex-
7	hept-
8	oct-
9	non-
10	dec-

Table 35.1

A saturated hydrocarbon is called an **alkane**. The names of all alkanes end in **-ane**. Therefore, a straight chain saturated hydrocarbon with six carbons is hexane. An unsaturated hydrocarbon, in which the site of unsaturation is a carbon-carbon double bond, is called an **alkene**. All alkenes end in **-ene**. Thus, a three carbon hydrocarbon with one double bond is propene. An unsaturated hydrocarbon, in which the site of unsaturation is a carbon-carbon triple bond, is called an **alkyne**. All alkynes end in **-yne**. Thus, a three carbon hydrocarbon with one triple bond is propyne. When the site of unsaturation is a ring, the prefix **cyclo-** is added to the name of the compound. A five membered ring consisting of otherwise saturated carbons would be named cyclopentane. A five membered carbon ring with one double bond would be named cyclopentene.

Hydrocarbon groups may also be substituents on other atoms. When this occurs, these groups are termed **alkyl groups**. All alkyl groups end in **-yl**. A four-carbon, saturated alkyl group is called a **butyl group**. A four carbon alkyl group containing a double bond is called a butenyl group, in which the -en- indicates the presence of the double bond.

Please solve this problem:

- The compound C_9H_{20} is a straight chain alkane.
The name of this compound is:

A. nonane.
B. nonene.
C. nonyne.
D. nonyl.

Problem solved:

The correct answer is A. From the problem or from the formula (no sites of unsaturation), we know that this compound is an alkane. Since all alkanes end in –ane, the correct name is nonane.

35.1.2.2 Branched Molecules

When hydrocarbons are branched, the base nomenclature is determined from the longest carbon chain present in the molecule. All substituents on the longest chain are named as alkyl substituent groups. The molecule:

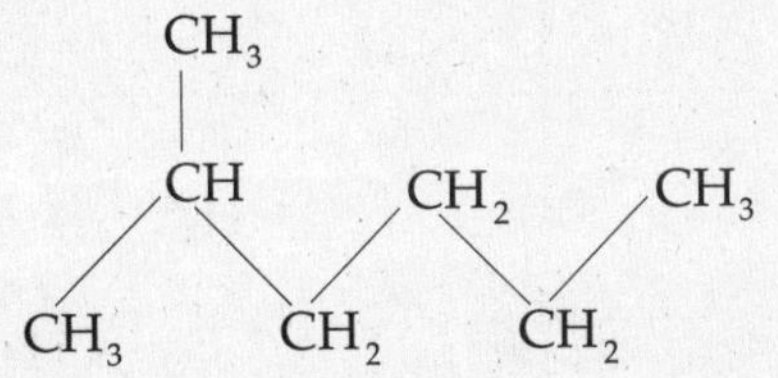

is called **2-methylhexane**. The 2 indicates that the methyl group is on the second carbon from the beginning of the chain. In a branched molecule without points of unsaturation, the carbons are numbered by beginning at the end that gives the substituent(s) the lowest numbers possible.

The Molecule:

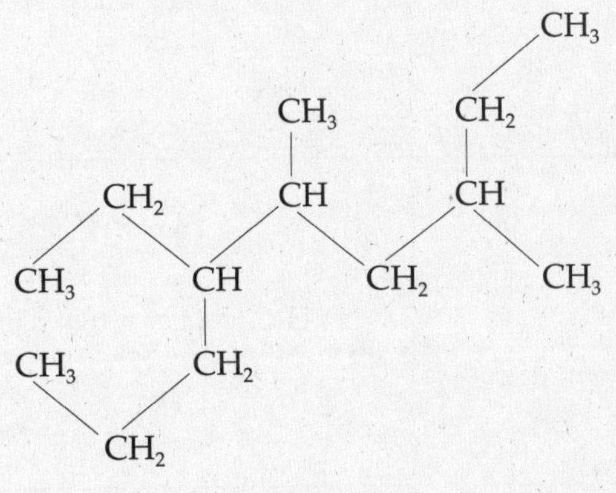

is named **6-ethyl-3,5-dimethylnonane**. The reason that, although the methyl groups are attached to groups earlier in the carbon chain, they are listed second in the compound name is that when substituents are not identical, they are ordered alphabetically.

Certain branched structures containing three to five carbons have common names with which you must be familiar. These are summarized in Table 35.2.

Name of Substituent Group	Structure
isopropyl	H_3C $\quad\ \ \diagdown$ $\qquad CH-$ $\quad\ \ \diagup$ H_3C
sec-butyl	$\qquad H_3C$ $\qquad\quad \diagdown$ $\qquad\qquad CH-$ $\qquad\quad \diagup$ CH_3-CH_2
iso-butyl	H_3C $\quad\ \ \diagdown$ $\qquad CH-CH_2-$ $\quad\ \ \diagup$ H_3C
tert-butyl	$\qquad\quad CH_3$ $\qquad\qquad \mid$ H_3C-C- $\qquad\qquad \mid$ $\qquad\quad CH_3$

Table 35.2

Please solve this problem:

- Name the following compound:

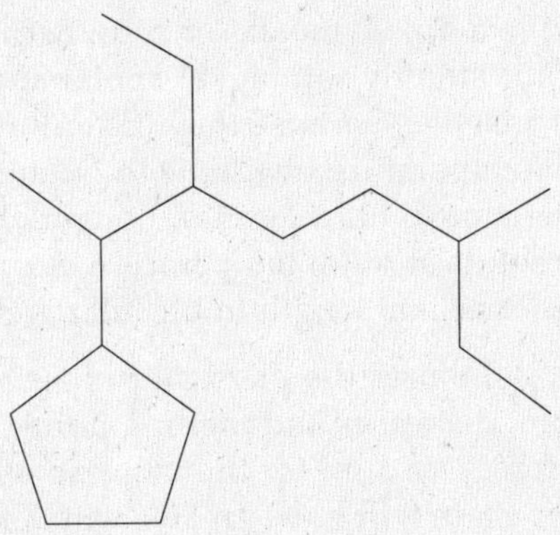

Problem solved:

The correct answer is 2-cyclopentyl-3-ethyl-6-methyloctane.

35.1.3 PHYSICAL PROPERTIES OF HYDROCARBONS

35.1.3.1 Saturated Hydrocarbons (Alkanes)

Alkanes are nonpolar and have a dipole moalxt of zero. Because of this lack of polarity, alkanes are either insoluble or only slightly solublcyê™ polar and ionic solvents. Alkanes also tend to be relatively chemically inactive, because they contain no functional groups. Short chain alkanes are gases at room temperature (methane to butane). Medium chain alkanes are liquids at room temperature (pentane to hexadecane). Longer chain alkanes (more than 17 carbons in a straight chain) are solids at room temperature. So, as you can see, both melting point and boiling points increase as chain length (molecular weight) increases.

Another imortant factor that influences the physical properties of alkanes is branching. As branching increases, boiling point decreases and melting point, though not as predictable, often increases. Van der Waals forces account for the increase in boiling and melting point as chain length increases—a longer chain will have greater van der Waals forces. Van der Waals forces also account for the configuration trends seen with branching. A branched molecule, unlike a straight chain molecule of the same molecular weight, cannot be configured in a way that will put much of its total surface area in contact with itself, and it is this surface-to-surface contact that gives rise to Van der Waals forces. A decrease in Van der Waals forces will lower the force needed to achieve a liquid-to-gas phase change. A decrease in surface area also allows molecules to arrange themselves more easily into a solid form from the liquid form. Thus, a decrease in surface area leads to an increase in melting point. To keep these concepts straight, compare them to the colligative properties of boiling point elevation and freezing point depression.

Please solve this problem:

- The compound with the highest boiling point is:

    A. *n*-pentane.
    B. 3-methylpentane.
    C. 2-methylbutane.
    D. 2,3-dimethylbutane.

Problem solved:

The correct answer is B. First, we must organize the choices based on molecular weight. The *n*-pentane has five carbons, 3-methylpentane has six carbons, 2-methylbutane has five carbons, and 2,3-dimethylbutane has six carbons. From this, we can eliminate choices A and C.

Now, we must choose the compound that is least branched. (Remember, branching lowers boiling point.) 2,3-Dimethylbutane is branched twice, and 3-methylpentane is only branched once. The methylpentane has a higher boiling point than the dimethylbutane.

35.1.3.2 Ring Conformations: Boat and Chair

For the MCAT, it is important to understand the fundamentals of hydrocarbon rings that contain from three to six carbons.

It is possible to form a three-membered ring; however, this creates huge angle strain between the participating atoms. A three-membered ring has internal C—C—C angles of 60°. These angles would prefer to be their normal tetrahedral conformation, with all bond angles equal to 109.5°. When angles are strained, the orbitals forming these bonds become more p-like. That is, they have greater than the 75% p-character found in the normal sp^3 hybrid orbital. This leaves less p-character available for the C—H bonds in the molecule, so they possess less than the 75% p-character found in the normal sp^3 hybrid orbital. It is important to recognize that an s–s bond is much stronger than a p–p bond (a double bond is always stronger than a single bond, because a double bond consists of an s–s bond and a p–p bond). Therefore, as the amount of p-character of a bond orbital (and thus the bond) increases, the strength of the bond decreases. As the amount of p-character of a bond decreases, the strength of the bond increases.

Rings of three, four, and five carbons possess ring strain. The C—C bonds that form these rings contain a higher p-character than a typical sp^3 hybrid orbital. Therefore, the bonds in these rings are weaker than the bonds in the open chain forms of these same molecules. The strength of the bonds in the rings increases in the order: three-membered < four-membered < five-membered, as ring strain is alleviated. As bond strength increases and ring strain decreases the ring becomes more stable. In a six-carbon ring, the carbons are able to adopt a configuration that allows for the complete elimination of ring strain.

There are two configurations available to the cyclohexane ring that minimize ring strain: the boat configuration and the chair configuration.

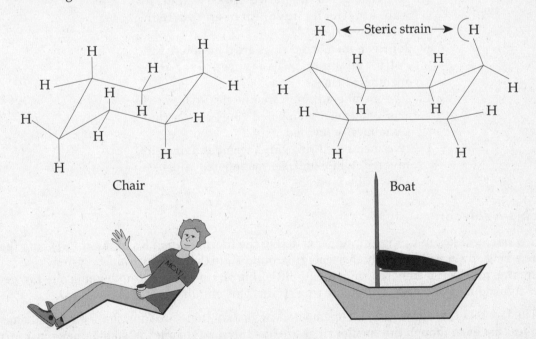

Chair

Boat

The chair is more stable than the boat because, in boat form, the hydrogens on the 1 and 4 carbons experience steric strain. Cyclohexane ring systems on the MCAT will always be in the chair form. In this configuration, we can see that there are two different types of hydrogens, a type that is in the "bumpy plane" of the ring and a type that is perpendicular to the ring.

Hydrogens that are perpendicular to the ring are **axial groups**, while hydrogens located "in plane" are **equatorial groups**. If a substituent is placed on a cyclohexane ring, it will adopt the equatorial position whenever possible, to avoid steric interaction with the axial hydrogens. This configuration is shown below, in which equatorial hydrogens are denoted H_e and axial hydrogens are denoted H_a. Notice that the t–butyl group adopts an equatorial orientation.

Please solve this problem:

- Five-membered rings suffer from more ring strain than do fourteen-membered rings. The most likely explanation for the occurrence of a greater number of five-membered rings than fourteen-membered rings in nature is:

    A. five-membered rings are thermodynamically and kinetically favored over fourteen-membered rings.

    B. fourteen-membered rings are thermodynamically and kinetically favored over five-membered rings.

    C. five-membered rings are kinetically favored, while fourteen-membered rings are thermodynamically favored.

    D. five-membered rings are thermodynamically favored, while fourteen-membered rings are kinetically favored.

Problem solved:

The correct answer is C. Ring strain is related to the thermodynamics of the ring. A ring that suffers ring strain will have a higher energy ground state than an unstrained system. Therefore, fourteen-membered rings—with little ring strain—are thermodynamically favored over five-membered rings—with more ring strain. This eliminates choices A and D.

The fact that there are more five-membered rings than there are fourteen-membered rings implies that even though the smaller rings are less thermodynamically stable, they must form at a more rapid rate—this is kinetics. Five-membered rings are kinetically favored over fourteen-membered rings. The reason for the kinetic preference of five-membered rings over fourteen-membered rings is that in the fourteen-membered rings the ends have difficulty "finding" each other.

35.1.4 CHEMICAL BEHAVIOR OF HYDROCARBONS

35.1.4.1 Alkanes

35.1.4.1.1 HALOGENATION AND THE ALKYL FREE RADICAL

Alkanes can react with halogens in the presence of ultraviolet light (uv) to form alkyl halides:

$$RCH_3 + Br_2 \rightarrow RCH_2Br + HBr$$

in which R designates the organic part of the molecule that does not contain any functional groups of interest to the reaction under consideration. For example, in the reaction above, if R were equal to a methyl group, the whole reaction, written without notation, would be:

$$CH_3CH_3 + Br_2 \rightarrow CH_3CH_2Br + HBr$$

The **halogenation** of alkanes proceeds via a free radical, and consists of three steps: **initiation**, **propagation**, and **termination**.

(1) Initiation—the formation of a free radical reactant:

$$Br\text{–}Br \rightarrow Br\bullet + Br\bullet$$

(2) Propagation—the radicals react with nonradicals to produce new radicals and new nonradicals:

$$Br\bullet + RCH_2\text{–}H \rightarrow H\text{–}Br + RCH_2\bullet$$

(3) Termination—the radicals are consumed:

$$Br\bullet + RCH_2\bullet \rightarrow RCH_2\text{–}Br$$

The relative reactivity of alkanes to free radical substitution is in the order:

$$tertiary\ (3°) > secondary\ (2°) > primary\ (1°) > methyl$$

This order is due to the relative stability of a tertiary carbon radical. Radical stability in alkanes is:

$$3° > 2° > 1° > methyl$$

Please solve this problem:

- The major product of the reaction of chlorine gas with 2,2,3-trimethylpentane is:

    A. 1-chloro-2,2,3-trimethylpentane.
    B. 2-chloro-2,2,3-trimethylpentane.
    C. 3-chloro-2,2,3-trimethylpentane.
    D. 4-chloro-2,2,3-trimethylpentane.

Problem solved:

The correct answer is C. The 2,2,3-trimethylpentane molecule can form a primary radical at the 1 carbon, a tertiary radical at the 3 carbon, a secondary radical at the 4 carbon, or a primary radical at the 5 carbon. Since the 2 carbon is already tetrasubstituted, radical formation at this carbon is precluded. This eliminates choice B.

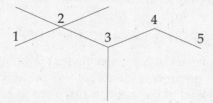

The major product is expected to come from the most stable carbon radical, which is the tertiary radical. Therefore, the correct answer is 3-chloro-2,2,3-trimethylpentane.

35.1.4.1.2 COMBUSTION

The only other important reaction involving alkanes is the **combustion reaction**. In a combustion reaction, a molecule is burned in oxygen gas to yield water and carbon dioxide. The general reaction equation for a combustion reaction of an alkane is:

$$C_nH_{2n+2} + \left(\frac{3n+1}{2}\right)O_2 \rightarrow nCO_2 + (n+1)H_2O$$

All combustion reactions are exothermic.

Please solve this problem:

- The complete combustion of $C_{24}H_{50}$ will produce:

    A. 24 moles of carbon dioxide and 25 moles of water.
    B. 24 moles of carbon dioxide and 51 moles of water.
    C. 50 moles of carbon dioxide and 25 moles of water.
    D. 50 moles of carbon dioxide and 51 moles of water.

Problem solved:

The correct answer is A. For every carbon in the molecular formula of the alkane, one mole of carbon dioxide will be produced. Therefore, this combustion will produce 24 moles of carbon dioxide. This eliminates choices C and D. For every two hydrogens in the molecular formula of the alkane, one mole of water will be produced. Therefore, 50 ÷ 2 = 25 moles of water will be produced.

35.1.4.2 Alkenes

35.1.4.2.1 CIS AND TRANS ISOMERIZATION

Consider 2-butene. This molecule may exist in one of the two following forms:

$$H-C=C-H \qquad H-C=C-CH_3$$

The form on the left is termed the **cis isomer** because both of its constituent methyl groups are on the same side. The form on the right is called the **trans isomer** because its methyl groups are on opposite sides. The trans isomer is also called the **E isomer** (E for *entgegen*, German for "opposite"), and the cis isomer is also called the **Z isomer** (Z for *zusammen*, German for "together"). To determine whether a tri- or tetrasubstituted double bond is E or Z, we compare the relative locations of the higher priority groups (again, using the same rules of priority as for stereochemistry).

The cis (Z) and trans (E) isomers of alkenes may chemically behave in drastically different ways. It is important to recognize which isomer you're dealing with when you're performing a reaction, and it is equally important to recognize which isomer will be formed in a reaction that yields an alkene.

Please solve this problem:

- An overall molecular dipole moment exists in ONLY:

  A. *cis*-2-butene.
  B. *trans*-2-butene.
  C. *trans*-1,3-dimethylcylcobutane.
  D. ethene.

Problem solved:

The correct answer is A. To solve this problem, we must first recognize that in certain cases rings, and even single bonds, may exhibit cis/trans isomerism. The four structures drawn out are:

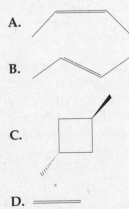

A.

B.

C.

D.

We can see that the two methyl groups on the cyclobutane ring are trans to one another: one is above the plane of the ring, the other is below the plane of the ring.

From an inspection of the symmetry of the above structures, it should be clear that the individual bond dipoles within each molecule cancel one another in all cases, except for the cis double bond. The correct answer is the choice that contains the cis arrangement: Choice A. The direction of the molecular dipole moment is:

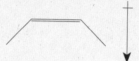

35.1.4.2.2 ELECTROPHILIC ADDITION

The only general reaction of alkenes that is of interest for the MCAT is electrophilic addition. In an **electrophilic addition**, a small ionic or polar covalent molecule is added across a double bond to form a substituted alkane. The general equation is:

$$R^2\ \ \ \ R^3 \qquad\qquad\qquad\qquad R^2\ \ R^3$$
$$\diagdown\!\!\diagup\qquad\qquad\qquad\qquad\qquad \mid\ \ \ \mid$$
$$C\!=\!C \quad + \quad AX \longrightarrow A-C-C-X$$
$$\diagup\ \ \ \ \diagdown \qquad\qquad\qquad\qquad\quad \mid\ \ \ \mid$$
$$R^1\ \ \ \ R^4 \qquad\qquad\qquad\qquad R^1\ \ R^4$$

in which A is the electropositive part of AX, and X is the electronegative part. Again, the R's refer to general groups that are not involved in the reaction.

In this reaction, the double bond serves as a nucleophile and attacks the electropositive A, to form a **carbocation**:

$$R^2\ \ \ \ \ \ \ \ R^3 \qquad\qquad\qquad\qquad R^2\ \ R^3$$
$$\diagdown\qquad\quad\diagup\qquad\qquad\qquad\qquad\qquad \mid\ \ \ \mid$$
$$C\!=\!C \quad + \quad AX \longrightarrow A-C-C+\ +X^-$$
$$\diagup\qquad\quad\diagdown\qquad\qquad\qquad\qquad\quad \mid\ \ \ \mid$$
$$R^1\qquad\qquad R^4 \qquad\qquad\qquad\qquad R^1\ \ R^4$$

A carbocation is formed on the most highly substituted carbon, since carbocations increase in stability in the order: Me < 1° < 2° < 3°. Once the carbocation is formed, it is consumed by X⁻ and the product is formed. The observation that the more substituted carbocation is formed and then subject to nucleophilic attack is called Markovnikov's addition, and when substitution occurs such that the least substituted carbon receives the nucleophile, this is called anti-Markovnikov addition.

Please solve this problem:

- The major product in the electrophilic addition of hydrochloric acid to 4-methyl-3-heptene is:

    A. 3-chloro-4-methyl-3-heptene.
    B. 4-chloro-4-methyl-3-heptene.
    C. 3-chloro-4-methyl-heptane.
    D. 4-chloro-4-methyl-heptane.

Problem solved:

The correct answer is D. In an electrophilic addition to an alkene, the carbons that bear the double bond are attacked. This eliminates choices A and B, which are still alkenes. Also, we know that an electrophilic addition to an alkene follows Markovnikov's rule: the electronegative atom attaches to the most substituted carbon of the double bond. Prior to the addition, the 3 carbon is monosubstituted, and the 4 carbon is disubstituted. Therefore, we expect the chlorine to attach to the 4 carbon, giving 4-chloro-4-methyl-heptane.

35.1.4.3 Alkynes

The reactions of alkynes are similar to those of alkenes. In an electrophilic addition, the electronegative group will attach to the more substituted carbon, just as we saw for alkenes (Markovnikov's rule). However, since we are making an alkene, we need to be concerned with the relative stereochemistry (cis or trans) of the addition process. Due to steric interactions, trans addition is almost exclusively favored in all electrophilic additions to alkynes. A trans addition implies that the two groups (A and X, below) are added in a fashion that places them trans to one another. A trans addition *does not guarantee* the formation of a trans product. The general equation for an electrophilic addition across an alkyne is:

$$R_1 - C \equiv C - R^2 + AX \longrightarrow \begin{array}{c} A \quad\quad R^2 \\ C=C \\ R^1 \quad\quad X \end{array}$$

35.1.5 AROMATICITY AND AROMATIC COMPOUNDS

Certain compounds that contain both rings and multiple bonds are stabilized by an additional factor. This factor is termed **aromaticity**. A compound is aromatic when it is additionally stabilized because of a cyclic overlap of alternating double bonds. The most familiar example of an aromatic compound is the compound benzene. (For the MCAT, discussions of aromaticity are generally limited to benzene and its derivative compounds.) These compounds will be discussed with regard to the functional group(s) on the benzene ring. At this time, our discussion will be limited to electrophilic additions to benzene.

When a benzene ring is not substituted, it is reasonably resistant to electrophilic addition. The presence of certain groups on a benzene ring tends to either activate or deactivate the ring to electrophilic addition reactions. Substituent groups will also tend to cause addition at certain carbons on the ring in preference to other ring carbons. To understand these trends, we must first define the relative positions on a benzene ring.

The carbon to which a substituent is attached is termed the **ipso carbon**. One carbon away from the substituent group, on either side, are the **ortho carbons**. Two carbons away, on either side, are the **meta carbons**, and the carbon opposite the substituent group is termed the **para carbon**. This is illustrated for toluene below:

CH_3

i

o   o

m   m

p

toluene

in which

i = ipso,

o = ortho,

m = meta,

p = para.

Electron-withdrawing substituents on a benzene ring are meta directors; that is, they direct the incoming electrophile to one of the two meta carbons. Electron-donating substituents on a benzene ring are ortho, para directors. The only exception to these rules is halogens, which are electron-withdrawing groups, but direct electrophiles to ortho and para positions.

To summarize:

- All *electron-withdrawing* groups, except the halogens, are *meta* directors

- All *electron-donating* groups are *ortho, para* directors

- The *halogens* are *ortho, para* directors

Substituents on benzene rings influence their susceptibility to further electrophilic addition reactions:

- *Electron-withdrawing* groups are *ring-deactivating*.

- *Electron-donating* groups are *ring-activating*.

Please solve this problem:

- The addition of a nitro group to bromobenzene will:

    A. proceed more rapidly than the addition of a nitro group to benzene, to yield primarily 1-bromo-3-nitrobenzene.

    B. proceed more slowly than the addition of a nitro group to benzene, to yield primarly 1-bromo-3-nitrobenzene.

    C. proceed more rapidly than the addition of a nitro group to benzene, to yield primarily 1-bromo-4-nitrobenzene.

    D. proceed more slowly than the addition of a nitro group to benzene, to yield primarily 1-bromo-4-nitrobenzene.

Problem solved:

The correct answer is D. Bromine, like all electron-withdrawing groups, somewhat deactivates a benzene ring. Therefore, we would expect the addition of a substituent to proceed more slowly than the addition of the same group to an unsubstituted benzene. This eliminates choices A and C. Bromine (a halogen) is an ortho, para director. Therefore, we expect the 1,4-disubstituted (para) product, *not* the 1,3-disubstituted (meta) product. This eliminates choice B, leaving only choice D.

35.2 MASTERY APPLIED: SAMPLE PASSAGE AND QUESTIONS

Passage

The addition of a hydrogen halide to an unsymmetric alkene will lead to a halogenated product in which the halide is on the more substituted carbon, or to a product in which the halide is on the less substituted carbon. The former addition is said to follow Markovnikov's rule. The latter is said to be an example of an anti-Markovnikov addition. If only one of these two possible products is formed in the reaction, the reaction is said to be **regiospecific**. If a mixture of the two products is formed, with a predominance of one product, the reaction is said to be **regioselective**.

The addition of a hydrogen halide across a double bond also has the potential to create two chiral centers, one at each of the former sp^2 carbons. If both the hydrogen and the halide add on the same side of the plane containing the double bond, this is termed **syn addition**. When one adds from the above the plane and the other adds from below the plane, this is termed **anti addition**.

1. When reacted with HBr, 3-methyl-2-hexene will most likely undergo:
   A. Markovnikov syn addition.
   B. Markovnikov anti addition.
   C. anti-Markovnikov syn addition.
   D. anti-Markovnikov anti addition.

2. The addition of HCl to 1,2-dimethylcyclohexene is anti at room temperature; however, syn addition dominates at −78°C. Which of the following statements best describes this observation?
   A. The activation energy for formation of the intermediate of syn addition is less than the activation energy for formation of the intermediate of anti addition.
   B. The activation energy for formation of the intermediate of syn addition is more than the activation energy for formation of the intermediate of anti addition.
   C. The syn addition involves a discrete two-step mechanism in which a carbocation intermediate is formed.
   D. The anti addition involves a discrete two-step mechanism in which a carbocation intermediate is formed.

3. The rate law for addition of HBr to most simple alkenes may be approximated as rate = k [alkene][HBr]^2. This rate law indicates all of the following EXCEPT:
   A. the reaction is second order in hydrogen halide.
   B. the reaction involves the alkene and one HBr in an irreversible step, followed by the intermediate formed from the first step reacting with a second HBr in the rate-determining step.
   C. the reaction is a single step, involving two HBr molecules for every one alkene molecule.
   D. the reaction is third order.

4. Which of the following would be the best solvent for the addition of HCl to 3-hexene?

   A. H_2O
   B. CH_3OH
   C. CH_3CO_2H
   D. $CH_3CH_2OCH_2CH_3$

5. Which of the following would show the LEAST regioselectivity after HBr addition?

   A. $CH_3HC=C(CH_3)CH_2CH_3$
   B. $(CH_3)_2C=CHCH_2CH_3$
   C. $(CH_3)_2C=C(CH_3)CH_2CH_3$
   D. $H_2C=C(CH_3)CH_2CH_3$

6. Rank the halides in order of increasing rate of addition to 3-hexene in a non-polar, aprotic solvent:

   A. HCl < HBr < HI
   B. HCl < HI < HBr
   C. HBr < HCl < HI
   D. HI < HBr < HCl

35.3 MASTERY VERIFIED: ANSWERS AND EXPLANATIONS

1. *The correct answer is B.* We know that HBr adds Markovnikov, which enables us to eliminate choices C and D. The information in the passage about syn and anti addition and steric considerations alone should allow you to pick choice B over choice A.

2. *The correct answer is C.* A carbocation intermediate will be stabilized by the lower temperature. Therefore, it makes sense that the mechanism that predominates at −78°C goes through a carbocation intermediate. We now know that the syn addition goes through a carbocation intermediate. The formation of a carbocation intermediate indicates at least a two-step mechanism. This leads us to choice C while eliminating choice D. We must also eliminate choices A and B, by realizing that we do not know, nor care, about the relative values of the activation energies.

3. *The correct answer is B.* The given rate law indicates that the reaction is second order in HBr, so choice A is true. The rate law also indicates that the reaction is overall third order, so choice D is true. Choice C is a statement of the rate law, so it is also true. The rate law does not indicate whether the first step of the mechanism is irreversible, nor does the rate law give information on the number of steps, or which is rate determining. While choice B may or may not fit this rate law, there are other possibilities which are clearly true. Choice B is the least true of the four answer choices.

4. *The correct answer is D.* This is the only solvent choice that does not compete with the desired reaction (the other three are all potential nucleophiles).

5. *The correct answer is C.* In choice A, the possible carbocations are secondary and tertiary; the tertiary carbocation would clearly be favored. In choice B, the possible carbocations are tertiary and secondary; as in choice A, the tertiary carbocation would clearly be favored. In choice C, the possible carbocations are both tertiary; in this distractor, it is not clear which carbocation would be favored. In choice D, the possible carbocations are primary and tertiary, and as in choices A and B, the tertiary carbocation would clearly be favored.

6. *The correct answer is D.* Chloride (Cl^-) is the best nucleophile, followed by bromide (Br^-), followed by iodide (I^-).

CHAPTER 36

ALCOHOLS, PHENOLS, AND ETHERS

36.1 MASTERY ACHIEVED

36.1.1 STRUCTURES AND PROPERTIES OF ALCOHOLS

The most basic alcohol is **methanol** (Me), and more complex alcohols are called **primary** (1°), **secondary** (2°), or **tertiary** (3°). The general form of each of these is:

$$\underset{\text{Me}}{\overset{\displaystyle H}{\underset{\displaystyle H}{H-C-OH}}} \qquad \underset{\text{1°}}{\overset{\displaystyle R}{\underset{\displaystyle H}{H-C-OH}}} \qquad \underset{\text{2°}}{\overset{\displaystyle R}{\underset{\displaystyle H}{R-C-OH}}} \qquad \underset{\text{3°}}{\overset{\displaystyle R}{\underset{\displaystyle R}{R-C-OH}}}$$

where R represents an **alkyl group**.

The physical properties of alcohols are attributable to their hydroxyl groups. Since the oxygen in a hydroxyl group is highly electronegative and possesses two lone pairs of electrons, it is capable of **hydrogen bonding** with the hydrogen of the hydroxyl group of other alcohol molecules, or any other molecule that is capable of hydrogen bonding.

All alcohols are capable of hydrogen bonding.

The hydrogen atom of the hydroxyl group of all alcohols is acidic because of the presence of the electron-withdrawing oxygen atom.

Because the carbon atom to which a hydroxyl group is attached is made partially positive by the electron-withdrawing oxygen atom, the carbon is often subject to nucleophilic attack.

The hydrogen-bonding capacity of alcohols increases their boiling and melting points in relation to ordinary hydrocarbons. Thus, methanol has a higher boiling point and a higher melting point than methane. Likewise, *t*-butyl alcohol has a higher boiling point and a higher melting point than *t*-butane.

As we discussed in Chapter 35, branching tends to decrease van der Waals' forces, which decreases the boiling point. The boiling point of alcohols with identical molecular weights would be expected to increase in the order: 3° < 2° < 1°.

Alcohol molecules are **polar**; they possess a permanent **molecular dipole moment**. As a result of this, all alcohols are soluble in polar solvents. Solubility is decreased by increasing chain length and by branching, since both of these effects serve to lessen the dipole moment (and, thus, the polarity) of the alcohol.

The oxygen atoms of alcohol groups can serve as bases and accept protons from stronger acids (those compounds with lower pK_a's).

$$R-\underset{\underset{R}{|}}{\overset{\overset{R}{|}}{C}}-O \ + \ HA \longrightarrow R-\underset{\underset{R}{|}}{\overset{\overset{R}{|}}{C}}-\overset{+}{O}\underset{H}{\overset{H}{\diagup}} \ + \ A$$

This transforms the alcohol group into a good leaving group—hydroxide is a poor leaving group—and makes the carbon more susceptible to nucleophilic attack.

The alcohol group can also serve as an acid, donating protons to stronger bases (bases with higher pK_b's—or lower pK_a's):

$$R-\underset{\underset{R}{|}}{\overset{\overset{R}{|}}{C}}-OH \ + \ B: \longrightarrow R-\underset{\underset{R}{|}}{\overset{\overset{R}{|}}{C}}-O^- \ + \ BH^+$$

Please solve this problem:

- The compound with the highest boiling point is:

  A. 3-methylhexane.
  B. 3-methyl-1-hexanol.
  C. 3-methyl-2-hexanol.
  D. 3-methyl-3-hexanol.

Problem solved:

The correct answer is B. Since alcohols have higher boiling points than their analogous alkanes, 3-methylhexane has the lowest boiling point. Therefore, choice A is eliminated. The compound in choice B is a primary alcohol; the compound in choice C is a secondary alcohol; the compound in choice D is a tertiary alcohol. We expect analogous alcohols to increase in boiling point in the order: $3° < 2° < 1°$. Therefore, the primary alcohol (3-methyl-1-hexanol) is expected to have the highest boiling point.

36.1.2 CHEMICAL BEHAVIOR OF ALCOHOLS

36.1.2.1 Acidity of Alcohols

There are two important factors that contribute to the acidity of alcohols: **branching** (1° versus 2° versus 3°) and the presence of **substituent groups** elsewhere in the molecule.

Earlier, we showed you that branching decreases molecular polarity, and should be clear that branching also decreases acidity.

Alcohol acidity increases in the order: $3° < 2° < 1°$.

It should also be clear that increasing molecular weight tends to decrease alcohol acidity.

Other functional groups within the alcohol molecule will influence the acidity of the alcoholic hydrogen. A group that withdraws electron density from the alcohol carbon will increase the acidity of the alcohol, while a group that donates electron density to the carbon will decrease the acidity of the alcohol.

Electron-withdrawing groups increase alcohol acidity.

Electron-donating groups decrease alcohol acidity.

An electron-withdrawing group increases alcohol acidity by stabilizing the alkoxy anion (RO$^-$) that results from the deprotonation. An electron-donating group destabilizes this anion.

Please solve this problem:

- The most acidic alcohol is:

  A. 2-propanol.
  B. 2-methyl-2-propanol.
  C. 2-amino-2-propanol.
  D. 2-nitro-2-propanol.

Problem solved:

The correct answer is D. The order of acidity of these compounds is: 2° alcohol with electron-withdrawing group > 2° alcohol > 3° alcohol > 2° alcohol with electron-donating group. Or, 2-nitro-2-propanol > 2-propanol > 2-methyl-2-propanol > 2-amino-2-propanol. Or, D > A > B > C. We know that 2-methyl-2-propanol is a stronger acid than 2-amino-2-propanol, since the methyl group is a weaker electron donor than the amino group.

36.1.2.2 Dehydration Reactions: E_1 and E_2

Alcohols may lose water to form alkenes via **dehydration reactions**:

$$
\begin{array}{c}
\underset{R^3}{\overset{R^4}{H-C}}-\underset{R^2}{\overset{R^1}{C}}-OH \longrightarrow \underset{R^3}{\overset{R^4}{C}}=\underset{R^2}{\overset{R^1}{C}}
\end{array}
$$

This reaction may occur by either a two-step mechanism (E_1) or a one-step mechanism (E_2). The mechanism nomenclature E_x means elimination (E), x-molecular. The molecularity of a mechanism indicates the number of molecules that are involved in the **rate-determining step**. Therefore, an E_1 reaction is a **unimolecular elimination**, with one molecule (a carbocation) involved in the rate-determining step. An E_2 reaction is a **bimolecular elimination**, with two molecules involved in the rate-determining step. You should know that alcohols are not the only substrates that undergo elimination reactions; alkyl halides and other substrates in which there is a proton on the carbon adjacent to the cationic carbon that can be attacked by a nucleophile also undergo eliminations.

E_2 reactions are favored in reactions involving primary alcohols, while E_1 reactions are favored in reactions that involve tertiary alcohols.

$$E_2: 1° > 2° > 3°$$

$$E_1: 3° > 2° > 1°$$

Secondary substrates can react by either an E_1 or an E_2 mechanism—usually the elimination reaction mechanism of secondary alcohols is E_2, but this does not necessarily apply to all eliminations of secondary substrates (i.e., nonalcohols).

Tertiary alcohols are dehydrated under acidic conditions to yield the most highly substituted alkene. The mechanism is E_1. The two steps are given below:

Step 1: carbocation formation

Step 2: formation of the more substituted alkene

An E_1 reaction exhibits overall first-order kinetics. The rate-determining step is the first step, or the formation of the **carbocation intermediate**. Therefore, substrate concentration is an important consideration in an E_1 reaction.

An E_1 reaction is first-order in substrate concentration.

Primary alcohols (and most secondary alcohols) require harsher conditions for dehydration than tertiary alcohols. The most common alcohol-dehydrating agent for primary and secondary alcohols is phosphorus oxychloride ($POCl_3$). The product is the most highly substituted alkene unless the formation of this product is precluded by steric considerations, and the mechanism of the elimination is E_2. While the overall mechanism involves two steps, the first step is not part of the elimination process. Only the second step is the E_2 mechanism.

Step 1: formation of the good leaving group $PO_2Cl_2^-$

Step 2: E_2 elimination

An E_2 reaction exhibits overall second-order kinetics. The rate-determining step is the only step. Therefore, the substrate concentration and effectiveness, and the incoming acid concentration and effectiveness, must *both* be considered in an E_2 reaction.

An E_2 reaction is first-order in substrate concentration *and* first-order in nucleophile concentration, so the overall reaction is second-order.

Comparing E_1 and E_2 reactions:

- Tertiary alcohols react via an E_1 mechanism.

- Primary alcohols react via an E_2 mechanism.

- Secondary alcohols may react via either pathway, but generally will react via an E_2 mechanism.

- E_1 reactions exhibit first-order kinetics.

- E_2 reactions exhibit second-order kinetics.

- E_1 reactions depend only on the nature and concentration of the substrate.

- E_2 reactions depend on the nature and concentration of both the substrate and the nucleophile.

Please solve this problem:

- The dehydration of 2,3-dimethyl-3-pentanol will proceed via an:

  A. E_1 mechanism to give 2,3-dimethyl-2-pentene as the major product.
  B. E_2 mechanism to give 2,3-dimethyl-2-pentene as the major product.
  C. E_1 mechanism to give 3,4-dimethyl-2-pentene as the major product.
  D. E_2 mechanism to give 3,4-dimethyl-2-pentene as the major product.

Problem solved:

The correct answer is A. 2,3-Dimethyl-3-pentanol is a tertiary alcohol. It will, therefore, undergo dehydration via an E_1 mechanism. This eliminates choices B and D. Dehydration via an E_1 mechanism results in the predominant formation of the most highly substituted alkene. The double bond in 2,3-dimethyl-2-pentene is tetrasubstituted. The alkene in 3,4-dimethyl-2-pentene is trisubstituted. The predominant product must, therefore, be 2,3-dimethyl-2-pentene.

36.1.2.3 Oxidation Reactions

Primary and secondary alcohols can be oxidized to form **aldehydes**, **ketones**, or **carboxylic acids**. The product that results from the oxidation of an alcohol depends on the structure of the alcohol and the nature of the oxidizing agent.

A simple rule for the organic chemistry on the MCAT is that if a reagent's molecular formula ends in "O," it is an **oxidizing agent**; if a reagent's molecular formula ends in "H," it is a **reducing agent**. This will save you the time and effort of memorizing a series of oxidizing and reducing agents. Using the above rule, we know that CrO_3 is an oxidizing agent, because it ends in "O." Likewise, we know that $NaBH_4$ is a reducing agent, because it ends in "H."

Primary alcohols may be oxidized to aldehydes or to carboxylic acids. Some common oxidizing agents are CrO_3, $KMnO_4$, $K_2Cr_2O_7$, and H_2CrO_4. The oxidation of a primary alcohol to a carboxylic acid is actually the oxidation of a primary alcohol to an aldehyde, followed by an oxidation of the aldehyde to a carboxylic acid. It is often difficult to prevent the oxidation from proceeding to the carboxylic acid. For this reason, you may assume on the MCAT that the oxidation product of a primary alcohol is a carboxylic acid unless you are told otherwise.

aldehyde   carboxylic acid

A secondary alcohol may be oxidized to a ketone in a two-electron oxidation that is analogous to the oxidation of a primary alcohol to an aldehyde. After this initial oxidation, there are no hydrogens remaining on the former alcoholic carbon (now the ketonic carbon), so no further oxidation will occur:

Ketone

Tertiary alcohols cannot be oxidized, since a hydrogen must be present on the alcoholic carbon for oxidation to proceed.

Carboxylic acids can be reduced to aldehydes of primary alcohols and ketones can be reduced to secondary alcohols.

Just to satisfy your curiosity, we'll provide a reaction mechanism for the oxidation of a secondary alcohol to a ketone by chromic oxide. You will NOT need to memorize reaction mechanisms for the MCAT—these are provided solely to help you understand the reactions.

Please solve this problem:

- The oxidation of a secondary alcohol gives:

    A. a carboxylic acid.
    B. a ketone.
    C. an aldehyde.
    D. a secondary alcohol—they cannot be oxidized.

Problem solved:

The correct answer is B. The complete oxidation of a primary alcohol gives a carboxylic acid. The partial oxidation of a primary alcohol gives an aldehyde and its complete oxidation gives a carboxylic acid. Tertiary alcohols cannot be easily oxidized.

Please solve this problem:

The most likely product of the reaction:

Problem Solved:

The correct answer is C. The reactant is a secondary alcohol. Secondary alcohols are oxidized to ketones, so B and D are wrong. (Notice D also has a carbon with five bonds.) The reason that the oxidation of a secondary alcohol stops at the ketone stage is because further oxidation would require the breaking of the carbon-carbon bond. Thus A is wrong and C is correct.

36.1.2.4 Nucleophilic Substitution Reactions: S_N1 and S_N2

A **nucleophile** is a species that is electron-rich and seeks an electron-deficient species, called an electrophile. Nucleophiles are usually represented as Nu^-.

Alcohols (and some other substrates) may undergo nucleophilic attack at the alcoholic carbon and lose water to form the corresponding substituted alkane via a substitution reaction. This is shown for the reaction of an alcohol with the general nucleophile Nu^-:

$$ROH + HNu \rightarrow RNu + H_2O$$

This reaction may occur by either a one-step mechanism (S_N2) or a two-step mechanism (S_N1). S_NX denotes substitution (S), nucleophilic (N), X-molecular. As was the case for elimination reactions (**36.1.2.2**), the molecularity of the mechanism indicates the number of molecules that are involved in the rate-determining step. Therefore, an S_N1 reaction is a unimolecular nucleophilic substitution with one molecule involved in the rate-determining step. An S_N2 reaction is a bimolecular nucleophilic substitution with two molecules involved in the rate-determining step.

Similar to elimination reactions (E_1 and E_2), S_N2 reactions are favored for primary alcohols,

Similar to elimination reactions (E_1 and E_2), S_N2 reactions are favored for primary alcohols, and S_N1 reactions are favored for tertiary alcohols:

$$S_N2: \ 1° > 2° > 3°$$

$$S_N1: \ 3° > 2° > 1°$$

Secondary substrates undergo nucleophilic substitution by either an S_N1 or an S_N2 mechanism—but usually the mechanism for substitution of secondary alcohols is S_N2.

Tertiary alcohols are easily substituted under acidic conditions to yield the substituted alkane. The mechanism is S_N1, and the two steps are given below:

Step 1: carbocation formation

$$R^1{-}\overset{\displaystyle R^3}{\underset{\displaystyle R^2}{C}}{-}O + HNu \longrightarrow R^1{-}\overset{\displaystyle R^3}{\underset{\displaystyle R^2}{C^+}} + H_2O + Nu^-$$

Step 2: nucleophilic attack

$$R^1{-}\overset{\displaystyle R^3}{\underset{\displaystyle R^2}{C^+}} + Nu^- \longrightarrow R^1{-}\overset{\displaystyle R^3}{\underset{\displaystyle R^2}{C}}{-}Nu$$

An S_N1 reaction exhibits overall first-order kinetics. The rate-determining step is the formation of the carbocation intermediate (first step). Therefore, the substrate concentration and its strength are the only considerations in an S_N1 reaction; the concentration and strength of the incoming nucleophile are unimportant.

An S_N1 reaction is first-order in substrate concentration.

Primary alcohols (and most secondary alcohols) require harsher conditions for substitution than tertiary alcohols, and the mechanism of their substitution is S_N2:

$$R^1{-}\overset{\displaystyle H}{\underset{\displaystyle H}{C}}{-}OH + HNu \longrightarrow R^1{-}\overset{\displaystyle H}{\underset{\displaystyle H}{C}}{-}Nu + H_2O$$

An S_N2 reaction exhibits overall second-order kinetics; the rate-determining step is the only step. Therefore, the substrate concentration and effectiveness *and* the incoming nucleophile concentration and effectiveness, must *both* be considered in an S_N2 reaction.

An S_N2 reaction is first-order in substrate concentration *and* first-order in nucleophile concentration. The overall reaction is second-order.

Comparing S_N1 and S_N2 reactions:

- Tertiary alcohols will react via an S_N1 mechanism.

- Primary alcohols will react via an S_N2 mechanism.

- Secondary alcohols may react via either pathway, but will generally react via an S_N2 mechanism.

- S_N1 reactions exhibit first-order kinetics.

- S_N2 reactions exhibit second-order kinetics.

- S_N1 reactions depend only on the nature and concentration of the alcohol (substrate).

- S_N2 reactions depend on the nature and concentration of both the alcohol (substrate) and the nucleophile.

In terms of stereochemistry, since an S_N1 reaction involves a planar carbocation intermediate, this reaction experiences racemization of a chiral alcohol. Since an S_N2 undergoes a one-step mechanism in which the nucleophile attacks as the protonated hydroxide leaves, this reaction accompanies inversion of stereochemistry at the chiral carbon of a chiral alcohol.

Please solve this problem:

- The reaction of (R)-1-methoxy-1-ethoxy-ethanol with bromide under conditions that result in the formation of water and 1-methoxy-1-ethoxy-ethylbromide goes via an:

  A. S_N1 mechanism, with inversion of stereochemistry.
  B. S_N1 mechanism, with racemization of stereochemistry.
  C. S_N2 mechanism, with inversion of stereochemistry.
  D. S_N2 mechanism, with racemization of stereochemistry.

Problem solved:

The correct answer is C. This is a primary alcohol, so it is expected to follow an S_N2 mechanism. Because the S_N2 mechanism is concerted (nucleophile comes in as leaving group goes out), the stereochemistry of the chiral carbon is inverted in this reaction.

36.1.3 PHENOLS

A **phenol** is an aromatic alcohol. The structure of an unsubstituted phenol is:

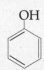

The chemistry of phenols is a combination of the chemistry of **benzene** (see **35.1.5**) and the chemistry of alcohols. A key feature in the chemistry of phenols is the acidity of the phenolic hydrogen. Along with carboxylic acids, phenols are the major acids of organic chemistry. Certain characteristics of phenols should be kept in mind:

- Phenols are acids.

- Electron-withdrawing groups in the meta position will decrease the acidity of a phenol.

- Electron-withdrawing groups in the ortho or para position will increase the acidity of a phenol.

- Electron-donating groups in the meta position will increase the acidity of a phenol.

- Electron-donating groups in the ortho or para position will decrease the acidity of a phenol.

Please solve this problem:

- Which of the following is the most acidic phenol?

  A. 3-nitrophenol
  B. 3-aminophenol
  C. 4-nitrophenol
  D. 4-aminophenol

Problem solved:

The correct answer is C. The nitro group is an electron-withdrawing group. An electron-withdrawing group in the meta position decreases the acidity of a phenol. This eliminates choice A. An electron-withdrawing group in the para position increases the acidity of a phenol. This makes choice B possible. The amino group is an electron-donating group. An electron-donating group in the meta position increases the acidity of a phenol. This makes choice C possible. An electron-donating group in the para position decreases the acidity of a phenol. This eliminates choice D. We must now decide between the electron-donating amino group in the meta position and the electron-withdrawing nitro group in the para position. The nitro group is a much stronger electron withdrawer than the amino group is an electron donater. Therefore, the 4-nitrophenol will be more acidic than the 3-aminophenol. All four choices are ranked in order of decreasing acidity as follows: 4-nitrophenol > 3-aminophenol > 4-aminophenol > 3-nitrophenol.

36.1.4 ETHERS

Ether groups consist of two alkyl groups bonded to an oxygen atom: R-O-R′, but three-membered ring cyclic ethers are termed **epoxides**:

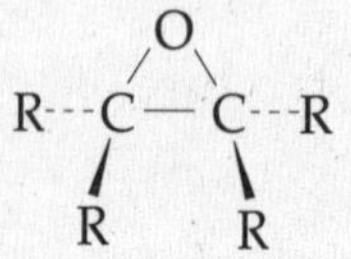

All other cyclic ethers are simply ethers. Epoxides are given a separate name designation because of their unique chemical properties. We will not discuss the chemistry of epoxides here, as it is not germane to the MCAT.

Ethers are polar, and can form hydrogen bonds with other polar molecules that contain hydrogen. (Note that ethers cannot hydrogen bond to themselves, since they have no appropriate hydrogens.)

Ethers are fairly chemically inert, although they can act as weak Lewis bases. Because of their stable chemistry, polarity, and hydrogen-bonding abilities, ethers are often used as solvents in organic chemistry. Whenever a question is posed on the MCAT about solvents, the answer is likely to be an ether.

Because of the polarity of ether molecules, they are expected to have higher boiling points than analogous hydrocarbons. However, since they cannot hydrogen bond with themselves, they are expected to have lower boiling points than analogous alcohols.

Ethers are susceptible to nucleophilic attack on their C-O carbons; however, the reactivity of ethers is significantly less than that of alcohols. In general, ethers may be considered unreactive unless there are no other molecules present.

Please solve this problem:

- Ethers are often used as solvents in organic chemistry. This is because:

    A. ethers can hydrogen bond to other molecules.
    B. ethers are reasonably chemically inert.
    C. ethers generally have low boiling points.
    D. all of the above.

Problem solved:

The correct answer is D. Ethers have many advantages as solvents. Because they can participate in hydrogen bonding, they are able to solubilize a wide range of compounds. Because they are not prone to undergo reaction, they are not likely to interfere with reactions. The low boiling points of ethers also make them ideal as solvents. After a reaction is complete in an ether solvent, the ether may be easily removed by the application of a low heat.

36.2 MASTERY APPLIED: SAMPLE PASSAGE AND QUESTIONS

Passage

An undergraduate chemistry student was given an alkyl halide and asked by his professor to create an alkene using a first-order reaction. The product would later be used as a precursor in a complex synthesis. The student combined his alkyl halide with ethanol and placed the solution over heat. He heated the reaction for a short period of time at a relatively low temperature. When he analyzed the products, he found a small amount of alkene and a large amount of an unknown product. The student realized a competing reaction had occurred. The following week, his professor started with the same alkyl halide but chose a very bulky base. The professor chose to heat the reaction for a long period of time at a high temperature. The resulting product consisted almost entirely of the desired alkene product. The initial alkyl halide used was *t*-butyl bromide.

1. The competing reaction in the student's experiment was:
   A. second-order elimination.
   B. first-order elimination.
   C. second-order nucleophilic substitution.
   D. first-order nucleophilic substitution.

2. The major product of the student's experiment was:
   A. an ether.
   B. an alcohol.
   C. a ketone.
   D. an ester.

3. The best solvent for a first-order elimination reaction is:
   A. a polar solvent that is a good nucleophile.
   B. a polar solvent that is a poor nucleophile.
   C. an apolar solvent that is a good nucleophile.
   D. an apolar solvent that is a poor nucleophile.

4. Dehydrohalogenation occurs to form the major product in:
   A. the student's reaction, because it is a substitution.
   B. the student's reaction, because it is an elimination.
   C. the professor's reaction, because it is an elimination.
   D. the professor's reaction, because it is a substitution.

5. Which of the following is the major product of the student's reaction?
   A. 2-methylpropene
   B. 1-methylpropene
   C. *t*-butyl ethyl ether
   D. *t*-butyl methyl ether

6. Which of the following is the major product of the professor's reaction?

   A. 2-methylpropene
   B. 1-methylpropene
   C. *t*-butyl ethyl ether
   D. *t*-butyl methyl ether

7. A bulky base was used by the professor because:

   A. a bulky base is more reactive than a small base.
   B. it would act as an excellent nucleophile, promoting an elimination.
   C. it would be too bulky to act as a nucleophile, promoting the elimination reaction.
   D. it would be too bulky to act as a nucleophile, promoting the substitution reaction.

36.3 MASTERY VERIFIED: ANSWERS AND EXPLANATIONS

1. *The correct answer is D.* The student was trying to create an alkene with an alkyl halide. This is most effectively accomplished by performing an elimination reaction. Because the student failed to heat the reaction sufficiently and chose a base that could act as a nucleophile, a substitution reaction was competing. Because the alkyl halide was on a tertiary carbon, we know that the reaction must be first-order. Second-order substitution reactions will not take place on a tertiary carbon.

2. *The correct answer is A.* As discussed in the previous question, the competing reaction that dominated the experiment was a first-order substitution reaction. Because ethanol was used, it must be assumed that ethanol acted as a nucleophile, attacking the carbocation formed after the halide left. The hydrogen on the oxygen of ethanol would quickly deprotonate to stabilize the molecule, resulting in an ether.

3. *The correct answer is B.* For both first-order substitution and first-order elimination reactions, a good ionizing solvent will be required to stabilize the carbocation formed in the first step of the reaction. Apolar solvents are not good ionizing solvents and will not help to stabilize the carbocation. Therefore, choices C and D are eliminated. We know that nucleophiles are used in substitution reactions. For an elimination reaction, we want to minimize the competing substitution reactions by decreasing the nucleophilicity of the solvent. Therefore, a solvent that acts as a poor nucleophile is preferred.

4. *The correct answer is C.* The professor's reaction was primarily an elimination reaction, while the student's was mostly a substitution. Knowing this, choices B and D are eliminated. The next question to ask is: "Is dehydrohalogenation associated with a substitution or an elimination?" The process of dehydrohalogenation involves the ionization of an alkyl halide which results in a carbocation intermediate. The intermediate quickly loses a proton to create an alkene. The process described is elimination.

5. *The correct answer is C.* The student conducted a substitution reaction by mistake while attempting an elimination. Knowing that an elimination was not involved in the formation of the major product, the alkene answer choices can be eliminated. The initial solvent was ethanol, not methanol, so the product of the substitution reaction must be *t*-butyl ethyl ether and not *t*-butyl methyl ether.

6. *The correct answer is A.* The thought process involved in solving question 6 is the same as it was for question 5. It is essential to recognize that the professor carried out a reaction that yielded primarily elimination products. Knowing that elimination results in an alkene, choices C and D are eliminated. The closest available hydrogens for deprotonation in the formation of the double bond are on the first carbon. Thus, the double bond forms on the first carbon, and the methyl group remains on the second carbon. The answer must be A.

7. *The correct answer is C.* The professor's reaction was mostly an elimination reaction. In order to promote an elimination reaction, nucleophilic effects must be reduced. Choices D and B can be eliminated immediately. Choice A is false. There are many small nucleophiles that are more reactive than bulky ones. The more bulky a base, the more difficult it is to move into a position to undergo substitution. Thus, a bulky base will reduce substitution products and increase elimination products.

CHAPTER 37

ALDEHYDES AND KETONES

37.1 MASTERY ACHIEVED

37.1.1 STRUCTURE OF ALDEHYDES AND KETONES

Aldehydes and **ketones** are defined by the presence of the **carbonyl** group $C{=}O$. Aldehydes usually have one alkyl or aryl group and a hydrogen attached to the carbonyl carbon. Ketones possess a second alkyl or aryl group in place of the carbonyl hydrogen of aldehydes. The general structures of aldehydes and ketones are depicted below.

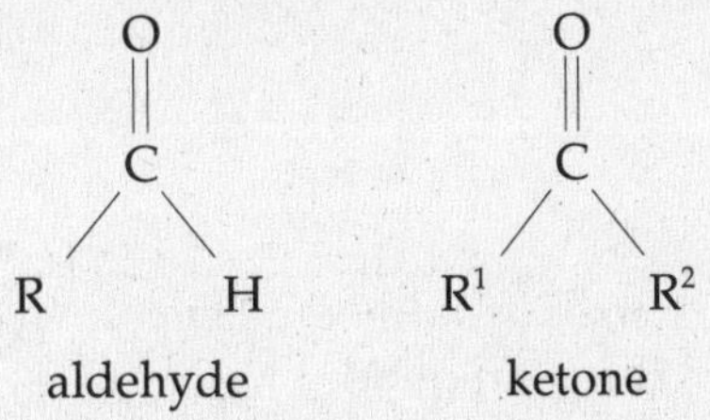

A ketone may exist as a ring structure; in fact, cyclic ketones are quite common. Because an aldehyde must have at least one carbonyl hydrogen, aldehydes are never enclosed within rings.

The special case of a carbonyl compound that bears no alkyl groups is the simplest aldehyde, formaldehyde.

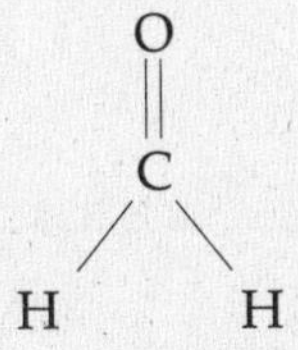

Please solve this problem:

- An aldehyde typically differs from a ketone in that:

  A. an aldehyde contains two alkyl groups, while a ketone contains only one.

  B. an aldehyde contains one alkyl group, while a ketone contains two.

  C. an aldehyde contains two carbonyl groups, while a ketone contains only one.

  D. an aldehyde contains one carbonyl group, while a ketone contains two.

Problem solved:

The correct answer is B. An aldehyde usually consists of an alkyl group and a hydrogen bonded to a carbonyl group. A ketone consists of two alkyl groups bonded to a carbonyl group.

37.1.2 NOMENCLATURE OF ALDEHYDES AND KETONES

In naming aldehydes, the final *e* in the name of the analogous hydrocarbon is dropped, and the suffix -al is added. Ketones are named in a similar manner, with the suffix -one added instead of -al.

In numbering the carbons of an aldehyde according to the IUPAC system, the carbonyl carbon is designated carbon 1 and the subsequent carbons of the longest carbon chain are then numbered. Thus the compound:

is named 2-ethyl-pentanal.

For ketones, the longest carbon chain is numbered such that the carbonyl group receives the lowest possible number. Thus the compound:

is named 4-ethyl-3-heptanone.

When a carbonyl group must be named as a substituent, the term oxo- is used. Thus, the compound:

is named 3-oxo-butanal.

Please solve this problem:

- Name the following compound:

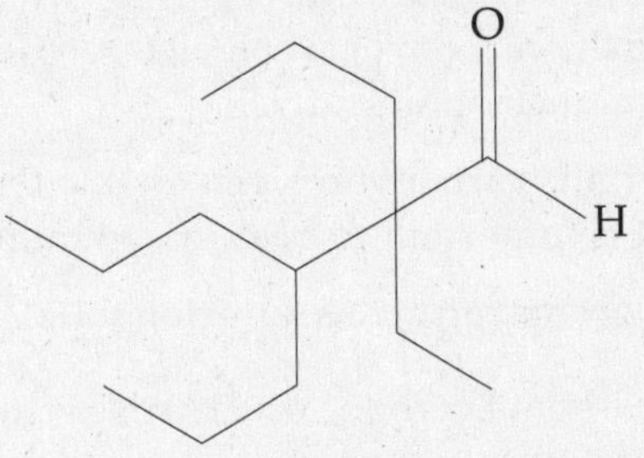

Problem solved:

The longest carbon chain in the compound is 6 carbons long and numbered as shown, beginning at the carbonyl carbon:

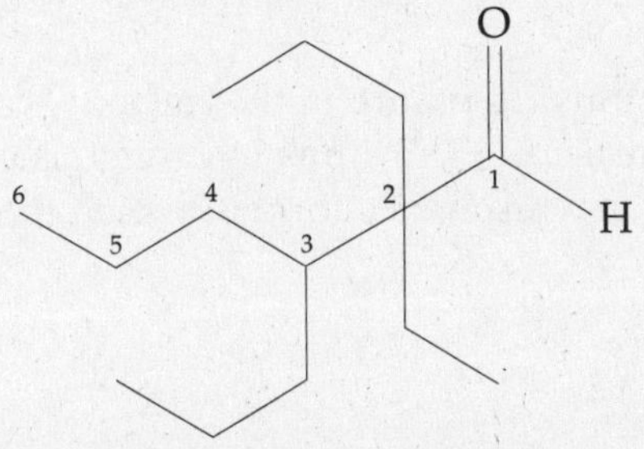

Thus, the correct answer is 2-ethyl-2,3-dipropyl-hexanal.

Using the common system of nomenclature, carbons attached to the carbonyl carbons of aldehydes and ketones are designated with Greek letters according to their distance from the carbonyl group. A carbon immediately adjacent to the carbonyl carbon is termed **alpha** (α).

Moving away from the carbonyl group, the next carbon is a **beta** (β) **carbon**, followed by **gamma** (γ), **delta** (δ), and so on. Likewise, the hydrogens attached to the alpha carbon are termed alpha hydrogens, those on beta carbons are beta hydrogens, and so on. The hydrogen attached to the carbonyl group of an aldehyde is *not* an alpha hydrogen—it is termed the **aldehyde hydrogen**, or the **aldehydic hydrogen**.

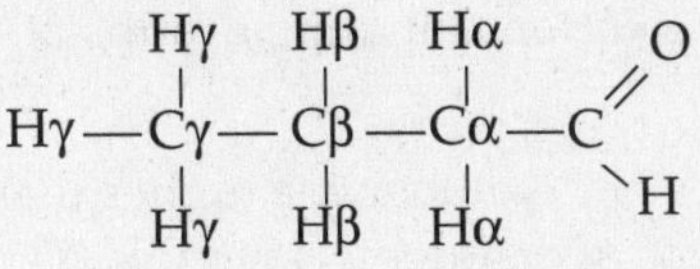

37.1.3 PHYSICAL PROPERTIES OF ALDEHYDES AND KETONES

The physical properties of both aldehydes and ketones are determined by the polarity of the carbonyl group. Since oxygen is highly electronegative, it withdraws electron density from the carbonyl carbon. This makes the carbonyl carbon electron deficient—or partially positive—and thus susceptible to nucleophilic attack.

The two lone electron pairs on the carbonyl oxygen enable the oxygen to function as either a Lewis base or a nucleophile. It is important to bear this in mind:

- The oxygen of a carbonyl group can act as a nucleophile.

The sp^2 hybridization of the carbonyl carbon, which arises from the double-bonding of carbon and oxygen, causes the molecule to be planar along the carbonyl group. Because of this planar configuration, an incoming nucleophile is as likely to approach the carbonyl carbon from one direction as it is from the other direction. Therefore, nucleophilic additions to carbonyls will not show any stereochemical preference unless there are other factors at play— such as a chiral center at the alpha carbon that sterically directs the nucleophile to one face or the other.

Because of the electron-withdrawing nature of the carbonyl oxygen, aldehydes and ketones that contain alpha hydrogens are acidic. The alpha hydrogen is easily extracted by base and the resulting anion is stabilized in a resonance form in which the oxygen bears the negative charge.

While alpha hydrogens are acidic, it is important to note that aldehydic hydrogen is not acidic. Aldehydes are more acidic than ketones because the second alkyl group on a ketone has more electron-donating character than does the corresponding hydrogen of an aldehyde. Aldehydes and ketones are not as acidic as alcohols, but they are more acidic than analogous alkynes. The addition of electron-withdrawing groups at the beta carbon will enhance the acidity of alpha hydrogens, while the addition of electron-donating groups at the beta carbon will decrease the acidity of alpha hydrogens.

The boiling points of aldehydes and ketones are higher than those of analogous hydrocarbons, but lower than those of analogous alcohols. The polarity of the carbonyl group accounts for their higher boiling points relative to hydrocarbons, and their inability to form hydrogen bonds accounts for their lower boiling points relative to alcohols.

37.1.4 CHEMICAL BEHAVIOR OF ALDEHYDES AND KETONES

37.1.4.1 Keto-Enol Tautomerism

As discussed in **37.1.3**, the alpha hydrogens of carbonyl compounds are acidic. When an acidic alpha proton is lost, the dominant resonance structure of the resultant anion is the enolate form:

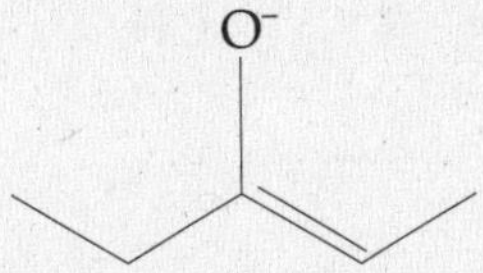

Proton transfers are extremely rapid, and an acidic proton will be continually lost and regained by an aldehyde or a ketone. When the proton is regained, it may be regained at *either* the carbonyl oxygen or the alpha carbon. The protonated enolate form of a carbonyl compound is called the **enol** form (**en** for double bond, **ol** for alcohol). Aldehydes exist in a constant equilibrium between the aldehyde (**keto**) form and the enol form. Likewise, ketones exist in a constant equilibrium between the keto and enol forms. The difference between the keto and enol forms is in the location of the proton and the double bond. The keto and enol forms, which are identical in chemical composition (formula), and are readily interconverted via proton movement, are **tautomers**. Thus, two structures are tautomers of one another if they meet the criteria of compositional equivalency and rapid interconvertibility. The equilibrium between the keto and enol forms of carbonyl compounds is termed **keto-enol tautomerization**. (Note that the term keto-enol tautomerization applies to both ketones and aldehydes.)

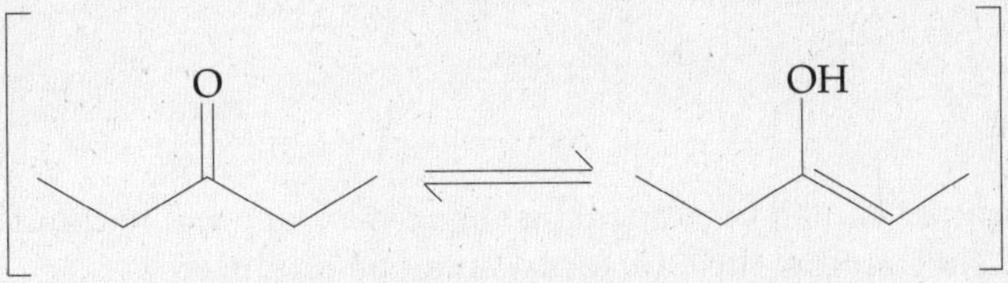

Keto form   Enol form

Carbonyl compounds are generally drawn in the keto form.

Please solve this problem:

- Which of the following molecules does NOT exhibit keto-enol tautomerization?

  A. 3,3-dimethyl-2-butanone
  B. 2,6-dimethyl-cyclohexanone
  C. 2,2-dimethyl-propanal
  D. 4,5-dimethyl-3-hexanone

Problem solved:

The correct answer is C. The structures of the compounds in question (with acidic and aldehydic hydrogens shown) are:

A.

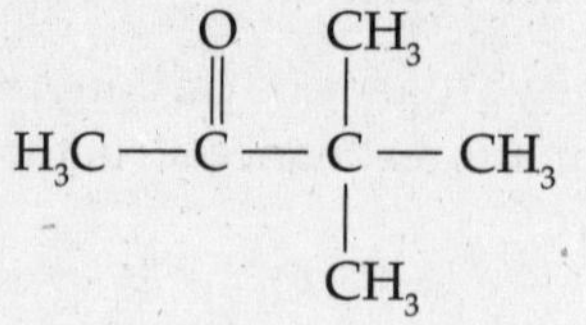

$$H_3C - \overset{\overset{\displaystyle O}{\|}}{C} - \overset{\overset{\displaystyle CH_3}{|}}{\underset{\underset{\displaystyle CH_3}{|}}{C}} - CH_3$$

B.

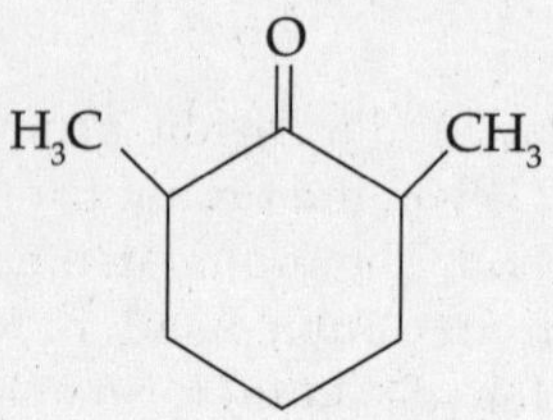

$$H_3C \quad \overset{O}{\diagdown\hspace{-0.3em}\diagup} \quad CH_3$$

C.

not acidic →

$$H - \overset{\overset{\displaystyle O}{\|}}{C} - \overset{\overset{\displaystyle CH_3}{|}}{\underset{\underset{\displaystyle CH_3}{|}}{C}} - CH_3$$

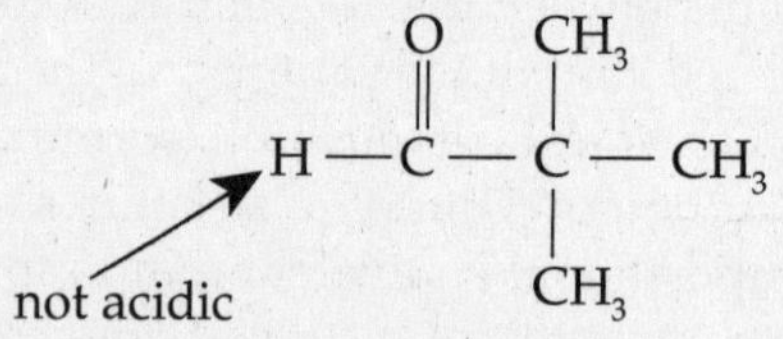

D.

$$CH_3CH_2 - \overset{\overset{\displaystyle O}{\|}}{C} - \overset{\overset{\displaystyle CH_3}{|}}{\underset{\underset{\displaystyle H}{|}}{C}} - \overset{\overset{\displaystyle H}{|}}{\underset{\underset{\displaystyle CH_3}{|}}{C}} - CH_3$$

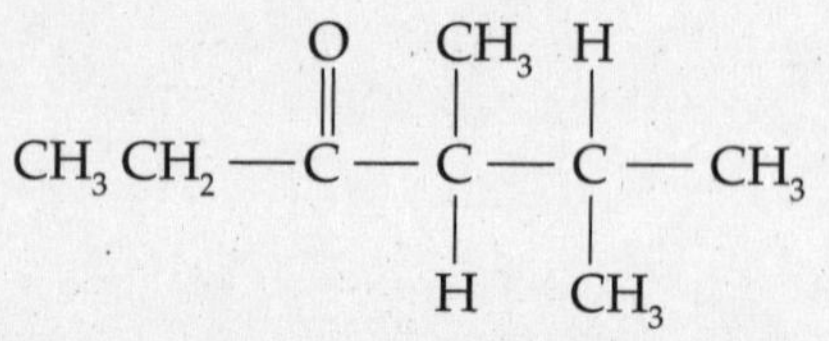

Thus, we can see that 2,2-dimethyl-propanal is the only compound without an acidic proton to lose. Without this acidic proton, the enol form cannot be produced.

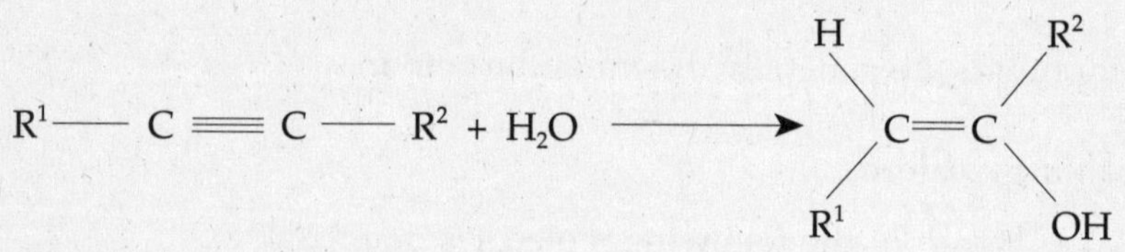

$$R^1 - C \equiv C - R^2 + H_2O \longrightarrow \quad \overset{\displaystyle H}{\underset{\displaystyle R^1}{\diagdown}} C = C \overset{\displaystyle R^2}{\underset{\displaystyle OH}{\diagup}}$$

$$\overset{\displaystyle H}{\underset{\displaystyle R^1}{\diagdown}} C = C \overset{\displaystyle R^2}{\underset{\displaystyle OH}{\diagup}} \quad \rightleftharpoons \quad R^1 \diagup \underset{CH_2}{\overset{\overset{\displaystyle O}{\|}}{C}} \diagdown R^2$$

ketone product

37.1.4.2 Electrophilic Addition

Attraction of a proton to the carbonyl oxygen of the keto form, or to the alpha carbon of the enol form of an aldehyde or a ketone, represents a special case of electrophilic activity. An **electrophile** is a species that seeks to gain electron density; it is represented by E^+. The general reaction between a ketone enolate and an electrophile is provided below.

Ketone   Keto form   Enol form

This general reaction is also valid for aldehydes, where R = H.

Alkyl halides are a convenient source of electrophiles in organic chemistry. An alkyl halide will add to an enolate either at the oxygen, which produces an unsaturated ether, or at the alpha carbon, which produces an alkyl-substituted carbonyl compound (a ketone or aldehyde). In general, O-alkylation is kinetically favored (it is faster) over C-alkylation, but C-alkylation is thermodynamically favored because it provides a lower-energy product. Production of a desired product may be controlled through the reaction temperature. If the desired product is the kinetically-favored product, the reaction should be run at a very low temperature (typically –78°C). If the desired product is the thermodynamic product, the reaction should be run at a higher temperature (usually room temperature).

Please solve this problem:

- A student ran the reaction between methyl bromide and the enolate of 3-pentanone at room temperature, while her professor ran the same reaction at –78°C. Each got a mixture of two products. Which of the following would be the predicted outcome of the experiments?

  A. The student's product was primarily the methyl ether of pent-2-en-3-one. The professor's product was primarily 2-methyl-pentanone.

  B. The student's product was primarily 2-methyl-pentanone. The professor's product was primarily the methyl ether of pent-2-en-3-one.

  C. Both products were primarily the methyl ether of pent-2-en-3-one.

  D. Both products were primarily 2-methyl-pentanone.

Problem solved:

The correct answer is B. The student ran her reaction under thermodynamic conditions, and therefore would expect to form primarily the C-alkylated product: 2-methyl-pentanone. The professor ran her reaction under kinetic conditions, and therefore would expect to form primarily the O-alkylated product: the methyl ether of pent-2-en-3-one.

37.1.4.3 Organometallic Reagents and Nucleophilic Addition

The general reaction between a ketone and a nucleophile is provided below.

This general reaction is also valid for aldehydes, where R = H.

Many nucleophilic species are readily obtainable, such as Br^-, Cl^-, or CN^-. The most convenient forms of carbon nucleophiles are organometallic reagents, specifically organolithium reagents, RLi, and the Grignard reagents, RMgBr. Here are the reaction mechanisms for the reduction of a ketone or aldehyde by two organometallic reagents. As we mentioned previously, you do not need to memorize mechanisms for the MCAT—these are provided solely for your understanding.

where X = a halogen, usually Br

As you can see, the first step in the addition reaction of this type is the combination of the aldehyde or ketone with the organometallic reagent, and the second step is the addition of water, which produces the alchohol. It is very important that water be added in a second step, because if it were present in Step 1 it would destroy the organometallic reagent, for instance:

$$R - Mg - X - H - OH \longrightarrow R - H + HO - Mg - X$$

37.1.4.4 Addition of Alcohols: Acetals and Ketals

The addition of an alcohol to an aldehyde or a ketone is a special case of nucleophilic addition. The addition of one equivalent of an alcohol to an aldehyde results in the formation of a **hemiacetal**. The addition of a second equivalent of alcohol results in the formation of an **acetal**. The addition of one equivalent of an alcohol to a ketone results in the formation of a **hemiketal** and the addition of a second equivalent of alcohol results in the formation of a **ketal**.

hemiacetal (R^1 = H)   acetal (R^1 = H)
hemiketal (R^1 = alkyl)   ketal (R^1 = alkyl)

Please solve this problem:

- An acetal is:

  A. a secondary ether alcohol.
  B. a tertiary ether alcohol.
  C. a secondary diether.
  D. a tertiary diether.

Problem solved:

The correct answer is C. Choice A describes a hemiacetal. Choice B describes a hemiketal. Choice C describes an acetal. Choice D describes a ketal.

37.1.4.5 The Aldol Condensation

The most important reaction of aldehydes and ketones for the MCAT is the **aldol condensation**. In an aldol condensation, an aldehyde, or ketone, acts as both a nucleophile and an electrophile in the same reaction. A simple aldol condensation occurs between two molecules of the same aldehyde. This is termed an aldol condensation because the product, a β-hydroxy aldehyde, is both an aldehyde (ald) and an alcohol (ol). Aldol condensations are catalyzed by either acid or base; one example of an aldol condensation is:

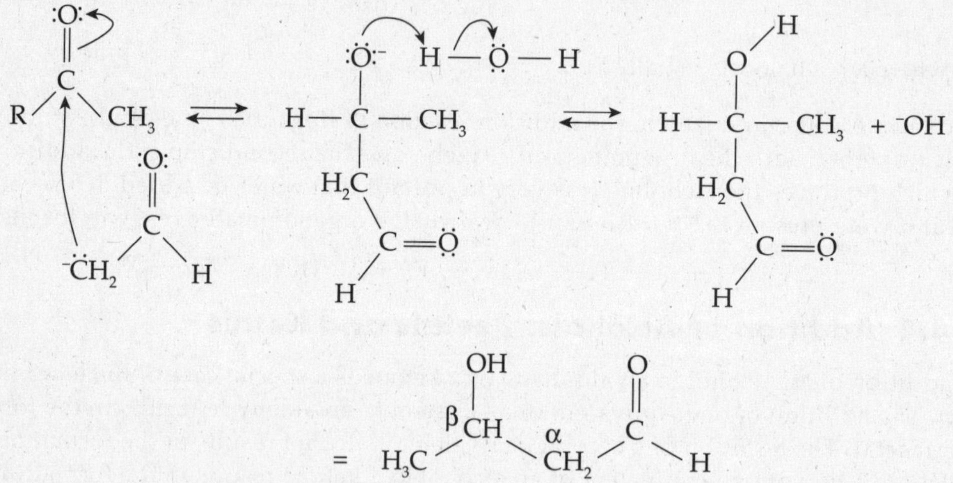

Aldol—a β-hydroxy aldehyde

Ketones with acidic alpha hydrogens will also undergo self (or simple) aldol condensations to give β-hydroxyketones (ketols). When two different carbonyl species are present in a solution, mixed aldol condensations may occur. In a mixed aldol condensation, one carbonyl compound will serve as the nucleophile and the other will serve as the electrophile. The compound that contains the more acidic alpha hydrogen will serve as the electrophile. This is easy to remember if you think <u>e</u>lectrophile = <u>a</u>cid, n<u>u</u>cleophile = <u>b</u>ase (the vowels go together, the consonants go together). Therefore, in the case of an aldehyde mixed with a ketone, the aldehyde will serve as the electrophile and the ketone will serve as the nucleophile to yield a β-hydroxyaldehyde (aldol).

In many instances, the aldol product is unstable. If a second acidic alpha hydrogen exists in this molecule, the molecule will generally dehydrate to form the more stable α,β-unsaturated carbonyl compound.

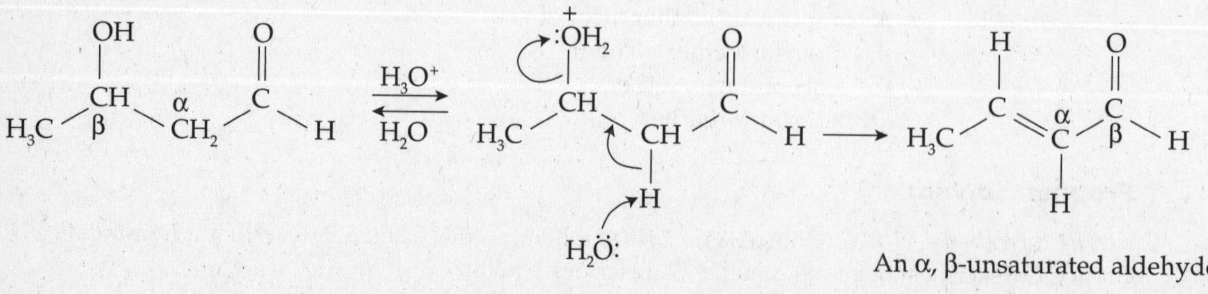

An α, β-unsaturated aldehyde

Please solve this problem:

- An aldol condensation between acetone (2-propanone) and 2-butanone will give rise to:

    A. a single product.
    B. two products.
    C. three products.
    D. four products.

Problem solved:

The correct answer is C. Since these are both ketones with similar pK_a's, we cannot say that one will exclusively act as the nucleophile and the other as the electrophile. We must consider that either ketone may act as the nucleophile, which would result in at least two products; this allows us to eliminate Choice A. We must also consider the number of possible nucleophiles (enolates) that can be formed. Acetone is symmetric about its carbonyl group, so it will form only one nucleophilic enolate:

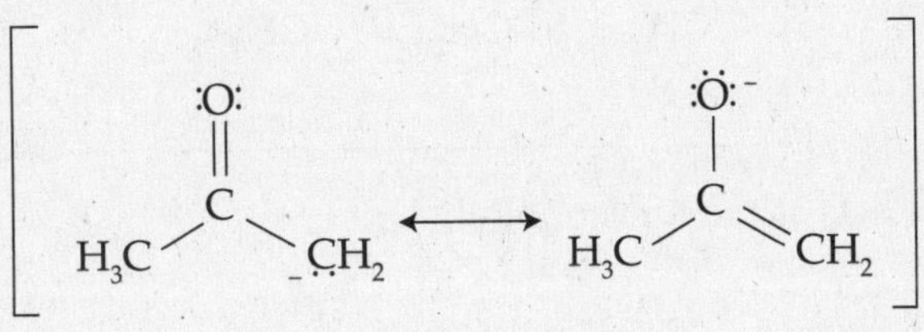

2-Butanone, however, is not symmetric about its carbonyl carbon. It therefore will form two nucleophilic enolates:

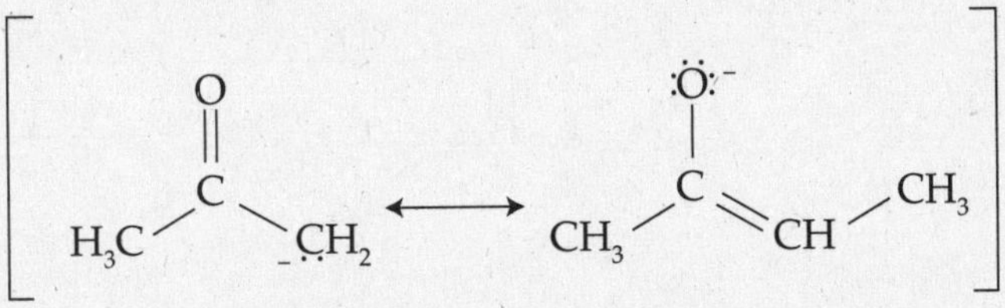

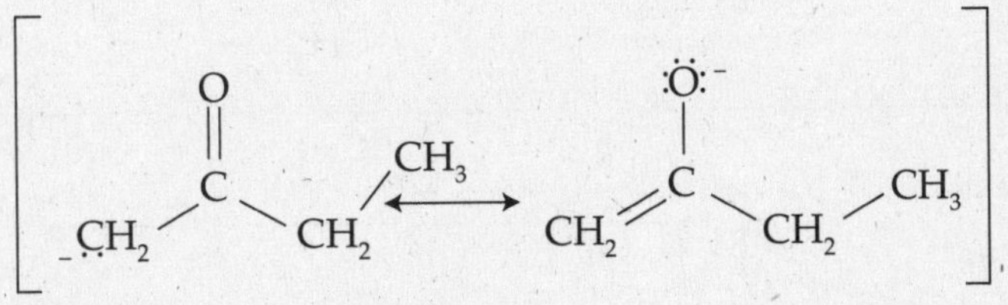

Each of these three enolates will form a single product. The three products are 4-hydroxy-4-methyl-2-hexanone, 5-hydroxy-5-methyl-3-hexanone, and 4-hydroxy-3,4-dimethyl-2-pentanone.

1.

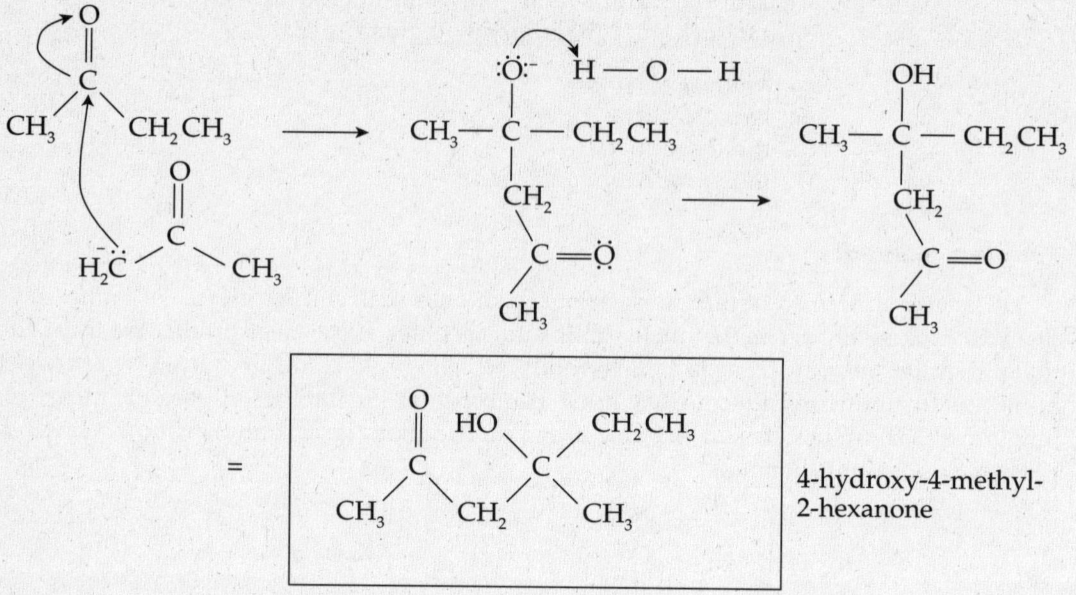

$$= \boxed{\begin{array}{c} \text{4-hydroxy-4-methyl-} \\ \text{2-hexanone} \end{array}}$$

4-hydroxy-4-methyl-
2-hexanone

Here acetone acts as the nucleophile!

2.

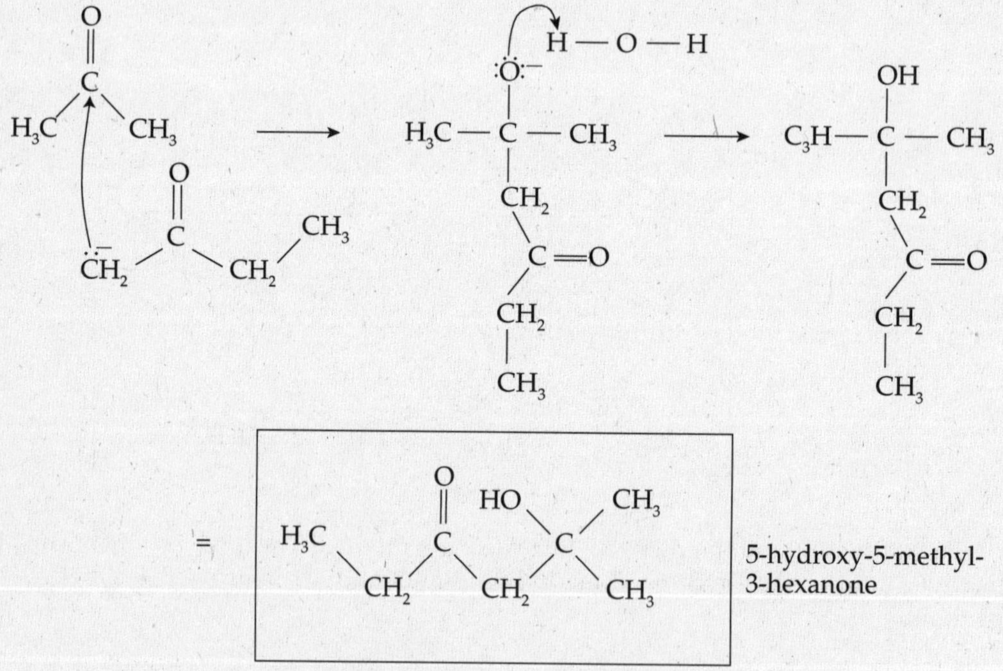

$$=$$

5-hydroxy-5-methyl-
3-hexanone

Here 2-butanone acts as the nucleophile!

3.

4-hydroxy-3,4-dimethyl-2-pentanone

37.2 MASTERY APPLIED: SAMPLE PASSAGE AND QUESTIONS

Passage

Efficient alkylation of aldehydes and ketones requires essentially quantitative formation of their respective enolates. When a low concentration of the enolate ion is formed it reacts more competitively with the parent ketone or aldehyde relative to the alkyl halide. This self-condensation is known as the aldol condensation. The reaction may also occur between two different carbonyl-containing moieties, in which case, the reaction is termed a mixed aldol condensation. The aldol condensation is often followed by a dehydration phase that gives an α, β-unsaturated carbonyl as product.

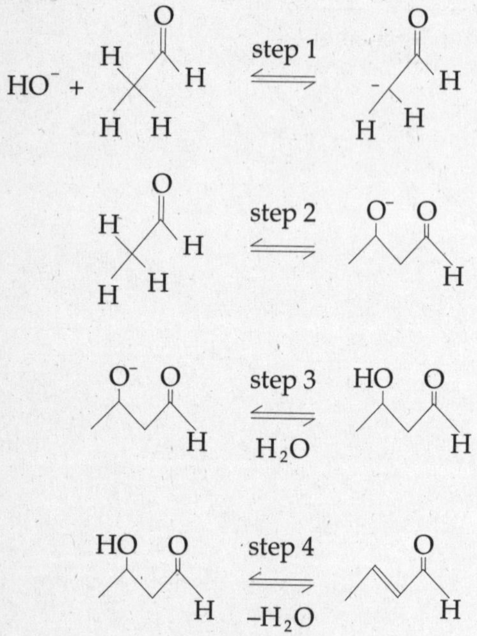

Figure 1

In certain cases, it is possible for a single molecule, which contains two carbonyl groups, to undergo an intramolecular aldol condensation. When available, this reaction is kinetically favored relative to intermolecular aldols. An example of a synthetically useful intramolecular aldol condensation,

followed by dehydration, is the **Robinson annulation**.

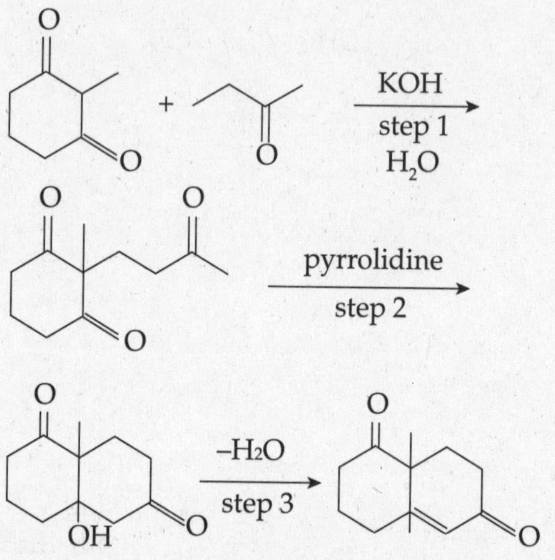

Figure 2

In general, the reactions in the addition phase of both the acid-catalyzed and the base-catalyzed condensations are readily reversible. The equilibrium constant for the addition phase is generally unfavorable for acyclic ketones and favorable for aldehydes and cyclic compounds. On the other hand, the equilibrium constant for the dehydration phase is generally favorable since the resulting product is stabilized by resonance. Therefore, even under conditions that are unfavorable for addition, the reaction may be driven to completion by the favorability of dehydration, which is not usually reversible.

Aldehydes that have no hydrogens attached to the alpha carbon undergo oxidation and reduction in the presence of strong alkali. This reaction, known as the Cannizzaro reaction, is a consequence of the fact that an aldehyde is intermediate in the oxidation-reduction pathway from primary alcohol to carboxylic acid. The steps of this reaction are presented below.

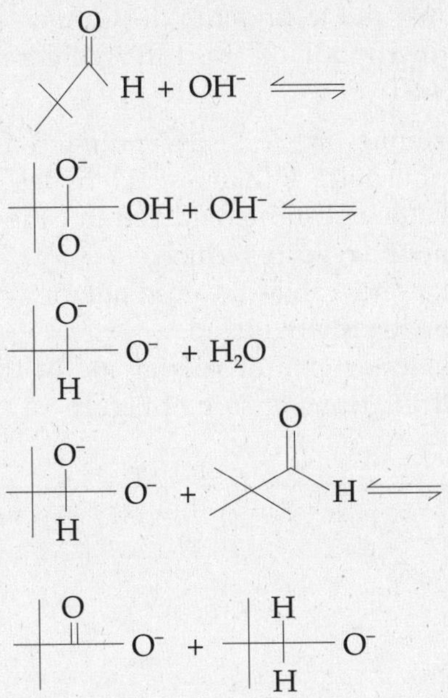

Figure 3

1. Based on the information in the passage, which of the following is the most likely product of the reaction between propanal and 2-propanone, in the presence of base?

A.

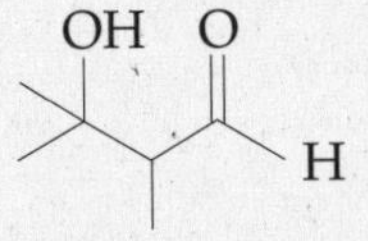

B.

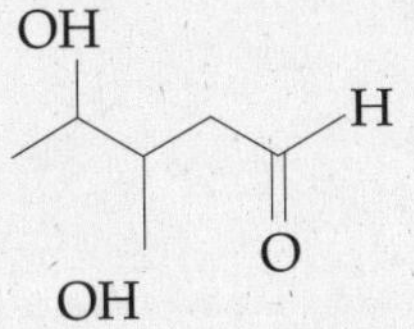

C.

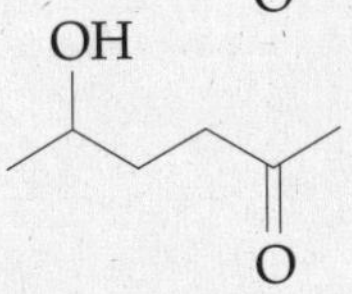

D.

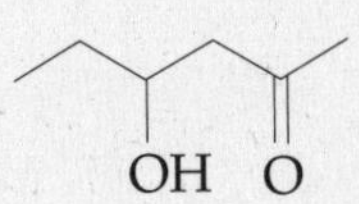

2. An aldehyde and a ketone are placed together in the presence of an acid and a mixed aldol condensation takes place. The nucleophile:

A. will be the aldehyde, giving a single product.
B. will be the ketone, giving a single product.
C. will be both the aldehyde and the ketone, giving two different products.
D. cannot be determined from the information provided.

3. Which step of the scheme presented in Figure 2 corresponds to the intramolecular aldol condensation?

A. Step 1
B. Step 2
C. Step 3
D. none of the steps

4. Comparing molecules A and B below:

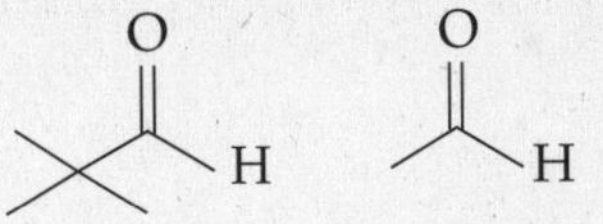

A   B

A. A will undergo aldol condensation, and B will not.
B. B will undergo aldol condensation, and A will not.
C. Both will undergo aldol condensation, but A will react faster.
D. Both will undergo aldol condensation, but B will react faster.

5. When the Cannizzaro reaction is carried out in D_2O, it is expected, based on Figure 3, that:

   A. both the alcohol and the carboxylic acid will incorporate deuterium.
   B. only the alcohol will incorporate deuterium.
   C. only the carboxylic acid will incorporate deuterium.
   D. neither the alcohol nor the carboxylic acid will incorporate deuterium.

6. Which of the following statements regarding propanal and 2,2-dimethylpropanal is true?

   A. Both would undergo the Cannizzaro reaction.
   B. Together they would undergo a crossed Cannizzaro reaction.
   C. Propanal would undergo the Cannizzaro reaction, while 2,2-dimethylpropanal would not.
   D. 2,2-Dimethylpropanal would undergo the Cannizzaro reaction, while propanal would not..

7. Ketones fail to undergo the Cannizzaro reaction for all of the following reasons EXCEPT:

   A. ketones are less susceptible to nucleophilic attack than are aldehydes.
   B. ketones can be oxidized but they cannot be readily reduced.
   C. ketones can be reduced but they cannot be readily oxidized.
   D. ketones cannot participate in the hydride transfer step of Figure 3.

37.3 MASTERY VERIFIED: ANSWERS AND EXPLANATIONS

1. *The correct answer is D.* Choices B and C should be instantly eliminated because they are not aldol products (β-hydroxycarbonyls). Choice D represents the aldol product of the nucleophilic attack of the ketone (2-propanone) on the aldehyde (propanal). Choice A represents the aldol product of the nucleophilic attack of the aldehyde on the ketone. In a mixed aldol between an aldehyde and a ketone, the ketone serves as the nucleophile and the aldehyde serves as the electrophile—aldehydes are more acidic than ketones.

2. *The correct answer is B.* The α-hydrogen of an aldehyde is more acidic than the α-hydrogen of a ketone. Therefore, the conjugate base (the enolate) of a ketone is a stronger base than the conjugate base of an aldehyde. Strong bases are strong nucleophiles— as long as they are not sufficiently strong that they would rather work as a base than as a nucleophile. Therefore, the enolate of the ketone is expected to nucleophilically attack the carbonyl of the aldehyde to give a single product. This answer also follows from the answer to question 1.

3. *The correct answer is B.* The first step is a base-catalyzed nucleophilic addition. The second step is the intramolecular aldol condensation. The third step is a dehydration to form the α,β-unsaturated ketone.

4. *The correct answer is B.* Molecule A cannot undergo an aldol condensation because it does not possess any α-hydrogens. Molecule B will certainly undergo an aldol condensation since it possesses three α-hydrogens.

5. *The correct answer is A.* From Figure 3, it is clear that both products must gain a proton to become the acid and the alcohol—the mechanism presented in the passage left them as the carboxylate and the alkoxide ion. The source of these protons would be the solvent (D_2O). Therefore, both products would become deuterated. When this reaction is actually performed, the alcohol product does not incorporate deuterium, but this is not what we would expect from the figure presented in the passage.

6. *The correct answer is D.* Propanal has α-hydrogens; therefore, under the conditions stated it would undergo an aldol condensation, not the Cannizzaro reaction. This eliminates choices A, B, and C, leaving only choice D. Furthermore, since 2,2-dimethylpropanal has no α-hydrogens it *will* undergo the Cannizzaro.

7. *The correct answer is B.* Choice A is a true statement. Choices B and C cannot both be true, since they are opposites of one another (therefore one has to be the correct answer). Choice D is also a true statement. From our knowledge of the behavior of ketones, we know that ketones are reduced to secondary alcohols, but ketones are not readily oxidized. Therefore, choice B is false and choice C is true. Since choice B is the only false statement, it is the correct answer.

CHAPTER 38

CARBOXYLIC ACIDS

38.1 MASTERY ACHIEVED

38.1.1 STRUCTURE OF CARBOXYLIC ACIDS

A **carboxylic acid** is any carbon chain or ring with a terminal **carboxyl group**. The carboxyl group is sometimes designated—COOH, and is schematically depicted as follows:

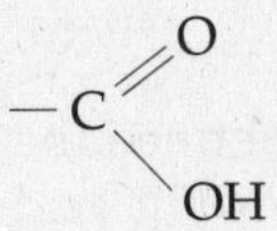

$$-C\overset{O}{\underset{OH}{\diagup}}$$

Carboxyl Group

The remainder of the carboxyl-containing molecule is sometimes designated as R or Ar. If the substituent group on the carbon of the carboxyl group is an aliphatic chain, it can be designated as R. **Aliphatic carboxylic acids** are named according to the nature and placement of the substituents within the aliphatic chain. If the substituent group on the carbon of the carboxyl group is a substituted benzene ring, the designation is **Ar,** for **aromatic**.

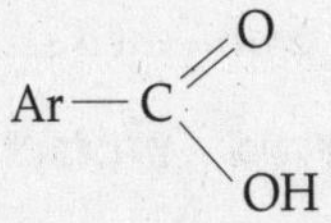

$$Ar-C\overset{O}{\underset{OH}{\diagup}}$$

Aromatic Carboxylic Acid

The simplest aliphatic carboxylic acid, in which the R group is a single hydrogen, has the common name *formic acid*. The IUPAC name for formic acid is methanoic acid. This molecule is depicted below. You should be familiar with both the IUPAC name and the common name for

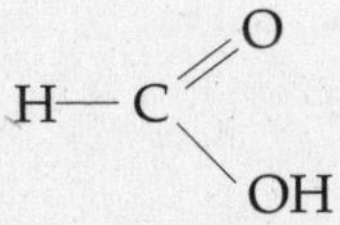

$$H-C\overset{O}{\underset{OH}{\diagup}}$$

Methanoic Acid
(Formic Acid)

The simplest aromatic carboxylic acid is benzoic acid:

Benzoic Acid

The carboxyl group contains a **carbonyl group** (such as ketones and aldehydes) and a **hydroxyl group** (as in alcohols).

The carbon atom of the carboxyl group is termed the **carboxylic carbon**. This carbon is always designated as carbon 1 when naming carboxylic acids.

The carboxyl group is polar; the carbon carries a slight positive charge, while the oxygens carry a slight negative charge.

As noted in Chapter 33, the carboxyl group is acidic. On deprotonation it leaves the carboxyl anion RCO_2^-, which experiences resonance stabilization.

38.1.1.1 Dicarboxylic Acids and Tricarboxylic Acids

The terms **dicarboxylic acid** and **tricarboxylic acid** refer to molecules that have two or three carboxyl termini, respectively.

Oxalic Acid (Ethanedioic Acid)

Malonic Acid (Propanedioic Acid)

Citric Acid (Tricarboxylic Acid)

38.1.1.2 Nomenclature of Carboxylic Acids

Nomenclature of carboxylic acids is not tested on the MCAT. Ordinarily, passages or questions that refer to carboxylic acids will provide the names. Nonetheless, it may be helpful to understand how carboxylic acids are named.

Carboxylic acids are named using the IUPAC system; however, many common carboxylic acids also have common names (as in the cases of formic, oxalic, and malonic acids). An aliphatic carboxylic acid is assigned its IUPAC name by eliminating the terminal "e" from the name of the aliphatic compound and substituting it with the suffix "oic acid." In the case of a dicarboxylic acid, the appropriate suffix is "dioic acid," and for a tricarboxylic acid the suffix is "trioic acid."

The aliphatic chain is identified by counting the longest continuous chain of carbon atoms that includes the carboxylic carbon (in the case of diacids—both carboxyl groups must be included in the chain). The carboxyl carbon is labeled carbon 1.

Consider this molecule:

$$\text{(CH}_3)_2\text{CHCH}_2\text{CH}_2\text{C}\overset{\overset{\displaystyle O}{\displaystyle \|}}{\text{OH}}$$

The longest carbon chain that includes the carboxyl group is comprised of five carbon atoms. To name this molecule use the following steps:

- Note that a five carbon chain is a pentane.

- Drop the "e" and replace it with "oic acid."

- Note that the molecule is a substituted form of pentanoic acid.

- Note that a methyl group is bound to carbon 4.

- Name the compound, therefore, 4-methyl pentanoic acid.

Consider this molecule:

$$\text{CH}_3\text{CHCH}_2\overset{\overset{\displaystyle \text{CH}_3\text{CH}_2}{\displaystyle |}}{\text{CH}}\text{CH}_2\underset{\underset{\displaystyle F}{\displaystyle |}}{\text{CH}}\text{C}\overset{\overset{\displaystyle O}{\displaystyle \|}}{\text{OH}}$$

The longest carbon chain that includes the carboxyl group is comprised of seven carbon atoms. To name the molecule use the following steps:

- Note that a seven carbon chain is a heptane.

- Drop the "e" and replace it with "oic acid."

- Note that the molecule is a substituted form of heptanoic acid.

- Note that a fluorine atom is bound to carbon 2, another fluorine atom to carbon 6, and an ethyl group to carbon 4.

- Name the compound, therefore, 4-ethyl 2, 6-difluoroheptanoic acid.

The following table shows a variety of carboxylic acids together with their IUPAC names. Common names are listed as well; however, it is not necessary to memorize them.

	IUPAC Name	Common Name	
HCOOH	methanoic	formic	
CH_3COOH	ethanoic	acetic	
CH_3CH_2COOH	propanoic	propionic	
$CH_3(CH_2)_2COOH$	butanoic	butyric	
$CH_3(CH_2)_3COOH$	pentanoic	valeric	
$CH_3(CH_2)_4COOH$	hexanoic	caproic	
$CH_3(CH_2)_6COOH$	octanoic	caprylic	
$CH_3(CH_2)_8COOH$	decanoic	capric	
$CH_3(CH_2)_{10}COOH$	dodecanoic	lauric	
$CH_3(CH_2)_{12}COOH$	tetradecanoic	myristic	
$CH_3(CH_2)_{14}COOH$	hexadecanoic	palmitic	Fatty
$CH_3(CH_2)_{16}COOH$	octadecanoic	stearic	acids
$CH_3(CH_2)_7CH=CH(CH_2)_7COOH$	(Z)-9-octadecenoic	oleic	

Table 38.1

38.1.1.3 Hydrogen Bonding in Carboxylic Acids

Carboxylic acids undergo hydrogen bonding. In fact, two carboxylic acid molecules may be involved in *two* hydrogen bonds. For two carboxylic acid molecules (1 and 2), the terminal OH group of molecule 1 forms a hydrogen bond with the terminal oxygen atom of molecule 2, and the terminal OH group of molecule 2 forms a hydrogen bond with the terminal oxygen atom of molecule 1.

Molecule 1   [structure diagram]   Molecule 2

Such "double" hydrogen bonding causes carboxylic acids to have boiling points that are even higher than the boiling points of alcohols (which also undergo hydrogen bonding).

Please solve this problem:

- The RCO_2^- anion results from:

  A. the low boiling point of carboxylic acids.
  B. resonance stabilization of carbonyl groups.
  C. hydrogen bonding between carboxylic acids.
  D. deprotonation of a carboxyl group.

Problem solved:

D is the correct answer. The carboxylate anion remains when a carboxylic acid loses a hydrogen ion—when it is deprotonated. Choice A is incorrect because in relation to the question it is nonsensical. Choice B describes resonance stabilization of a carbonyl group. However, it is the carboxylate anion, not the carbonyl group, that experiences resonance stabilization. Choice C refers to hydrogen bonding between two carboxylic acids. Such bonding does occur, but it does not contribute to the stability of the carboxylate anion.

Please solve this problem:

- Carboxylic acids have higher boiling points than might be predicted primarily because of:

    A. hydrogen bonding.
    B. resonance stabilization.
    C. nonpolarity of carbonyl and O–H bonds.
    D. unsaturation of carbon chains.

Problem solved:

A is the correct answer. Hydrogen bonding tends to hold atoms together in the liquid state, and to increase the energy required to move them into the gaseous state. As noted in the text, carboxylic acids may undergo hydrogen bonding at *two sites*. That phenomenon confers on them a higher boiling point than would otherwise be predicted on the basis of their structure. Resonance stabilization (choice B) does not affect boiling point; it affects the stability of the carboxylate anion. Choice C is an incorrect statement. The carbonyl and OH bonds that compose the carboxylic groups *are* polar. In the OH group, hydrogen is relatively positive and oxygen is relatively negative; this polarity produces the hydrogen bonding. Choice D refers to unsaturation of carbon chains, which is irrelevant to the question. The question concerns carboxylic acids generally. The carbon chain (R) component of a carboxylic acid may be saturated or unsaturated.

Please solve this problem:

- Carboxylic acids resemble ketones in that they:

    A. possess an OH group.
    B. possess a carbon double bonded to an oxygen.
    C. are highly acidic.
    D. show pronounced hydrogen bonding.

Problem solved:

B is the correct answer. As noted in the text, the carboxyl group of a carboxylic acid contains a carbonyl group (carbon double bonded to an oxygen). In that way, carboxylic acids resemble ketones. All of the characteristics listed in choices A, C, and D apply to carboxylic acids but not to ketones. Ketones do not necessarily contain OH groups, nor are they highly acidic, nor do they show pronounced hydrogen bonding.

38.1.2 ACIDITY OF CARBOXYLIC ACIDS

38.1.2.1 Aliphatic Acids

A carboxylic acid's acidity derives from its relative readiness to part with a proton (hydrogen ion). To a considerable degree, the carboxylic group owes its acidity—its readiness to lose a proton—to the relative stability of the carboxylate anion RCOO⁻, which owes its stability to its resonance structure (see Chapter 33). The anion's surplus electron is delocalized, encircling the nuclei of both of the remaining oxygen atoms (with the the concomitant result that both the remaining carbon-oxygen bonds have partial double bond character).

$$R - C \Big\langle \begin{array}{c} O_\delta^- \\ O_\delta^- \end{array} \Big\rangle \ominus$$

Because the carboxylate ion is so stable, carboxylic acids are more acidic than alcohols, phenols, aldehydes, and ketones. Among carboxylic acids, aryl alcohols, water, and non-aryl alcohols, the order of acidity is (1) carboxylic acids, (2) aryl alcohols, (3) water, and (4) alcohols: RCOOH > ArOH > HOH > ROH.

Factors that enhance the carboxylate anion's stability enhance the acidity of the corresponding acid. Conversely, factors that tend to destabilize the carboxylate anion tend to lessen the acidity of the corresponding acid.

Consider a molecule of 2-chloro-3-phenyl propanoic acid:

2-chloro-3-phenyl propionic acid

Note that the carbon adjacent to the carboxyl carbon is called the **alpha carbon**. If a halogen atom is bound to the carboxylic acid's alpha carbon, the corresponding carboxylate ion is stabilized. This is because the halogen atom is electrophilic. It is sometimes called an **electron-withdrawing group**, because it tends to "absorb" some of the anion's negative charge. Any group that tends to have the opposite effect—to repel electrons—is termed an **electron-donating group**. An electron-donating group that's bound to the alpha carbon tends to destabilize the corresponding carboxylate anion and lessen the acid's acidity. The effects of electron-withdrawing and electron-donating groups are called **inductive effects**.

Consider, for example, this molecule of 2-methyl -3-phenyl propanoic acid:

2-methyl-3-phenyl propanoic

It differs from the molecule just discussed in that the alpha carbon carries a methyl group instead of a chlorine atom. The methyl group is an electron-donating group; it has a tendency to repel electrons. It therefore also has a tendency to destabilize the corresponding carboxylate anion.

The table below lists a variety of carboxylic acids with their pK_a values. The lower the pK_a, the greater the acidity.

Structure	pK_a (H_2O, 25°)
CH_3COOH	4.75
CH_3CH_2COOH	4.87
$(CH_3)_2CHCOOH$	4.84
$(CH_3)_3CCOOH$	5.03
$CH_3(CH_2)_{16}COOH$ (*stearic acid*)	4.89
$ClCH_2COOH$	2.85
$BrCH_2COOH$	2.96
ICH_2COOH	3.12
$CH_3CHCOOH$ $\quad\vert$ $\quad OH$	3.08

Table 38.2

The table shows that substitution at the alpha carbon with electron-withdrawing groups increases acidity. Substitution with electron-donating groups decreases acidity.

Remember, in particular, that *halogens and oxygen are strongly electrophilic*. If bound to a carboxylic acid's alpha carbon they tend to stabilize the carboxylate anion and increase acidity. Aliphatic groups (methyl groups, ethyl groups, propyl groups, etc) are electron-donating, and if bound to the alpha carbon tend to decrease acidity.

38.1.3 SYNTHESIS OF CARBOXYLIC ACIDS

38.1.3.1 Synthesis by Oxidation

Carboxylic acids may be formed by **oxidation**. The oxidation of a primary alcohol—an aldehyde, an alkene, an alkylbenzene, or a methyl ketone—yields a carboxylic acid in the presence of appropriate oxidizing agents.

The oxidation of a primary alcohol in the presence of the oxidizing agent potassium permanganate ($KMnO_4$) yields a carboxylic acid according to this generic reaction:

$$RCH_2OH \xrightarrow[\text{heat}]{\substack{(1)\ KMnO_4, OH^- \\ \\ (2)\ H_3O^+}} RCO_2H$$

The oxidation of an aldehyde in the presence of the oxidizing agent silver oxide (Ag_2O) yields a carboxylic acid according to this generic reaction:

$$R\text{--}CHO \xrightarrow[\text{(2)}\ H_3O^+]{(1)Ag_2O\ \text{or}\ Ag(NH_3)_2{}^+OH^-} RCO_2H$$

The oxidation of an alkylbenzene in the presence of the oxidizing agent potassium permanganate yields a carboxylic acid according to this generic reaction:

$$\text{C}_6\text{H}_5-\text{CH}_3 \xrightarrow[\substack{\text{heat} \\ (2)\ \text{H}_3\text{O}^+}]{(1)\ \text{KMnO}_4,\ \text{OH}^-} \text{C}_6\text{H}_5-\text{CO}_2\text{H}$$

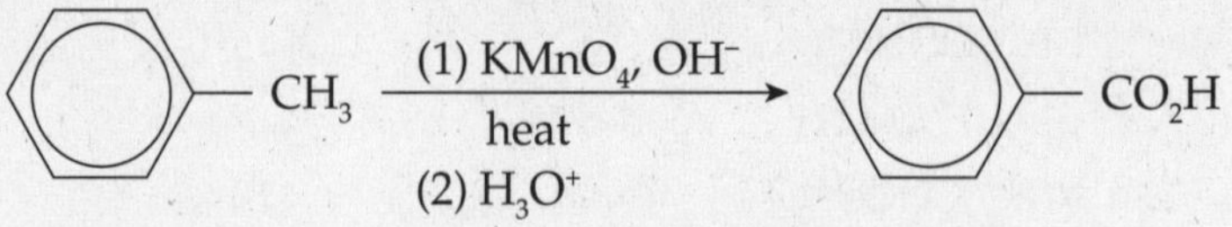

The oxidation of methyl ketones in the presence of a halide and sodium hydroxide generates a carboxylic acid according to the haloform reaction:

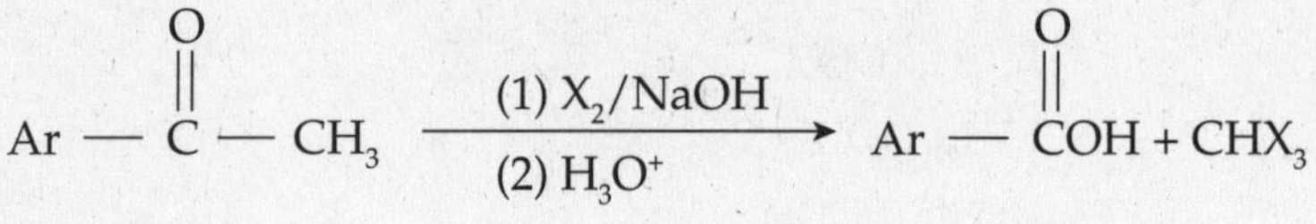

$$\text{Ar}-\overset{\overset{\displaystyle O}{\|}}{\text{C}}-\text{CH}_3 \xrightarrow[(2)\ \text{H}_3\text{O}^+]{(1)\ \text{X}_2/\text{NaOH}} \text{Ar}-\overset{\overset{\displaystyle O}{\|}}{\text{C}}\text{OH} + \text{CHX}_3$$

where X = Br, Cl, I, or F

38.1.3.2 Grignard Reaction

The reaction of an alkyl or aryl halide with magnesium produces a Grignard reagent according to this generic reaction:

$$\text{Mg}+\text{R–X} \xrightarrow[\text{diethyl ether}]{} \text{RMgX}$$

If a Grignard reagent is then reacted with carbon dioxide (carbonation), the result is a carboxylic acid according to this generic reaction:

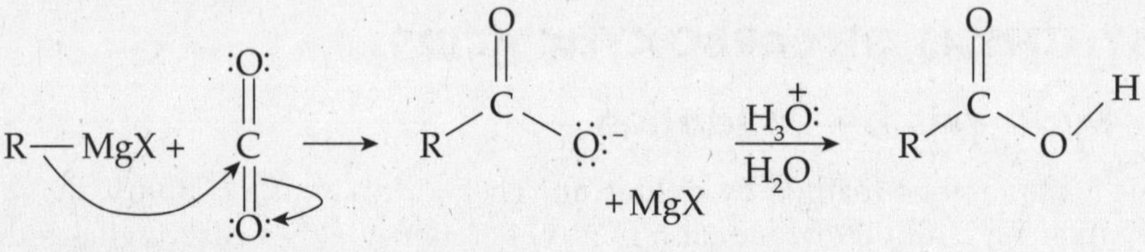

38.1.3.3 Hydrolysis of Nitriles

Nitriles can be hydrolyzed by strong acids or bases to yield carboxylic acids according to this generic reaction:

The reaction mechanisms for these conversions are very complicated, so we won't reproduce them here. (Remember—there are no reaction mechanisms on the test!) If you're curious, look it up in an old textbook.

Please solve this problem:

- In order to produce a carboxylic acid, each of the following requires the presence of an oxidizing agent, EXCEPT:

  A. an alkylbenzene.
  B. an aldehyde.
  C. a nitrile.
  D. a primary alcohol.

Problem solved:

C is the correct answer. The principal oxidative pathways through which carboxylic acids are generated begin with primary alcohols, aldehydes, alkyl benzenes, and methyl ketones. The oxidizing agents are silver oxide for aldehydes, and potassium permanganate for primary alcohols and alkylbenzenes. The oxidation of a methyl ketone proceeds via the haloform reaction, as discussed in the text. Only nitriles may generate carboxylic acids through hydrolysis in the presence of a strong acid or base.

Please solve this problem:

- Which of the following does NOT accurately characterize the Grignard reagent?

  A. Its reaction with carbon dioxide produces a carboxylic acid.
  B. Its organic component must not contain an aromatic ring.
  C. It has a metallic component.
  D. It may be prepared from an alkyl halide.

Problem solved:

B is the correct answer. The Grignard reagent is prepared from an alkyl or aryl halide and magnesium (a metal). Its combination with carbon dioxide under appropriate conditions produces a carboxylic acid, the latter process is called the Grignard reaction. Choices A, C, and D, therefore, are accurate statements. Because the progenitor to the Grignard reagent may be an alkyl or aryl halide, its organic component may contain an aromatic ring. Choice B, therefore, makes a false statement and is the correct answer.

Please solve this problem:

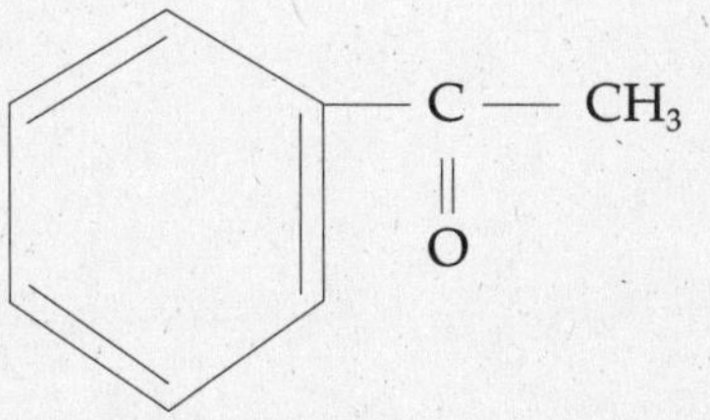

- The molecule depicted above might generate a carboxylic acid via which of the following processes?

  A. Oxidation
  B. The haloform reaction
  C. Both A and B
  D. Neither A nor B

Problem solved:

C is the correct answer. The pictured molecule is a an aryl methyl ketone and, as noted in the text, generates a carboxylic acid through oxidation via the haloform reaction. Hence, both choices A and B are correct.

Please solve this problem:

- Which of the following statements does NOT accurately characterize the formation of a carboxylic acid from a primary alcohol?

    A. It requires the presence of halide and sodium hydroxide.
    B. It requires the presence of an oxidizing agent.
    C. Both A and B
    D. Neither A nor B

Problem solved:

A is the correct answer. The formation of a carboxylic acid from a primary alcohol is an oxidation reaction and requires the presence of a strong oxidizing agent, such as potassium permanganate. Choice B, therefore, is an *accurate* statement and is incorrect. Choice A is an inaccurate statement; the presence of a halide and sodium hydroxide apply to the haloform reaction, from which methyl ketones generate carboxylic acids.

38.1.4 GENERATION OF CARBOXYLIC ACID DERIVATIVES

Carboxylic acids serve as key points of initiation in the synthesis of **carboxylic acid derivatives.** The most important derivatives fall within five categories: (1) primary alcohols, (2) halogenated alkanes, (3) the carboxylate ion itself, (4) acid halides, and (5) the products of nucleophilic substitution.

38.1.4.1 Reduction to Yield Primary Alcohols

Carboxylic acids can be reduced to primary alcohols. The reduction requires a powerful reducing reagent, such as lithium aluminum hydride or borane (BH_3).

$$RCOOH \xrightarrow{LiAlH_4} RCH_2OH$$

The mechanism looks like this:

38.1.4.2 Decarboxylation to Yield Halogenated Alkanes

Carboxylic acids can be **decarboxylated** to yield halogenated alkanes through a process called the **Hunsdiecker reaction**. Decarboxylation denotes the loss of a CO_2 molecule and means that the number of carbon atoms on the resulting molecule will be one less than that of the original carboxylic acid.

$$RCO_2H \xrightarrow[\text{heat}]{Br_2,\ HgO} RBr\ +\ CO_2$$

38.1.4.3 Deprotonation to Yield the Carboxylate Ion

One of the essential characteristics of carboxylic acids is that they can deprotonate to produce a proton and a carboxylate anion. Recognize that the carboxylate anion is itself a useful intermediate and reagent in a number of reactions (that need not be listed or memorized).

38.1.4.4 Alpha Substitution

A carboxylic acid undergoes **alpha substitution** when, at its alpha carbon, a hydrogen atom is replaced by some other substituent. In most circumstances germane to the MCAT, alpha substitution of carboxylic acids refers to the replacement of a hydrogen atom by a **halide** at the alpha carbon according to this generic reaction:

$$RCH_2COOH \xrightarrow[\text{H}_2O]{Br_2,\ PBr_3} RCHBrCOOH$$

38.1.4.5 Nucleophilic Substitution

With respect to carboxylic acids, nucleophilic substitution may produce **acid chlorides**, **acid anhydrides**, **amides**, and **esters**. The nucleophilic substitution reaction begins when a nucleophile attacks the carbonyl carbon and forms a tetrahedral intermediate. The intermediate loses a nucleophilic substituent, and another nucleophile replaces it.

If, under appropriate conditions, a carboxylic acid is treated with thionyl chloride ($SOCl_2$) or phosphorous trichloride (PCl_5), it will lose its –OH group and it will be replaced with a chlorine atom.

$$RCO_2H + SOCl_2 \text{ or } PCl_5 \longrightarrow \overset{\displaystyle O}{\overset{\displaystyle \|}{R}}CCl$$

A carboxylic acid may be converted to an acid anhydride, which might be conceived of as two carboxylic acids joined together.

$$RCO_2H + \text{excess } (CH_3C)_2O \longrightarrow R\overset{O}{\overset{\|}{C}}O\overset{O}{\overset{\|}{C}}R$$

If a carboxylic acid is reacted with an alcohol under appropriate conditions it will produce an ester (RCOOR'). A carboxylic acid might also give rise to an ester if it is first converted to produce an acid chloride and then reacted with an alcohol.

$$RCO_2H + R'OH \xrightarrow{H^+} RCO_2R'$$

$$\overset{\displaystyle O}{\underset{\displaystyle \|}{RCCl}} + R'OH \longrightarrow RCO_2R'$$

If a carboxylic acid's hydroxyl (OH) group is replaced with a nitrogen substituent, an amide is formed.

$$\overset{\displaystyle O}{\underset{\displaystyle \|}{(RC)_2O}} + HNR_2' \longrightarrow \overset{\displaystyle O}{\underset{\displaystyle \|}{RCNR_2'}}$$

$$RCO_2R' + NH_3 \longrightarrow \overset{\displaystyle O}{\underset{\displaystyle \|}{RCNH_2}}$$

Please solve this problem:

- The production of a primary alcohol from a carboxylic acid requires the presence of which of the following?

  A. A reducing agent
  B. Potassium permanganate
  C. Both A and B
  D. Neither A nor B

Problem solved:

A is the correct answer. It was noted in section **38.1.3** that a carboxylic acid might be produced by oxidation of a primary alcohol. Similarly, a primary alcohol might be generated by reduction of a carboxylic acid. The process requires the presence of a reducing agent. Choice A, therefore, is an accurate statement. Choice B, on the other hand, is not. It refers to potassium permanganate, the *oxidizing agent* often used in the formation of carboxylic acids from primary alcohols.

Please solve this problem:

- Nucleophilic substitution at the carbonyl carbon of a carboxylic acid may produce which of the following choices?

  A. An acid anhydride
  B. An ester
  C. Both A and B
  D. Neither A nor B

Problem solved:

C is the correct answer. As noted in the text, nucleophilic substitution at the acid's carbonyl carbon may generate acid chlorides, acid anhydrides, amides, and esters. Choices A and B are both correct, making choice C the answer.

Please solve this problem:

- Which of the following is NOT produced from nucleophilic substitution at a carboxylic acid's carbonyl carbon?

    A. An acid chloride
    B. An amide
    C. A halogenated alkane
    D. An ester

Problem solved:

C is the correct answer. All of the named compounds may arise from nucleophilic substitution at the carbonyl carbon except a halogenated alkane. The halogenated alkane arises from decarboxylation through the Hunsdiecker reaction.

Please solve this problem:

- If an aliphatic carboxylic acid bearing eight carbon atoms is subjected to the Hunsdiecker reaction in order to produce a halogenated alkane, how many carbons will be on the resulting molecule?

    A. 6
    B. 7
    C. 8
    D. 9

Problem solved:

B is the correct answer. As noted in the text, the Hunsdiecker reaction involves decarboxylation—the loss of a carbon dioxide moiety—and consequently the loss of a carbon atom. The number of carbon atoms on the halogenated alkane resulting from the Hunsdiecker reaction is one less than the number carried by the original carboxylic acid: $8 - 1 = 7$.

38.1.5 HYDROLYSIS OF ACID CHLORIDES, ANHYDRIDES, AMIDES AND ESTERS

The nucleophilic substitution reactions described in the preceding section may undergo *reversal through hydrolysis.* Hence, acid chlorides, acid anhydrides, amides, and esters (all of which are formed from carboxylic acids by nucleophilic substitution) may be hydrolyzed to carboxylic acids.

An acid halide, for example, may be hydrolyzed to generate a carboxylic acid according to this generic reaction:

$$\text{acid halide:} \quad \overset{\overset{\text{O}}{\|}}{\text{RC}}-\text{X} + \text{H}_2\text{O} \xrightarrow{\text{H}^+ \text{ or OH}^-} \text{RCO}_2\text{H} + \text{X}^-$$

An anhydride may undergo hydrolysis to regenerate two carboxylic acids according to this generic reaction:

$$\text{anhydride:} \quad \overset{\overset{\text{O}\quad\text{O}}{\|\quad\|}}{\text{RC}-\text{OCR}'} + \text{H}_2\text{O} \xrightarrow{\qquad\qquad} \text{RCO}_2\text{H} + \text{HO}_2\text{CR}'$$

An amide may undergo hydrolysis to generate a carboxylic acid and an amine or ammonia according to this generic reaction:

$$\text{amide:} \quad \overset{\overset{\text{O}}{\|}}{\text{RC}}-\text{NR}_2' + \text{H}_2\text{O} \xrightarrow{\text{H}^+ \text{ or OH}^-} \text{RCO}_2\text{H} + \text{HNR}_2'$$

An ester may undergo hydrolysis to generate a carboxylic acid according to this generic reaction which is sometimes called **alkaline hydrolysis** or **saponification**:

$$\text{ester:} \quad \overset{\overset{\text{O}}{\|}}{\text{RC}}-\text{OR}' + \text{H}_2\text{O} \xrightarrow{\text{H}^+ \text{ or OH}^-} \text{RCO}_2\text{H} + \text{HOR}'$$

Please solve this problem:

- Which of the following may generate a carboxylic acid on hydrolysis?

  A. An anhydride
  B. An amide
  C. Both A and B
  D. Neither A nor B

Problem solved:

C is the correct answer. The carboxylic acid derivatives that arise from nucleophilic substitution (see section **38.1.4**) are all susceptible to hydrolytic reactions that regenerate carboxylic acids. When an anhydride is subjected to hydrolysis it regenerates the two carboxylic acids from which it arose. When an amide is subjected to hydrolysis it regenerates a carboxylic acid and ammonia or an amine.

38.2 MASTERY APPLIED: SAMPLE PASSAGE AND QUESTIONS

Passage

The commonly used analgesic (pain killing) agents include acetylsalicylate (aspirin), indomethacin, ibuprofen, and acetaminophen. The structure of each of these compounds is shown in Figure 1.

Acetylsalicylic acid is a derivative of salicylic acid, which is synthesized according to the *Kolbe reaction* in which a phenol salt is treated with carbon dioxide. This results in the phenyl ring losing a hydrogen atom which is then replaced by a carboxyl group, as shown in Figure 2.

Aspirin, indomethacin, and ibuprofen have independent analgesic and anti-inflammatory properties. Therefore, they are often prescribed for pain that is due to inflammation (for example, arthritis). The anti-inflammatory effects of aspirin and indomethacin are chiefly due to their inhibition of prostaglandin synthesis.

In some patients, acetylsalicylate, indomethacin, and ibuprofen cause gastric disturbance. In such patients, prolonged use may lead to gastric ulcer. Acetylsalicylate and indomethacin tend to cause such effects more frequently than does ibuprofen. Acetaminophen tends not to produce such effects at all.

An investigator wishes to find an explanation for the adverse gastric effects of acetylsalicylate, indomethacin, and ibuprofen, and to explore the reasons acetaminophen exerts no such effects.

Experiment

From 100 patients diagnosed with osteoarthritis, four groups of twenty-five are assembled and identified as Groups 1, 2, 3, and 4. Each group is treated daily with one of the analgesic agents described above: group 1 with aspirin, group 2 with indomethacin, group 3 with ibuprofen, and group 4 with acetaminophen. All subjects are evaluated bi-weekly for reports of pain relief and objective manifestations of reduced inflammation at previously inflamed joints. Results are shown in Table 1.

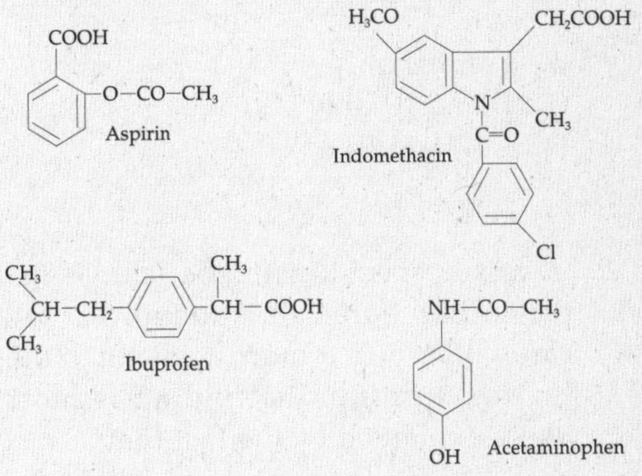

Figure 1

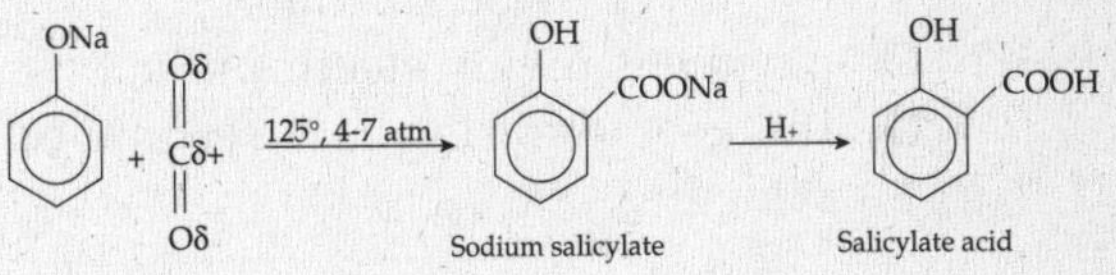

Figure 2

Group	Pain Relief	Reduced Inflammation
1	++	+
2	++	+
3	++	+
4	+	O

Key: ++ very significant + significant O not significant

Table 1

1. Figure 1 and Table 1 indicate that acetaminophen differs from aspirin in that:

    I. it has no significant analgesic effect.
    II. it has no significant anti-inflammatory effect.
    III. it is not a carboxylic acid.

    A. I only
    B. I and II only
    C. II and III only
    D. I, II, and III

2. If, with respect to salicylic acid, as depicted in Figure 2, it is found that the carboxyl group is more acidic than the hydroxyl group, the finding is most likely explained by the fact that:

    A. the carboxyl anion is stabilized by charge delocalization.
    B. the carboxyl anion is destabilized by charge delocalization.
    C. oxygen is highly electrophilic.
    D. the aromatic ring is a resonance structure.

3. An investigator finds that the Kolbe intermediate (sodium salicylate), as depicted in Figure 2, has some analgesic effect, but that the effect is less than that of salicylic acid or aspirin. She tentatively hypothesizes that the analgesic effect is negatively correlated with pKa. Is the hypothesis plausible?

    A. No, because the precursor to salicylic acid is not acidic.
    B. No, because the data in Table 1 are inconsistent with the hypothesis that analgesic effect is related to acidity.
    C. Yes, because sodium salicylate and acetaminophen likely have lower pKa values than do the other analgesics under investigation.
    D. Yes, because neither acetaminophen nor sodium salicylate are carboxylic acids.

4. With respect to the four medications under study, which among the conclusions is supported by the data in Table 1?

    I. Gastric disturbance is associated with acidity.
    II. Acidity is essential to anti-inflammatory effects.
    III. Anti-inflammatory effects and analgesia are unrelated.

    A. I only
    B. I and II only
    C. II and III only
    D. I and III only

5. If the investigator wished to determine whether acetaminophen is a relatively less effective pain reliever due to its failure to reduce inflammation, which of the following experimental procedures would be most advisable?

   A. Treat one group of osteoarthritic patients with acetaminophen alone. Treat another group with acetaminophen and an anti-inflammatory that has no independent analgesic properties, to determine whether pain relief approximates that which is observed with the other three medications under study.

   B. Administer acetaminophen to two groups of patients, each with separate painful conditions that do not relate to inflammation to determine if the two groups differ as to the degree of pain relief they experience.

   C. Select four different animal species with four different forms of arthritis, and treat each species with one of the four agents under study to determine whether the acidic agents provide greater relief than acetaminophen.

   D. Prepare isomeric forms of the acidic agents under study and determine whether in some isomeric conformations the analgesic properties are preserved while the anti-inflammatory properties are lost.

6. Which among the following distinguishes acetaminophen from aspirin?

   A. Aspirin does not inhibit prostaglandin synthesis.

   B. Acetaminophen does not inhibit prostaglandin synthesis.

   C. Aspirin offers no independent analgesic effect.

   D. Acetaminophen offers no independent analgesic effect.

38.3 MASTERY VERIFIED: ANSWERS AND EXPLANATIONS

1. *C is the correct answer.* Table 1 shows that patients treated with aspirin show marked reduction in their pain, and that those treated with acetaminophen show some significant reduction in their pain. Statement I, therefore, does not describe a difference between the two drugs. Table 1 also shows that aspirin produces a marked anti-inflammatory effect, but that acetaminophen does not. Therefore, statement II is accurate. Figure 1 shows that aspirin is a carboxylic acid (bearing a COOH group), but that acetaminophen is not. Statement III, therefore, is accurate. Since statements II and III are accurate and I is not, choice C is correct.

2. *A is the correct answer.* The question asks only that the student understand a principle emphasized in the text. The carboxyl anion RCOO⁻ has particular stability because it is a resonance structure. Resonance is one form of charge delocalization; the negative charge with which the ion is "burdened" is shared among the two oxygen atoms bound to the carboxyl carbon (with the consequence, also, that there is partial double bond character between the carbon atom and each of the oxygen atoms). Choice B is incorrect. Choice C is a true statement; oxygen is electrophilic. That fact, however, would tend to *promote* the acidity of the OH group and would not explain the finding that the OH group showed less acidity than the COOH group. Choice D also makes a true statement; the aromatic ring is a resonance structure. As noted in the text, however, that fact does not enhance acidity of an aromatic carboxylic acid.

3. *D is the correct answer.* Figure 1 demonstrates that acetaminophen is not a carboxylic acid; it does not conform to the prototypical structures RCOOH (aliphatic carboxylic acid) or ArCOOH (aromatic carboxylic acid). Sodium salicylate is a salt, not a carboxylic acid. It conforms to the structure ArCOONa, not ArCOOH. Choice A makes a correct statement, but is not relevant to the question. The fact that sodium salicylate's precursor is not an acid does not bear on the investigator's hypothesis. Choice B is incorrect. The data in Table 1 *are* consistent with the investigator's hypothesis. Among the medications tested, acetaminophen is the only one that is not an acid and it shows the least degree of analgesic effect. Choice C is incorrect as well. Acetaminophen and sodium salicylate are not acids. They most likely have higher pK_a's than the other substances under study.

4. *B is the correct answer.* According to Table 1, the only group of patients to be free of gastric disturbance were those treated with acetaminophen, which is the only one of the four tested agents that is not an acid. Statement I, therefore, represents a correct response. That same group of patients is the only group to show no significant reduction in inflammation. Statement II also reflects a correct response. Statement III is not justifiable. Acetaminophen seems to produce no anti-inflammatory effects and shows less analgesic effect than the other three agents. The data do not support the conclusion that the anti-inflammatory effects and analgesia are unrelated.

5. *A is the correct answer.* The MCAT frequently presents questions like this one, which require the student to apply logical reasoning in connection with experimental science. The question does not draw on any substantive knowledge with respect to carboxylic acids.

The investigator has observed (Table 1) that acetaminophen produces a smaller degree of pain relief than aspirin, indomethacin, and ibuprofen. She has noted also that acetaminophen is the only one of the four agents that does not produce anti-inflammatory effects. She postulates that the additional pain relief produced by the other three drugs might be a direct consequence of the fact that they have a separate anti-inflammatory effect.

In order to test her hypothesis, she would like to administer an agent that is identical to acetaminophen except that it has an independent anti-inflammatory property. If such an agent produces the level of pain relief associated with the other three agents she will have support for her hypothesis. If it does not, she will not.

In order to simulate an agent that is identical to acetaminophen but has a separate anti-inflammatory effect, the investigator might administer acetaminophen together with an anti-inflammatory agent that does not itself have an independent analgesic effect. She could then assess the level of pain relief it affords, precisely as described in choice A.

Choices B, C, and D do not describe any processes logically connected to the investigator's objective. These may seem attractive to students who assume that two experimental groups are better than one, or that animal experiments are more "science-like" than others, or that creation of isomers is more in the nature of "real organic chemistry."

6. *B is the correct answer*. The question calls for careful reading of the passage's third paragraph, which states that "aspirin, indomethacin and ibuprofen have independent analgesic and anti-inflammatory properties." It appears, therefore, that acetaminophen has no such property, which is consistent with the data reported in Table 1. The passage also states that "the anti-inflammatory properties of aspirin and indomethacin are attributable to their capacity to inhibit the synthesis of prostaglandins..."

It appears, therefore, that acetaminophen, lacking an anti-inflammatory property, does not inhibit prostaglandin synthesis. (The passage does not describe the mechanism by which ibuprofen exerts its anti-inflammatory effect.)

Choice A is incorrect because aspirin does inhibit prostaglandin synthesis. Choices C and D are also inaccurate statements. Both aspirin and acetaminophen exert analgesic effects, and in the case of aspirin such effects are independent of anti-inflammatory effects.

CHAPTER 39

AMINES, AMINO ACIDS, AND PROTEINS

39.1 MASTERY ACHIEVED

39.1.1 AMINES

The **ammonia** molecule has the formula NH_3 and is normally depicted as follows:

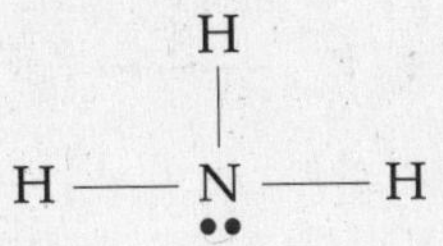

An **amine** normally arises from alkylation or multiple alkylation of an ammonia molecule, so that one or more hydrogen atoms are replaced by an alkyl or aryl group. If one hydrogen atom is replaced, the amine is **primary**. If two hydrogen atoms are replaced, the amine is **secondary**. If three hydrogen atoms are replaced, the amine is termed **tertiary**.

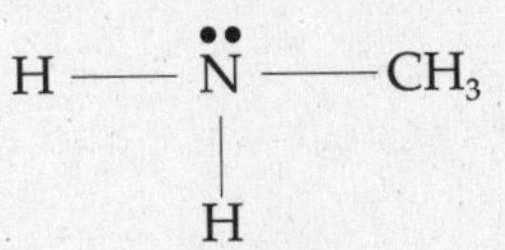

1° Amine 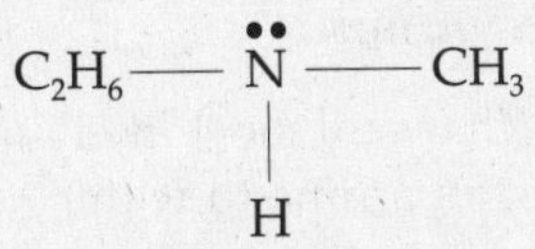   2° Amine

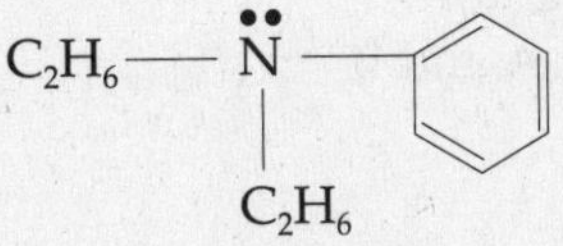

3° Amine

Amines are polar molecules, because nitrogen generally has a higher electronegativity than hydrogen and most other alkyl or aryl substituents. The polarity means, among other things, that primary and secondary amines exhibit hydrogen bonding; tertiary amines do not because they bear no lone hydrogen.

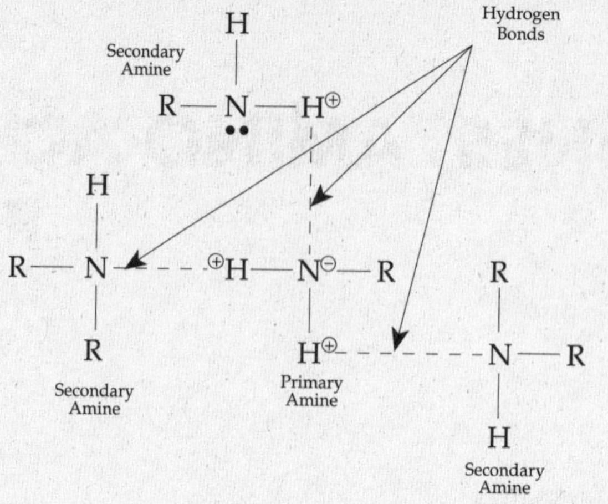

The fact that an amine features an unshared pair of electrons (like the ammonia molecule from which it derives) makes it a Lewis base; it has a tendency to donate an electron pair.

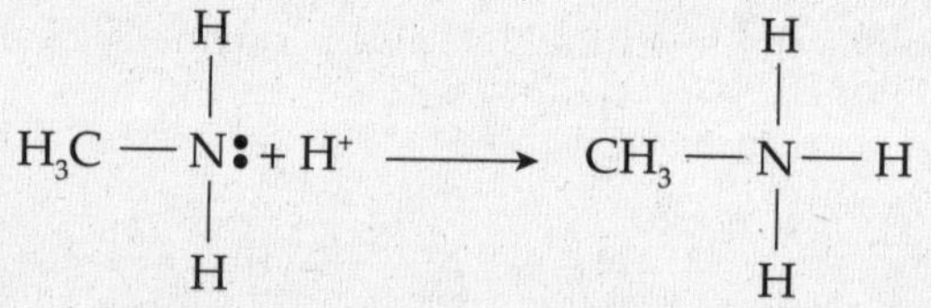

An amine's acidity is affected by the nature of its substituents. If a hydrogen atom is replaced by an aliphatic chain, the resulting amine tends to be more basic than ammonia. If a hydrogen atom is replaced by an aryl group, the resulting amine tends to be less basic than ammonia.

Please solve this problem:

- What will most likely be the effect of the addition of an amine to water?

  A. Reduce pH
  B. Increase pOH
  C. Both A and B
  D. Neither A and B

Problem solved:

D is correct. Amines, like ammonia itself, are basic. The fact that they feature a lone pair of electrons allows them to easily donate an electron pair. In aqueous solution, therefore, an amine molecule has a tendency to take up a hydrogen ion (proton), thereby decreasing the solution's hydrogen ion concentration (increasing pH) and increasing the solution's hydroxy (OH) ion concentration (decreasing pOH). Choices A and B are both false statements.

Please solve this problem:

- A primary amine bearing an ethyl group is likely to be:

  A. more acidic than hydrochloric acid.
  B. more acidic than acetic acid.
  C. more basic than ammonia.
  D. more basic than sodium hydroxide.

Problem solved:

C is correct. Ammonia is a weak base—meaning that in aqueous solution it does not ionize completely. (Sodium hydroxide, on the other hand, is a strong base—meaning that in aqueous solution it does ionize completely.) An amine in which a single hydrogen atom is replaced by an aliphatic chain is also a weak base, but tends to be more basic than ammonia. Choice A suggests that an amine is a strong acid and choice B raises the possibility that an amine is a weak acid. Both suggestions are false. Choice D suggests that an amine is a strong base. That too is false.

Please solve this problem:

- Does a tertiary amine exhibit hydrogen bonding?

    A. Yes, because it is a polar molecule.
    B. Yes, because it is a nonpolar molecule.
    C. No, because it has no hydrogen atoms bound to its central nitrogen atom.
    D. No, because only the water molecule exhibits hydrogen bonding.

Problem solved:

C is correct. Hydrogen bonding occurs when a polar molecule bearing a hydrogen atom with partial positive charge opposes another molecule of the same species. The partial positive charge on the hydrogen atom interacts with the corresponding partial negative charge. That process occurs with ammonia itself and with primary and secondary amines, because they each have at least one hydrogen that carries a partial postive charge. A tertiary amine, on the other hand, is one in which all three hydrogen atoms that belong to an ammonia molecule have been replaced by alkyl or aryl substituents. The resulting molecule has no hydrogen atoms bound to its central nitrogen atom and so cannot exhibit hydrogen bonding. Choice A reflects, in part, a true statement. A tertiary amine is polar, but that does not mean it undergoes hydrogen bonding. Choice B reflects an incorrect statement because it characterizes an amine as nonpolar. Choice D is also incorrect. While water does undergo hydrogen bonding, it is not the *only* molecule to do so.

39.1.2 STRUCTURE AND NOMENCLATURE OF AMINO ACIDS

On the MCAT, the most important ammonia derivative is the **amino acid**. Generically, the amino acid is depicted as follows:

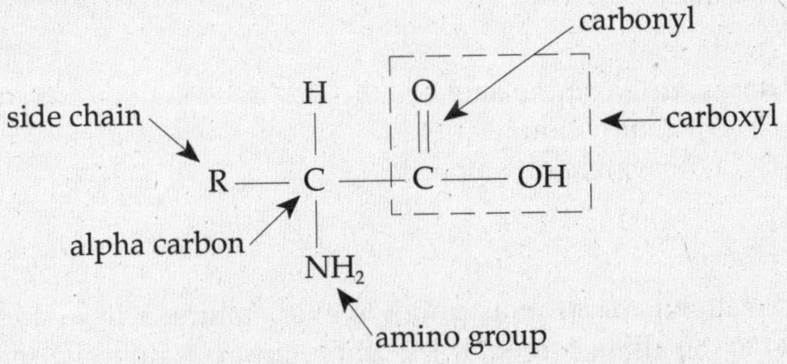

The NH_2 moiety represents the **amino group** and is a constituent of all amino acids. The COOH moiety represents the **carboxyl group** (see Chapter 38), and is also a constituent of all amino acids. The R group represents the **side chain** and is the molecule's **variable portion**; it makes each amino acid distinct from every other.

Most amino acids of biological significance are called **alpha amino acids**, meaning that the amino group is bound to the alpha carbon—the carbon that is adjacent to the carbonyl carbon (see Chapter 38).

39.1.2.1 Chirality of Amino Acids

Chirality, the chiral center, and associated phenomena of stereoisomerism are discussed in Chapter 34. For most biologically significant amino acids, *the alpha carbon is chiral*. That is, it bears four different substituents: (1) the side chain; (2) the amino group; (3) the carboxylic acid group; and (4) a hydrogen atom.

The amino acid **glycine** is an exception. Its side chain is a lone hydrogen atom; the alpha carbon, therefore, carries two hydrogen atoms (plus a carboxylic group and an amino group).

Since each substituent is not different from every other, the alpha carbon is not chiral.

Please solve this problem:

- Which of the following do most biologically significant amino acids exhibit?

  A. Enantiomerism
  B. Chirality
  C. Both A and B
  D. Neither A nor B

Problem solved:

C is correct. The text notes that for most biologically significant amino acids, the alpha carbon is chiral, and the molecule itself is chiral as well. All chiral molecules exhibit enantiomerism. That is, none are superimposable on the molecule that represents their mirror images (see Chapter 34). Choices A and B both make accurate statements.

Please solve this problem:

- An amino acid in which the amino group is bound to carbon 3 is NOT:

  A. an acid.
  B. an alpha amino acid.
  C. covalently bound.
  D. a derivative of ammonia.

Problem solved:

B is correct. The term alpha amino acid applies to every amino acid in which the amino group (NH_2) is bound to the alpha carbon. If the amino group is bound elsewhere, then the amino acid is not an alpha amino acid. Most amino acids of biological significance *are* alpha amino acids. Choices A, C, and D make false statements. All amino acids are acids (due to the presence of the COOH group), all are covalently bound, and all are derivatives of ammonia.

Please solve this problem:

- Which one of the following choices confers on each alpha amino acid its own identity?

  A. Placement of the carboxyl group relative to the amino group
  B. Variability of the R group
  C. Presence or absence of a hydrogen atom bound to the alpha carbon
  D. Orientation of N-H bonds within the amino group

Problem solved:

B is correct. In alpha amino acids the alpha carbon carries an amino group (NH_2), a hydrogen atom, and a carboxyl group (COOH). Amino acids differ from each other because of the fourth substituent bound to the alpha carbon. That substituent is known, generically, as the R group and affords each amino acid its own identity. For glycine, the R group is a single hydrogen atom. For the amino acid threonine, for example, the R group is CH_3CHOH.

$$
\begin{array}{c}
COOH \\
| \\
H_2N\!-\!C\!-\!H \\
| \\
H\!-\!C\!-\!OH \\
| \\
CH_3
\end{array}
$$

Threonine

Please solve this problem:

- Which one of the following choices is NOT true of most alpha amino acids?

  A. They exhibit stereoisomerism.
  B. They tend to generate a carboxyl anion in a basic environment.
  C. They exist as dextrarotatory and levarotatory isomers.
  D. They are optically inactive.

Problem solved:

D is correct. The question addresses the phenomenon of chirality as it applies to amino acids. As noted in the text, most biologically significant amino acids are alpha amino acids, and most of these are chiral. If a molecule is chiral it is optically active. Choice D is a false statement and is therefore correct. Choices A, B, and C are true statements. Chiral molecules exist as enantiomers, and enantiomers represent a form of stereoisomerism. Moreover, for any pair of enantiomers one member represents the dextrarotatory ("d"/+) isomer and the other the levarotatory("l"/−) isomer. All amino acids carry the carboxyl (COOH) group and tend, therefore, to shed a proton, especially in a basic environment.

39.1.3 CLASSIFICATION OF AMINO ACIDS

The side chain (R group) affords each amino acid its identity. Amino acids are classified on the basis of *commonalities* among side chains. As already noted, all amino acids carry one carboxyl group and are, therefore, carboxylic acids. Some amino acids carry a *second* carboxyl group on their side chain and are known as **acidic amino acids**. While all amino acids are acidic since all carry a COOH group, the term "acidic" amino acid refers to an amino acid that carries two carboxyl groups.

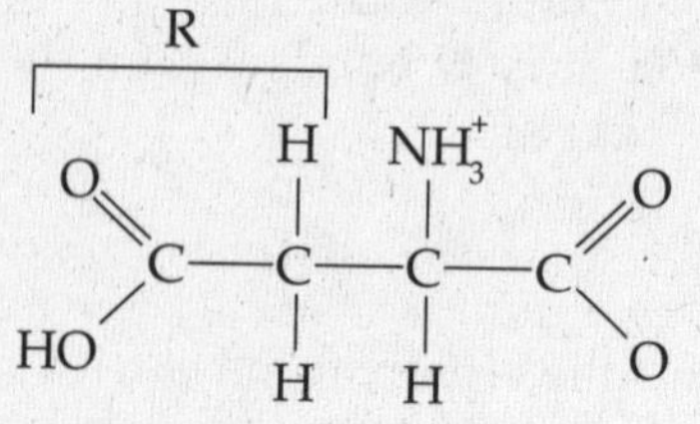

Aspartic acid

A **basic amino acid** has an amino group on its side chain, in addition to the one attached to its alpha carbon.

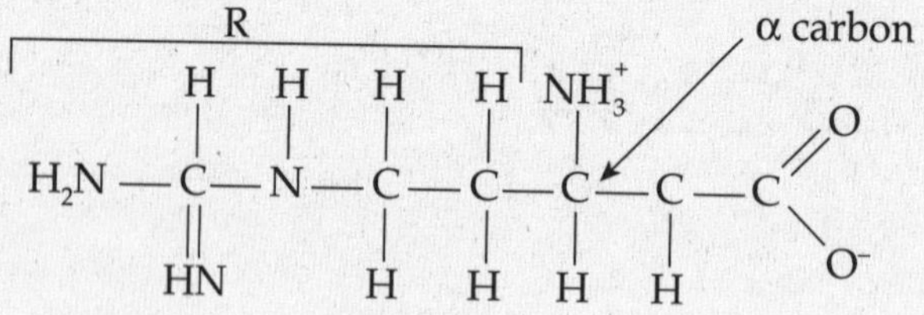

Arginine

A **neutral amino acid** has neither a carboxyl acid group nor an amino group on its side chain. It is neither acidic nor basic, as those terms have just been described.

A **polar amino acid** is one whose side chain features polarity in its bonding patterns. Polar amino acids are hydrophilic and are relatively soluble in water. Examples include neutral serine and threonine.

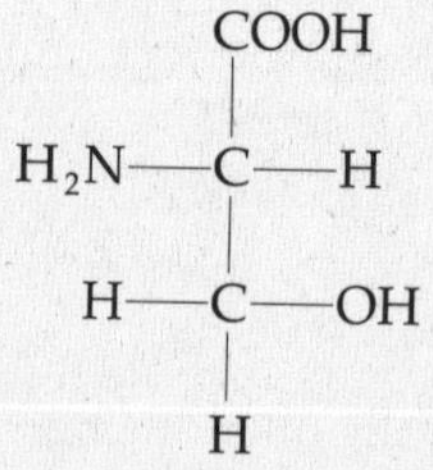

Serine

A **nonpolar amino acid** is one whose side chain is not polar. Such amino acids generally have side chains that are saturated hydrocarbons. Nonpolar amino acids are hydrophobic and are relatively insoluble in water. Examples include alanine and valine.

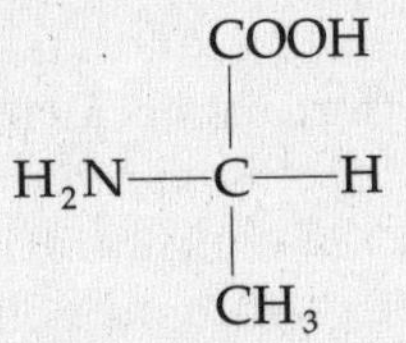

Alanine

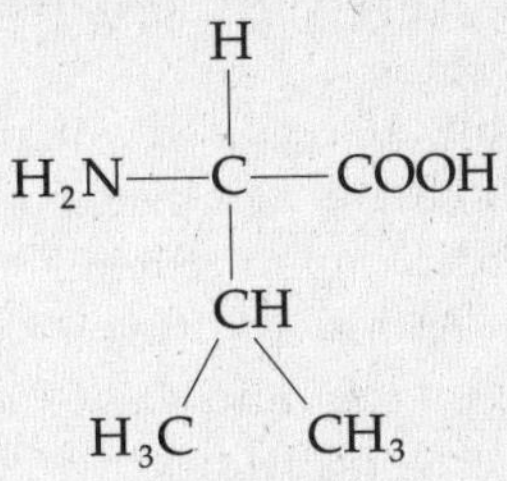

Valine

Acidic or basic amino acids tend to have charged side chains, since an acidic amino acid's side chain tends to lose an H+ ion and a basic amino acid's side chain tends to acquire one. Acidic and basic amino acids are therefore considered polar—their side chains carry charge. They are also hydrophilic and dissolve with relative ease in water.

39.1.3.1   Sulfur-Containing Amino Acids

Three of the 20 amino acids encountered in proteins contain sulphur in their side chains. They are methionine, cysteine, and cystine. Cystine is formed from two molecules of cysteine linked by a **disulfide bridge**.

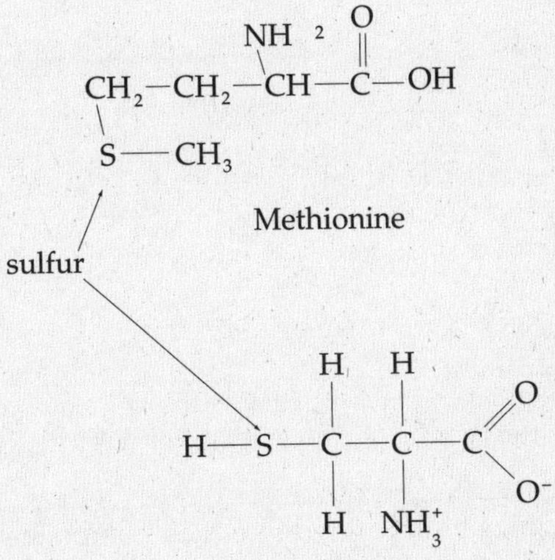

Methionine

sulfur

Cysteine

disulfide bridge

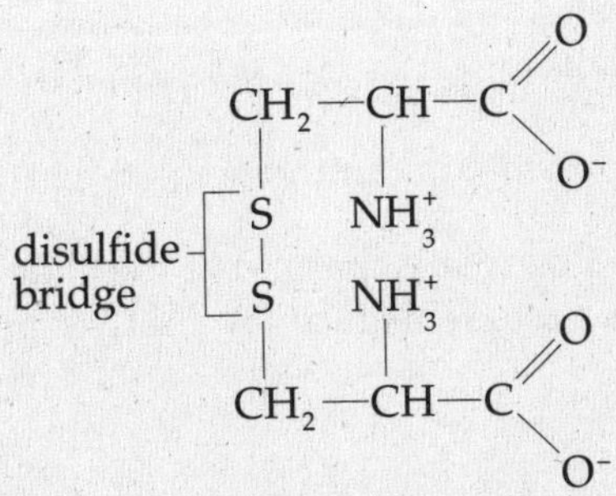

Cystine

39.1.3.2 Amino Acids as Zwitterions; Isoelectric Point

Generally, a **zwitterion**, also called a **dipolar ion**, is an ion that has both a positive and a negative "end." Amino acids can give rise to zwitterions because they carry a basic moiety (NH_2) and an acidic moiety (the COOH group). Consider simple equilibrium and Le Chatelier's principle. At low pH (high hydrogen ion concentration) the NH_2 group will tend to acquire a hydrogen ion, and the COOH group will tend not to release one. At high pH (low hydrogen ion concentration) the COOH group will tend to release an H^+ ion, and the NH_2 group will tend not to acquire one.

For every amino acid there is some mid-level pH at which the COOH group will deprotonate and the NH_2 group will acquire a proton. This mid-level pH is termed the amino acid's **isoelectric point**. At its isoelectric point an amino acid carries both a positive and a negative charge and is, therefore, a zwitterion.

Zwitterion

The isoelectric points for the twenty amino acids of biological significance fall within the range 5.0–6.5.

A mixture of amino acids may be separated into their component species according to isoelectric point using the following procedure:

1. The mixture of amino acids is placed near the center of a paper strip, then wetted and buffered at a known pH.

2. Electrodes are attached to the ends of the paper strip.

3. An electric field is applied, and amino acids migrate along the strip.

4. Amino acids that are positively charged at the chosen pH migrate toward the negative end, and amino acids that are negatively charged at the chosen pH migrate toward the positive end.

Please solve this problem:

- If an amino acid carries a carboxyl group on its side chain, it acquires which of the following labels?

    A. Basic
    B. Acidic
    C. Polar
    D. Nonpolar

Problem solved:

B is correct. All amino acids carry one carboxyl group; that is why they are designated acids. Some amino acids have a second carboxyl group on their side chain. These amino acids are called acidic amino acids.

Please solve this problem:

- Which of the following amino acids features sulfur in its side chain?

    A. Cysteine
    B. Cystine
    C. Both A and B
    D. Neither A nor B

Problem solved:

C is correct. Cystine and cysteine both contain sulfur in their side chains. Cystine is comprised of two molecules of cysteine, linked by a disulfide bridge, as illustrated in the text.

Please solve this problem:

- At very acidic pH, a neutral alpha amino acid is likely to carry:

    A. a positive charge on its amino moiety.
    B. a negative charge on its carboxyl moiety.
    C. both A and B
    D. neither A nor B

Problem solved:

A is correct. A neutral alpha amino acid is one that does not carry either a carboxyl moiety or an amino moiety on its side chain. It does carry both such moieties on its alpha carbon. In a very acidic environment, proton concentration is high. According to Le Chatelier's principle, the molecule's amino group will tend to acquire a proton and its carboxyl group will tend not to lose one. Thus, the molecule will be positively charged.

Please solve this problem:

- At very basic pH, a neutral alpha amino acid is likely to carry:

    A. a positive charge on its amino moiety.
    B. a negative charge on its carboxyl moiety.
    C. both A and B
    D. neither A nor B

Problem solved:

B is correct. The reasoning is identical to that of the preceding problem. In a basic environment hydrogen ion concentration is low. According to ordinary equilibrium dynamics, the carboxyl group will tend to lose a proton and thereby acquire a negative charge. The amino group will tend not to acquire a proton and will remain neutral.

Please solve this problem:

- At its isoelectric point, a neutral alpha amino acid is likely to carry:

    A. a positive charge on its amino moiety.
    B. a negative charge on its carboxyl moiety.
    C. both A and B
    D. neither A nor B

Problem solved:

C is correct. With respect to deprotonation of an amino acid's carboxyl group and protonation of its amino group, the isoelectric point represents an intermediate pH. It is that pH at which the carboxyl group deprotonates and the amino group acquires a proton. At its isoelectric point, therefore, the amino group carries a positive charge (NH_3^+) and the carboxyl group carries a negative charge. Each amino acid has its own isoelectric point. As noted in the text, for the alpha amino acids of biological significance, isoelectric points fall within the range 5.0–6.5.

39.1.3.3 Amino Acids as Amphoteric Species

Because an amino acid is both an acid and a base (depending on ambient pH), it can, depending on environment and reaction medium, react as either. That fact groups amino acids among chemistry's **amphoteric species**—species that may react as acids or bases.

39.1.3.4 Relative Acidity of Carboxyl and Amino Groups

At pH's well below its isoelectric point, an amino acid carries a positive charge on its amino group and no charge on its carboxyl group; the carboxyl group does not deprotonate. If the ambient pH is raised (by the addition of a base, for example), both the carboxyl group and the protonated amino group (NH_3^+) will tend to deprotonate so that the carboxyl group acquires a negative charge and the amino group becomes neutral. The student should remember that for any alpha amino acid, the carboxyl moiety is more acidic than the protonated amino moiety.

When pH is raised, the carboxyl group will deprotonate before the charged amino group does. Conversely, when pH is lowered (so that hydrogen ion increases) the carboxyl anion and the neutral amino group (NH_2) will tend to acquire protons. Because the carboxyl group is more acidic than the amino group, the amino group will acquire a proton before the carboxyl group does.

Please solve this problem:

- For a given neutral alpha amino acid, X, the iso-electric point is 5.6. At pH 5.0, both the carboxyl group and the amino group are protonated. As pH is raised:

    A. the carboxyl group will deprotonate first, and the amino group will then deprotonate.
    B. the amino group will deprotonate first, and the carboxyl group will then deprotonate.
    C. the amino group and the carboxyl group will deprotonate simultaneously.
    D. neither the amino group nor the carboxyl group will deprotonate.

Problem solved:

A is correct. The carboxyl moiety is more acidic than the amino moiety. When pH is well below the isoelectric point of a neutral alpha amino acid, both the carboxyl group and the amino group will be protonated, as indicated in the question. As pH is increased (ambient proton concentration reduced), equilibrium phenomena will tend to deprotonate both moieties. However, because the carboxyl group is more acidic than the amino group, the carboxyl group will be first to deprotonate; it is more "eager" to lose a proton.

Please solve this problem:

- For a given neutral alpha amino acid, X, the iso-electric point is 5.2. At pH 5.8, both the amino group and the carboxyl group are deprotonated. As pH is lowered:

    A. the amino group will protonate first, and the carboxyl group will then protonate.
    B. the carboxyl group will protonate first, and the amino group will then protonate.
    C. the amino group and the carboxyl group will protonate simultaneously.
    D. neither the amino group nor the carboxyl group will protonate.

Problem solved:

A is correct. Once again, because the carboxyl moiety is more acidic than the amino group, it is more "willing" to part with a proton and less "willing" to acquire one. Therefore, as pH is lowered, with equilibrium dynamics tending to "push" a proton on both groups, the carboxyl group will be the last to protonate.

39.1.4 SYNTHESIS OF AMINO ACIDS: DIRECT AMMONOLYSIS, STRECKER SYNTHESIS, REDUCTIVE AMINATION

Among the processes through which amino acids are synthesized, the most significant is **direct ammonolysis** of an alpha-bromo or alpha-chloro carboxylic acid (which can be prepared through a process called the **Hell-Volhard-Zelinsky** halogenation of unsubstituted acids).

$$CH_3CH_2COOH \xrightarrow{Br_2, P} CH_3CHCOOH \xrightarrow{NH_3^+ (excess)} CH_3CHCOO^-$$

Propionic acid

α - Bromopropionic acid (Br)

Alanine (NH$_3^+$)
70% yield

The process tends to produce a racemic mixture of dextro and levo isomers. Other procedures commonly used to produce amino acids are the **Strecker synthesis** and **reductive amination of a keto-acid** (which need not be discussed further for MCAT preparation). The student should recognize, however, that *all such processes tend to produce racemic mixtures—* enantiomeric mixtures in which D- and L-isomers are present in equal concentration (see Chapter 34).

Please solve this problem:

- A sample of amino acid is prepared according to the Strecker synthesis. Polarimetry will most likely reveal that:

  A. the sample rotates the plane of polarized light to the right.
  B. the sample rotates the plane of polarized light to the left.
  C. the sample rotates the plane of polarized light to the right and then the left alternatively.
  D. the sample does not rotate the plane of polarized light to left or right.

Problem solved:

D is correct. Amino acids that are prepared through direct ammonolysis, the Strecker synthesis, or reductive amination of a keto-acid produce racemic mixtures. A racemic mixture is one in which D- and L-enantiomers are present in equal concentrations. Such a mixture does not rotate the plane of polarized light at all; it is optically inactive. Choice A would be correct if the sample contained predominantly the D-isomer, and choice B would be correct if the sample contained predominantly the L-isomer. Choice C is nonsensical. No mixture of enantiomers would produce the result it describes.

39.1.5 FORMATION OF POLYPEPTIDES FROM AMINO ACIDS

Two amino acids may join by the formation of a **peptide bond**. The peptide bond is formed through **dehydration synthesis,** in which the OH group from the carboxyl terminus of one molecule and a hydrogen atom from the amino group of the other are removed to form a molecule of water, and a bond is formed between the carbonyl carbon of the first amino acid and the amino nitrogen of the second.

peptide bond

Two amino acids thus linked are called a **dipeptide**. The dipeptide may in turn form additional peptide bonds with other amino acids to produce a long chain of peptides called a polypeptide. A protein is a long polypeptide, or a combination of polypeptides bound together by cross-links. The amino acid constituents of a polypeptide are sometimes called **amino acid residues,** which means, simply, amino acid constituent.

Hydrolysis breaks peptide bonds, and might be pictured as the reciprocal of dehydration synthesis. In the process of hydrolysis, a molecule of water is interposed between a peptide bond. The OH moiety bonds to the carbonyl carbon of one amino acid and the hydrogen atom bonds to the nitrogen atom of another.

A process called the **Edman degradation** constitutes a controlled means of conducting a series of peptide hydrolyses in order to ascertain the sequence of amino acids that compose a particular polypeptide. One performs the Edman degradation by treating a polypeptide with phenyl isothiocynanate and then subjecting it to mild acid hydrolysis. The process removes amino acids sequentially, one by one, from the nitrogen terminus of the polypeptide. Each amino acid thus removed from the polypeptide chain can be identified according to a variety of mechanisms. (Further details of the Edman degradation will not be tested on the MCAT unless the relevant information is provided by the test writers.)

Please solve this problem:

- The formation of a protein from its constituent amino acids involves which of the following?

    A. Multiple episodes of hydrolysis
    B. Dehydration synthesis
    C. Both A and B
    D. Neither A nor B

Problem solved:

B is correct. As noted in the text, the binding of two amino acids to make a dipeptide involves a dehydration synthesis in which a molecule of water is removed, and the nitrogen terminus of one amino acid is bound to the carbonyl carbon of another. The manufacture of a protein (one or more polypeptides) involves repetition of this process. Choice A describes hydrolysis, the process through which peptide bonds are broken.

Please solve this problem:

- The Edman degradation involves which of the following?

    A. Multiple episodes of hydrolysis
    B. Dehydration synthesis
    C. Both A and B
    D. Neither A nor B

Problem solved:

A is correct. As noted in the text, the Edman degradation is a process in which polypeptide chains are separated into their constituent amino acids. It constitutes an orderly sequence of hydrolyses and permits the investigator to ascertain the sequence of amino acids that compose a given polypeptide.

Please solve this problem:

- Direct ammonolysis of a keto-acid involves which of the following?

    A. Multiple episodes of hydrolysis
    B. Dehydration synthesis
    C. Both A and B
    D. Neither A nor B

Problem solved:

D is correct. Direct ammonolysis of a keto-acid is a manner in which *amino acids* (not polypeptides) are synthesized. It does not involve dehydration synthesis (through which peptide bonds are formed) or hydrolysis (through which peptide bonds are broken).

39.1.6 PROTEINS

39.1.6.1 Structure

The terms "protein" and "polypeptide" are not quite synonymous. This is because some proteins consist of a single polypeptide and others consist of more than one polypeptide.

A protein may be conceived in terms of its primary structure, secondary structure, tertiary structure, and quaternary structure.

Primary structure refers to the sequence of amino acids that make up the protein. To describe a protein's primary structure is to list, in sequence, the amino acids that compose it.

Secondary structure refers to the manner in which the polypeptide chain(s) that compose a protein fold and curl. To describe a protein's secondary structure is to describe in some graphic detail, the manner in which its polypeptide chain(s) folds.

Tertiary structure refers to the way in which a protein folds and curls in three dimensions.

Quaternary structure refers only to proteins composed of *more than one polypeptide chain*. To refer to such a protein's quaternary structure is to refer to the way its several polypeptide chains form bonds and cross-links between and among one another.

Please solve this problem:

- A biochemist subjects a protein to the Edman degradation and discovers both the identity of the amino acids that compose it and the sequence in which they are arranged. He has, therefore, discovered the protein's:

  A. primary structure.
  B. secondary structure.
  C. tertiary structure.
  D. quaternary structure.

Problem solved:

A is correct. The question asks only that the student understand the meaning of the term "primary structure" as it relates to a protein. It refers to the identity and sequence of the amino acids that compose it.

Please solve this problem:

- A biochemist works with protein Y that is composed of several polypeptide chains. He studies and ascertains the manner in which the several chains are bound together. He has thus discovered the protein's:

  A. primary structure.
  B. secondary structure.
  C. tertiary structure.
  D. quaternary structure.

Problem solved:

D is correct. The question asks that the student understand the meaning of quaternary structure as it pertains to proteins. The phrase refers to proteins composed of more than one polypeptide chain and, more particularly, to the way the separate chains are bound together.

39.1.6.2 Proteins as Enzymes

Proteins serve as structural components of cells and tissues and as **enzymes**. As noted in some detail in chapter 28, enzymes are organic catalysts, which serve to lower the activation energy of biochemical reactions. So vital are enzymes to the function of the organism that it is *their* synthesis for which the genome is principally responsible. That is, an individual's genes govern the enzymes it manufactures and, therefore, the chemical reactions its system will conduct.

The student should be very familiar with the role of enzymes in lowering **activation energy**. Many, if not all, chemical reactions (even if exothermic) require a supply of energy to initiate activity. That initial energy is called activation energy. For any given reaction, an effective catalyst lowers the activation energy and so allows the reaction to proceed more swiftly. In the realm of biological/organic reactions, all catalysts are made of protein, and in this context are termed "enzymes."

In one form or another, the figure most commonly used to demonstrate the enzyme's role in lowering activation energy is the following:

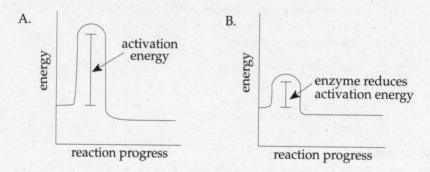

Figure 39.1

Comparison of Activation Energies of a Reaction
Without (A) and With (B) Enzymes

Note that the depicted reaction is in fact exothermic—the energy of its products is less than that of its reactants. Nonetheless, in order for the reaction to proceed, an activation energy must be required. The enzyme (like all catalysts) acts to reduce the activation energy. Further detail is provided in chapter 28.

Please solve this problem:

- For a reaction that it catalyzes, an enzyme serves, principally, to:

    A. shift the equilibrium state of a reversible reaction to the right.
    B. convert endothermic processes to exothermic processes.
    C. convert exothermic processes to endothermic processes.
    D. reduce activation energy demands.

Problem solved:

D is correct. The question requires that you understand the enzyme's principal function—to reduce activation energy. In choice D the phenomenon is described as a reduction of "initial energy demands." Choices A, B, and C are inaccurate statements. An enzyme does not alter a reaction's equilibrium dynamics; neither does it affect the reaction's status as exothermic or endothermic. An enzyme is not consumed during the course of a reaction it catalyzes. It emerges intact at the reaction's completion and is free to catalyze additional reactions.

39.2 MASTERY APPLIED: PASSAGE AND QUESTIONS

Passage

Adult human hemoglobin, a protein, is the basis of oxygen transport in erythrocytes. It is built of four polypeptide chains which may be thought of as existing in pairs; two chains are of the alpha type and two are of the beta type. (1 percent to 3 percent of adult hemoglobin also features a third type of polypeptide termed the delta chain, which in that small proportion of molecules replaces the beta chains.) Alpha chains feature 141 amino acid residues and beta chains feature 146. Chains are linked together by noncovalent forces.

Fetal hemoglobin is distinct from adult hemoglobin. It consists of two zeta chains and two epsilon chains. As fetal development proceeds, zeta chains are gradually replaced by alpha chains and epsilon chains are gradually replaced by beta chains to form adult hemoglobin. The timing of the replacements is depicted in Figure 1.

The sequence of amino acids in the polypeptide chains of the hemoglobin molecule varies among different species. Hemoglobin, therefore, does not represent a single substance, but rather a class of substances. The hemoglobin molecule is highly folded and coiled and, in particular, the amino acid constituents in the internal aspects of the molecule vary considerably across species. Yet, in most species residues located on the internal aspect of the molecule are nonpolar. On the surface of most hemoglobin molecules, the amino acid constituents do not show particular patterns of constancy in terms of nonpolarity or polarity, nor of basicity or acidity.

Notwithstanding the variations just described, however, certain positions of the hemoglobins that have been studied show constancy as to the amino acids that occupy them. These are listed in Table 1. Research suggests that the invariance of these amino acid residues means that they play a role in hemoglobin's central physiologic purpose.

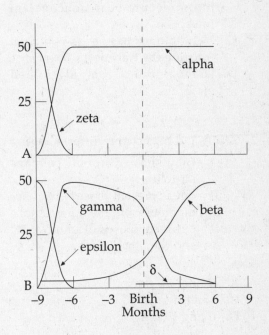

Figure 1

Invariant Amino Acid Residues in Hemoglobins	
Position	Amino acid
F8	Histidine
E7	Histidine
CD1	Phenylalanine
F4	Leucine
B6	Glycine
C2	Proline
HC2	Tyrosine
C4	Threonine
H10	Lysine

Table 1

1. Which of the following facts is most directly applicable to hemoglobin's quaternary structure?

    A. Its polypeptide chains are of different types.
    B. The various chains of the hemoglobin molecule bear noncovalent links.
    C. Hemoglobin has as its principal function the transport of oxygen.
    D. Hemoglobin is a highly folded molecule.

2. Alpha and beta chains differ in that:

    I. they show different primary structures.
    II. one is present in early fetal hemoglobin and the other is not.
    III. one is composed of amino acids and the other is not.

    A. I only
    B. II only
    C. I and II only
    D. II and III only

3. If an investigator wishes to ascertain the composition of the zeta chain of fetal hemoglobin, which of the following would be the most appropriate first step for her procedure?

    A. Isolate the chain and perform dehydration synthesis.
    B. Isolate the chain and perform direct ammonolysis.
    C. Isolate the chain and perform the Edman degradation.
    D. Isolate the chain and perform Strecker synthesis.

4. An investigator hypothesizes that the internal aspects of hemoglobin molecules must be largely nonpolar in order for the molecule as a whole to remain in solution while coursing through the blood. Is the hypothesis plausible?

    A. Yes, because nonpolar amino acids are relatively insoluble in water.
    B. Yes, because water is, itself, a nonpolar molecule.
    C. No, because solubility of the hemoglobin molecule would tend to be governed by the solubility properties of residues on the outer aspect.
    D. No, because polarity and nonpolarity do not affect solubility in blood.

5. If one amino acid residue is isolated from a zeta chain and noted to be a neutral alpha amino acid, which of the following would NOT apply to it?

    A. It carries a negative and positive charge at its isoelectric point.
    B. It carries an amino group on its side chain.
    C. Its carboxyl group is more acidic than its charged alpha amino group.
    D. It is positively charged at extremely low pH.

6. According to Figure 1, the replacement of an epsilon chain by a beta chain has, as an intermediate step:

    A. overproduction of epsilon chains.
    B. elimination of all alpha chains.
    C. conversion of epsilon chains to beta chains.
    D. replacement by a gamma chain.

7. Among the following amino acids, which is (are) most likely necessary to the role of hemoglobin as oxgyen carrier?

    I. Histidine
    II. Leucine
    III. Cysteine

    A. I only
    B. I and II only
    C. I and III only
    D. I, II, and III

39.3 MASTERY VERIFIED: ANSWERS AND EXPLANATIONS

1. *B is correct.* The passage indicates that the four polypeptide chains of adult hemoglobin are bound together by noncovalent links. The linking and bonding among several chains of a single protein relate to its *quaternary structure*. Choices A and C make true statements about hemoglobin, but do not answer the question regarding quaternary structure. Choice D also makes a true statement, but bears on secondary and tertiary structure which refer, respectively, to the manner in which a single chain is folded generally, and to the way in which protein is folded in three dimensions.

2. *A is correct.* The text indicates that alpha and beta chains—both of which belong to adult hemoglobin—are different and, in particular, that they differ in the number of amino acid residues (constituents) of which they are composed. Alpha chains carry 141 residues and beta chains carry 146. That means that the two chain types differ in primary structure, which refers to the type, number, and sequence of amino acid residues. Statement I, therefore, is accurate. Statement II is not accurate. Alpha and beta chains do not appear in early fetal hemoglobin, as indicated in the text and in Table 1. Statement III is clearly inaccurate. All polypeptides are composed of amino acids. Since statement I is accurate and statements II and III are not, the correct answer is A.

3. *C is correct.* As noted in the text, the Edman degradation represents an orderly process of hydrolysis, in which peptide bonds are sequentially broken so that each amino acid residue can be removed from a polypeptide and identified. Since the investigator wishes to ascertain the identity and sequence of the residues that compose the zeta chain, she should first perform the Edman degradation. Choice A refers to dehydration synthesis—a process in which polypeptides are formed, not broken. Choices B and D refer to processes through which amino acids (not proteins) are formed (not degraded). They are, therefore, incorrect.

4. *A is correct.* The passage states that "in most species residues located on the internal aspect of the molecule are nonpolar." As noted in this chapter, nonpolar amino acids tend to be relatively insoluble in water. If the nonpolar species were located on the hemoglobin molecule's outer surface they would impair solubility in water and hence in blood (whose fluid base is, of course, water). One can speculate, therefore, that the fact that the hemoglobin molecule's nonpolar residues are sequestered from the molecule's surface is what makes the molecule soluble in water. Choice B is inaccurate statement: water is most certainly a polar molecule. Choice C is a correct statement in that solubility is, probably, governed by the solubility properties of the molecule's outer constituents. That observation, however, does not justify the answer "no." Choice D is incorrect. As noted in the text, polarity and nonpolarity are important determinants of solubility properties.

5. *B is correct.* A neutral amino acid is one that is neither acidic nor basic, meaning that it carries neither a carboxyl group nor an amino group *on its side chain*. If an alpha amino acid carries an amino group on its side chain it is not neutral. The statement made in choice A is true of all alpha neutral amino acids. The isoelectric point is that pH at which the carboxyl group is deprotonated (carrying a negative charge) and the amino group is protonated (carrying a positive charge). The statements in choices C and D are also true of all alpha neutral amino acids. The carboxyl group is more acidic than its charged alpha amino group. At extremely low pH the amino group will be protonated (thus carrying a positive charge), as will the carboxyl group (to make it neutral).

6. *D is correct*. You must examine Figure 1 without fear. The lower portion of the figure depicts a decline in the quantity of epsilon chain, closely coupled with an increase in a gamma chain (not mentioned in the passage). It then shows a decline in the quantity of gamma chain closely correlated with an increase in the quantity of beta chain. It is reasonable to conclude, therefore, that as an intermediate event between the elimination of epsilon chains and the emergence of beta chains gamma chains are formed. Choice A refers to overproduction of epsilon chains, and neither portion of the graph gives any evidence of such an event. Choice B is contrary to what is seen in the upper portion of the figure. As the quantity of epsilon chains diminishes, the quantity of alpha chains increases. Choice C speaks of "conversion" of epsilon chains to beta chains. The trends shown in the lower portion of the figure are not consistent with the statement. As epsilon chains disappear, beta chains do not *contemporaneously* appear. At time = (-)6 months, for example, epsilon chains have virtually disappeared and the quantity of beta chains remains at very near zero. If epsilon chains were *converted* to beta chains, the beta chain curve would rise as the epsilon chain curve fell.

7. *B is correct*. The question requires that you carefully read the passage's last paragraph and examine Table 1. The last paragraph states that "certain positions of the hemoglobins that have been studied show constancy as to the amino acids that occupy them. These are listed in Table 1. Research suggests that the invariance of these amino acid residues means that they play a role in hemoglobin's central physiologic purpose." Hemoglobin's central physiologic purpose is *oxygen transport*, and Table 1, therefore, likely indicates the amino acids that are crucial to that purpose. Among the acids listed in I, II, and III, only histidine and leucine appear on Table 1. Cysteine does not. Therefore, according to the information in the passage and table, histidine and leucine—but not cysteine—likely play a key role in allowing hemoglobin to conduct oxygen transport.

CHAPTER 40

CARBOHYDRATES

40.1 MASTERY ACHIEVED

40.1.1 STRUCTURE OF CARBOHYDRATES

Carbohydrates are sugars; sugars are **polyhydroxy aldehydes** or **ketones** with the general formula $(CH_2O)_n$. Carbohydrates vary in size, from structures containing only a few carbons to vast polymeric molecules, such as glycogen. Biosynthetically, all sugars of importance for the MCAT derive from (+)-**glyceraldehyde**.

The (+) in the name (+)-glyceraldehyde indicates that this enantiomer of glyceraldehyde rotates plane-polarized light in a clockwise direction. The positive sign tells only the direction of the rotation of plane-polarized light; it does not indicate the actual spatial arrangement of atoms attached to the chiral carbon. As it happens, (+)-glyceraldehyde is the *R* **enantiomer**; therefore, (–)-glyceraldehyde is the *S* **enantiomer**. The designations of (+) and (–) are indicators of the optical rotation of a molecule, they do not signify the arrangement of bonds. These are, therefore, relative configurations; anything that rotates plane-polarized light in a clockwise direction is (+), anything that rotates plane-polarized light in a counterclockwise direction is (–). The designations *R* and *S* are absolute configurations. They represent the configuration of bonds around a chiral center. There are other designations with which you should also be familiar.

The designations D and L are identical to the designations (+) and (–), respectively. D indicates that the compound is dextrorotary (involves clockwise rotation of plane-polarized light). L indicates that the compound is levorotary (involves counterclockwise rotation of plane-polarized light). These designations are now out of date, but they occasionally still appear in use.

The designations d and l should not be confused with the common carbohydrate designations D and L. A sugar is designated as a D sugar if that sugar has a similar configuration to (+)-glyceraldehyde at a comparable carbon. The designations D and L do not relate to the direction in which plane-polarized light is rotated, just as *R* and *S* designations do not relate to light rotation.

Sugars may be depicted in several ways. On the MCAT, sugars are commonly illustrated as **Fischer projections**. The Fischer projections of some common **monosaccharides** are given in Figure 40.1.

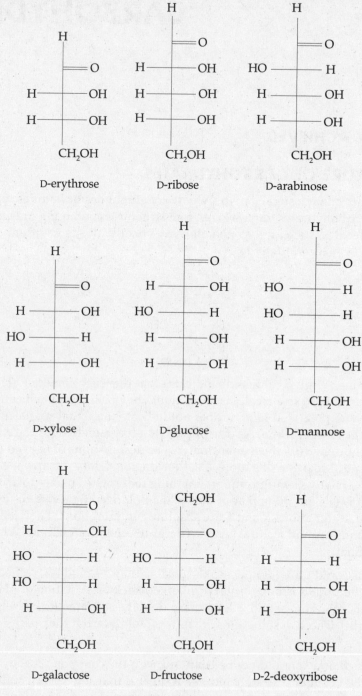

Figure 40.1

In a Fischer projection, it is assumed that the vertical components of a projection are pointing into the paper, while the horizontal components of the projection are pointing out of the paper.

Please solve this problem:

- The relationship between D-galactose and D-mannose is:

    A. enantiomeric.
    B. diastereomeric.
    C. anomeric.
    D. epimeric.

Problem solved:

The correct answer is B. The relationship between D-galactose and D-mannose is that of diastereomers. These compounds are geometric isomers that are not mirror images of one another. Geometric isomers that are non-superimposable mirror images of one another are enantiomers. Anomers and epimers are discussed in section **40.1.3**.

40.1.2 CLASSIFICATION AND NOMENCLATURE OF CARBOHYDRATES

Carbohydrates are named, in part, based on their relationship to either (+)- or (–)-glyceraldehyde. Apart from the D or L designation, sugars are classified in other ways. A carbohydrate that cannot be broken down into simpler units by the performance of hydrolysis is termed a monosaccharide, or simple sugar. A carbohydrate that is broken down into simpler units upon hydrolysis is termed a **complex sugar**. Complex sugars are further classified by the number of simple sugars of which they are comprised. A **disaccharide** is a sugar that is composed of two monosaccharide units. A **trisaccharide** is composed of three monosaccharides. **Polysaccharides** are composed of many monosaccharides.

Monosaccharides are categorized as **aldoses** or **ketoses**. An aldose is a monosaccharide that contains an aldehyde group. A ketose is a monosaccharide that contains a ketone group. Aldoses and ketoses are further categorized by the number of carbons contained in their backbone structure. The major monosaccharides are **trioses** (three carbons), **tetroses** (four carbons), **pentoses** (five carbons), and **hexoses** (six carbons). The two most common examples of simple sugars are glucose and fructose. Glucose is an **aldohexose**. Fructose is a **ketohexose**.

Please solve this problem:

- The structure of D–lyxose is:

$$
\begin{array}{c}
\text{H} \\
| \\
\text{==O} \\
| \\
\text{HO} \text{---} \text{H} \\
\text{HO} \text{---} \text{H} \\
\text{H} \text{---} \text{OH} \\
| \\
\text{CH}_2\text{OH}
\end{array}
$$

What type of sugar is this?

    A. Aldopentose
    B. Aldohexose
    C. Ketopentose
    D. Ketohexose

Problem solved:

The correct answer is A. Lyxose is an aldehyde, not a ketone. This eliminates choices C and D. Lyxose has a five-carbon backbone, therefore it is a pentose.

40.1.3 MONOSACCHARIDES

Monosaccharides can exist either in an **open chain form** (as depicted by the Fischer projection of glucose in **40.1.1**) or as a **ring structure**. Ring structures result from the intramolecular nucleophilic attack of a hydroxyl functional group on the carbonyl carbon in the sugar. An aldohexose will form a six-membered ring in which one atom in the ring is an oxygen. Such a structure is termed a **pyranose**. The suffix -ose indicates that the structure is a sugar.

The ring structure of glucose is termed **glucopyranose**. The formation of glucopyranose from the open chain form of glucose is depicted in Figure 40.2. The jagged line indicates a lack of knowledge of the stereochemistry at this carbon.

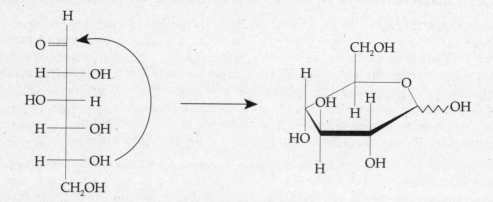

Figure 40.2

A ketohexose, such as fructose, will form a five-membered ring in which one atom in the ring is an oxygen. Such a structure is termed a **furanose**—furan is a five-membered ring.

The ring structure of fructose is termed **fructofuranose**. The formation of **fructofuranose** from the open chain form of fructose is depicted in Figure 40.3.

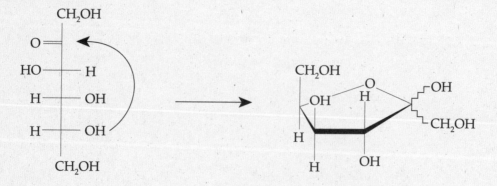

Figure 40.3

In each of these ring structures, an additional chiral carbon has been produced—the carbonyl carbon becomes tetrasubstituted when it is attacked by the hydroxyl group. This carbon is referred to as the **anomeric carbon**. The two possible **diastereomers** that could result from the ring formation are termed **anomers** of one another. Anomers are a special class of **epimers**, which are a special class of diastereomers.

Stereoisomers that are not mirror images of one another are termed diastereomers (see Chapter 35). Epimers are diastereomers that differ from one another in only one of many chiral centers within the molecule. Anomers are carbohydrate epimers that differ only in the stereochemistry of a potential carbonyl carbon in the ring form.

The anomeric carbon of a sugar is a carbonyl carbon in the open chain form and a **hemiacetal** (for aldoses) or a **hemiketal** (for ketoses) in the ring form. The two possible anomers of glucose are depicted in Figure 40.4. α-Glucose is the anomer in which the hydroxyl group of the anomeric carbon is pointing down. β-Glucose is the anomer in which the hydroxyl group of the anomeric carbon is pointing up.

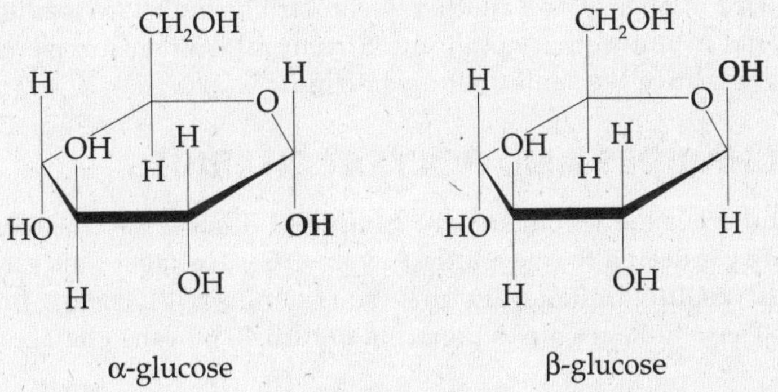

Figure 40.4

Ring structures drawn in this fashion are termed **Hayworth projections**. These structures can also be drawn in the chair form. The alpha form is on the left, the beta form is on the right.

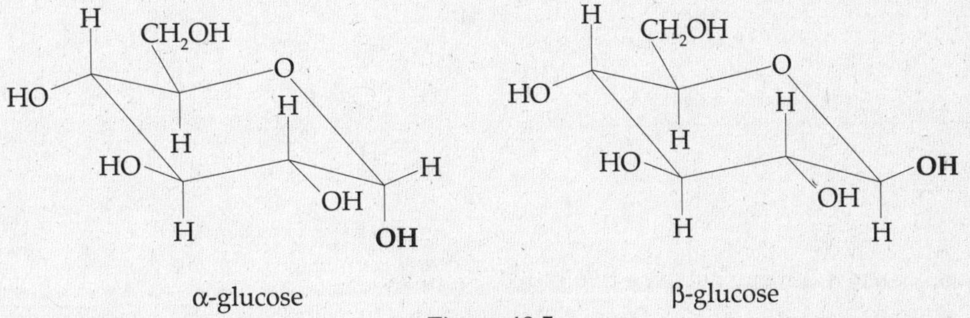

Figure 40.5

Monosaccharides react chemically according to the functional groups that they contain. Hydroxides, ketones, aldehydes, carboxylic acids, esters, ethers, hemiacetals, hemiketals, acetals, and ketals are the most common functional groups of sugars.

Please solve this problem:

- Which one of the following does NOT describe an anomer?

  A. Diastereomer
  B. Enantiomer
  C. Epimer
  D. Geometric isomer

Problem solved:

The correct answer is B. A pair of anomers is a pair of epimers that differ in stereochemistry only at the anomeric (hemiacetal or hemiketal) carbon. A pair of epimers is a pair of diastereomers that differ in stereochemistry at only one of many possible chiral centers. D-glucose is epimeric with both D-mannose and D-galactose. Diastereomers are optical that are not mirror images of one another. Enantiomers are geometric isomers that are non-superimposable mirror images of one another. Geometric isomers are isomers that differ only in stereochemistry, not in connectivity of atoms. Structural isomers are isomers that differ in atomic connectivity but have the same chemical formula.

40.1.4 DISACCHARIDES AND POLYSACCHARIDES

Disaccharides and other higher sugars, are composed of monosaccharides. The monosaccharides are connected to one another by an **ether linkage**. This ether linkage in sugars is termed a **glycosidic linkage**, and may be either an α-glycosidic linkage or a β-glycosidic linkage. These linkages are depicted in Figure 40.6 in the chair form.

α-1,4-glycosidic linkage between two glucose molecules

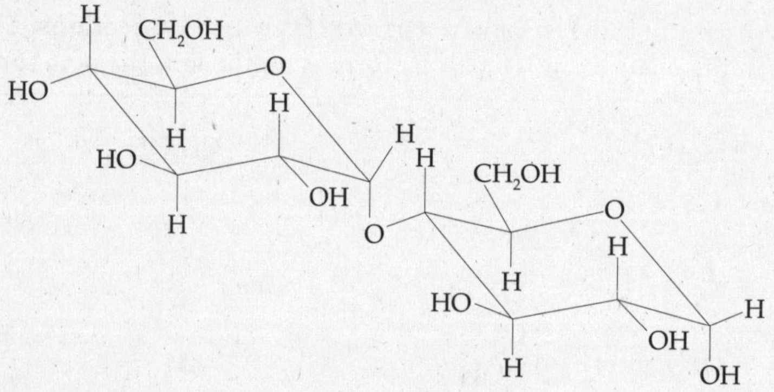

β-1,4-glycosidic linkage between two glucose molecules

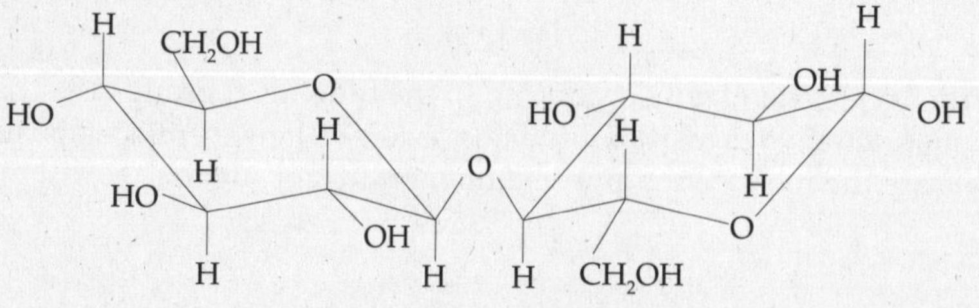

Figure 40.6

The top structure, containing the α-glycosidic linkage, is **maltose**. The bottom structure, containing a β-glycosidic linkage, is **cellobiose**. Both of these sugars are composed of two glucose units; however, only maltose may be metabolized by humans (and most other higher animals). This is because the human digestive system contains enzymes that specifically cleave α-glycosidic linkages. The enzyme maltase, for example, cleaves the glycosidic linkages of maltose. The human digestive system does not contain enzymes that are capable of cleaving β-glycosidic linkages.

Another important disaccharide is **sucrose** (table sugar). Sucrose is composed of one glucose unit linked to one fructose unit via a bond that is α-glycosidic from the first carbon of glucose and β-glycosidic from the fourth carbon of fructose.

Starch is a polysaccharide that is broken down completely into glucose by the enzyme maltase. Starch can be fractionated into two different kinds of molecules: **amylose** and **amylopectin**. Amylose is a polysaccharide with a simple structure consisting entirely of glucose units connected via α-1,4-glycosidic linkages. Amylopectin, the major component of starch, is a more complicated polysaccharide that consists of glucose units connected via α-1,4- and α-1,6-glycosidic linkages.

Please solve this problem:

- Gentiobiose is an indigestible disaccharide found in many natural products. Gentiobiose is composed of two glucose units, but it is structurally distinguishable from both maltose and cellobiose. The glucose units in gentiobiose are most likely linked by:

  A. an α-1,4 linkage.
  B. an α-1,6 linkage.
  C. a β-1,4 linkage.
  D. a β-1,6 linkage.

Problem solved:

The correct answer is D. To solve this problem, we must first recall that it is beta glycosidic linkages that render saccharides indigestible. Since we are told that gentiobiose is indigestible, it must contain beta linkages. This eliminates choices A and B. We are also told that gentiobiose is structurally distinguishable from another indigestible disaccharide—cellobiose. Since we know that cellobiose consists of glucose linked by β-1,4 bonds, we know that gentiobiose cannot contain these same bonds and yet be structurally distinguishable from cellobiose. This eliminates choice C, leaving only choice D.

40.2 MASTERY APPLIED: SAMPLE PASSAGE AND QUESTIONS

Passage

Epimers are diastereomeric compounds that differ in only one of several possible chiral centers. D-Mannose and D-galactose are both epimers of D-glucose. D-Mannose and D-glucose are epimeric at carbon 2. D-Glucose and D-galactose are epimeric at carbon 4.

The conversion of glucose to fructose is an important step in glycolysis. This transformation is believed to proceed via an enolization reaction, the steps of which are given below.

This reaction can also proceed back to the glucose starting material.

glucose

Or, a third pathway leads to a different sugar.

1. The product of the third pathway represented in the passage is:

    A. D-mannose.
    B. D-galactose.
    C. L-glucose.
    D. L-sucrose.

2. The relationship between D-mannose and D-galactose is:

    A. anomeric.
    B. epimeric.
    C. enantiomeric.
    D. diastereomeric.

3. D-Fructose and D-glucose are:

    A. enantiomeric.
    B. diastereomeric.
    C. geometric isomers.
    D. structural isomers.

4. D-Fructose and D-mannose are:

    A. enantiomeric.
    B. diastereomeric.
    C. geometric isomers.
    D. structural isomers.

5. When glucose is placed into a solution containing dilute NaOH, the reaction produces 70 percent glucose, 20 percent fructose, 1 percent mannose, and the remainder goes to decomposition products. In the body, the conversion of glucose to fructose is nearly quantitative. Which of the following choices offers the best explanation for this discrepancy?

    A. Biological systems are more efficient than man-made systems.
    B. In the body, the fructose produced is consumed; in the experiment, it is not.
    C. The body does not contain pure glucose in dilute alkali, as the experiment did.
    D. At the location of glycolysis within the body the base concentration is much higher than in the experiment.

6. When the reaction in the passage is run using D_2O instead of H_2O, we would expect deuterium to incorporate:

    A. only in the glucose.
    B. only in the fructose.
    C. at carbon 1 of the glucose and carbon 2 of the fructose.
    D. at carbon 2 of the glucose and carbon 1 of the fructose.

40.3 MASTERY VERIFIED: ANSWERS AND EXPLANATIONS

1. *The correct answer is A.* We know from the passage that glucose is epimeric with mannose at carbon 2. The product of the third pathway differs from glucose only at carbon 2. It must, therefore, be D-mannose.

2. *The correct answer is D.* From the passage, we know that D-mannose differs from D-glucose at carbon 2 and that D-galactose differs from D-glucose at carbon 4. Therefore, D-mannose and D-galactose must differ from one another at both carbon 2 and carbon 4. The difference in these two chiral centers makes these two molecules diastereomeric.

3. *The correct answer is D.* D-Fructose and D-glucose have the same chemical formula ($C_6H_{12}O_6$), so they are isomers of one another. D-Fructose is a ketohexose; D-glucose is an aldohexose. Since one contains a ketone group and the other contains an aldehyde group, they cannot be more than structural isomers.

4. *The correct answer is D.* D-Fructose and D-mannose have the same chemical formula ($C_6H_{12}O_6$), so they are isomers of one another. D-Fructose is a ketohexose, D-mannose is an aldohexose. Since one contains a ketone group and the other contains an aldehyde group, they cannot be more than structural isomers.

5. *The correct answer is B.* As fructose is produced during glycolysis it is also consumed. Based on Le Chatelier's principle, this will drive the equilibrium of the interconversion of glucose to fructose to the product side, causing the production of more fructose.

6. *The correct answer is D.* Considering the reaction mechanism as presented in the passage, it is clear that all three products will incorporate deuterium from D_2O. Fructose will incorporate the deuterium at carbon 1 since this is the carbon that becomes protonated from the enolate. Similarly, glucose and mannose will both incorporate deuterium at carbon 2.

CHAPTER 41

SEPARATION AND IDENTIFICATION OF ORGANIC COMPOUNDS

41.1 MASTERY ACHIEVED

41.1.1 SEPARATION AND PURIFICATION TECHNIQUES

41.1.1.1 General Principles

Separations rely upon the differences in the physical properties of the substances to be separated. Several of these properties have been covered elsewhere: solubility (Chapter 18), boiling point (Chapter 20), melting point (Chapter 20), acid/base properties (Chapter 21) and bonding properties (Chapter 14).

41.1.1.2 Extraction

Extraction is the process of removing a solute from one solvent through the use of a second solvent. The efficacy of extraction is controlled by the immiscibility of the two solvents and the solute's higher affinity for (solubility in) the second solvent.

When the solvents are thoroughly mixed, the solute will distribute itself between the two solvents. The **partition coefficient** indicates the *relative* concentrations of solute in each solvent at equilibrium. It is more efficient to extract with several small volumes of the second solvent than to extract with one large volume of the second solvent. This is because the partition coefficient is independent of total solute concentration. Each extraction will result in a partition coefficient ratio at equilibrium. Therefore, a greater total percentage of solute will be removed via consecutive extractions.

The solubility characteristics and intermolecular forces of a substance are used to determine which components of a solution can be differentially extracted (and with which solvents). Most often, the properties involved in the choice of an extraction solvent are polarity and acid/base properties.

Please solve this problem:

- Extraction separates substances based on the principle of:

    A. polarity.
    B. solubility.
    C. molecular weight.
    D. acid/base properties.

Problem solved:

The correct answer is B. Choices A and D are properties that must be considered in the selection of an extraction solvent, not the principles on which extraction is itself based.

41.1.1.3 Recrystallization

Recrystallization is a technique for isolating one solid substance from a mixture containing other solids, other liquids, or both. Recrystallization is an inefficient process. Significant amounts of the desired material are often lost in the process of recrystallization.

Recrystallization differs from simple precipitation in two important ways. First, recrystallization is a slow process that requires several hours and sometimes days, while precipitation is a rapid process that takes only seconds. Recrystallization, on the other hand, increases the purity of the desired substance by eliminating impurities. Precipitation increases the amount of impurities in the desired substance (in solid phase), since precipitation occurs around nucleation sites which are generally impurities in the mixture.

Recrystallization solvents are often difficult to determine. Such a solvent should possess a low affinity for the substance to be recrystallized at low temperatures, but a much higher affinity for the substance at higher temperatures. In other words, the solubility of the substance to be recrystallized should approach zero at low temperatures, but should be fairly high at higher temperatures. Additionally, the melting point of the recrystallant must exceed the boiling point of the recrystallization solvent. When a recrystallant is allowed to melt within a recrystallization solvent the end result is an oil, rather than the desired solid product. A final quality of the recrystallization solvent is a high vapor pressure at low temperatures. This solvent volatility makes for the easy removal of the solvent from the crystals once they have formed.

A recrystallization solvent will also exhibit a higher affinity for impurity molecules than for the desired substance, particularly at low temperatures. The lower the percentage of impurities present in the initial mixture, the higher the probability of a successful recrystallization.

Please solve this problem:

- When considering a recrystallization solvent, the best solvent will have:

  A. a boiling point higher than the melting point of the recrystallant.
  B. a boiling point lower than the melting point of the recrystallant.
  C. a boiling point higher than the boiling point of the recrystallant.
  D. a boiling point lower than the boiling point of the recrystallant.

Problem solved:

The correct answer is B. In order to avoid "oiling out," the boiling point of the recrystallization solvent must be lower than the melting point of the solute to be recrystallized. While choice D must also be true, it is not sufficient to solve the problem at hand.

41.1.1.4 Distillation

Distillation is a separation method based on boiling point differences. Two important distillation techniques are **simple distillation** and **fractional distillation**.

A simple distillation is a one-step process in which the mixture is heated to the boiling point of the liquid for which recovery is sought. The liquid is then allowed to vaporize and then condense into a separate flask (the receiving flask).

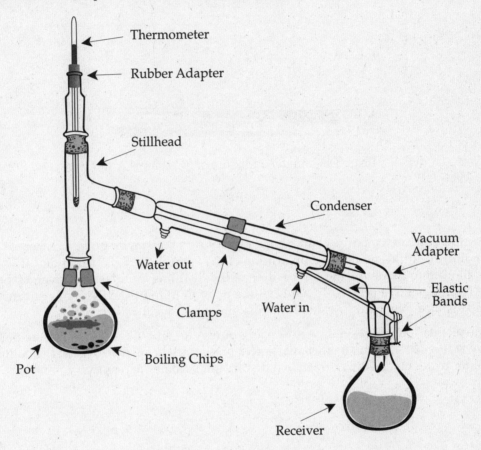

Apparatus for Simple Distillation

Figure 41.1

The phase diagram for a mixture containing liquids A and B, in which substance A is to be isolated, is given in Figure 41.2.

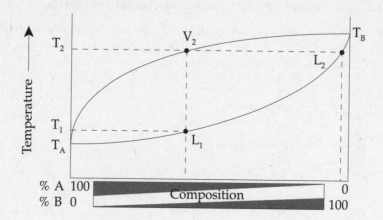

Phase Diagram for a Mixture of Substances A and B

Figure 41.2

The temperature of a mixture containing a ratio of A to B given by point L_2 is heated to its boiling point, T_2. At this point, the composition of the vapor is that given by point V_2. As the vapor is allowed to condense, the composition of the distilling liquid is that given by point L_1. T_A is the boiling point of pure A, T_B is the boiling point of pure B. The figure reveals that some B has also distilled over with A; a simple distillation cannot yield 100 percent A.

Simple distillation will result in a reasonably pure A for a liquid A with a boiling point that differs by at least 20°C from all other substances present in the mixture. When the boiling points differ by less than 20°C, a fractional distillation becomes necessary.

A fractional distillation is a series of simple distillations carried out in a single apparatus. A fractional distillation requires the addition of a fractionating column between the distilling flask and the condenser.

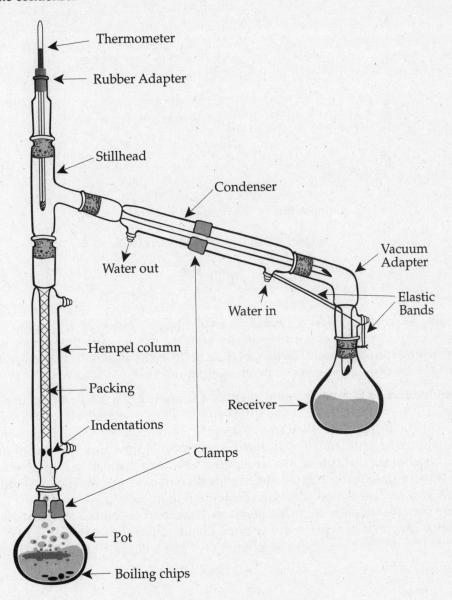

Apparatus for Fractional Distillation

Figure 41.3

In a fractionating column, several distillation steps occur, as shown in Figure 41.4.

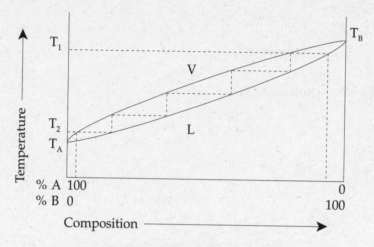

Stepwise Distillation of Substances A and B

Figure 41.4

In this case, the distilling flask is heated to temperature T_1; however, within the fractionating column a series of purifications occur as the temperature drops prior to the distillate reaching the condenser. The temperature at the condenser is T_2; therefore, the composition of the distillate is given at this temperature.

Vacuum distillation is a modification to either a simple distillation or a fractional distillation. In a vacuum distillation, the still is attached to a pump which lowers the pressure inside the still. As the pressure is lowered, the temperature required to reach the boiling point of the substance to be distilled is also lowered—remember, a substance boils when its vapor pressure is equal to the pressure of its surroundings. Vacuum distillation is often employed in organic chemistry since many organic compounds decompose upon boiling (at standard pressure). A vacuum distillation allows the compound of interest to boil at a much lower temperature than the decomposition temperature. The modification to a simple distillation apparatus that is necessary to perform a vacuum distillation is shown in Figure 41.5.

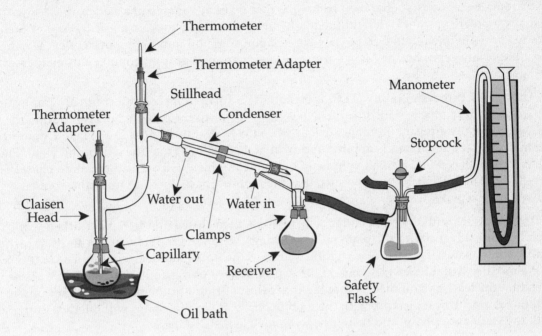

Apparatus for Vacuum Distillation

Figure 41.5

Please solve this problem:

- A fractional vacuum distillation should be performed when:

    A. substances to be separated differ in boiling points by less than 20°C and the substances decompose on heating.
    B. substances to be separated differ in boiling points by more than 20°C and the substances decompose on heating.
    C. substances to be separated differ in boiling points by less than 20°C and the substances do not decompose on heating.
    D. substances to be separated differ in boiling points by more than 20°C and the substances do not decompose on heating.

Problem solved:

The correct answer is A. A fractional distillation (rather than a simple distillation) is indicated when the substances to be separated differ in boiling points by less than 20°C. A vacuum distillation is most often carried out when the substances to be distilled are heat sensitive. Therefore, choice A contains the criteria for both a vacuum distillation and a fractional distillation.

41.1.1.5 Chromatography

Chromatography is a separation technique that takes advantage of a *stationary phase* (usually a polar substance) that differentially adsorbs substances from a *mobile phase* (solvent). The many types of chromatography are based upon common underlying principles. The three most important types for the MCAT are: thin-layer chromatography, column chromatography, and gas chromatography.

Thin-layer chromatography (TLC) is essentially a small-scale column chromatography. In TLC, a stationary phase is adsorbed to a glass plate prior to the experiment. The stationary phase is typically a polar substance such as silica (SiO_2) or alumina (Al_2O_3). A small amount of the mixture to be separated is applied approximately one inch from the end of the plate. The plate is then placed into a small volume of the solvent which will act as the mobile phase. The depth of the mobile phase must be such that the mobile phase does not wash the applied solvent off the plate.

The container with the plate and mobile phase is then closed and left undisturbed while the mobile phase advances up the plate via a "wicking" action. As the solvent advances, it carries with it those materials that are not tightly bound to the polar stationary phase. The substances in the mixture will interact differently with the stationary phase and with the mobile phase such that the least polar molecule (having the lowest affinity for the polar stationary phase) will move the farthest distance with the mobile phase. Polar molecules will interact strongly with the stationary phase, and therefore, will move lesser distances.

In **column chromatography**, the stationary phase is packed into a vertical column through which the mixture is eluted by the mobile phase. In **gas chromatography** the mixture is vaporized and eluted through a solid stationary phase by a carrier gas (mobile phase).

Solvent (mobile phase) selection is based on the polarity of the substances in the mixture and the expected solubilities of the substances in the mixture. Preferably, all mixture components will be soluble in the mobile phase. Table 41.1 lists several common TLC solvents in order from least to most polar. Table 41.2 lists the common organic functional groups from least to most polar.

Relative Polarities of TLC Solvents	
Petroleum ether	least polar
Cyclohexane	
Carbon tetrachloride	
Benzene	
Chloroform	
Methylene chloride	
Methyl ether	
Ethyl acetate	
Acetone	
Pyridine	
Ethanol	
Water	
Acetic acid	most polar

Table 41.1

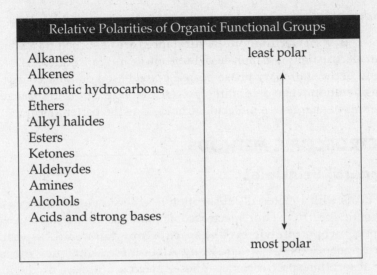

Table 41.2

Please solve this problem:

- Thin layer chromatography (TLC) separates substances based on the principle of:

    A. polarity.
    B. solubility.
    C. molecular weight.
    D. acid/base properties.

Problem solved:

The correct answer is A. In TLC, substances are adsorbed by a polar stationary phase and eluted by a less polar mobile phase.

41.1.1.6 Electrophoresis

Electrophoresis is similar to chromatography except in the means of separation. Whereas chromatography separates components of a mixture based on differences in polarity, electrophoresis separates mixture components based on electric charge. One end of a plate is supplied with a positive charge, the other with a negative charge. Solutes move along the plate, towards one pole or the other, based on the laws of electrostatics. Since amino acids and proteins have different charge characteristics at differing pHs, electrophoresis is used extensively as a separation method for these compounds.

Please solve this problem:

- Electrophoresis separates substances based on the principle of:

    A. polarity.
    B. molecular weight.
    C. acid/base properties.
    D. electric charge.

Problem solved:

The correct answer is D. In electrophoresis, substances are adsorbed by a stationary phase through which an electric field is established. Substances migrate either towards the positive or the negative end of the stationary phase-coated plate, based on their charge characteristics. Choice C is a consideration when determining electric charge, but acid/base reactions are not the sole determinants of charge in a molecule. Choice D is the better answer.

41.1.2 SPECTROSCOPIC METHODS

41.1.2.1 General Principles

Spectroscopy deals with a material's absorption or emission of energy in a defined portion of the electromagnetic spectrum. Four spectroscopic methods are outlined in the following sections: mass spectroscopy, ultraviolet (UV) spectroscopy, infrared (IR) spectroscopy, and nuclear magnetic resonance (NMR) spectroscopy. All of these techniques, except mass spectroscopy, are absorption spectroscopies. These spectroscopies are used, either together or separately, to determine the identities of unknown chemical substances.

41.1.2.2 Mass Spectroscopy

Mass spectroscopy is employed to determine the molecular weight of a substance. In this spectroscopic method, the substance to be analyzed is placed in a chamber where it is bombarded by a stream of high-energy electrons. The substance is broken into smaller pieces by this bombardment. Some of the small pieces take a negative charge, some take a positive charge, and some remain neutral—depending on the particular bond cleavage processes. Once these ions are formed, they are subjected to a magnetic field that serves to filter out the neutral molecules and negatively charged ions, leaving only the positively charged ions. These positively charged ions are then dispersed based on their mass to charge ratio (m/z) and focused on a detector. The result is a mass spectrum, a pattern of peaks corresponding to structural features of the sample substance.

The mass spectrum provides information about the initial molecular weight of the substance and gives insight into the structure of the molecule, since certain peaks are indicative of certain structures.

The mass spectrum of methyl bromide (CH_3Br) is given in Figure 41.6.

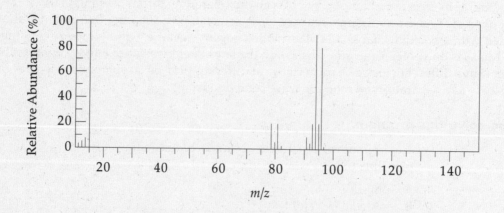

Figure 41.6

For the MCAT, it is not important to be an expert at determining structures from mass spectra; it is important to understand the underlying principles of the technique.

Please solve this problem:

- In a typical mass spectrometer, the particles that are detected are:

    A. neutral molecules.
    B. positive ions.
    C. negative ions.
    D. all of the above.

Problem solved:

The correct answer is B. Although a mass spectrometer may be set up to record either positive ions or negative ions, the typical experiment records positive ions. Neutral molecules or not detected in either experimental set up.

41.1.2.3 Ultraviolet Spectroscopy

In **ultraviolet spectroscopy**, a sample is irradiated with a continuous source of UV radiation of varying wavelength. The energy associated with the UV portion of the electromagnetic spectrum coincides with the difference in energy levels between molecular orbitals. When a molecule is subjected to a UV wavelength that "matches" the difference in energy between an occupied molecular orbital and an unoccupied molecular orbital, this UV radiation is absorbed—causing an electron to move from the ground state (occupied orbital) to an excited state (the previously unoccupied orbital).

In UV spectroscopy, the sample is placed between the UV source and a detector. If no radiation is absorbed, the amount of UV radiation emitted by the source is the amount of radiation detected at the detector. However, when UV energy is absorbed by the sample, these two amounts differ. It is the difference that allow for the "construction" of a UV spectrum.

The important concept for the MCAT, in relation to UV spectroscopy, is that double bonds absorb UV radiation. Isolated double bonds absorb weakly, while conjugated double bonds and aromatic systems absorb strongly in the UV energy region.

Please solve this problem:

- All the following are expected to be UV active (i.e., produce peaks in the UV spectrum) EXCEPT:

    A. 1,2-dichloroethylene.
    B. 1-propyne.
    C. cyclopentadiene.
    D. 1,3-dibromoethane.

Problem solved:

The correct answer is D. The three compounds in choices A, B, and C each contain at least one site of unsaturation other than a ring (a double bond or a triple bond). 1,3-Dibromoethane is a saturated compound and, therefore, it is expected to be UV inactive.

41.1.2.4 Infrared Spectroscopy

Infrared spectroscopy involves the absorption of energy in the IR region of the electromagnetic spectrum. Energy in this region coincides with vibrational modes within a molecule—such as the bond stretching and the bond angle bending that occurs in all molecules at temperatures above absolute zero. Vibrational frequencies are highly indicative of functional groups within a sample. Therefore, the primary use of IR spectroscopy is the identification of functional groups within a sample.

IR spectral units are most often reported in wave numbers. A wave number is the reciprocal of the wavelength. The range of IR wave numbers is from approximately 625 cm^{-1}, corresponding to 16 μm, to 4000 cm^{-1}, corresponding to 2.5 μm. The IR spectrum of N-cyclohexylformamide is provided in Figure 41.7.

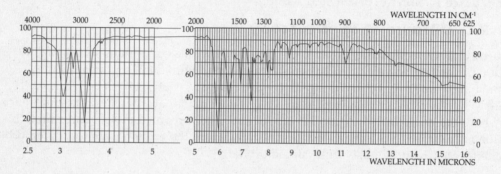

Figure 41.7

The structure of this compound is:

Bond Type	Stretch (cm^{-1})	Bend (cm^{-1})
C–H alkane	2,960–2,850	1,470–1350
C–H alkene	3,080–3,020	1,000–675
C–H aromatic	3,100–3,000	870–675
C–H aldehyde	2,900 & 2,700	
C–H alkyne	3,300	
C–C alkyne	2,250–2,100	
C–N nitrile	2,260–2,220	
C=C alkene	1,670–1,620	
C=C aromatic	1,600–1,440	
C=O ester	1,750–1,735	
C=O acid	1,725–1,700	
C=O aldehyde	1,740–1,710	
C=O ketone	1,725–1,705	
C=O aryl ketone	1,700–1,680	
C=O amide	1,690–1,650	
O–H alcohol (non-H bonded)	3,650–3,580	
O–H alcohol (H bonded)	3,600–3,200	
O–H acid	3,000–2,500	
N–H amine	3,500–3,300	1,620–1,590
N–H amide	3,500–3,350	1,650–1,510
C–O	1,300–1,000	
C–N amine	1,220–1,010	
C–N aromatic amine	1,360–1,250	
NO$_2$	1,560–1,515 & 1,385–1,345	

Table 41.3

On the MCAT, questions about IR spectra will be accompanied by information resembling Table 41.3. Each of the IR bands produced by the stretching or bending of bonds represents the characteristic absorption ranges of the corresponding functional group.

Please solve this problem:

- The reaction between methanol and propanyl chloride to form methyl propanoate could best be followed by:

    A. the appearance of an IR peak at 1800 cm^{-1} and the appearance of an IR peak at 1740 cm^{-1}.
    B. the disappearance of an IR peak at 1800 cm^{-1} and the appearance of an IR peak at 1740 cm^{-1}.
    C. the appearance of an IR peak at 1800 cm^{-1} and the disappearance of an IR peak at 1740 cm^{-1}.
    D. the disappearance of an IR peak at 1800 cm^{-1} and the disappearance of an IR peak at 1740 cm^{-1}.

Problem solved:

The correct answer is B. The IR peak at 1800 cm^{-1} coincides with the stretching wave number of the carbonyl group of an acid chloride. The peak at 1740 cm^{-1} coincides with the stretching wave number of the carbonyl group of an ester. This level of detail, however, is not necessary for the MCAT.

To solve this problem, we must first recognize that both peaks referred to in all four choices are in the carbonyl range. Next, we must recognize the difference between the carbonyl group (or groups) in the reactants and the carbonyl group (or groups) in the products. Knowing that only one carbonyl group is in the reactants, we can eliminate choice D—there would have to be two carbonyl groups in the reactants in order for two carbonyl peaks to disappear. Likewise, since there is only one carbonyl group in the products, we can eliminate choice A— there would have to be the formation of two carbonyl groups for us to see two peaks in the carbonyl region.

To decide between B and C, we must determine which will have a higher wave number—an acid chloride carbonyl or an ester carbonyl. Table 41.3 reveals the general trend of increase in wave number as the electron-withdrawing capacity of the substituent groups attached to a carbonyl increases. Therefore, an acid chloride should absorb at a higher wave number than would an ester. Since 1800 cm^{-1} is the acid chloride, choice B is the correct answer.

41.1.2.5 Nuclear Magnetic Resonance (NMR) Spectroscopy

Nuclear magnetic resonance spectroscopy uses wavelengths in the **radio frequency** (rf) **region** of the electromagnetic spectrum to measure the magnetic field produced by atomic nuclei as they spin (recall that any moving or changing electric field produces a magnetic field, and that a moving positive charge creates a changing electric field). An atom's nucleus is, of course, positively charged.

When there is no external magnetic field, the magnetic fields of the nuclei in a molecule are randomly oriented and cancel each other out. When a large external magnetic field is applied to a sample, the individual nuclei within the sample will align either with the field or in opposition to the field. Nuclei that align with the field are termed **low spin state nuclei**. Nuclei that align opposite the field are called **high spin state nuclei**. The application of rf waves causes nuclei in the low spin state to absorb this radiation and "flip" into the high spin state. The absorption of this spin flip energy is measured and recorded as an NMR spectrum.

Not all nuclei show activity under NMR. In order for a nucleus to be NMR active, it must have an odd mass number, or have an even mass number and an odd atomic number. Two common isotopes used in organic chemistry are ^{1}H and ^{13}C. The proton (^{1}H) NMR spectrum of p-ethoxybenzaldehyde is given in Figure 41.8 and the carbon-13 (^{13}C) NMR spectrum of 3-methyl-2-butanone is given in Figure 41.9.

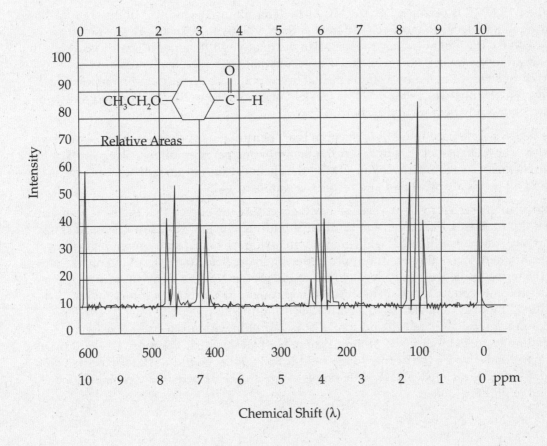

Figure 41.8

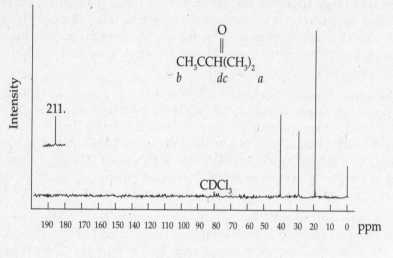

Chemical Shift (• •

Figure 41.9

Carbon-13 NMR is presented on the MCAT in determining the number of different carbons appearing in a molecule (since each different carbon will give rise to a peak at a distinct chemical shift). It is not necessary to memorize the relative shift values of various carbons. It is important to remember, however, that a molecule that possesses symmetry may have several carbons represented by a single peak. For example, 2,2-dimethyl propane {$(CH_3)_4C$} will give rise to only two carbon-13 NMR peaks—one from the central carbon and one from the other four equivalent methyl carbons.

The relative scale used in NMR is the ppm (part per million). A chemical shift of one ppm coincides with a change in the applied rf frequency of one part per million. The standard for organic chemistry is tetramethylsilane (TMS): the chemical shift of this substance is set as 0 ppm, and all peaks are measured and recorded relative to TMS.

Progressing from left to right along an NMR spectrum, the energy that is absorbed to cause the spin flip increases. This condition is called **shielding**. Nuclei with a low chemical shift (upfield) are said to be shielded, while nuclei with a high chemical shift (downfield) are said to be **deshielded**. While these terms apply to the magnetic field strengths of the nuclei, we can apply the terms "shielded" and "deshielded" to the proton NMR in terms of acidity. The more acidic a proton becomes, the more deshielded it becomes. As a proton becomes more deshielded, it moves to the left on the NMR spectrum (higher ppm, downfield). The most acidic proton would be a "naked" proton: that is, a proton with no electron density surrounding its nucleus. A naked proton is completely deshielded. The more shielded (more basic) a proton becomes, the further to the right it will appear on the NMR spectrum (lower ppm, upfield). Characteristic NMR shift values for protons in different environments are provided in Figure 41.10.

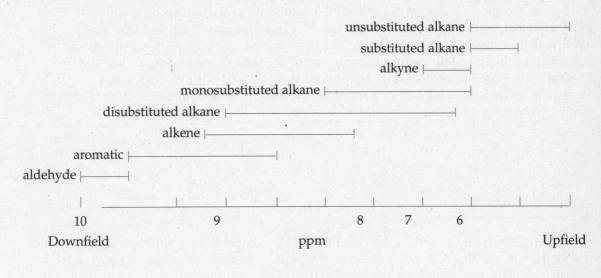

Figure 41.10

For a proton NMR spectrum, the area under each peak gives the relative abundance of the protons contributing to that peak. Therefore, in the NMR spectrum of chloroethane ($ClCH_2CH_3$), we expect to see two peaks—one with an integration area of two, the other with an integration area of three. Integration areas are extremely useful for the determination of the total number of hydrogens in a molecule (or contributing to a single peak). However, care must be exercised in that integration areas are *relative* areas, not absolute areas. Therefore, a molecule with symmetry may appear to have fewer hydrogens than it actually does. Consider the NMR spectrum of propane ($CH_3CH_2CH_3$). The two methyl groups are equivalent. Thus, they cause a single peak, with an integration area of three. The methylene group causes a second peak, with an integration area of one.

A final consideration in the interpretation of proton NMR spectra is a phenomenon known as spin-spin splitting (or spin-spin coupling), symbolized J. It is important to recognize that a magnetic field will be affected by any other magnetic (or electrical) field that is placed in proximity to the original field. For this reason, the magnetic fields of some nuclei are affected by the magnetic fields of other nuclei which are located within the same molecule. This can get extremely complicated; however, the MCAT is only concerned with coupling that occurs between nearest neighbor hydrogens ($J_{1,3}$ coupling).

$J_{1,3}$ coupling occurs when two nonequivalent protons are separated from one another (within the same molecule) by two other atoms. For example, if the hydrogens H_A and H_B are chemically nonequivalent, they will experience $J_{1,3}$ coupling; whereas, H_C and H_D will not couple (according to the MCAT).

One peak arises for each nonequivalent proton in the NMR spectrum. When the proton giving rise to one of these peaks is split by a neighboring proton, the peak is split into ($n + 1$) peaks, where n equals the number of protons that are splitting the proton. One peak represents the proton itself, and one additional peak arises for each proton that splits it. Consider, again, the NMR spectrum of propane ($CH_3CH_2CH_3$). As we saw earlier, the two methyl groups are equivalent. Thus, they cause a single peak, with an integration area of three. The methylene group causes a second peak, with an integration area of one. Labeling these two types of hydrogen as H_E and H_F, we see:

$$H_E \underset{\underset{H_E}{|}}{\overset{\overset{H_E}{|}}{C}} \underset{\underset{H_F}{|}}{\overset{\overset{H_F}{|}}{C}} \underset{\underset{H_E}{|}}{\overset{\overset{H_E}{|}}{C}} H_E$$

From the above discussion, we can see that the H_E's on the left are split by the two H_F's, as are the H_E's on the right. This causes the methyl peak to be split into three ($n + 1$, where $n = 2$) peaks—or a triplet. Likewise, we can see that the H_F's are split by all six H_E's. This causes the methylene peak to be split into seven ($n + 1$, where $n = 6$) peaks—or a septet.

What if the hydrogens on the left and right carbons are not equivalent? Consider the NMR spectrum of 1-chloropropane:

$$Cl \underset{\underset{H_X}{|}}{\overset{\overset{H_X}{|}}{C}} \underset{\underset{H_Y}{|}}{\overset{\overset{H_Y}{|}}{C}} \underset{\underset{H_Z}{|}}{\overset{\overset{H_Z}{|}}{C}} H_Z$$

Here, we expect peaks at three distinct chemical shifts (H_X, H_Y, and H_Z). The peak for H_X will be a triplet (split by the two H_Y's). The peak for H_Z will also be a triplet (split by the two H_Y's). The peak for H_Y will be split into a triplet by the two H_X's and into a quartet by the three H_Z's. The resultant peak is a quartet of triplets—NOT a sextet.

NMR splitting for:		Type:
H_x	⋀⋀	Triplet
H_z	⋀⋀	Triplet
H_y	⋀⋀ ⋀⋀ ⋀⋀ ⋀⋀	Quartet of triplets

Table 41.4

Please solve this problem:

- The proton NMR of 1-bromo-4-chlorocyclohexane will have:

    A. two doublets of triplets and one pentet.
    B. four doublets of triplets and one pentet.
    C. two doublets of triplets and two pentets.
    D. four doublets of triplets and two pentets.

Problem solved:

The correct answer is C. To solve this problem, we must first recognize the symmetry of the molecule. 1-bromo-4-chlorocyclohexane has a mirror plane that runs through both the 1 and 4 carbons and through the bromine and chlorine atoms (as well as the hydrogens on the 1 and 4 carbons). Once you see this mirror plane, you should recognize that there are only four sets of peaks in the NMR spectrum—one for each of the four types of hydrogen.

Knowing that there are four sets of peaks, we can eliminate all choices except C—choice A has 3 sets, choice B has 5 sets, and choice D has 6 sets. H_a and H_d will be split into pentets by their four hydrogen neighbors. H_b will be split into a triplet by H_c and into a doublet by H_a—giving a doublet of triplets. H_c will be split into a triplet by H_b and into a doublet by H_a—giving a second doublet of triplets.

41.2 MASTERY APPLIED: SAMPLE PASSAGE AND QUESTIONS

Passage

A wide variety of techniques can be used to separate and identify compounds. Most of these techniques are based on differences in physical properties. Procedures differ in their specific mode of action, each of which may separate or help to identify a compound based on a different characteristic of the unknown sample. Extraction separates solutions by drawing chemicals with similar properties into aqueous solution. A series of extractions are used in a solution with many components. Distillation is based on differences in boiling points. This technique can only be used when the vapor pressures are far enough apart to allow one substance to be completely removed without boiling out the others simultaneously. Frequently, a technique is used that involves purification and separation through a process of solvation. This procedure is known as recrystallization. When dealing with substances of significantly different polarity, thin layer chromatography (TLC) can reveal different elution distances as a result of differences in polarity of the unknown components of the solution. A similar technique is electrophoresis. This procedure is commonly used in genetic sequencing. DNA is broken down and its components are drawn through a gel based on the attraction of opposite charges. Different negatively charged nucleotides arrive at a positively charged plate at varying times, revealing the nucleotide sequence of the sample. Other methods of identification include methods of spectroscopy. Proton nuclear magnetic resonance and infrared spectroscopy are the most common. The former identifies compounds based on differing magnetic environments of protons, while the latter compares absorption frequencies of electromagnetic energy.

1. Which of the following techniques would be best for distinguishing compounds of differing dipole moments within a solution?

   A. Electrophoresis
   B. Extraction
   C. Thin layer chromatography
   D. Distillation

2. In the process of recrystallization, why must the desired solute, relative to the solvent, have high solubility at high temperatures and low solubility at low temperatures?

   A. The desired solute must be in the liquid phase at high temperatures, otherwise it would melt.
   B. The solubility must be high at high temperatures to allow the desired solute to pass into solution and ultimately be purified, but low at low temperature so that the purified solute can recrystallize upon cooling.
   C. The solubility must be high at high temperatures so impurities will remain in their solid form to be removed by filtration.
   D. The solubility must be high at high temperatures and low at low temperatures so that the solute can pass into solution and the two compounds can be boiled off and recondensed at different times.

3. Why would a chemist NOT run an IR on an unknown most likely to be identified as hexane?

 A. An IR would not be effective because all the protons in hexane have the same magnetic environments.

 B. An IR would not be effective because there are no stretching frequencies between carbon and hydrogen in hexane.

 C. An IR would not be effective because it typically distinguishes compounds based on functional groups.

 D. An IR would not be effective because hexane would not absorb electromagnetic energy.

4. Which of the following describes the proton NMR pattern seen for 2-chloropropane?

 A. Two singlets
 B. A doublet and a septet
 C. A singlet and a septet
 D. A doublet and a sextet

5. An extraction is performed in which a substance is separated out with the addition of sodium bicarbonate. Which of the following would *definitely* be removed by the extraction?

 A. Methane
 B. An amino acid
 C. An ether
 D. Acetic acid

6. Immediately following the extraction described in the previous question, a second extraction is performed in which an amine is removed after passing into the aqueous phase. What compound was used to extract the amine?

 A. Diethyl ether
 B. $NaHCO_3$
 C. HCl
 D. NaOH

7. In a distillation process involving two components, an impurity soluble in the less volatile component is added after the first component is removed. What effect will this have on the process relative to when it is performed without the addition of the impurity?

 A. The boiling point of the second solution will be higher than the boiling point of the first because it's boiling point is raised with the addition of solute.

 B. The process will not be affected by the addition of an impurity because a given substance has a constant boiling point.

 C. The boiling point of the second solution will be closer to that of the first because the addition of the impurity will lower it's boiling point.

 D. The effect cannot be determined based on the information provided.

8. Which of the following procedures breaks up compounds by bombarding them with high-energy electrons to yield information regarding mass/charge ratio?

 A. NMR
 B. Mass spectroscopy
 C. IR
 D. Electrophoresis

41.3 MASTERY VERIFIED: ANSWERS AND EXPLANATIONS

1. *The correct answer is C.* To speak of dipole moments is to imply polarity. Thin layer chromatography uses polarity to differentiate between components of a solution. More polar substances tend to remain in the stationary phase while less polar substances will elute further in the mobile phase. Distillation involves boiling points and extraction involves solubility. Electrophoresis requires charge, which is not necessary for polarity.

2. *The correct answer is B.* The basis of recrystallization is that a substance can be purified when heated and solvated, and will *recrystallize* upon cooling. Choice A implies that melting point is the critical factor, which it is not. Although filtration (choice C) may occur at some point in the process, it does not explain why the solvent requires certain characteristics. Choice D implies that boiling point is the determining factor in choosing a solvent. While boiling point may be a factor, it does not explain why solubility must change at different temperatures.

3. *The correct answer is C.* Infrared spectroscopy is based on absorption frequencies of functional groups with different dipole moments. Hexane has no functional groups. Choice A describes NMR. Choices B and D are incorrect; C-H stretches do exist for hexane, and electromagnetic energy would be absorbed.

4. *The correct answer is B.* The single proton on the central carbon would be split by six neighboring carbons (three from each attached methyl group). The two methyl groups would be split by the single proton on the central carbon. According to the $n + 1$ rule, there would be a doublet and a septet.

5. *The correct answer is D.* Extraction removes substances by separating them from an ether solution to an aqueous solution. The components that react with, or are soluble in, the added compounds will pass into aqueous solution. In this case a base, sodium bicarbonate, will interact with an acid. The only definite acid among the answers is acetic acid. Although many amino acids (choice B) are acidic, some are basic.

6. *The correct answer is C.* Again, the same principles apply as in question five. This is simply the opposite situation. Here, we are extracting an amine, which is a base. The most likely compound added would be an acid, which would react with the base and pass into aqueous solution. The only acid given is HCl.

7. *The correct answer is A.* There are two critical factors to consider in order to solve this problem. First, distillation involves boiling points. Knowing this would eliminate choices B and D. Second, boiling point is elevated with the addition of solute. Since the component with the lower boiling point is removed prior to the addition of the solute, and the solute raises the boiling point of the second component of the solution, the result must be a greater temperature difference between the first and second boiling point relative to the circumstance in which the solute had not been added.

8. *The correct answer is B.* NMR involves magnetic environments. Electrophoresis is a separation and identification technique based on movement of charged particles. Infrared spectroscopy involves absorption frequencies of various bonds within a molecule. Mass spectroscopy is the only process that yields information regarding mass/charge ratio.

CHAPTER 42

MASTERING VERBAL REASONING

The MCAT verbal reasoning section sets forth 9 passages, each accompanied by approximately 6-9 questions. The test-taker is allowed 85 minutes to read the passages and answer the questions. Students vary widely as to the degree to which they find this portion of the examination challenging; it has proven especially challenging for those test-takers whose native language is not English. Nonetheless, the verbal reasoning portion of the MCAT is susceptible to *strategy*.

To begin, the student should not make the *passage* the central focus of his effort. He must remember that scores follow from the number of *answers marked "correct."* If he is able to apply a strategy that allows him to maximize the number of correct answers he selects he should do so, even if it means he does not truly comprehend the passage in its entirety. The test-taker who performs most successfully on the MCAT verbal reasoning section is the one who (a) recognizes that the passages are in a sense "secondary" to his task, and (b) approaches his task strategically.

Most students who sit for the MCAT exam have developed good study habits in secondary school and college, and most have produced high cumulative grade-point averages throughout their undergraduate years. For this sort of student, the suggestion that passages laden with fact, theory, and information represent *obstacles* to their success on this exam will probably be very difficult to accept. Good students do not usually look to avoid reading, learning, or understanding. Certainly, successful medical students will not wish to shortchange their professors, their future patients, or themselves by seeking "shortcuts" around the challenging reading assignments that characterize the study of medicine.

However, in medical *school*, you are not obliged to read under the same time restrictions that apply to the MCAT. The tasks one is asked to complete on this section of the MCAT are unlike the academic challenges met in college, and unlike those to be faced in medical school. You should not, therefore, be averse to approaching the MCAT's verbal reasoning section with something akin to shortcuts and strategies. Our recommendation that you do so is based on our wish to see you achieve a high score. *We make no such recommendation in respect to medical school itself*; nor indeed in respect to any serious scholarly endeavor.

42.1 PASSAGES AND QUESTIONS IN GENERAL

The Verbal Reasoning Section presents nine passages, each followed by several (usually 6-9) questions. Like all multiple-choice questions, verbal reasoning questions feature a *stem* (the portion that precedes the answer choices), and answer choices.

Passages might concern almost any topic at all. Each test usually presents 1-2 passages addressing some topic of mathematics or natural science (other than those that properly belong to the physical and biological science MCAT syllabi). The remaining passages concern the social sciences, history, public policy, the humanities, literature, philosophy, religion, or a writer's personal account of her own experience or perspective.

Passages that concern mathematics or the natural sciences usually feature substantial amounts of factual information, conceptual distinctions, and technical explanations. For illustration, consider this passage segment.

Excerpt 42A

The "knot problem," as it has been called, relates largely to the difficulties associated with classifying knots. In mathematical terms, a knot is any closed curve in three dimensional space, a curve that never passes more than once through the same point of space and that may be thought of as starting at a point S and ultimately returning to S.

Any two knots belong to the same knot class if a continuous deformation of space carries one of them into the position initially held by the other. If a knot should belong to the same class as a circle, it is *considered* unknotted. The reason pertains to cognitive convenience. Just as it is conceptually helpful to view a straight line as one particular species of curve, so is it mentally useful to consider an unknotted curve as one subtype of knot.

Curves with a reasonable degree of regularity are ordinarily conceived of as threads, twisted and tangled in such a manner as to have their ends sealed to each other. According to this conception the "knot problem," in some minds, asks for a description of the conditions under which the process of stretching, shrinking, and bending will allow one twisted...

For passages concerning mathematics or the natural sciences, many (but not all) questions require you to recognize a statement that paraphrases technical information set forth in the passage. Consider this simulated MCAT question:

1. According to the passage, a knot is characterized by a curve whose **STEM**   beginning point:

   A. represents a spot on an arbitrary circle.
   B. generates a curve with a reasonable degree of regularity.
   C. coincides with the point of its own ending.
   D. fails to approximate its own endpoint.

Some of the questions associated with natural science passages require not a direct and immediate understanding of the text, but (1) extrapolation, (2) abstraction, and/or (3) application of the text to a seemingly unrelated subject. Consider the "knot" passage and read this simulated MCAT question:

2. When celestial navigators work their calculations, they find it practical **STEM** to envision the earth as the center of an orbit through which the sun moves. This manner of thought most closely parallels which of the following views described in the passage?

   A. A knot cannot conveniently be conceived as embodying a straight line.
   B. The "knot problem" is not susceptible to any single solution but is instead understandable from a variety of perspectives.
   C. A knot never passes through the same point twice.
   D. A knot belonging to the same class as a circle is considered "unknotted."

Humanities and social science passages *sometimes* ask the student to recognize statements that paraphrase the text. More often, they call for the kind of extrapolation and abstraction depicted in question 2 above. At times they call for an understanding of the author's tone or attitude. Frequently they require the student to understand the sense of a word or phrase that appears in the passage.

Consider this simulated MCAT passage segment and the questions that follow it:

Excerpt 42B

In ancient times, the spiritual life of an individual remained tethered to a vibrant, intricate and vivid natural world. Humans required a means by which their own actions might achieve control and mastery over "reality". Despite great diversity and variation among the myriad ancient civilizations that developed and declined during the ages, this objective reality retained certain unchanging elements. For example, virtually all cultures confronted the need to protect themselves from dangerous and nihilistic external powers. Common throughout antiquity was the strategic use of animism and anthropomorphism to constrain climactic, cosmological and natural phenomena within familiar and readily understood paradigms.

By conjuring forces imagined more dark and more brutal even than the "real" phenomena beyond human influence—which nearly always appeared antithetical to the goals and aspirations of individuals and societies—"magic" provided a systematic method for acquiring supernatural leverage. As human theology matured, the dark forces lost cultural favor, and communities appointed priests to petition benevolent potencies for protection against menace and destruction.

Cultural history gradually transformed these benevolent potencies into deities of creation and gods of healing, and the ancient Greek hierarchy, for example, bestowed upon them a more exalted position than it accorded the evil powers. If a community faced a period of cultural waning, however, and passed through a crisis of confidence, foreign cabals and alien sects of tremendous variety would become prominent and popular. Despite governmental sanctions, these exotic cults offered novel perspectives and esoteric rituals for a population dissatisfied with displaced traditions and dissipated spiritual conceptions.

1. According to the passage, early human cultures resorted to **STEM** animism and anthropomorphism because:

    A. sorcery threatened to disrupt their communities.

    B. animal sacrifice relieved stress on scarce food resources.

    C. priests became involved in tribal political struggles.

    D. simple models of reality mollified their sense of vulnerability.

2. As used in the second paragraph, the word "dark"
   most nearly **STEM** means:

   A. unenlightened.
   B. invisible.
   C. threatening.
   D. benighted.

As further illustration, consider *this* passage segment and the questions that follow it:

Excerpt 42C

Playwrights of the naturalist school believed in representationalism, rather than expressionism, as the most appropriate mode for dramaturgy. This belief translated in practice to constraining their dialogues and actions to forms they observed in everyday life. Such a strategy proved facile for writers whose interests delved no more deeply than the superficial interactions of human affairs: ordinary discussions of jobs and meals and mating mishaps required no expressionistic elaboration to articulate the pauses and silences that punctuate normal human discourse.

The more significant playwrights, however, wished to explore weightier themes relating to the entire experience of the human condition, but not at the expense of their artistic commitment to naturalistic dialogue. Out of this dilemma evolved the recourse to "symbolism", through which many of our most accomplished playwrights—Chekhov, Ibsen, and Strindberg, for instance—enlisted visual metaphors to convey a substantial portion of the dramaturgical gist. Thus, by restricting their dialogue to the patterns and rhythms of normal conversation, the naturalists uncovered a wealth of theatrical representation in the visual dimension.

1. According to the passage, naturalist playwrights:
   STEM

   A. confined themselves to depictions of superficial matters.
   B. used expressionistic metaphors to convey weighty themes.
   C. rejected dialogue devices that stylized the ordinary tempos and syntax of conversation.
   D. considered symbolism to be a mark of sophistication.

2. Suppose a naturalist playwright wants an audience to perceive **STEM** that a particular character is experiencing grief over the loss of a loved person or object. Among the following, the playwright would LEAST likely attempt to achieve that goal by:

A. creating dialogue in which the character describes the grief he feels and the reasons for which he feels it.
B. conveying the character's sense of grief through a conversation that concerns ordinary daily affairs.
C. introducing a symbolic representation of grief.
D. conveying the concept of grief through visual imagery.

For passages that describe a personal experience one or two questions might require that the reader search the passage for factual details, but most ask that she abstract, extrapolate, interpret. Some, ask that she apply *simple logic*. Consider this excerpt from a simulated MCAT passage and the questions that follow:

Excerpt 42D

In my adolescence and adulthood, I went through experiences that I could only describe as supernatural interventions, such episodes varying from visual manifestations and audible voices to the feeling that animals conceived a special—and extraordinary—communicability with me. On one occasion, I even received physical, serendipitous manna falling from the providential skies. Raised in an agnostic tradition by loving parents who never openly professed a belief in a divine being, I did not know exactly how to incorporate my formative understanding of the world and the human condition with these undeniably odd perceptions and unworldly contacts.

Did all these episodes occur under the direction of a beneficent God? I yearned for the certainty that some of my friends declared, friends who had devoted their childhood Saturdays and Sundays to religious services; absent that, I considered the likelihood of the Oz explanation: that some human agency possessing a vast, secret, futuristic technology could transmit graphic holograms and microradiowaved sounds to my brain. Somehow, it seemed more plausible than the possibility that a divine being would take the time and the interest to communicate with and watch out for me especially. Nonetheless, the Oz explanation was terribly frightening, too, and I knew better than to speak openly of it outside private and trusted circles. After all, people were diagnosed as schizophrenic—and stowed away in locked hospital wards—just for talking about such ideas!

1. Based on this passage, the author's feelings about himself **STEM** are best characterized as demonstrating:

   A. self-hatred and obsession
   B. conceit and narcissism
   C. humility and self-doubt
   D. apathy and self-destruction

2. Suppose a person believes that his misfortunes are the **STEM** result of evil spirits that have placed themselves within his body. Given the discussion of the "Oz explanation," the author would most likely advise this person to:

   A. consider his observations as serendipitous, but not truly providential.
   B. exercise caution when choosing the people in whom he confides his belief.
   C. seek psychotherapy in order that he better understand his feelings and impulses.
   D. ask himself whether there is a more plausible explanation for his sensations.

42.1.1 QUESTIONS ON THE PERIPHERY

In 1995, the MCAT verbal reasoning section began to present questions that might be termed "peripheral." Such questions bear only a tenuous relationship to the passage and are usually answerable with little or no reference to its text. Consider this question, which might easily follow Excerpt 42B above.

> A medical historian once wrote, "Early man first confronted **STEM** illness as pain. Knowing that other *persons* could willfully inflict pain on him, he first concluded that a willful living agency was responsible for his illness—that cure would come with the appeasement or defeat of that agency." Which of the following practices, if followed by early humans, would most strengthen the historian's view?
>
> **A.** Using herbs, tonics, and vapors to cleanse the sick of atmospheric poisons
> **B.** Applying various nematodes to the bodies of the sick to suction the blood that carries illness
> **C.** Appealing to deities of goodness in order that the sick might be healed
> **D.** Conducting ceremonies over the sick in order to destroy the evil spirits within them

Together with the student's own facility for logic, the stem presents all of the information necessary to selecting an answer. The question, therefore, is peripheral to the passage. It requires little or no review of the passage's text.

First, the question introduces a medical historian not mentioned in the passage. According to the historian's view, early humans thought illness was caused by willful beings ("agencies"). On the basis of that information alone, the student is expected to select choice D as representing a practice which, if followed, would strengthen the historian's view. (Choice C is incorrect because the historian refers not to the solicitation of willful agencies that might cure disease, but to the appeasement or defeat of those that *cause* it.)

Consider this question which might follow Excerpt 42C above.

> A drama professor recently wrote, "No so-called drama **STEM** belongs on the stage if its author constructs some symbol, label, or artifice that signals the audience as to a character's nature or experience." Among the following, the professor would LEAST like a play in which:
>
> **A.** a conceited character is named "James Boast."
> **B.** characters speak with foreign accents.
> **C.** all the major players are children.
> **D.** dialogue is carefully constructed with cadence and rhythm.

The question is peripheral to the passage. The student is to answer on the basis of her own capacity for logic, fueled by information provided in the *stem* (not the passage). The drama professor dislikes symbols, labels, and artifice that inform ("signal") the audience of a character's personality or feelings. The professor would, therefore, dislike a play in which a boastful character is named "Boast." Choice A is correct, and the passage has little to do with it.

Frequently a peripheral question presents *incorrect* answer choices that use words and phrases set forth in the passage. When students read words and phrases drawn directly from the passage they sometimes (1) forget that the question is peripheral, (2) lose sight of the stem, and (3) revisit the passage in search of an answer not to be found there. *Peripheral questions are answerable on the basis of (a) the stem, and (b) the student's own resources of knowledge and logic.* When facing a peripheral question, do not let an answer choice send you back to the passage on a wasteful wild goose chase. Focus on the stem, think logically, answer the question, and move on.

Having discussed, in very general terms, passages and questions, we move now to discuss, *only generally*, the selection of a correct answer. (More detailed discussions appear in chapters 43 and 44.)

42.2: THE RIGHT ANSWER: UNMASKING DISGUISES

Many MCAT verbal reasoning questions offer answer options that represent information or assertions from the associated passage—*expressed in different words*. For example, the phrase "a convincingly communicated insight" conveys very much the same meaning as "a perception articulated with persuasion". One primary "skill" that this MCAT section evaluates is your ability to recognize textual meaning "dressed up" in verbal disguise.

Consider this sentence:

> In accordance with the nature of healthcare work and the character of those who enter the field, most dedicated healthcare professionals, regardless of ethnicity or gender, are known to derive substantial gratification when their therapeutic efforts lead to positive patient outcomes.

Based on this one sentence, choose the one most appropriate answer to the following question:

1. Which of the following assertions best reflects the author's belief about the way medical workers feel regarding patient care:

   A. doctors and nurses largely prefer to recommend medical treatments rather than surgical measures.
   B. interns and residents enjoy emergency room rotations more than they do other hospital duties.
   C. dedicated healers find substantial gratification from positive outcomes.
   D. sensitive physicians don't discuss their patients' private records.

Option B is clearly correct, and very few students would have a problem identifying it as such. Options A, C, and D present possible answers which in and of themselves are not necessarily nonsensical or erroneous statements, but they represent ideas nowhere to be found in the passage. Option B, conversely, reiterates several of the author's exact words.

Rarely will the MCAT offer an answer option that exactly duplicates words from the passage. Frequently, however, one answer option will set forth the author's meaning in paraphrase. The option might at first appear incorrect, but you should be sensitive to the questioners' tendency to paraphrase. You should not rely on your first impression. Consider again this sentence and then the question that follows.

In accordance with the nature of healthcare work and the character of those who enter the field, most dedicated healthcare professionals, regardless of ethnicity or gender, are known to derive substantial gratification when their therapeutic efforts lead to positive patient outcomes.

Which of the following assertions best reflects the author's belief about the way medical workers feel regarding patient care:

A. doctors and nurses largely prefer to recommend medical treatments rather than surgical measures.
B. interns and residents enjoy emergency room rotations more than they do other hospital duties.
C. devoted caregivers garner meaningful satisfaction from successful therapeutic interventions.
D. sensitive physicians don't discuss their patients' private records.

Without a doubt, option C remains the appropriate answer, even though the assertion has been reworded. Test-takers who understand that verbal disguise is one main tactic used by the MCAT producers will much less likely be confused by the paraphrase. After all, "most dedicated healthcare professionals...are known to derive substantial gratification when their therapeutic efforts lead to positive patient outcomes"

means very much the same thing as

"devoted caregivers garner meaningful satisfaction from successful therapeutic interventions."

In terms of the particular words that comprise them, these two statements are completely dissimilar. Examined closely, however, it is easy to recognize that:

"dedicated healthcare professionals"
is disguised as
"devoted caregivers"

"substantial gratification"
is disguised as
"meaningful satisfaction"

"positive patient outcomes"
is disguised as
"successful therapeutic interventions."

The author's questioned assertion is represented *in disguise* in answer option C.

You should master a few simple techniques designed to help you penetrate disguises. Several very brief examples of MCAT-like paraphrases are offered below. You should:

- read the selections

- attentively consider the meaning of the text

- mindful of that meaning, think about each response option

- decide which option best reflects a *disguised* version of the author's original meaning

The realities of life lend themselves to myriad interpretations, and not infrequently one's personal orientation and attitude colors one's subjective experience. Life is not so much what it is—but rather, what it seems.

According to the passage, one's subjective experience of life:

A. is appropriate subject matter for literature and art.
B. depends on an individual's perspective and disposition.
C. varies according to the season of the year.
D. depends on parental teachings and values.

The author's meaning is that the way a person perceives the hazards and vicissitudes that constitute the human condition can affect the way he or she thinks and feels about life. The author believes that two different people might experience an identical phenomenon, and because of the difference in the way they view things, their respective sense of what had happened to them might be remarkably distinct. Mindful of that, the student should analyze each answer option and identify the one that represents the author's message—in disguise.

Choice A means that an individual's life experiences provide good material for artistic representation. Although this sounds like a sensible statement, it is not anything like the statement conveyed by the passage. Choice B means approximately the same thing as the text, only presented to the test-taker in paraphrase:

"colors"
is disguised as
"depends on"

"perspective"
is disguised as
"orientation"

"attitude"
is disguised as
"disposition"

Option C refers to the idea that people's sense of their experiences can change with the seasons. The passage says nothing close to that in meaning. Option D indicates that an individual's experience of life may be greatly determined by his or her formative upbringing. This idea is certainly not a silly one, however it is not related to the author's message. Option B is the only one of the four suggested options that seems similar to the author's meaning: It is the only answer that represents the author's meaning in disguise.

Powerful politicians and important statespersons have arisen from origins tremendously diverse in terms of the social, economic and educational conditions of their respective lives.

The student of history must conclude from this observation that political greatness stems from individual traits of personality and inner character.

> The text implies that successful political careers are due to:
>
> A. the ability of individuals to educate themselves.
> B. a lack of sophistication on the part of the voting public.
> C. strategic intervention at crucial historical moments.
> D. human characteristics unrelated to cultural or pecuniary circumstance.

To begin with, the author's text conveys the view that regardless of an individual's background, history has demonstrated that he or she can achieve political success given the right combination of personal attributes.

Option A states that a politician's success depends on his or her level of autodidacticism. While this notion seems intriguing, and may even have relevance to the author's point, it is not really what was said in the passage. Option B implies that only in the context of a population which is uneducated, uninterested, uninformed, or easily misled can politicians achieve success. Although historians might enjoy debating this idea, it is not in the least similar to the author's passage. Option C focuses on a particular aspect of a politician's activities, the ability to anticipate political trends and manage crises adroitly. Again, the assertion appears coherent and logical; the author, however, does not mention it. Option D, on the other hand, very closely approximates the significance of the text, by presenting the author's idea in disguise:

> "individual traits of personality and inner character"
> *is disguised as*
> "human characteristics"
>
> "social, economic and educational conditions"
> *is disguised as*
> "cultural or pecuniary circumstance"

Hence, answer D is correct.

People's willingness to believe in tales of extraterrestrial visitations and flying saucer abductions reveals a fundamental dearth of fulfillment in their daily experience: thus, the invention of extraordinary activities and involvements to convince themselves of their own importance.

The author contends that experiences of extraterrestrial contacts derives from:

A. the intellectual desire to integrate new astronomical findings with daily experience.

B. the moral need to believe in deliverance from human problems.

C. an underlying lack of satisfaction with their lives.

D. a basic conviction that technologies on other planets are more advanced than those on Earth.

The author asserts that in order to compensate for the ordinariness and tedium of their everyday lives, some people profess to have been visited by or witness to manifestations of creatures from outer space. Option A states that stories of space alien exploits stem from a wish to incorporate daily life with recent scientific discoveries. Nothing like this sentiment appears in the passage. Option B refers to a spiritual hunger for salvation from the dilemmas of mortal humanity as the motive behind reports of extraterrestrial phenomena. Although as a psychological thesis this notion may prove feasible, it reflects nothing of what this author wrote. Option C concerns a basic dissatisfaction with daily routine and circumstance as the cause of people's accounts of extraterrestrial activity. On reflection, that is quite similar to the author's meaning:

"fundamental dearth of fulfillment"
is disguised as
"underlying lack of satisfaction"

"in their daily experience"
is disguised as
"with their lives"

Option D cites a suspicion that extraterrestrial civilizations have invented far more sophisticated technologies than humans on Earth have developed as the reason for descriptions of alien sightings. The author did not refer to such a concept. Option C is the only one of the four that paraphrases the author's original text. It is correct.

CHAPTER 43

VERBAL REASONING DISTRACTERS

43.1 DISCARDING WRONG ANSWERS

In the field of standardized testing, incorrect answers are called "distracters." Question writers devise them to mislead, to confuse, and, regrettably, to trick the student. Distracters may be so artfully composed as to derail even those who read and comprehend the passages with diligence.

Approach the MCAT's verbal reasoning section by understanding how its distracters are designed. There are four identifiable types. Learn how each operates, and turn that learning to your advantage.

43.2 DISTRACTER TYPE 1: THE MANGLER

The most common distracter type is the "mangler." It copies actual language from the associated passage, and simultaneously distorts its meaning. Such answer options mangle the author's message. Please read this sentence:

> "Whenever Alice was feeling lonely, it always seemed to rain."

It is easy to imagine a number of sentences that (a) feature the words "Alice," "lonely," and "rain" as used in the statement, and yet (b) alter the original meaning, subtly or obviously:

> "Every time it rained, Alice felt lonely."

> "Alice thought the rain always sounded lonely."

> "Lonely as she was, Alice liked the rain."

None of these statements really reflects the sense of the first sentence. On the contrary, each one mangles the original sense by duplicating some of the language in an entirely different context. Still, a quick reading of them could generate apparent echoes of the original, because many of the words are identical.

These are good examples of the manner in which MCAT question writers introduce error into answer options. A passage that included the statement, "Whenever Alice was feeling lonely, it always seemed to rain," might be followed by this question:

Which of the following assertions best reflects the author's description of Alice?

A. Every time it rained, Alice felt lonely.
B. Rain seemed to fall whenever Alice found herself in a lonely mood.
C. Alice thought the rain always sounded lonely.
D. Lonely as she was, Alice liked the rain.

Each of the answer options A, C, and D includes words copied directly from the original passage. However, option B is the only one that repeats the original significance (*in disguise*, as usual).

Learn to spot manglers. Examine the examples that follow according to the instructions. Five statements follow each of the four excerpts from MCAT-like passages. Of those five, only three correctly represent the original intent of the author; the other three are mangled distracters.

Consider this natural science excerpt:

Insomnia, a sleep disorder characterized by inadequate or non-restful sleep under conditions that should allow normal sleep, is a virtually universal experience for adults at some time in their lives.

What is the author's message?

• Insomnia prevents people from getting restful sleep.

• It occurs under conditions that would normally be appropriate for restful sleep.

• It is experienced by nearly all adults at some point.

Please read these five statements. Identify those that mangle and those that do not.

1. Insomnia disturbs conditions that usually allow people to sleep normally.

2. Insomnia occurs in circumstances that are generally conducive to good sleep.

3. Insomnia affects people with universal severity.

4. Insomnia afflicts most people at one or another time in their lives.

5. Almost all adults sleep normally under restful conditions.

Assertions 1, 3, and 5 mangle the original statement's significance. The statement did not indicate that:

• normal sleep conditions are disturbed by insomnia.

• all people are affected to the same extent by insomnia.

• nearly every adult enjoys restful sleep under appropriate circumstances.

Assertions 2 and 4 do not mangle. The original statement indeed points out that:

- normal sleep conditions are present when insomnia occurs.

- At some time in their lives, most adults will suffer insomnia.

Consider this social science excerpt:

Excerpt 43A

Keeping in focus the multitudes of children who enter school under the tyranny of totalitarian values and authoritarian compulsion, or, inversely, surrounded by an uncaring, dysfunctional, or disrupted familial structure, it becomes incumbent upon educators to discover methodologies to overcome the social and political suppression of such individuals' intrinsic intellectual capacities. As more than one authority has emphasized, absent the development of cognitive aptitudes, a child in school might readily assume the form of a robot, with inflexible behavioral and ethical restrictions, and the absolute impossibility of liberty.

What is the author's message?

- Many children grow up in repressive political or dysfunctional familial conditions which suppress their intellectual aptitudes.

- Educators must figure out how to liberate students from such suppression.

- When one does not develop innate cognitive abilities, the resulting existence is devoid of freedom, and suffers from intractable limitations on conduct and attitudes.

Among the following assertions, identify those that mangle the author's meaning, and those that do not:

1. Tyrannical political systems prevent educators from discovering effective teaching methodologies.

2. Children with suppressed intellectual capacities develop into uncaring and nonsupportive parents.

3. The challenge for educators is to develop techniques useful for developing the full potential of children who grow up in circumstances that would not otherwise permit it.

4. Many authorities have developed robotic behavioral limitations.

5. With the failure to develop innate intellectual abilities, the possibility of real human freedom disappears.

Assertions 1, 2, and 4 mangle the original statement. The language resembles the language in the original statement, but it conveys some very different meanings. The statement did not indicate that:

- Oppressive political conditions make it impossible for educators to develop adequate pedagogical techniques.

- Youngsters whose potentials are never developed themselves become dysfunctional parents.

- Many authorities suffer from automaton-like conduct.

Assertions 3 and 5 do not mangle. The original statement points out that:

- The professional task of educators is to find ways of unlocking the cognitive aptitudes of intellectually suppressed children.

- No chance for human liberation exists unless the suppressed individual is empowered to develop intrinsic mental aptitudes.

Consider this excerpt from a simulated MCAT passage about personal experience:

Excerpt 43B

Despite my certain belief—more than belief, really: understanding, knowledge—that cigarette smoking leads inexorably to substantial impairments of health, I found myself seemingly helpless to rid my life of the noxious habit. "I ought to know better!" I scolded myself on occasions as frequent as the number of half-smoked, extinguished butts in my ashtrays. "Do those butts symbolize my life?" I pondered. "Will my very existence be prematurely ground out in the choking smog of nicotine oxidation?"

My friends and family had begged me to join SmokeBeaters, or Q.U.I.T., to get help with my poisonous addiction. Sometimes I tired of their insistence, of their intrusion. "Obviously, I'm getting *something* out of it," I shouted at my brother one evening, following his offer to provide the name of a hypnotist who specialized in substance abuse problems. But I knew they meant well, and in the privacy of my thoughts I did not fault them.

What is the author's message?

- She smokes cigarettes.

- She has no doubt that smoking is detrimental to her health.

- She criticizes herself for maintaining the habit.

- She muses about her smoking's effect on her own longevity.

- Friends and family have counseled her to end the habit.

- Her brother suggested the name of a specialist in hypnosis.

- She becomes irritated at the constant nagging and advice.

- Despite her annoyance, in her heart she does not condemn those who want only to help her.

Please read these five statements. Identify those that mangle and those that do not.

1. The author realizes that she has a habit which might cost her substantial health impairments in the future.

2. The author found herself helpless to rid her life of people's constructive suggestions.

3. The author wonders if cigarettes symbolize the meaning of life.

4. The author shouted at her brother because he threw away her cigarettes.

5. When she was honest with herself, she recognized the truth of her family's concerns.

Assertions 2, 3 and 4 mangle the original meaning. Some of the language comes directly from the original statement, but it's significance is altered. The statement did not indicate that:

- The author was at a loss as to how to stop her friends and family from making their suggestions about her smoking.

- The author believed that cigarettes stood for her life's significance.

- The author yelled at her brother because he discarded her tobacco.

Assertions 1 and 5 do not mangle. The original passage indeed points out that:

- The author is aware of the serious risks to her health posed by continued smoking.

- She understood, and recognized the justice and compassion of her family's interest in having her quit smoking.

Consider this humanities excerpt:

> Although not considered a mystic herself, Sor Juana, Mexico's finest colonial poet, created verse comparable in greatness to that of the Peninsular mystic poets. The illegitimate daughter of a Spanish colonizer and his Creole lover, Juana Inés Asbaje melded her multicultural origins in her artistic consciousness, and from them forged her beautiful rhymes. Inheriting the diverse attitudes of her Old World father and New World mother, she integrated them in her original vision to become the outstanding pioneer of Mexican poetry.

In one of her most famous works, *The Divine Narcissus*, she identifies Christian leitmotifs in the pre-Colombian sacrifice and eating sacrament of the Mexican God of Corn. In suggesting that long prior to the arrival of the Spanish conquistadors and their Catholic missionaries, the indigenous people's ancient theology had developed such modern sophistication as rituals of divine communion, Sor Juana offended the sensibilities of the ecclesiastical authorities. The girl who educated herself in childhood and adolescence through the resources of her grandfather's extensive book collection, swimming from her earliest years against the tides of tradition and prejudice, became the adult woman eventually chastised and condemned as a heretic for her verse and polemics.

What is the author's message?

- Sor Juana was Mexico's finest colonial poet, and a pioneer of her art.

- She is not considered a mystic.

- She was the offspring of a union between a Spanish man and a Creole woman.

- Her poetry grew from the composite nature of her origins.

- Her work, *The Divine Narcissus*, identifies Christian themes in pre-Colombian religion.

- Never confined by social convention, she came under attack by church authorities for her writings.

Please read these five statements. Identify those that mangle and those that do not.

1. The mysticism of the Spanish Peninsular poets is comparable in greatness to that of Sor Juana.

2. Sor Juana's artistic consciousness forged her rhymes without relation to her parental roots.

3. Sor Juana is considered the preeminent originator of Mexican verse.

4. Sor Juana maintained that the Christian ritual motif of a central beneficent god resurrected in the form of comestible nourishment, is anticipated in ancient Mexican worship.

5. Sor Juana trained in her adolescence as a marathon swimmer.

Assertions 1, 2 and 5 mangle the original significance. Although some of the language in these choices is exactly duplicated from the overlying text, it appears in assertions that bear no relation to the text's meaning. The passage did not indicate that:

- Sor Juana, like the Spanish writers before her, was also a mystic poet.

- Sor Juana's poetry developed without significant relation to the multicultural influences of her parents.

• Sor Juana was schooled during her teens as a water athlete.

Assertions 2 and 3 do not mangle. The original passage indeed points out that:

• Scholars identify Sor Juana as the mother of Mexican poetry.

• Her work depicted the communion rite of some Christian traditions as being predated in certain ancient Mexican Indian religions.

In the last analysis, think of a mangler as a distracter that (1) borrows words from the passage, and (2) *misuses* them by presenting them out of context, and/or miscombining them to form inappropriate connections among and between ideas. The result is an answer choice that *seems* to draw on the passage but actually misstates the author's message. You will practice further with manglers (and all forms of distracters) in chapter 45.

43.3 DISTRACTER TYPE 2: THE SEDUCER

A second type of distracter used on the verbal reasoning section is one we call a "seducer." Seducers make statements that *seem* entirely appropriate, proper, and sensible, even though they fail to (1) reflect the passage's meaning, and/or (2) logically follow the stem. Seducers tempt those test-takers who fail to *keep the stem and passage in mind* and are thus vulnerable to incorrect answers that "just sound good," or "seem right."

Some seducers "sound good" because they echo statements or sentiments with which the student is familiar. Others "seem right" because they parrot prevailing cultural doctrine. Consider these statements of which seducers might readily be made.

> In the last analysis, people are the governors of their own fate.

> Community standards are crucial, but they should not constrain the freedom of the individual.

> Majority rules, and in the long run the majority usually knows what is best for its nation.

These three statements seem so logical and reasonable that many test-takers assume they "just must be right." Usually, however, they are not.

Please consider the following excerpt from a simulated MCAT personal experience passage, and the questions that follow it:

> Despite my generally scientific cast of mind, I had always recognized in myself a fascination with the mystical and inexplicable. Besides, why should any human entity equipped with advanced technological powers expend resources on maintaining round-the-clock electronic surveillance of, and communication with, *me*? Talk about your paranoid ideation! Through the mental ether it waggled like a cheap perfume. And anyway, I'd bounced around these seemingly unresolvable questions as restlessly as a hard rubber ball in a four-walled squash court. No, unless I wished to accept the mind-boggling implications of paranoid schizophrenia, I would have to opt for mystery. Mystery! Now there was an answer!

For each of the questions that follows, three choices have been removed and one—*a seducer*—remains for your inspection.

1. The author was drawn to the notion of existential mystery

   A. —
   B. —
   C. Faith requires an acceptance of the fact that one cannot understand everything.
   D. —

Choice C is seductive. It suggests a cogent and persuasive explanation foq.the author's thinking, but nothing in the passage indicates that the author turned to the concept of mystery because she wished to accept the fact she did not understand everything. In the final three lines of the passage the author makes it explicit that her thought process was as much a turning away from psychosis as it was a turn toward "mystery."

Some seducers "sound good" and "seem right" because they appear, *on their surface*, to reflect statements or positions set forth in the relevant passage. Consider this question.

2. In the last paragraph the author most likely writes that she has "bounced around" in order to express:

   A. —
   B. her determination to understand her psyche in fully rational terms.
   C. —
   D. —

Choice B is a seducer. Superficially understood, the author seems to be determined about *something*, and the word "determination" tempts the unwary. Furthermore, it seems, generally, a "good thing" to understand one's environment in rational terms. That too makes choice B seductive. Yet, choice B does not reflect the author's sentiments and fails correctly to complete the stem. This author is *not* determined to understand her environment in rational terms. She settles on "mystery" as an answer to her questions.

Whatever may be the root of their appeal, seducers have in common these three features: (1) they "seem right," (2) they fail accurately to reflect the passage's meaning, and (3) *they fail logically to follow or complete the stem.* Avoid seducers by remembering this simple truth: However sensible, appealing, attractive, or superficially appropriate it might seem, an answer choice is "correct" only in relation to the relevant passage and stem. Forget that fact and you might fall prey to seducers. *Avoid seducers by keeping your mind on the stem and the passage.* Practice further with seducers (and all forms of distracters) in chapter 45.

43.4 DISTRACTER TYPE 3: THE IRRELEVANT TRUTH

A third form of MCAT distracter is what we call the "irrelevant truth." It traps students by *diverting their attention from the stem* with a statement that seems fully and genuinely to repeat one of the author's messages. When considered in light of the stem, the irrelevant truth makes an inaccurate statement. Look again, for example, at excerpt 43A and the question that follows:

Excerpt 43A

Keeping in focus the multitudes of children who enter school under the tyranny of totalitarian values and authoritarian compulsion, or, inversely, surrounded by an uncaring, dysfunctional, or disrupted familial structure, it becomes incumbent upon educators to discover methodologies to overcome the social and political suppression of such individuals' intrinsic intellectual capacities. As more than one authority has emphasized, absent the development of cognitive aptitudes, a child in school might readily assume the form of a robot, with inflexible behavioral and ethical restrictions, and the absolute impossibility of liberty.

The author seems to believe that some children fail to learn well because, before beginning school:

A. they grow accustomed to excessive amounts of liberty.
B. they have been taught to reject all authority and discipline.
C. they readily assume the form of robots.
D. they have lived in broken homes.

Some students *lose sight of the stem* and select choice C because it seems directly to repeat a statement presented in the passage. But choice C is an irrelevant truth. Considered *in light of the stem*, its statement is <u>incorrect</u>. The author does not believe that children readily assume the form of robots *before they begin* school. (Choice D is correct. Examine the author's reference to dysfunctional and *disrupted* familial structure. Taken in light of the stem, choice D accurately restates the author's view—*in disguise*.)

Avoid selecting irrelevant truths by keeping your mind on the stem. Practice further with irrelevant truths (and all forms of distracters) in chapter 45.

43.5 DISTRACTER TYPE 4: THE ABSOLUTE

Less common in recent administrations is a fourth type of MCAT distracter: the "absolute." Words such as "always," "universally," "never," and "without exception" should alert you to the possible presence of an *absolute* distracter. Other key words enlisted in this effort to mislead test-takers are: "entirely," "completely," and "perfectly."

The reason absolutes are usually incorrect is that they lend themselves rather easily to dispute. For instance:

Excellent physicians never make mistakes.

Certainly, such an assertion seems to make such implicit sense, that were it to appear as an answer option on the MCAT, one would pass it by only with the greatest of reluctance. The unfortunate truth, however, is that in any field even the best of the best are susceptible to human error. The absolute nature of the assertion should warn you to "stay away." Please read this statement:

It is universally true, that the harder one works, the more one earns.

Mostly true. Usually true. Nearly always true. Difficult to think of an exception. Nevertheless, the mere appearance of "universally" should sound an alarm. It imports an absolute.

Without reference to any particular passage, consider the following questions and identify the absolute:

> The author's discussion of suiting the therapeutic modality to the individual circumstance leads to her conclusion that:
>
> A. Recovery from substance abuse syndromes requires a positive attitude.
> B. Breaking a chronic smoker's habit takes great effort.
> C. Alcohol abusers can overcome their addiction only under ideal circumstances.
> D. Cases of positively adaptive behavioral changes involve multiple psychological factors.

Option C sets forth an absolute. The suggestion that something or someone must be "ideal," or "perfect," or "precisely accurate," or "totally mistaken" indicates that an absolute is likely operating.

Identify the absolute(s) contained in the following option set:

> The author believes that an individual's self-image:
>
> A. cannot possibly be improved by self-hypnotic techniques.
> B. is hopelessly dependent on childhood traumas.
> C. is subject to rational analysis of past misconceptions.
> D. ought to be considered in many abusive situations.

Assertions A and B are framed as absolutes. Phrases such as "cannot possibly" or "hopelessly dependent" represent situations at the extreme. In nine cases out of ten, such absolute statements will be incorrect answers.

As earlier noted, the MCAT writers seem lately not to be writing absolute distracters. Furthermore, an absolute might occasionally constitute a *correct* answer. If and when confronted with an absolute, exercise much caution before selecting it as your answer.

CHAPTER 44

SYSTEMATIC IDENTIFICATION OF CORRECT ANSWERS

The fact that MCAT verbal reasoning passages seem difficult has less to do with your abilities than with the conditions under which you are tested. A medical student who wishes to learn basic medical science, for example, ought not to read one short fragment from one subject—say, physiology—and two minutes later leap to a brief clipping from a second—say, microbiology. To be sure, the medical sciences are fundamentally and profoundly interrelated, but one cannot comprehend the whole without a preliminary understanding of its parts. Rushed, disconnected readings, with no unifying direction, will never afford a medical student the sort of detailed understanding that only hours of organized, focused study can provide.

But the MCAT is *not* medical school. You are assessed on your ability first to immerse yourself for fractional minutes in disconnected parcels of unrelated text, and then to select the particular shred of minutiae that yields a correct answer. Whereas a medical student enrolled in a full-time course of study understands the problem of the task, knows where to direct his or her attention, and what to look for, MCAT candidates on the verbal reasoning skills section find myriad bits of information clamoring for attention, with little way to decide which ones matter.

Raising your MCAT verbal reasoning score requires systematic efficiency. Building on chapters 42, and 43, *this* chapter presents a five-step process that will help you strategically to process the passage, read the questions, and select your answers.

44.1 MAPPING THE PASSAGE

To begin with, remember this: A typical passage is 600-900 words long. Most of its paragraphs, words and sentences do *not* give rise to questions. Whole bodies of text filled with names, dates, and data may be entirely unrelated to the relatively few questions that follow the passage. *Attempting at the outset to understand the whole passage in detail is counterproductive.* Your purpose is to score points in the time allowed you—not to waste time in an attempt to understand arcane material unrelated to the questions you must answer.

Your first step is to skim the passage and create a map of its paragraph's main ideas. Don't read closely. Don't try to understand thoroughly. Read each paragraph quickly. Very quickly. Skim it. Sift it. In the margins, record a few words that remind you of its central topic. This will likely cause you to feel anxious and "out of control." For sure, this is no way for a serious medical student to read—once he or she is *in* medical school. But it *is* the way to approach an MCAT verbal reasoning passage. Minutes later, when you begin to answer questions, you'll read *certain portions* of the passage closely, for detail. The questions and your map will direct you to those parts of the passage that require your careful attention. But your *first* reading should be quick and sketchy. It should generate not understanding, but—a map.

Develop a "sifting mentality." Ask yourself, "What is the paragraph about?" Your answer should require only a few words jotted in the margins.

Please look at these several paragraphs from a humanities passage that follow.

Map it.

Excerpt 44A

Embracing the four decades between 1494 and 1530, the Italian Renaissance achieved its artistic pinnacle and suffered its spiritual, social, and political collapse within that interval. One could not remain alive and cognizant during that swiftly passing span of years and emerge unchanged by the influences and events that defined it: notions regarding Humanity's rightful place in the Universe, and conceptions of the community's relationship with the individual and the proper role and prerogatives of each, underwent radical modification. The moral essence of the period evolved through a four-stage process, each stage being embodied by one great cultural authority of the era.

Fascinated by Nature's anarchy, the Renaissance individual came to understand the inevitable vengeance of unleashed Cosmic license: the sheer hazard of fortune dangled over one's life like the sword of Damocles. Destiny's permutations lay beyond the reach and outside the control of the individual. Such a spiritual predicament provoked the quest for faith, and four seers arose in turn who whispered private terrors and bequeathed revelatory prophecies each to the next. One wishes to confer upon them the title of lawgivers, because history tells us that like parched horses mustering towards water, their peers and contemporaries rallied to the ideas promulgated, and the causes championed, by this quartet of greatness.

In retrospect, the four definitive Renaissance figures—Savonarola, Machiavelli, Castiglione, and Aretino—loom larger than life over the cultural evolutions they influenced. In their lives, these progressions become highlighted, foreshadowed and manifest. Locating the precise center of life, respectively, in the spirit, in the intellect, in culture and in instinct, each one encountered the core truth of earthly existence in harmony with his personal essence: be it in theology, politics, gentility, or sensuality. The tours of status and leverage conducted by their respective oracles counterbalance one another like coherent and sensible sequels.

Savonarola's spartan humility, Machiavelli's resourceful expediency, Castiglione's courtly congeniality, and Aretino's primitive hedonism: each represents an eternal response to life, respectively, that of one who dreads life, who assents to it, who settles with it, and who surrenders to it. As the centuries have barreled by, their perspectives on human experience and their perceptions of the human condition—the beliefs and understandings which informed and directed their lives—have today achieved the stature of truisms. If the cocoon of time, however, has metamorphosed their vital truths into well-learned platitudes, these are platitudes essentially undulled by the fleeting years; and for being basic, they are no less primary.

Paragraph 1:

The paragraph discusses the individual and social changes that occurred during four decades of the Italian Renaissance. In the margin you might write:

4 decades>>radical changes

Paragraph 2:

This second paragraph describes the sense of existential dread which apparently afflicted people during this period, and the consequent search for faith and spiritual authority which elevated four Renaissance figures. In the margin you might write:

spiritual terrors>>4 seers

Paragraph 3:

This paragraph focuses on the individual authorities of interest to the author, and identifies each one's intellectual propensity. In the margin you might write:

intellectual essence of the 4

Paragraph 4:

The excerpt's final paragraph further elaborates on the attitudes and orientations of the four individuals, and observes that their teachings have endured through the centuries to become commonplaces of wisdom in our own times. In the margin you might write:

their perceptions>>truisms

You can learn to map a typical MCAT-like passage in approximately one minute. Chapter 45 will give you practice.

44.2 DIRECTIONAL ARROWS

While skimming a passage, look for words or phrases that signal direction. Certain words indicate that a point just made might be confirmed, or shifted, or conditioned, or reversed, or undercut, or otherwise modified. Words like, "therefore," "hence," and "thus"—signal that a conclusion will be drawn.

Look at the twenty words and phrases listed below. Each is a directional arrow.

> Accordingly
> But
> Consequently
> Conversely
> Despite
> Hence
> However
> In this connection
> In spite of
> Ironically
> Nonetheless
> Notwithstanding
> On the contrary
> On the other hand
> Rather
> Regardless
> Still
> Therefore
> Unfortunately
> Yet

While making your map, look for words and phrases like these. Circle them. When, later, you return to the passage to read closely *some* of its text, the circled words will help you understand it and answer questions.

Consider the last sentence of excerpt 44A:

If the cocoon of time, however, has metamorphosed their vital truths into well-learned platitudes, these are platitudes essentially undulled by the fleeting years; and for being basic, they are no less primary.

"However" is a signal. How does it help you? It helps you see the author's point which is this: The insights described in the passage might be platitudes. Nonetheless, they are as valid now as they were when first set forth.

44.3 SETTLING ON CORRECT ANSWERS

After mapping the passage and noting directional arrows, you are ready to answer questions according to this system:

1. Read the question.

2. Ask yourself, "Is it peripheral?" (See chapter 42.) If the answer is yes, answer it on the basis of the stem and your own resources of logic. Don't revisit the passage. If the answer is no, then

3. Read your map, and locate the relevant text in the passage.

4. Carefully read the relevant sentences.

5. Return to the question and consider the answer options.

At this point, one answer choice may "leap out," and look right. But be skeptical of your first instinct. Be wary. Distracters are everywhere. Look for manglers, seducers, and irrelevant truths. Discard them. Look for absolutes. If you find them, determine whether they are so exaggerated as to exceed the author's meaning. With some distracters thus eliminated, study those one or two that remain. Remember, as noted in chapter 42, that *the right answer is often disguised*. The answer choice that initially seemed least promising might be right. Find it, select it, and move on.

Sometimes you may read the stem, revisit the passage, scrutinize the answer choices and still—nothing will seem correct. When that happens the reason is usually that

(1) The question is peripheral and you have failed to realize it, or

(2) the "disguise" continues to fool you.

Ask yourself, *again*, "Is this question peripheral?" If the answer is yes, know that the answer will not come from the passage but from (1) the stem and (2) your own resources of logic and understanding. If the answer is no, repeat steps 4 and 5. Carefully reread the relevant text and return to the answer options. Among the choices not yet eliminated, look for a correct answer *in disguise*. You will probably find it. If not, make your best guess and move on.

44.4: SPECIAL CONSIDERATION: AUTHOR'S ATTITUDE

Occasionally, an MCAT question will ask the student to characterize the author's attitude, feeling, or state of mind. Frequently, the options are limited to single adjectives:

1. Regarding...etc., etc., etc.,...the author's attitude was:

   A. disapproving
   B. incredulous
   C. open-minded
   D. intrigued

2. In this passage, the author's basic feeling was one of:

   A. security
   B. relief
   C. confidence
   D. anticipation

Consider this excerpt from a simulated MCAT passage:

> Having concluded that I would probably never come fully to comprehend the nature of the force— or forces?—responsible for these strange visitations in her life, I at last found in my imagination a meta-

phor that made sense to me, and for some reason afforded me a measure of tranquillity. I'd lately been struck with the idea that somehow, for some mysterious motive, a window had been shown to me. Whether this window opened onto another dimension, another world, a top-secret governmental apparatus, the angelic operations of the divine, or the diabolic enterprise of the demon, I did not know, could not know, might never know, it seemed. I looked to my *only hope* and took from it a positive feeling. I had to decide that whatever the source and motive of these powers clearly beyond my knowledge and well beyond my control, I'd best not ignore them, and intending my moral relativist's level best, would do my best to understand their purpose and their meaning.

The author's decision as to how best to deal with her perceptions and experiences left her feeling:

A. knowledgeable.
B. empty.
C. hopeful.
D. exuberant.

For questions like this, distracters are particularly confusing. Convert the question into a true/false statement:

TRUE OR FALSE: The author was left feeling _____.

Make four sentences by completing the blank with each of the answer options. One sentence will likely seem more sensible and accurate than the other three. That sentence reveals the correct answer.

Apply the technique to the question above:

TRUE OR FALSE: The author was (left feeling) <u>knowledgeable</u>

TRUE OR FALSE: The author was (left feeling) <u>empty</u>

TRUE OR FALSE: The author was (left feeling) <u>optimistic</u>

TRUE OR FALSE: The author was (left feeling) <u>exuberant.</u>

Option C sounds most likely. Was the author knowledgeable? On the contrary, she writes, "...I did not know, could not know, might never know, it seemed..." Was she therefore feeling empty? No. Was she exuberant? Not quite. A good case could probably be made for both of those! Nonetheless, the question wants to know how she was *left feeling* after her decision? The relevant information is found in the final sentence:

I looked to my *only hope* and took from it a positive feeling. I had to decide that whatever the source and motive of these powers clearly beyond my knowledge and well beyond my control, I'd best not ignore them, and intending my moral relativist's level best, would do my best to understand their purpose and their meaning.

Below, a social sciences passage is presented for the student to practice the special technique for author's attitude questions:

Over the past decade, the line between news and entertainment has become increasingly blurred. When Norman Lear's *All In The Family* opened its hugely successful tenure as a prime-time situation comedy in the early seventies, it pioneered the entertainment vehicle as a forum for discussion of the critical social issues of the day, questions which until that time had remained entirely within the province of the news divisions. Around the same time, television news underwent a quantum evolution: from something akin to a prudent parrot of government propaganda, it developed almost overnight into a powerful, non-partisan, independently-thinking entity devoted to an honest, objective exploration of government, society, and the world.

A decade after Watergate, however, the media's objectivity began to blur its focus in the intoxicating ether of the freewheeling eighties. Where once a noble quest for truth and reason had defined the goal, the new programmers, driven by a lust for economic supremacy, now fixated and obsessed on the bottom line. Profitability became the primary organizational principle, and ratings represented the golden gate to profits. Whatever excited, whatever entertained, whatever titillated, whatever sold: these fields of straw became the fecund yellow ground for journalists of the electronic media!

1. In these two paragraphs the author's attitude in reference to the media is most accurately described as:

   A. ironic
   B. approving
   C. congratulatory
   D. apathetic

The technique calls for the student to construct four TRUE/FALSE statements, one for each answer option.

About the media, the author remarked:

- the media's objectivity began to blur

- Whatever excited, whatever entertained, whatever titillated, whatever sold: these fields of straw became the fecund yellow ground for journalists of the electronic media!

TRUE OR FALSE: This person was (being) <u>ironic.</u>

TRUE OR FALSE: This person was (being) <u>approving.</u>

TRUE OR FALSE: This person was (being) <u>congratulatory.</u>

TRUE OR FALSE: This person was (being) <u>apathetic.</u>

Surely, option D sounds false. The author's tone in discussing the subject does not lack concern or energy. Some might argue that in the first paragraph of this excerpt the author enthusiastically applauds the media's coming-of-age:

- ...pioneered the entertainment vehicle as a forum for discussion of the critical social issues of the day....

- ...television news underwent a quantum evolution...into a powerful, non-partisan, independently-thinking entity devoted to an honest, objective exploration...

Accordingly, distracters B and C might tempt some test-takers with some justification. Nonetheless, the final paragraph casts those earlier observations into shadow, and the author concludes the essay on an ironic note. The correct answer is A.

CHAPTER 45

NINE SAMPLE
VERBAL REASONING PASSAGES

45.1 PASSAGE I

45.1.1 Passage and Questions

In the context of rising global competition for finite resources and trade, America approaches the 21st century confronting a broad agenda of perplexing policy questions.
5 Not only must we prepare ourselves to deal successfully with the realities of advanced technology, surging international expertise and international productivity, we must also design effective strategies to remedy the hard
10 social problems emerging from current domestic demographic trends. Because meeting these diverse national challenges will require a citizenry equipped with advanced knowledge and superior skills, the need for
15 higher education and professional training becomes greater than perhaps at any period in our history.

In times of economic cutbacks and downsizing, however, when real wages for
20 most Americans continue to shrink even as the national economy grows, voters are wary of proposals to increase—or even maintain—current levels of government spending. They equate increased spending with increased
25 taxation. Yet recent studies make clear that over the long run, increased financial support for education combined with increased access for all citizens to the nation's colleges and universities will offer advantages to all
30 taxpayers, regardless of economic status.

Even among those who advocate cutting higher education's budget, few would question the immediate practical benefits of post-secondary schooling to the individual stu-
35 dent, or "consumer" of learning. Figures show, for example, that increases in individual earnings relate directly to educational achievement: the higher the level of education completed, the higher the income. Ac-
40 cording to White House data, the mean earnings of a college graduate in 1992 reached almost $40,000, 25% higher than those of persons who started college but did not finish, and more than 60% above that of indi-
45 viduals with no schooling at all beyond high school. This last group, in turn, earned 25% more than those who did not finish high school.

A similar correspondence occurs with
50 unemployment statistics: as years of schooling increase, the probability of joblessness diminishes. Thus, the 1993 unemployment rate for those who completed college was only 3.5%, less than half the 7.2% for high
55 school graduates with no college at all. Experiencing a joblessness rate just about midway between those levels, at 5.7%, as might be expected, were people with some college credits still short of graduation. High school
60 dropouts, meanwhile, again suffered most, with a 12.6% rate of unemployment, almost double that of high school graduates.

The more education one acquires, then, the more likely he or she is to find work, and
65 at a higher salary. Of course, as salaries increase, so do taxes. An individual who attains a higher degree of education also generally achieves a higher tax bracket. What might be less apparent, although critical for
70 determining policy, is that taking federal income tax revenues as a whole, the percentage paid by college graduates is considerably out of proportion with their numbers in the population.

75 A recent issue of the "Post-secondary Education Opportunity" research newsletter reported government statistics demonstrating that as of 1991, college graduates headed 23% of U.S. households which together ac-
80 counted for 43.2% of annual I.R.S. revenues. (Conversely, 54.9% of U.S. households that year were headed by individuals with no college at all, and they paid only 33.9% of all federal income taxes. Heads of households
85 with some college credit who did not attain a diploma made up the rest.)

These analyses further indicate that between 1970 and 1991, as the percentage of college-educated citizens increased among
90 the population so did the size of the middle class, and with it, the tax base of higher-wage earners as well. As one well-known Chicago business leader testified before the National Commission on Responsibilities for Financ-

ing Post-secondary Education (NCRFPE), "It
95 seems to me that the social costs of no education or miseducation may very well exceed
the finite costs of a sound, competitive education . . . I think we might demonstrate that
a strategic investment in education is a rela-
100 tive bargain."

1. A sociologist recently proclaimed, "It is
   sad but true that a college degree has lost
   much of its educational significance. An
   institution that calls itself 'college,'
   might receive government funding and
   yet offer courses on almost any topic at
   all, many of them unrelated to the sciences and humanities as we once knew
   them." This sociologist would probably
   want the government to fund only those
   colleges:

   A. at which professors enjoy significant
      autonomy in the design of their
      courses and curricula.
   B. whose curricula fall within objec-
      tively defined specifications.
   C. where students are required to con-
      centrate their studies on a relatively
      narrow body of subject matter.
   D. that prepare students for profitable
      professions and careers.

2. The author's statement that voters are
   wary of increased government expenditure on education suggests that such
   wariness:

   I.   represents concern over in-
        creased taxation.
   II. arises from their hesitancy to
        bear financial responsibility for
        the associated cost.
   III. reflects their belief that college
        education no longer serves any
        significant needs of the society at
        large.

   A. I only
   B. I and II only
   C. I and III only
   D. I, II, and III

3. What evidence does the author introduce to support his assertion that few
   would question the immediate practical
   benefits of post-secondary schooling to
   the individual student?

   I.   Students who continue educa-
        tion beyond high school enjoy a
        better economic status than
        those who do not.
   II. Most Americans experience a re-
        duction in real wages even
        though the nation's economy is
        expanding.
   III. Increases in salary correspond to
        increases in taxation.

   A. I only
   B. I and II only
   C. I and III only
   D. I, II, and III

4. Which of the following, if true, would
   best strengthen the author's view that
   America needs to promote higher education and professional training?

   A. Large numbers of American college
      students are foreign born and tend
      to return to their native countries
      after graduation.
   B. American colleges have become in-
      creasingly dependent on charitable
      donations from their alumni and
      other philanthropic donors.
   C. Most graduates of American col-
      leges do not pursue post-graduate
      or professional training.
   D. Foreign nations that invest in edu-
      cation consistently demonstrate in-
      creased economic growth and
      greater per capita income.

5. According to the passage, which of the following statements most accurately describes the relevance of technological advance to education?

   A. Rapid technological advances have no place in determining public education policy.
   B. Rapid technological advances have made it more difficult for students to make effective use of higher education.
   C. Rapid technological advances have made universal access to higher education a national objective.
   D. Rapid technological advances have made universal access to higher education a luxury generally reserved for the wealthy.

6. Analysts for the newsletter "Post-secondary Education Opportunity" reported that between 1970 and 1991:

   A. the percentage of college-educated citizens decreased among the population.
   B. the tax base of higher wage earners decreased among the population.
   C. the tax base of higher wage earners increased among the population.
   D. the size of the upper class increased among the population.

7. According to the passage, "current domestic demographic trends" will cause the society to experience:

   A. greater barriers to opportunity because of international competition.
   B. greater and more challenging social problems.
   C. social problems that are more easily remedied.
   D. the elimination of most educational barriers to opportunity.

8. According to the data presented in the passage, educational level correlates:

   A. positively with income level and unemployment.
   B. positively with unemployment and negatively with income level.
   C. negatively with tax payments and unemployment.
   D. positively with tax payments and negatively with unemployment.

9. The author's general attitude about the nation's future would best be described as:

   A. cynical.
   B. optimistic.
   C. concerned.
   D. apathetic.

45.1.2 PASSAGE I QUESTIONS ANSWERED

1. *B is correct.* The question is peripheral to the passage. It requires only that we first understand the sociologist's sentiment and then recognize it *in disguise*. The sociologist is concerned that an institution might receive government funding and yet call itself "college" regardless of the courses it offers. She would prefer that the government tie its funding to requirements regarding curriculum. Choice B sets forth that same sentiment *in disguise*. Choice A is a seducer; it "sounds good," but is not at all the sort of thing for which this sociologist would argue in view of the concern she expresses. Choice C is unresponsive to the stem. The sociologists expresses no concern about narrowness or breadth, but about curriculum and subject matter. Choice D is an irrelevant truth. The passage's author does express certain concerns regarding professions and economic advancement, but this sociologist does *not*.

2. *B is correct.* The relevant text is in paragraph 2, which concerns, generally, the reluctance of some citizens to favor increased expenditure for education. The paragraph's chief message is that (1) improved educational resources carry a cost, presumably in the form of taxation, and (2) that many citizens are resistant to increased taxation. Statements I and II reflect both those propositions. Statement III is not embodied in paragraph 2 and is *contradicted* by paragraph 3, in which the author states that even those who resist increased expenditure nonetheless acknowledge the practical benefit that would be associated with improved educational resources.

3. *A is correct.* The pertinent text is in paragraph 3 whose principal point is that education yields practical benefits. Among the data offered to support the point is that "This last group," meaning those whose education ends at high school graduation, "earned 25% more than those who did not finish high school." Statement II represents an irrelevant truth. It embodies a statement genuinely made in the passage (at paragraph 2), but it does not logically follow the stem. Statement III is a mangler. (If the last word were "earnings" and not "taxation," it might then correctly apply.) The author does state (at paragraph 5) that increased earnings produce increased taxation. She does not, however, offer that proposition as evidence that few would question the practical benefits of education for the student.

4. *D is correct.* The question is peripheral to the passage. It calls for (1) attention to the stem, and (2) logic. There is a meaningful logical connection between the propositions that (1) America will reap economic gain by investing in education, and (2) other countries have reaped gain by making that investment. Choice A does not logically follow from the stem. Choices B and C are seductive, but wrong. We might have heard that colleges are increasingly dependent on charitable donations and it might be our impression that most college students do not pursue formal education after they graduate. Accurate or not, such statements do not logically follow the stem.

5. *C is correct.* The relevant text is in the first paragraph. The author cites technological advance (among other matters) as a challenge that increases the need for higher education. The words "access" and "universal" tend to *disguise* the statement, but the statement closely reflects the author's meaning. Choice A is contrary to the author's view as expressed at paragraph 1. Choice B is a seducer. The passage addresses a problem, choice B seems to describe a problem, and superficial examination gives B a "ring" of plausibility. Yet the author makes no such statement as is made in choice B. Choice D is seductive as well, and the student who loses sight of the stem might be drawn to it. There *is* ongoing national concern over the availability of higher education to those who are not wealthy. But the author nowhere states that *technological advance* has produced such a problem.

6. *C is correct.* The question directs us to paragraphs 6 and 7, where the author refers to the newsletter and its analyses. In paragraph 7 she states that according to the newsletter analyses, the middle class has grown and the tax base of higher wage earners has increased. Choice A is seductive because it suggests that too few citizens attend college and the author seems to regard that as a problem. Yet the author nowhere refers to any such problem *in connection with the newsletter*. Choice B is a mangler; it presents the word "decreased" where it should present the word "increased" (as is correctly presented in choice C). Choice D is a mangler as well. The author refers to the increased size of the *middle* class and the increased *tax base* of higher wage earners.

7. *B is correct.* The relevant text is in paragraph 1. The author refers to a number of phenomena including technological advance, surging international expertise and productivity, and *current domestic trends*. All of these, the author writes, will produce society with "diverse national challenges." The phrase "greater and more challenging social problems," as set forth in choice B reflects the author's thinking with some *disguise*. Choices A and D are manglers. They resort to words and concepts within the passage like "opportunity" and "international," but combine them in a way that does not reflect the author's thinking or respond to the question stem. Choice C is contrary to the message set forth in paragraph 1.

8. *D is correct.* The relevant material is in paragraphs 4 and 5, whose principal messages are that education produces higher rates of employment (lower rates of <u>un</u>employment) and increased tax payments. The distracters A, B, and C are designed to make the student's head spin. If patiently, properly, and carefully read, each proves itself wrong. Choices A and B indicate that education correlates positively with <u>un</u>employment. Choice C indicates that it correlates *negatively* with tax payments.

9. *C is correct.* The question requires that we get a "feel" for the author's attitude and tone. The author describes a problem and urges that it be solved; she is *concerned*. She is not apathetic for that would suggest a *lack* of concern. She is worried, but not cynical. Neither is she particularly hopeful or optimistic.

45.2 PASSAGE II

45.2.1 Passage and Questions

The question of how forager honeybees communicate to their hivemates the exact location of new food sources has perplexed naturalists at least since Aristotle observed
5 the phenomenon in the fourth century BC. Only in this century have scientists determined that several characteristics of honeybee dances vary precisely according to the geographic relation between the nest and the
10 food source. Even more recently, experimenters have demonstrated that honeybee communication occurs along a multisensory pathway, of which some sensory channels appear to be more crucial than others.

15 After locating a new food source, a forager bee returns to the hive and initiates an intricate series of movements, including wiggles of the bee's body, as well as brief looping figure-eights over a circumscribed
20 area of the comb. Other bees observe this dance, and some observers follow the forager in her movements, as though learning the dance steps by rote imitation. In 1943, Karl von Frisch established an exact correlation
25 between the dancing bee's spatial orientation as she looped in eights—straight up, or angled to the left or right—and the sun's relation to the new food source. Furthermore, von Frisch concluded that the rate at which
30 the dance leader beats her wings supplies specific information about the hive-to-source distance. During the first half of this century, investigators believed that the visual spectacle of the forager bee's dance provided all
35 the signals necessary to inform the dance observers about the food location, and recruit them to it.

Despite the elegance of von Frisch's correlations, however, a nagging conundrum re-
40 mained: given the darkness of the interior hive, how could the bees see the dance movements? Researchers Wolfgang Kirchner, William Towne, and Alex Michelsen measured minute changes in air currents close to the
45 forager dance leader's body, and later deter-
mined that dance observers detect these changes in air flow as low-frequency sound, through Johnson's organ, a bilateral cluster of nerve cells on the second joint of each an-
50 tenna. By virtue of these vibratory sonic signals—the dancesong, so to say—honeybees can learn and follow the route to a new food site.

Other experiments added interesting
55 details to the process of honeybee dance communication, indicating that it rests on multisensory mechanisms. At certain points during the dance, for example, the dance attenders will press against the honeycomb
60 with their thoraxes, producing a quick squeaking noise. When the dance leader hears this sound, she pauses in her movements to distribute a bit of the food she has found as samples to her hivemates. On the
65 basis of these observations, Kirchner and Michelsen concluded that taste and odor also play a role in identifying a new food source to the hive. Later investigations showed, however, that bees with congenitally or sur-
70 gically shortened wings, who could not emit sonic signals in the dance, were not able to recruit nestmates to the food source, even though dance observers who were not given taste and odor samples did learn new loca-
75 tions based on the dancesong alone.

Without the dance, forager bees cannot inform their hivemates how to find food; without food, workers in the nest cannot provide sustenance for the Queen; without
80 sustenance, the Queen—and so, the hive—cannot survive. In describing his view of the rhythmic vitality of the universe, the groundbreaking English psychologist Havelock Ellis wrote: "Dancing . . . is no mere
85 translation or abstraction from life; it is life itself." However accurate that perception may be in general, it is absolutely true for honeybees.

10. Which of the following best describes the principal subject of the passage?

   A. Research techniques concerning communicative methods among honeybees
   B. The maintenance of social structure among honeybees
   C. The role of the honeybee's dance as a nonvisual form of communication
   D. An elucidation of the way in which honeybees communicate regarding the location of food

11. The fact that forager bees must perform a dance to direct their hivemates to a food source is used to support the author's point that:

   A. the queen cannot survive without well-nourished workers.
   B. honeybees perceive dance as changes in air flow.
   C. for the honeybee, dance is equivalent to life itself.
   D. honeybee communication occurs along a multisensory pathway.

12. In relation to the passage the word *elegance* (line 13) means:

   A. precision.
   B. tastefulness.
   C. gracefulness.
   D. propriety.

13. As described in the passage, the fact that bees with shortened wings are unable to communicate effectively most strongly suggests that:

   A. taste and odor signals are more important to communication than is the dancesong.
   B. the dancesong is more important to communication than are taste and odor signals.
   C. normal wings are not necessary to the emission of sonic signals.
   D. communication among honeybees is a multisensory phenomenon.

14. If the author were to write a critical assessment of researchers who have studied honeybee communication, he would most likely regard Karl von Frisch with:

   A. disapproval, because he did not address the issues with appropriate scientific thoroughness.
   B. indifference, because he added only slightly to that which Aristotle had reported in the fourth century BC.
   C. respect, because his work was refined and scientific even though it left certain questions unanswered.
   D. awe, because he correctly theorized that the dancesong was effective primarily as a visual signal.

15. The honeybee is traditionally described as a "social organism." If the author were to take note of that description in the passage, he would most likely do so in order to:

    A. prove that for many species the procurement of food requires interaction among individual members.
    B. illustrate the fact that the dancesong is ineffective without auditory and visual components.
    C. emphasize that the honeybee depends on communication for its survival.
    D. establish that honeybees live according to a hierarchy that includes a queen and foragers.

16. The author suggests that a forager bee communicates information about each of the following EXCEPT:

    A. the color of the flower at which food is located.
    B. the odor given off by food.
    C. the distance between a food source and the hive.
    D. the direction of a food source from the hive.

17. According to the information in the passage, which of the following statements is accurate?

    I. Bees cannot learn of food source locations without the ability to sense taste and odor.
    II. Bees can communicate food source locations by sound and movement alone.
    III. Bees can communicate food source locations by taste and odor alone.

    A. I only
    B. II only
    C. I and II only
    D. I, II, and III

45.2.2 PASSAGE II QUESTIONS ANSWERED

10. *D is correct*. The student should crudely characterize the passage's main topic. Roughly, the passage is about the honeybees' dancesong, which is the means through which they communicate regarding the location of food. Knowing that, the student should look among the choices for a phrase of like meaning. Choice D does not mention the dancesong explicitly, but among the choices it most closely mirrors the crude characterization just set forth. Choices A and B pertain to subjects on which the author does touch but not on that which represents the passage's *principal* subject. Choice C is not so good as Choice D, for it refers to the *role* of the honeybees' dance song, which is not the author's chief topic. The author discusses the dancesong in general—its role, the way in which it has been studied and understood, and the way in which it operates.

11. *C is correct*. The question *stem* does not direct the student to any particular portion of the passage, but the answer choices do. Choices A, C, and D point to paragraph 5, choice B to paragraph 3. To select among the four, the student must focus on and comprehend the *stem*. Ask: "which among the four choices reflects a point that the author supports by noting that the dancesong is essential to the location of food?" At the beginning of paragraph 5, we read that without the dancesong, the bees "cannot inform their hivemates how to find food . . ." The remainder of the paragraph builds from that observation toward a conclusion (a point) that, for the honeybee, *dance is life itself*. Choices A, B, and D direct the student's attention away from the stem. Each represents a statement made in the passage, but none responds sensibly to the stem.

12. *A is correct*. The stem clearly directs the student to the beginning of paragraph 3, where the "elegance" appears. The student must "read around" the word and determine which among the answer choices best restates its meaning in context. If the correct answer is not immediately evident, substitute the word tied to each answer choice into the sentence and determine whether it makes for sense and meaning. "Despite the *precision* of von Frisch's correlations . . ." is sensible and meaningful within the surrounding context. In paragraph 2 the author describes certain correlations and findings put forth by von Frisch and they might well be called precise. "Despite the *tastefulness* of von Frisch's correlations . . ." and "Despite the *gracefulness* of von Frisch's correlations . . ." create no sensible meaning. "Despite the *propriety* of von Frisch's correlations . . ." is not meaningless, but it is not well aligned with the author's meaning. The author intends to focus on the fact that von Frisch's experiments showed care, subtlety, refinement, and attention to detail.

13. *B is correct*. The stem points to paragraph 4 where the author writes of bees with surgically shortened wings. Reading closely the surrounding text we learn that taste and odor signals play a role in communication regarding food source. We learn further that bees with surgically shortened wings cannot emit sonic signals and thus lose their ability to communicate effectively, even if their "audience" are given taste and odor signals. On the other hand, in the absence of taste and odor signals a honeybee does communicate if its wings emit appropriate sonic signals. The point? The dancesong is more important to communication than are taste and odor signals. Choices A and C are contrary to the text. Choice D represents an irrelevant truth. The author does characterize honeybee communication as a multisensory phenomenon (at paragraphs 1 and 4), but that fact bears no logical relationship to the stem.

14. *C is correct*. The question points to paragraphs 2 and 3. At paragraph 2 the author describes von Frisch's work, and at paragraph 3 he calls the correlations elegant. The author's attitude toward von Frisch is *positive*, which eliminates A and B, leaving us to choose between C and D. In the first sentence of paragraph 3 the author describes von

Frisch's correlations as elegant, but notes that a "nagging conundrum remained..." Choice C expresses that same message *in disguise*. The words "refined" and "scientific" roughly reflect the meaning of "elegance." The phrase "it left certain questions unanswered" roughly reflects the "nagging conundrum" that "remained." Choice D is a mangler. It refers to "visual signal," a concept that does appear in the passage (at paragraph 2). Yet choice D distorts the author's meaning. Paragraph 3 teaches us that those who thought the dancesong to operate as a visual signal were <u>in</u>correct. Researchers who followed von Frisch demonstrated that it operated primarily as a *sonic* signal.

15. *C is correct.* The question is peripheral to the passage. To a degree it tests your understanding of "social." Consider the phrase and ask which of the answer choices best relates to it. The concepts of <u>soci</u>ality, and <u>soci</u>ety refer, generally, to cooperative interaction. All four choices bear, in some sense, on cooperative interaction. Choice B, however, is a mangler. The dancesong, we learn, does *not* operate as a visual cue. Sociality does not pertain specifically to food or to hierarchies but to cooperation and interaction *in general*. Pivoting on the word "communication," choice C is better than A or D.

16. *A is correct.* Notice the word "EXCEPT," and search among the answer options for the one form of information that the passage does NOT associate with honeybee communication regarding food source. Ask:
    For choice A, "Does the passage indicate that honeybee communication carries information regarding *flower color*?" Answer: **no**. A is correct.
    For choice B, "Does the passage indicate that honeybee communication carries information regarding *odor*?" Answer: yes, in paragraph 4
    For choice C, "Does the passage indicate that honeybee communication carries information regarding *distance*?" Answer: yes, in paragraph 2
    For choice D, "Does the passage indicate that honeybee communication carries information regarding *direction*?" Answer: yes, in paragraph 2. The phrase "sun's relation to the new food source" concerns direction.

17. *B is correct.* The relevant information is in paragraph 4. Reading it closely for meaning, we learn that the honeybee who cannot emit sound signals cannot communicate. Sound signal is vital to the communication. Furthermore, if "observers" receive no taste and odor cues they understand the dancer's communication through the dance alone. To understand the communication, observers *need* the dance, and that is *all* they need. Statement II is accurate. Statements I and III spin the student's head and mangle the author's meaning. Honeybees *can* learn of food source without taste and odor signals and they can<u>not</u> do so through taste and odor cues alone.

45.3 PASSAGE III

45.3.1 Passage and Questions

Perhaps the most salient artistic revelation generated by the Impressionist aesthetic is the inclusion of *movement* as a crucial element of human perception and experience.
5 Impressionist painters, for example, sought to portray on their canvases more than the mere form and beauty of the world before them: they needed to convey the transient quality of reality's composition, and of the
10 artist's individual observations of reality as well. In the world of literature, the Symbolist writers adopted the Impressionist commitment to transience by disdaining narrative exactitude and precision in favor of sug-
15 gestion and inference.

Wholesale transformations in the structure and function of social, economic, and political relationships impelled artists to abandon ideas of permanence, and to recog-
20 nize the ever-changing nature of the universe. The painters spurned a photographic imitation of reality as too static, and thereby untrue to human life. They developed new strategies of color and stroke to depict a vi-
25 sion of volume and shape actively shifting moment by moment, techniques which reached their zenith, perhaps, in the Pointillist school. Meanwhile, the Symbolist poets and novelists delved into the worlds
30 of dream, fantasy and myth for their visions, implying that the inner lens of the human spirit provided a truer representation of human perceptions than might a narrower, journalistic focus on events.

35 Where graphic artists forfeited realism to seize on perception, and writers surrendered verbatim description to immerse themselves in stream-of-consciousness and inner monologue, musical artists sacrificed
40 the formalistic restrictions and formulaic preconceptions of traditional techniques to emphasize and exalt sensation and feeling. Among the greatest of the Impressionist composers stands Claude-Achille Debussy,
45 who affirmed that in his music he wanted "to reproduce what I hear" in the world. His emphasis on the subjective sensation of his hearing over the aural, physical and mathematical structures of sound, drove him to
50 shed inhibitions, to revere spontaneity, and reclaim freedom. In part, his objective was to prevent his listeners from responding to his music on an intellectual plane, and so he purposefully ruptured their conventional
55 expectations by rejecting cliché and arbitrary limitations, aiming instead to liberate his audience with compositions that reproduced the textures and immediacy of improvisation.

60 To achieve his ambitious artistic goals, and in accordance with Impressionist priorities, Debussy engineered a thorough expurgation of major-minor key progressions, so rigid and inflexible in their rules and rela-
65 tionships; he explored and exploited the pentatonic scales for innovative approaches to harmony, while the seemingly haphazard meanderings of his melodies drew heavily on the eastern musical forms: arabesques,
70 and even whole-tone scales, so alien and incongruous to the western ear. Perhaps even more importantly, Debussy ushered in a new ascendancy for harmony, whose role until his era had always been decidedly subservient
75 to melody. Now harmony acquired an identity and a dimension all its own, no longer regimented and subjugated by a strictly controlled melodic tyranny, but free, willful and expressive of its own truth, its own sensa-
80 tions, constantly shifting the resonant background through and against which his melody wove.

Debussy's third great Impressionistic contribution consisted of the revolutionary
85 principles of orchestration he introduced. Where earlier composers had conventionally divided their musicians into distinctly compartmentalized and segregated sections—woodwind, brass, percussion and string—
90 Debussy conceived of his orchestra not by category, but instrument by instrument. Each

musician played a crucial and independent part, the flow and ebb of each instrument's timbre providing essential if fleeting detail
95 within the elusive whole, producing an overall effect of multilayered sensation and pointillist evanescence looming, dissipating, and emerging yet again within a multicolored matrix of continual flux and movement.

18. The central thesis of the passage is that:

   A. Impressionism evolved first in painting, and only later in the other arts.
   B. Impressionism was limited primarily to the avant-garde artists.
   C. Impressionism became popular in several art forms to communicate visions of change and movement.
   D. Impressionism represents the zenith of visionary artistic movements.

19. As used in the passage, the term *freedom* (line 51) refers to Debussy's wish to:

   A. separate his work from the restrictions imposed on the graphic arts and literature.
   B. create music that did not necessarily adhere to preexisting conventions of form and technique.
   C. teach his audiences that their lives should not be ruled by their intellects.
   D. mark the distinction between perception on the one hand and sensation and feeling on the other.

20. The author implies that the Symbolist writers differed from their predecessors in that they:

   A. preoccupied themselves with fact and exactitude.
   B. invested their writings with allusion and subtlety.
   C. rejected stream-of-consciousness techniques.
   D. believed that mythical imagery was better suited to painting than to novels.

21. According to the passage, Impressionism had which of the following effects on painters, writers, and composers?

   A. It gave them their first united vision of the human condition.
   B. It caused them to lose the approval of artists of earlier schools.
   C. It inspired them to depict reality as dynamic rather than stationary.
   D. It helped them to appreciate the essential similarities among their art forms.

22. The passage indicates that Debussy made use of the pentatonic scales primarily in order to:

    A. construct melodies that pleased his own ears.
    B. avoid the melodic chaos that had previously characterized his music.
    C. reveal himself to the artistic community as a composer with ambitious objectives.
    D. create music that was not constrained by the major-minor key relationships of his day.

23. The author mentions the Pointillist school in the second paragraph in order to illustrate:

    A. the Impressionists' tendency to have their paintings depict movement.
    B. the Impressionists' general disdain for photography.
    C. the analogy between Symbolist writing and Impressionistic painting.
    D. the interdependency of color and shape.

24. According to the author, which of the following contributed most directly to the development of Impressionism?

    A. The recognition by artists that truth could not be depicted by any one art form
    B. The rapid emergence of photographic technologies
    C. Significant changes in the society and its underpinnings
    D. The unwillingness of most people to value their own perceptions and sensations

45.3.2 PASSAGE III QUESTIONS ANSWERED

18. *C is correct.* The student should quickly and crudely characterize the passage's main topic. Roughly, the passage is about Impressionism, its focus on motion and change, and the way it affected a variety of art forms. Choice C offers a sentence of like meaning. Choices A and D are seducers. A student who fails to keep his mind on the stem and the passage might choose A simply because the author first describes Impressionist painters and then other kinds of artists. Choice D does not reflect the author's central thesis even though the author does seem to regard Impressionism favorably and to believe that Impressionist artists were innovative. Furthermore, choice D is a mangler. More than once, the author uses the word "vision" in connection with Impressionism, and in paragraph 2 the author notes that the Pointillist school constituted the "zenith" of certain techniques associated with Impressionism. Choice B is wild, setting forth a statement not made in the passage.

19. *B is correct.* The word "freedom" appears near the end of paragraph 3. Study its context. Learn that Impressionistic composers like Debussy "sacrificed the formalistic restrictions and formulaic preconceptions of traditional techniques." Debussy rejected "arbitrary limitations" imposed by convention and so "ruptured" "conventional expectations." Choice B consolidates such statements *in disguise.* Choice A is a mangler. The passage refers to a rejection of restrictions, to the graphic arts, and to literature. Nowhere, however, does it suggest that Impressionist composers sought to separate their work from restrictions imposed on other kinds of artists. Choice D, too, is a mangler, making inappropriate use of the words "perception," "sensation," and "feeling," all of which do appear in the passage. Choice C is both a mangler and a seducer. In paragraph 3 the author refers to "intellect," but nowhere speaks of lives being *ruled* by intellect. Yet the student who loses sight of the stem might think "it sounds good—people should not let intellect *rule* their lives. Emotion is important as well." Attractive or not, that idea does not respond to the stem.

20. *B is correct.* The author discusses symbolist writers (poets and novelists) at the end of paragraph 2 and the beginning of paragraph 3. We learn that they probed the worlds of "dream and fantasy," surrendering "verbatim descriptions" in favor of "stream-of consciousness and inner monologue." Choice B attempts to make similar statements in disguise. If that is not evident, consider the distracters and eliminate them. Choices A and C borrow words from the passage but express a meaning opposite to the author's. Choice D is a mangler, using words from the passage to make a statement not made by the author.

21. *C is correct.* The stem concerns Impressionism and its effect on painters, writers, and composers (all three). Throughout the passage we learn that Impressionist artists rejected arbitrary limitations, narrative exactitude, mathematical precision, and somehow invested their art with movement. With its use of the words "stationary" and "dynamic," Choice C summarizes such statements *in disguise.* Choices A , B, and D are seducers. They all speak favorably of Impressionists as the author seems to do. The student who loses sight of the stem and the passage might easily conclude that a new artistic movement produced disapproval among more conservative artists. He might think well of a "united vision of the human condition." He might believe it a "good thing" that artists should appreciate the similarities of their work.

22. *D is correct*. The relevant text appears at the beginning of paragraph 4 where we learn that Debussy made an "expurgation of major-minor key progressions." As a part of that process he "explored the pentatonic scales." Choice D summarizes those statements in disguise. Choices A, B, and C are manglers. They misuse, respectively (A) the reference to Debussy's wish to "reproduce what I hear," (B) the appearance of the word "haphazard" in paragraph 4, and (C) the use of the phrase "ambitious goals" at the beginning of paragraph 4.

23. *A is correct*. In paragraph 3 the author describes the Pointillist school as the "zenith" of "new strategies" that depicted "volume and shape actively shifting moment by moment." Choice A summarizes that statement *in disguise*. Choices B and C represent irrelevant truths. It is true that (a) impressionist painters did not wish their art to resemble photography, and (b) the author analogizes Symbolist writing to impressionism. Neither of those truths pertains to the author's mention of the Pointillism. Choice D is a seducer. It is easy and tempting to believe that a painter sees an interdependency between color and shape. It "sounds right." Yet the author makes no such statement and, in any event, no such statement logically follows the stem.

24. *C is correct*. The relevant text is in paragraph 2. "Wholesale transformations in the structure and function of social, economic, and political relationships..." inspired impressionism. Choice C reflects that message *in disguise*. Choice A is a seducer. The student who loses sight of the stem and passage might be drawn to the open-minded attitude expressed in choice A. Choices B and D are manglers, misusing the passage's references to photography in paragraph 2, and the repeated appearance of the words "perception" and "sensation" throughout the passage.

45.4 PASSAGE IV

45.4.1 Passage and Questions

Among the many issues Norman Mailer seems to probe in *The Executioner's Song* is the question of personal courage: was Gary Gilmore's decision a courageous one? Does
5 it require great human courage to choose death over a life of infinite, daily psychological tortures? Of course, with life imprisonment Gilmore would always have had the possibility to escape. Or was his choice,
10 Mailer wants to ask, a convict's last ditch attempt to snub his nose at a system that had, in his own eyes, abused and belittled him all his life? Was Gilmore, unloved by a "rounder" of a father, acting out childhood
15 frustrations by demanding recognition from a substitute paternal authority—the judicial and penal system, equally insensitive and uncaring as his father—by pretending to be just as tough and callous as his real father
20 had been? Or was his unflinching confrontation with the unknown, with death, Gilmore's attempt to convert himself from villain to anti-hero?

After all, Gilmore was, for all his vicious-
25 ness, in other respects merely human: were the choice available, he certainly would have chosen escape over execution. Moreover, Gilmore, an individual of unusual intelligence and artistic ability, might have made
30 as productive and creative a life as possible within prison even without escape. Mailer seems to say, however, that in the end Gilmore decided on a mean, vengeful, and perhaps cowardly final course: execution at
35 the hands of a state firing squad: a death empty, insignificant, pitiful, and ultimately sordid.

Nonetheless, Gilmore assumes his burden, what he recognizes as his responsibil-
40 ity, and through the donation of his organs to the living he seeks to rectify his existential debt to the species; Mailer, however, does not quite permit the reader to feel that even this last act of sacrifice and charity can make
45 amends for Gilmore's cruelty, or balance the scales for the lives he destroyed. And

Gilmore, himself, is aware of that ultimate imbalance, for it forms a part of his final knowledge:

50 "'Vern, there's no use talking about the situation. I killed those men, and they're dead. I can't bring them back, or I would.'"

In the Mailerian orchestration, though, Gilmore's persona crescendoes to an eccle-
55 siastical dimension: martyred to a death of his own choosing, his 20th century "Church" is the established American media—television, magazines, newspapers, films and novels. His "disciples" are reporters, producers,
60 actors, authors, editors and publishers: and in particular, one Lawrence Schiller (together with his gnome-like collaborator, Barry Farrell), a reporter/producer who figures largely in the second part of the novel as col-
65 lator of Gilmore's inner life and marshall of his conscience. The "bible" for this church of the latter day American sinner, is, perhaps, Mailer's novel itself, *The Executioner's Song*.

According to this gospel, we cannot, like
70 Gilmore on parole, expect to be handed the good life as our due, simply for the asking; nor are we permitted, like Nicole, to rest content on survival by the pure charity of state welfare. Rather, like Schiller and Farrell, and
75 the thousand others who populate this novel in Salt Lake City, Denver, New York, Washington, Los Angeles, and points beyond, we must find the courage to strive and reason, plan and persevere, tread a careful line be-
80 tween enlightened self-interest and service to humankind, and wrest from a pressured, predatory environment—both human and natural—our good works, and our good name.

85 For nourishment in our human condition, our human life, Mailer seems to say, we find love: love for our fellow human, for our family, for our sexual partners, for ourselves. That nourishment provides our spiritual ne-
90 cessities, and enables us to accept our choices, our lives, our selves. And in that ac-

ceptance, in that discovery and sharing of self, and in the discovery of that sharing, we are transcendent, we are communed, and are
95 redeemed.

In this novel, above all, the gift of life is ours: ours to possess, ours to create, ours to take and to give. All the price already paid for life on this planet—all the frustration, the
100 loneliness, the ambivalence and the rigor of human life—notwithstanding, we remain indebted, we can never reimburse the value of this gift: we are in the red, we owe. And what we owe is love.

25. The author's main point is that:

   A. the courage to carry out the death sentence gives meaning to a lawful society.
   B. the courage to carry out the death sentence gives meaning to human love.
   C. executing a murderer evens the moral balance sheet.
   D. life's meaning rests in the obligation to love.

26. Given the views set forth in the passage, the phrases "paying a debt to society," "life is a matter of give and take," and "you have to give something back," are best interpreted to mean:

   A. daily life requires ongoing payment and repayment.
   B. the privilege of life comes with an obligation.
   C. human existence carries a price that few can afford to pay.
   D. human existence carries a price that many would rather not pay.

27. As described in the passage, Mailer's views regarding Gilmore's wish to be executed might be most relevant to:

   A. a psychology professor discussing the effects on children of indifferent and unloving parents.
   B. a criminologist exploring a murderer's motivation in taking life.
   C. a sociological economist considering the social costs and benefits of capital punishment.
   D. a political candidate who argues in favor of capital punishment as a deterrent to crime.

28. According to Mailer's view, as described in the passage, a convicted murderer who proclaims "I demand to die for my crime" may be attempting to achieve all of the following EXCEPT to:

   A. transform himself into an anti-hero.
   B. receive from society recognition withheld by his parents.
   C. restore the balance of right and wrong by sacrificing his own life.
   D. show contempt for a society he believed to be uncaring.

29. According to the author, Mailer's depiction of Gilmore's public image analogizes:

   I. a convicted criminal to a self-sacrificing hero.
   II. news reporters to martyrs.
   III. informational sources to a religious institution.

   A. I only
   B. II only
   C. I and II only
   D. I and III only

30. Based on the information in the passage, one might correctly conclude that Gilmore had:

    A. innate abilities that gave him the potential for a productive life.
    B. the capacity to become a charismatic religious figure.
    C. no chance for a successful life from the day he was born.
    D. no experience of love from another human being.

31. According to the passage, Mailer believes that the pressures of human life require that we:

    A. sacrifice the interests of others in order to preserve our own good names.
    B. take from the public sector the support to which we are entitled.
    C. carefully balance our own interests against the well-being of others.
    D. sacrifice spiritual nourishment in favor of practical necessities.

32. According to the passage, the "existential debt" (line 41) that Gilmore attempts to repay is owed to:

    A. himself as a spiritual being.
    B. other people in general.
    C. the surviving family members of his victims.
    D. his own family members.

45.4.2 PASSAGE IV QUESTIONS ANSWERED

25. *D is correct*. The question asks for a main point, but the passage is so dense and difficult as to make it hard to answer the question: "Roughly, what is this passage all about?" This question is more easily answered by examining all distracters and eliminating those that are clearly wrong. Choices A, B, and C are manglers. Choices A and B refer to courage which sends us to paragraph 1. "Courage" is introduced in connection with this question: "Was Gilmore's decision to die a courageous one?" It is limited to the assessment of Gary Gilmore as one who was or was not courageous and does not bear on the meaning of a lawful society or the meaning of love. Choice C directs us to paragraph 3 where the author uses the phrase "balance the scales." The phrase refers to Gilmore's decision to donate his organs. Choice C, too, is a mangler. We are left with choice D. It does coincide with the author's conclusion and best responds to the stem.

26. *B is correct*. All of the statements to which the stem refers build to the author's conclusion that life carries an obligation—the obligation to love. Choices A and D are seducers. One who loses sight of the stem ("Given the views set forth in the passage...") might easily be drawn to them. They "sound right." Choice C is a mangler. It borrows the word "price" from the last paragraph and makes a statement not at all supported by the passage.

27. *A is correct*. The question seems to go beyond the passage, yet it refers us to a particular portion of its text. Mailer's views regarding Gilmore's wish to be executed are discussed in the second part of the first paragraph. Focusing solely on that, as the question directs us to do, it is not terribly difficult to dismiss C, and D as by and large wild. Choice B is a mangler. The paragraph does not concern a murderer's motivation in *taking life* but Gilmore's motivation for *choosing death*. The paragraph does refer to the effects of indifferent and loving parents on Gilmore's mental processes, which leaves A as the best answer.

28. *C is correct*. The stem prominently presents the word "EXCEPT." The student should test all answer choices, searching for the one that does NOT apply. Choices A, B, and D all find support in paragraph 1, which concerns Gilmore's motivation for choosing death ("wanting" to die for his crime). The paragraph describes a speculation that Gilmore may want to convert himself from villain to anti-hero (choice A), "demand attention from a substitute paternal authority" (choice B), or "snub his nose" at a society that had not cared for him (choice D). Only Choice C is *lacks* support. The passage does refer to Gilmore's possible wish to donate organs as a means of righting his wrongs. That reference, however, does not logically follow the stem. The stem asks about a murderer's demand that he die for his crime, not his wish to donate organs.

29. *D is correct*. The applicable text is in paragraph 4. There, the author refers to an "ecclesiastic" crescendo, analogizing various aspects of the Gilmore case to participants in a church-related episode. Reading closely, we learn that the "church" is the media (Statement III), the "disciples" (not martyrs) are reporters, and the criminal is a "martyred" figure (Statement I). Note that statements I and III reflect the text in disguise. The phrase "self-sacrificing hero" stands for a "martyred" figure, "informational sources," stands for news media, and "religious institution" stands for church. Statement II is a mangler. According to the author Mailer would analogize news reporters to disciples, not martyrs.

30. *A is correct*. The answer is found in paragraph 2 which states that, "...Gilmore, an individual of unusual intelligence and artistic ability might have made as productive and creative a life as possible..." Choice B is a mangler, misusing the passage's reference to religion. Choice C is precisely contrary to the author's statements. Choice D is a tempting seducer. One who fails to focus on the stem and the passage might endorse the idea that murderers might likely be unloved persons. The author does state that Gilmore was unloved by his father, but he does not indicate that Gilmore's life was entirely devoid of love. (Choice C might be defended, however, were it not for the presence of choice A which is clearly and unambiguously correct.)

31. *C is correct*. The relevant text is in paragraph 5. Reading it carefully we learn that "...we must...tread a careful line between enlightened self-interest and service to humankind..." Choice C makes a similar statement *in disguise*. Choices A, B, and D are manglers. They abuse the author's references to our "good names" (choice A), to "charity of state welfare" (choice B), and to "sacrifice, and "nourishment" (choice D).

32. *B is correct*. In paragraph 3, the author refers to Gilmore's "existential debt to the species." "The species" means Gilmore's own species—human beings. Choice B restates the text *in disguise*. Choices A, C, and D are either wild or, perhaps, manglers in the extreme. Choice A grossly misuses the author's reference to "spiritual" necessities, and choices C and D misuse references to Gilmore's own family and to the "lives" that Gilmore "destroyed."

45.5 PASSAGE V

45.5.1 Passage and Questions

At precisely what point in their evolution human beings began to experience a spiritual dimension to their existence is difficult to specify. The archaeological record
5 makes clear, however, that modern religious practice developed out of what we, today, generally regard as a more "primitive" system of belief and ritual. Early humans relied on magical rites to maintain their healthy
10 and correct relationship with an animistic universe of spirits and natural forces.

As magic grew influential, amulets played an important part in the mediation between the daily life and physical needs of
15 human beings, and the influences on their general welfare that seemed emergent from an altogether different level of reality obviously beyond their control. Through the proper use of the appropriate amulet, the
20 tribe might assure themselves of reproductive fertility; the necessary incantation focused through the correct amulet might induce the unknown powers to provide food and drink, whether through hunting, gath-
25 ering or pillage; similarly, the magic of amulets could bestow upon the tribe and their descendants cunning and endurance in conflicts with other tribes or in the face of natural disasters.

30 As magic practice evolved, so did animistic theory, such that these powerful, otherworldly forces acquired personification in the form of deities. Amulets became the concrete media through which the deities'
35 made their magical power accessible to humans. The amulet was not viewed simply as a one-way conduit from the gods to humans; rather, amulets also enabled the deities to function, as though their own survival de-
40 pended on a human agency and complicity in their magic. The men and women who claimed to understand the significance and use of amulets gradually developed into a class of priests, who eventually came to rep-

45 resent themselves as especially gifted by the deities to bestow divine magic—and the benefits that flowed from it—on their tribesfolk.

Although the advent of monotheism included an official forbiddance of their use,
50 many sects and priests permitted amulets to their congregants as an expedience to help minify disruptions in the continuity of their spiritual practices, particularly as the fundamental theological concepts regarding rela-
55 tionships between the human and the divine underwent significant transformation. Even the official prohibitions against the traditions of magic, however, often served to stimulate the popularity of the sanctioned objects. It
60 should be remembered, too, that great craftsmanship had developed in the manufacture of amulets, and the distribution, barter and sale of these items was not unimportant to the economy of the time.

65 That amulets occupied a crucial and necessary place in ancient Egyptian and Babylonian religions appears beyond doubt. In the turbulent period between the end of VIth Dynasty and the emergence of Thebes
70 as a world power, large areas of ancient civilization came under the sway of the mideast potentate Khati. Khati, who ruled some three thousand years before the birth of Jesus Christ, set down religious teachings which
75 survive today in a St. Petersburg papyrus. According to this tract, Ra, the sun god, whom the Egyptians considered the Creator of humankind, invented magic and provided amulets for the advantage and profit of his
80 followers. "For...[the]...pleasure of the flocks and herds of God", Khati wrote, Ra "made heaven and earth...and dissipated the darkness of the primeval ocean...[and] made the breezes of life for their nostrils"; and "He
85 gave them the gift of magic...a weapon for resisting the force of unwanted occurrences and the terrors of the night and day."

33. The author's primary thesis is that:

    A. amulets led primitive societies into sorcery and devil worship.
    B. amulets allowed early humans to channel their need to influence forces beyond their control.
    C. amulets acquired magical power by virtue of their association with Nature deities.
    D. amulets acquired magical power by virtue of their association with the caste of priests.

34. About which of the following does the author express uncertainty?

    I. The ways in which amulets played a role in daily life
    II. The fact that amulets were vital to ancient religions
    III. The time at which spirituality became a part of human culture

    A. I only
    B. III only
    C. I and III only
    D. II and III only

35. The author states that otherworldly forces acquired "personification." In the context of the passage that word refers to:

    A. the practice of incantation by tribesfolk.
    B. the emergence of priests.
    C. the magical powers associated with inanimate objects.
    D. early conceptions of gods and spirits.

36. According to the ideas expressed in the second paragraph, amulets would LEAST likely be directed to which of the following uses?

    I. Curing a tribesperson who is ill
    II. Predicting the identity of the tribe's future ruler
    III. Producing rain during a drought

    A. I only
    B. II only
    C. I and II only
    D. I, II, and III

37. The author seems to believe that the "sanctioned" objects continued in use partly because of:

    A. monotheistic doctrine.
    B. political pressure.
    C. economic interests.
    D. disrespect for priests.

38. The author claims that official prohibitions against the traditions of magic stimulated the popularity of amulets. Which of the following, if true, would most WEAKEN the claim?

    A. Tribespeople of the time did not dare defy the official dictates of their priests.
    B. The artisans who produced amulets did not actually believe their products had magical properties.
    C. Some early monotheistic leaders themselves believed in the use of amulets.
    D. The prevailing economy did not depend on production of amulets or the trade they produced.

39. Some people today carry charms which they believe will bring them good luck. Such practices suggest that:

    A. modern society promotes a belief in chance over a belief in animism.
    B. modern society rejects the belief that amulets mediate connections with deities.
    C. some people have rejected modern religion and prefer more primitive systems of belief and ritual.
    D. the human impulse to rely on amulets persists even in the modern era.

45.5.2 PASSAGE V QUESTIONS ANSWERED

33. *B is correct.* The student should quickly and crudely characterize the passage's main topic. Roughly, the passage is about amulets and the way humans at one time relied on them to control their circumstances. Choice B offers a sentence of like meaning. Choice A is wild and Choice C represents an irrelevant truth. Choice D is a mangler, misusing the author's discussion of priests. Priests, the author states, arose from those men and women who claimed a special knowledge of how to use amulets.

34. *B is correct.* Read the passage's very first sentence. The author there reveals uncertainty regarding the time at which spirituality became a part of human culture. She nowhere expresses uncertainty as to (1) the fact that amulets played an important role in early religions, and (2) the ways in which amulets functioned in the daily lives of those who relied on them. (Perhaps she is not entirely certain on these points, but she *expresses* no uncertainty.)

35. *D is correct.* The word appears in paragraph 3. There, the author all but answers the question for us, writing that "...these powerful otherworldly forces acquired personification in the form of deities." Choice D substitutes the words "gods and spirits" for deities. Choices A and B are irrelevant truths. The reader who loses sight of the stem might select one of them. Choice C is a mangler, misusing the author's reference to "animistic" conceptions.

36. *B is correct.* Paragraph 2 provides the relevant text. Close reading reveals that amulets played an important part in respect of daily life and physical needs. Statements I and III apply. Statement II does not.

37. *C is correct.* The phrase "sanctioned objects" appears in paragraph 4. At the end of that paragraph the author observes that barter and sale of amulets was "not unimportant" to the economy. Choice A is a mangler. The author does mention monotheism, but nowhere states that *its* doctrine promoted the use of amulets (although it is stated that some continued to use amulets precisely because they were prohibited). Choices B and D are more or less wild, drawing on little or nothing set forth in the passage.

38. *A is correct.* In paragraph 4 the author notes that the priests' prohibition against the use of amulets sometimes stimulated their use. The question requires no detailed review of the passage beyond that. It presents a fairly simple test of logic. If it were true that tribespeople did not dare defy their priests then it could scarcely be true that they made use of amulets when priests had prohibited it. As a matter of simple logic choices B, C, and D fail to weaken the claim.

39. *D is correct.* The question calls for logic and extrapolation. The passage indicates that human beings have a deep-rooted tradition of relying on symbolic objects for their well-being. To carry a good-luck charm is, perhaps, to follow that tradition. Choices A, B, and C misdirect the student back to the passage on a "wild goose chase" for information, when the answer is within the reach of his own common sense.

45.6 PASSAGE VI

45.6.1 Passage and Questions

The Humanist Alliance for Curricular Integration and Awareness (H.A.C.I.A.) is an independent administrative entity which monitors foreign policy trends and develop-
5 ments with a special focus on related academic issues. Our primary concern is for foreign literature and language departments in our public universities where budgetary constraints and state admission requirements
10 often leave administrators overloaded—if not overwhelmed!—with their own daily paper process. Our purpose is to call attention to certain recent American foreign policy ramifications and evaluate their potential
15 implications for current and prospective curricular planning. We must emphasize that in no way do we seek to impinge on individual or institutional independence and autonomy: Our goal is simply to provide for-
20 mative perspectives to an understaffed and overburdened academy for appropriate consideration and planning.

Our world is changing and growing at such a dizzying pace these days that even
25 the cartographers are having trouble drawing all their "P's" and "Q's" in the proper places. New challenges present themselves everyday for the political scientist, the historian, the cultural studies experts, and the
30 mathematicians and natural scientists. Not only do nations around the globe transform and redirect themselves before our very eyes, but here at home new openness in cultural diversity and interdependent sensitivities
35 demand our good faith perception and efforts.

Among these global changes is the historic new initiative in North American relations. Now, Canada and Mexico have joined
40 together with the United States to form the North American Free Trade Agreement (NAFTA). The Canadians, of course, have always been vital economic and strategic partners in our best endeavors. For the first
45 time, however, the Mexicans are receiving

formal recognition for being friendly, supportive and constructive allies in our economic, political and intellectual purposes.

This new relationship with Mexico be-
50 hooves us to examine most carefully our own cultural assumptions and biases. We all love those dear romantic images of beautiful Old Mexico: the soulful "señoritas," and the strolling mariachis, and the poor but simple
55 sombreroed campesinos dancing and drinking late into the night (when not lounging idly but menacingly in a cantina doorway), with their quaintly casual notions of social responsibility and charmingly ambiguous in-
60 terpretations of personal punctuality. Unfortunately, all too many of our academic textbooks, on both the secondary and university levels, misinform their readers and convey those pictures of stereotypical Mexico as
65 though they were the reality of modern Mexico, a nation of nearly 70 million inhabitants and enormous natural resources.

Modern Mexico has about as much to do with strolling mariachis and simple
70 campesinos as today's America has to do with dance hall girls and drunken cowboys: sure, their contemporary equivalents are here with us still today, but no one in her right mind would dream of portraying, and
75 much less defining, the United States based on those anachronistic cultural stereotypes. Disgracefully, when it comes to Mexico, even at some of our finest Universities students are brainwashed with those unfortunate,
80 outdated, culturally and intellectually irrelevant images.

Modern Mexico, our nearest neighbor to the south, boasts an educationally sophisticated and numerically growing citizenry, a
85 developing, cosmopolitan technology, a vast consumer market and a diligent, energetic labor force within an exponentially expanding economy and a culturally advanced and intellectually fertile society. If we are ad-
90 equately to prepare our students for the chal-

lenges and opportunities they will face in the coming century we must impart to them a truthful image of the world they will live in: to continue to do otherwise would be both
95 intellectually corrupt and professionally irresponsible. Anachronistic and irrelevant stereotypes will not do the job. We owe our students our best efforts at illuminating the truth about these real concerns, so that their
100 futures in a competitive and interrelated global environment will be absolutely the brightest they can be.

Accordingly, and because present prognostications point to a significantly increased
105 demand for studious individuals with a solid preparation in Latin American culture—and specifically in that of our closest neighbor—we would urge college and university Spanish departments, at a *minimum*, to do noth-
110 ing to discourage their students, at either the undergraduate or graduate level, from exploring and studying the Latin American and Mexican literatures.

40. The author's belief that the world is changing rapidly, expressed in the second paragraph, is supported by:

A. textbook references to global transformations.

B. testimony from foreign language department administrators.

C. statements regarding the tasks of those who study social and natural sciences.

D. an economic analysis of NAFTA.

41. It is probably the author's view that a principal purpose of studying foreign language and literature is to afford students:

A. an appreciation of traditional images of foreign countries.

B. an understanding of their own culture in relation to others.

C. a knowledge of international relations.

D. a view of foreign countries based on modern realities.

42. According to the passage, which of the following characterizes modern Mexico?

I. It has a rapidly expanding economy.

II. It has a growing population.

III. It is actively developing its technological resources.

A. I only

B. II only

C. II and III only

D. I, II, and III

43. Given the information in the passage, if the H.A.C.I.A. is successful in achieving its goals, which of the following changes would most likely be effected in foreign literature and language departments of public universities?

    A. They would be less occupied with their own paperwork.
    B. They would be better prepared to plan their curricula.
    C. They would experience reduction in budgetary pressures.
    D. They would be pressured to conform to H.A.C.I.A. guidelines.

44. The author indicates that the scholastic pursuit of foreign languages and cultures is relatively unenlightening when it:

    A. relies on conventional notions of foreign civilizations.
    B. differentiates between romantic images and reality.
    C. includes a consideration of geopolitical developments.
    D. emphasizes the achievements of foreign civilizations.

45. Suppose an economic study indicates that Mexico presently lags behind the other North American nations in implementation of computer technologies. Such findings, if made, would most CHALLENGE the assertion that:

    A. many students who study Mexican literature and culture are misinformed.
    B. the relationships created by NAFTA are new and innovative.
    C. Mexico is prepared to serve as a partner in modern economic enterprise.
    D. United States relations with Canada are invariably advantageous.

45.6.2 PASSAGE VI QUESTIONS ANSWERED

40. *C is correct.* In paragraph 2 the author states that the world is changing rapidly. In support of that statement she writes that political scientists, historians, cultural studies experts, mathematicians, and social scientists face new challenges. Choice C reflects such references, in disguise. Choices A, B, and D are manglers, misusing the author's references to "global transformation," foreign language departments, and NAFTA. Note that the author's reference to NAFTA does support her point that the world is changing rapidly. But the author provides no *economic analysis* of NAFTA. Those two words make choice D incorrect.

41. *D is correct.* Toward the end of paragraph 4 the author bemoans the way in which high school and university courses depict Mexican culture. The depiction, says the author, is outdated. A small measure of extrapolation indicates that she would want such study to reflect modern realities. Choices A, B, and C are all seducers. They "sound nice." The student who loses sight of the stem and passage might be tempted to choose one of them.

42. *D is correct.* Modern Mexico is described in paragraph 6. The author tells us that it boasts a "numerically growing citizenry" (statement II), a "developing cosmopolitan technology" (statement III), and a "vast consumer market" with a "diligent labor force" (statement I). All three statements apply.

43. *B is correct.* The relevant information is in paragraph 1, where the author discusses H.A.C.I.A. The last three sentences describe its purpose, which is to identify American foreign policy trends that might have impact on curricular planning. Choice B reflects H.A.C.I.A.'s purpose as just described. Choices A and C are manglers. The author does note that foreign language and literature departments now experience budgetary constraints and burdensome paperwork. These concerns, however, do not underlie H.A.C.I.A.'s purpose. Choice D is contrary to the passage. The author writes that H.A.C.I.A. does *not* wish to intrude on institutional autonomy.

44. *A is correct.* The pertinent text is found in paragraphs 4 and 5. There, the author sharply criticizes educational institutions and textbooks for depicting Mexico in anachronistic stereotypical terms. Although the text refers particularly to Mexico, extrapolation indicates that the author would deem the study of any foreign language or culture unenlightening when it rests on conventional images and stereotypes. Choice A correctly characterizes her view. Choice B is a mangler, misusing the author's reference to romantic images and thus distorting her meaning. Choices C and D are by and large wild. They draw on little or nothing set forth in the passage and do not characterize the author's view.

45. *C is correct.* The question is peripheral to the passage. The author characterizes Mexico as a modern dynamic society, with technologies and sophistication that qualify it as a partner in modern economic activity. Simple logic indicates that if the nation were shown not yet to have "caught up" with modern day computer technologies it would not be quite so well qualified a partner. Choice A is an irrelevant truth. The author does believe that today's textbooks misinform their readers regarding the nature of Mexican culture, but that belief is unrelated to the stem. Choice B is by and large a seducer/ and to some extent an irrelevant truth. It makes a statement that is partially correct and, in any event, appealing. Yet it is unresponsive to the stem. Choice D constitutes an "absolute" of which the student should be wary.

45.7 PASSAGE VII

45.7.1 Passage and Questions

In June of 1963, five months before President Kennedy was shot and the world seemed to change forever for most Americans (certainly for those too young to know
5 the Axis horrors of World War II), I supervised production at Manhattan Braid and Lace Producers as assistant foreman. Our factory was located on Tenth Avenue, close to the west side piers. I ran the machines,
10 and repaired them when necessary; I drew designs for textile patterns in lace and nylon; from those blueprints, I built intricate arrays of chains and crosslinks which wove the cotton into delicate filigrees; I made sure
15 the beams spun straight and the knitters tended to their tasks. Many brides around the world came with their betrothed to trade their blessed altar vows dressed and fancied in our lace; and when they raised their shin-
20 ing faces and puckered newlywed lips for that first, unforgettable matrimonial kiss, the veils their grooms lifted proved the tender care in our looms.

The textile field boomed in the early six-
25 ties due mostly to overseas expansion and escalating foreign competition in Europe and Asia. And while that pleased retailers and consumers, who could get product in the market at lower cost, it turned out hard on
30 American textile workers. The American share of the business was draining down. Italy and Hong Kong began to take over. Put simply, the prospects in New York textile manufacture, which a scant decade earlier
35 had seemed incandescent, now dimmed significantly.

About that time the City of New York was slowly coming to the conclusion that if it was to provide effective law enforcement,
40 safe streets, and a livable social milieu for its decent, hard-working, law-abiding citizens, it would need to enhance the rewards and compensations offered to those charged with ensuring public safety and civil order.
45 There was talk then of raising the annual wages of peace officers—transit police, corrections officers, and city cops—up to ten thousand dollars, with retirement pensions after twenty years at 1/2 retirement grade
50 pay!

Now don't get me wrong: I liked being assistant foreman on the looms. We had some great times! As the machines hummed and buzzed and clanked and rang we workers
55 would among ourselves compose original songs, and down there by the docks, as we fed our looms, by God, we used to sing! Out loud! Like a Broadway chorus!

Every day at breathless pace
60 We spin the nylon and the lace
We twirl the links and knit the loops
So every handsome groom who swoops

His bride from earth's to heaven's
65 charms

Yet holds her close within his arms
Will gaze upon her white veiled face
And feel the love of pure embrace

But Manhattan Braid and Lace Produc-
70 ers paid me only seven thousand dollars a year, and that with considerable overtime, and they could promise only fifty dollars a month as pension to employees who survived in the company to sixty-five. Thirty-
75 four years old, married and father of two, I felt the push of present and future responsibilities.

In June, I sat for the Civil Service exam for peace officers, along with seven or eight
80 thousand others. I did not know then that it would be a full year before openings became available. Nor did I know for certain to which force the City might assign me, or if, indeed, I'd be assigned, or accepted, at all.
85 In those days wherever the need first arose, be it transit, corrections, or NYPD, was

where they sent the rookies. I did believe that I had at least one edge over most of the other applicants. In Korea, nine years earlier, I'd
90 served with the United States Army Combat Engineers and Signal Forces, and with the Airborne Special Forces. My experience under fire, behind enemy lines, performing difficult, dangerous, and sensitive missions,
105 might well prove attractive to my prospective employers.

46. Which of the following best summarizes the main idea of the passage?

   A. Unexpected changes in conditions sometimes cause us to change our life's course, but previous experience usually remains valuable.
   B. The New York City Police Department achieved its reputation for bravery and professionalism primarily due to its policy of hiring Korean War veterans.
   C. Lace manufactured in New York City has never been equaled in terms of its quality or worldwide popularity.
   D. The textile industry in America lost considerable ground to foreign competition during the decade of the '60s.

47. The author decided to leave his factory job for a position with the police force because he:

   A. was concerned about job stability.
   B. was weary of factory work.
   C. felt the lure of adventure.
   D. felt the need for better compensation.

48. In the context of the passage, the word *incandescent* (line 35) means:

   A. intensely hot.
   B. filamentous.
   C. bright.
   D. fluorescent.

49. Which of the following statements, if true, would most WEAKEN the author's claim that the textile boom of the 1960s pleased retailers?

   A. The decreased activity in the American textile industry occurred only in New York, not in other U.S. cities.
   B. The textile industry was not responsible for the majority of economic growth in either Italy or Hong Kong.
   C. Intense competition among wholesalers was limited primarily to domestic producers.
   D. Instead of creating competition among wholesalers, the boom created noncompetitive monopolies and oligopolies.

50. In giving advice to a gathering of young people about to enter the labor force, the author would most likely counsel them to:

  A. decide what they love to do, and follow their dream aggressively.

  B. choose a career path, and remain open and ready to adapt their goals to new realities.

  C. derive a good living wage from part-time jobs in diverse fields, recognizing that any one industry may founder.

  D. devote some time to the national military because soldiering is always salable.

51. A recent analysis of U.S. employment trends reported that "the labor market is a dog-eat-dog world" and that "life-time job security is a benefit much in demand among today's workers." If the author had cited these statements he would probably have done so in order to:

  A. support the notion that employees should work together harmoniously.

  B. illustrate his idea that employment is analogous to battle.

  C. emphasize his point that people should be realistic about job expectations.

  D. explain why an industry might at one time flourish and later falter.

45.7.2 PASSAGE VII QUESTIONS ANSWERED

46. *A is correct*. The student should quickly and crudely characterize the passage's main topic. Roughly, the passage is about a person who liked his work, experienced altered economic circumstance, and sought a change in career. Among the choices, choice A comes closest to making such a statement. (It adds material concerning the value of previous experience which refers to the writer's service in Korea.) Choices B and C are manglers. They misuse words and phrases drawn from the passage and, in any event, fail to identify the passage's main topic. Choice D is an irrelevant truth. One who loses sight of the stem and the passage might select it. It accurately restates information set forth in the passage but surely does not summarize the passage's central theme.

47. *D is correct*. The pertinent text is in paragraphs 2, 3, and 4. In those paragraphs we learn that New York's textile industry experienced downturn and that the writer felt the need to better his income by becoming a police officer. Choices A and C are seducers. Superficially examined they have an appeal. Yet, they are not supported by the passage. Choice B is thoroughly contrary to the passage. The writer speaks fondly of textile work and he seems never to have grown weary of it.

48. *C is correct*. Reread the appropriate text. The author writes that the prospects in New York textile manufacture...had seemed incandescent" but now "dimmed." Incandescence is contrasted with dimness. It is sensible to conclude, therefore, that it means "bright." Choices A, B, and D are wild. They relate neither to the passage nor the stem.

49. *D is correct*. The question calls for logical deduction and the relevant text is in the second sentence of paragraph 2. Retailers were pleased because foreign competition, apparently, caused wholesalers to reduce their costs. If that were *not* true, retailers would not have been pleased. Choice D reflects that observation. Choices A, B, and C present a sort of gibberish that offers no logical response to the stem. One who chooses them would likely do so by wild guess, not by rational design.

50. *B is correct*. The question calls for (1) an understanding of the passage's main idea, and (2) extrapolation. The writer reports that he chose and liked one occupation but decided to leave it in response to altered economic circumstance. He seems, moreover, to believe that he did the right thing. Choice B reflects the writer's experience and point of view. Choice A is a seducer. It "sounds good," but it has no support in the passage and is unresponsive to the stem. Choice C is wild; it bears no relation to passage or stem. Choice D is a mangler. The writer refers to his service in the military as an experience that might have helped him secure work on the police force. He nowhere states or implies that soldiering is *always* marketable.

51. *C is correct*. The question calls for (1) a general comprehension of the author's point of view, and (2) extrapolation. Yet, since no answer seems quite correct. we resort to process of elimination. Choice A is unresponsive to the stem. Choice B does not reflect the author's view. We are left with choices C and D. Choice C reflects, in its way, one of the author's implicit points and is responsive to the stem. Choice D does not respond to the stem; it relates to an industry, not to individual workers.

45.8 PASSAGE VIII

45.8.1 Passage and Questions

For many Native American societies, religious ideology and ritual expressed the intimacy their peoples experienced between humankind and nature. Their spiritual in-
5 stincts led them closer to an awareness of the wholeness of Creation, of the intact chain of life from the simplest forms to the most highly evolved. In fact, they achieved this awareness much earlier than did the Judeo-
10 Christian-Moslem traditions.

Centuries before Charles Darwin dared to risk the wrath of organized, institutional religion by declaring or implying a direct lineage from paramecium to humans, Native
15 American peoples acknowledged their connection to their animal ancestors, and also to more fundamental forces of Nature.

Whereas the testaments of the Bible and the Koran assign to God the creation of hu-
20 man beings in the story of Adam and Eve, the doctrines of the Wisconsin Menomini, for instance, which probably predate both Bible and Koran, teach that at the Great River's Mouth the Earth gave birth to two bears.
25 These bears, distinguished from each other by gender, transmogrified into the first man and woman. A brief analysis of this ancient Menomini revelation demonstrates its intuition of profound insights which western
30 societies only began to understand in relatively modern times .

In the Menomini creation, water provides the fount of land-based life, just as biologists today believe that the atoms of hy-
35 drogen and oxygen in water furnish the essential elements without which organic compounds—and the life forms they generate and sustain— will not form. Also, the story affirms that fecundated by the virile fluids
40 at the river mouth, the Earth itself—which today we recognize as a great carbon/nitrogen reservoir—serves as the uterus of animal creation. Still more strikingly, perhaps,

the Menomini intuited that human life owed
45 its origin ultimately to animal and elemental forebears.

Several Native American origin testaments did not limit themselves to the physical process itself, but included an important
50 moral dimension as well. Some indigenous societies in the northwest United States, for example, blame the development of community evils such as disease, famine, discord or infertility on the excessive selfishness of one
55 or more of its members. This belief roots in a vision of the beginnings in which chaos reigns supreme throughout the created universe until the hero figure initiates prosperity and order by the purposeful sharing of
60 resources and assets with the less fortunate. Without generosity as a founding principle, the lesson says, no individual can prosperously organize a commonwealth; and to maintain a healthy society, leaders must dis-
65 tribute tribal wealth fairly.

Moral edification, however, did not always eradicate selfishness (or, for that matter, other human traits deemed undesirable for the tribal well-being) from the commu-
70 nity. In such cases, the community needed a reference to guide them in dealing with moral offenses. Thus, the possibility of individual redemption found expression in certain creation doctrines of the Native Ameri-
75 cans, often through the metaphor of a dual creation.

The Iroquois, for example, teach that creation results from the efforts of not one, but two primordial hero-spirits, one of whom en-
80 genders the noble elements of human character, while the other begets the negative traits. Frequently, the two spirits are related, oftentimes brothers, and their opposite intentions inevitably lead to personal conflict
85 with each other. Some Iroquois teach, for example, that in this struggle the good

brother triumphs and threatens to destroy his evil twin. The evil brother can escape certain death only by vowing to endow humans
90 with the knowledge of medicine and guide them in the arts of healing. Such creation metaphors allow for the existence of human sin, moral conflict and ultimate redemption through a personal commitment to life ac-
95 tivity beneficial to self and community.

52. Given the ideas expressed in the passage, the author most likely describes the Iroquois doctrine of dual creation to suggest that some Native American religions:

I. resemble Western religions in their emphasis on moral conflict.
II. resemble Western religions in their recognition that one individual has the capacity for both good and evil.
III. differ from Western religions in that they deny sinners the hope of salvation.

A. I only
B. II only
C. I and II only
D. I, II, and III

53. As used in the passage, the word "virile" (line 39) probably refers most specifically to:

A. power.
B. speed.
C. richness.
D. fertility.

54. As evidence that Native American accounts of creation were not limited to physical phenomena, the author describes a cause and effect relationship between:

A. generosity and order.
B. heroism and chaos.
C. animals and humans.
D. animals and elements.

55. Among the following, the passage's overall description of Native American religious belief might be most useful to:

A. a religious philosopher who contends that all human beings have a basic tendency toward goodness.
B. a sociologist who postulates that unconnected peoples reach similar conclusions about their own beginnings.
C. a biologist who hypothesizes that Darwin's theories leave some evolutionary phenomena unexplained.
D. a poet analogizing the conflicts between siblings to those among members of a social community.

56. In the context of the passage the reference to Adam and Eve serves to:

A. emphasize the difference between those theories of creation that depend on deities and those that do not.
B. highlight the similarities among Judeo-Christian and Moslem teachings.
C. contradict the view that any one religious belief is superior to another.
D. support the view that Native American thought was in some sense ahead of Western thought.

45.8.2 PASSAGE VIII QUESTIONS ANSWERED

52. *C is correct.* At various points in the passage the author marks the similarities between the doctrines of Native American religion and those of modern Western religion and science. The Iroquois doctrine, as described in paragraph 7, recognizes (1) a conflict between good and evil (Statement I), and (2) that even the evil are capable of good (Statement III). Statement II is contrary to the Iroquois doctrine, as described in the passage. The Iroquois teaching *does* provide for "redemption" (salvation) through "personal commitment..."

53. *D is correct.* In paragraph 4 the author describes the Menomini view of creation and refers to the "virile" fluids at the river mouth. According to the Menomini, the fluids gave rise to life. The virility is intended to imply fertility. Choices A and B miss the mark but might tempt one who loses sight of the stem. The stem features the words "most specifically," and choice D is more specific to the meaning of paragraph 4 than are choices A and B. Choice C is by and large wild.

54. *A is correct.* The relevant information is in paragraph 5 where the author first notes that "Native American origin testaments did not limit themselves to the physical." The paragraph describes how, according to some Native Americans, a hero invested the world with order by sharing of resources (generosity). Choice A, therefore, correctly characterizes the text *in disguise*.

55. *B is correct.* One of the passage's chief themes is that Native American religious doctrine resembles the teachings of modern Western religion and science. In particular, the author focuses on creation (beginnings of life). Choice B, therefore, correctly characterizes the passage's central theme and, among the choices, properly identifies the professional to whom it would be most useful. Choices A, C, and D are all manglers. Out of context, each draws on and misuses one or more words or phrases used in the passage.

56. *D is correct.* The author mentions Adam and Eve at the beginning of paragraph 3. She goes on to describe the Menomini view of creation, which (1) recognizes two primal figures of opposite sex, and (2) "probably predates" the Bible. The author thus points out that Native American religious doctrine was, in its way, ahead of Western teaching. Choices A and B are manglers, each borrowing words and phrases from the text and reproducing them in distorted context. Choice C is a seducer. One who loses sight of the stem and the passage might be drawn to so appealing and "acceptable" a statement as is made in Choice C.

45.9 PASSAGE IX

45.9.1 Passage and Questions

Most people who have paid even minimal attention to health insurance issues are familiar with the concept of cost-shifting by health care providers. In hospitals, for example, patients with good insurance coverage—whose policies reimburse providers fully and adequately for the realistic costs of health care—wind up underwriting care for indigent, uninsured or underinsured patients. This sort of cost-shifting is fairly self-evident: One person's insurance may reimburse the hospital and doctors, say, five thousand dollars for a hernia reduction, while Medicaid might cover only a fraction of that expense for an indigent patient. Obviously, the average cost for a hernia reduction at that hospital lies somewhere between those two figures.

However, there is another sort of insurance cost-shifting that has received very little, if any, attention, although it stands to reason that such account juggling must occur within the industry: huge insurance conglomerates, and re-insurers, beset with tremendous losses from natural and human-made disasters—earthquakes, floods, wildfires, hurricanes, oil spills, riots, etc.—outrageously balance their profit margins by raising revenues from the one, guaranteed source with little or no clout to dispute price increases or seek redress: ordinary citizens, whose budgetary struggles to make everyday ends meet, must include the ever-rising monthly health insurance premiums for themselves and their families.

In this light, the so-called "health care crisis" becomes refocused as an "insurance industry crisis." Accordingly, the brunt of legislative remedies ought to be aimed at reforming the financial structure of the insurance industry, not that of a health care system which, until now, has been the envy of the world. Modest suggestions along these lines include prohibiting insurance companies and re-insurers doing business in the United States from mixing their revenues from health insurance premiums with other kinds of insurance receipts or payouts. This way, health care users will not be paying huge rate increases to provide relief to victims of earthquakes, floods and hurricanes, or to reimburse merchants burned out of business in a wildfire or civil riot, or to fund multi-million dollar judgments awarded by juries as penalties for corporate negligence.

Also too often ignored in the public debate is a second element crucial to the drive to improve health care. The media has devoted far too little discussion exploring the enormous expenditure of clinicians' time and office resources devoted to conflict with "utilization review" personnel of the insurance companies. Do Americans really want to require their trained, experienced, licensed physicians to partake of this costly and profligate procedure? Can there be any method more inefficient and potentially hazardous than to allow insurance personnel, buttressed only by a computer printout of actuarial statistics, to demand disputatious justification for—much less to overrule—an expert physician's clinical observations, clinical reasoning and clinical determinations?

It must be said, of course, that this sort of "review" very closely mirrors the educational process by which physicians are trained, first in medical school and later in hospital residencies, except that in the professional training experience the "reviewers" are not insurance company personnel—they are experienced, expert physicians themselves, as they must be, to shoulder such a serious responsibility as maintaining the standards and quality of sound clinical practice. Their experience has taught them certain medical truths not included in the curriculum of insurance accountants and database personnel: that each clinical case can be decided only on the facts and observations in the specific clinical situation, not on some formulaic basis of statistics and probabilities.

The logic of the insurance utilization review process, however, would seem to call
95 into question the very need for Professors of Medicine altogether: why not simply let a medical student, an intern or a resident read textbooks, examine patients, and phone in their findings and tentative diagnoses to in-
100 surance company clerks? Then let insurance company pharmacists, not highly trained clinical specialists, prescribe the most appropriate—read "cost-effective"—treatment. After all, that's the way things are beginning
105 to work in the real world of daily practice!

57. One expert in public health has proclaimed that "HMO's exert moderate pressure on primary care physicians to limit referrals. But the highly trained specialist must withhold certain treatments until obtaining approval from PPS utilization reviewers." This expert would most likely:

A. endorse legislation eliminating government regulation of health insurance policies.
B. favor a one-payer health care system in the U.S.
C. reject the belief that either HMO's or PPS's interfere with patients' access to physicians and care.
D. conclude that both HMO's and PPS's interfere with the physician/patient interaction, but PPS's to a greater extent.

58. The author of the passage would likely favor federal legislation that:

A. requires people to choose regional physician groups from whom they would receive all health care.
B. restricts patients' rights to appeal an insurance company decision affecting their health care.
C. denies insurance companies the final power to decide that they will or will not reimburse the cost of a particular treatment.
D. limits the number of per year specialist referrals for each patient.

59. The author believes that shifting insurance losses from home insurance policies and corporate liability settlements to health insurance premiums probably results in:

I. unjustifiably high health insurance costs.
II. inadequate health care for those who are underinsured.
III. unfair burdens to patients with relatively better health insurance.

A. I only
B. II only
C. II and III only
D. I, II, and III

60. Which of the following points is/are presented in the passage to argue that utilization review procedures are potentially problematic?

I. Utilization review personnel rely on statistical models rather than a specific clinical situation to approve or deny recommended treatment.
II. Patient outcomes under utilization review procedures are significantly worse than in their absence.
III. Utilization review procedures consume physician's time that could be more valuably used attending to patients.

A. I only
B. I and II only
C. I and III only
D. I, II, and III

61. Which of the following findings, if true, would best support the author's contention that health insurance pricing policies are unfair?

A. Many Americans cannot afford health insurance.

B. The increase in the cost of health insurance is far greater than the rise in actual health care claims paid by insurance companies.

C. Most Americans believe that if you maintain good nutritional and life style habits you will maintain good health.

D. Insurance company revenue from non-health insurance policies are greater than expenditures in those areas.

62. According to the passage, which of the following is likely to be true about the relationship between utilization review procedures and physicians' attendance to patients' needs?

A. The more review required, the less attendance to patients' needs.

B. The more review required, the greater attendance to patients' needs.

C. The less review required, the less attendance to patients' needs.

D. The passage does not indicate any connection between utilization review requirements and attendance to patients' needs.

45.9.2 PASSAGE IX QUESTIONS ANSWERED

57. *D is correct.* The question is peripheral to the passage. It calls for logic. The "expert" proclaims that (1) HMO's exert *moderate* pressure on primary care physicians but that (2) PPS's actually forbid specialists to administer certain treatment without permission. According to the expert, therefore, the HMO's impose some interference with physician/patient interaction and the PPS's create greater interference. Choices A and B are in their way seducers. They have little to do with the passage and nothing to do with the stem. A student who disregards passage and stem might select A or B because the statements appeal to him. Choice C contradicts the sense of the stem.

58. *C is correct.* The question requires little or no review of the passage. A first and fast reading of paragraphs 4, 5, and 6 reveals the author's attitude. He generally opposes the interference by insurance companies with the physician's medical decision making. Choice C closely summarizes his view. Choice A is a seducer, reflecting in part the health care plan put forth by the Clinton administration. It is irrelevant to passage and stem. Choices B and D are contrary to the author's views.

59. *A is correct.* The relevant information is set forth in paragraph 2. According to the author, insurance companies raise the cost of health insurance in order to compensate for the claims they pay on other forms of insurance. He characterizes the practice as outrageous. Statement I, therefore clearly applies. Statement II is a seducer. It seems clearly to make a true statement but it is unrelated to the stem. Statement III is, in its way, a mangler. It loosely refers to the cost-shifting described in the *first paragraph*. It is, however, unresponsive to the stem, which concerns the cost-shifting described in the *second* (which at the beginning of paragraph 2, the author describes as "another sort" of cost-shifting).

60. *C is correct.* In paragraph 4 the author begins his criticism of utilization review. He asks, rhetorically, whether trained, experienced, physicians to partake of this costly and profligate (wasteful, extravagant) procedure (statement III). He refers to the inefficiency and danger that arise when insurance personnel make decisions on the basis of actuarial statistics, overruling the physician's determinations based on clinical reasoning (statement I). Statement II is wild. It relates to nothing in the passage or the stem.

61. *B is correct.* The question requires little or no review of the passage. First and fast reading of the second paragraph indicates that the author opposes the sort of cost-shifting under which insurance companies raise health care premiums in order to cover claims paid on other forms of insurance. The author's view would be supported and confirmed if it were shown that the increase in health insurance premiums exceeds insurance claims paid for health care. Choices A and C are seducers. They make what many believe to be true statements, but they are unrelated to the passage or stem. Choice D is a mangler. Out of context, it borrows and misuses the author's discussion of non-health insurance policies.

62. *A is correct.* In criticizing utilization review at paragraphs 4, 5, and 6 the author expresses a view that utilization review generally impairs the quality of health care (disguised in choice A as "patient needs") by (1) consuming physicians' time, and (2) allowing insurance personnel to make decisions that properly belong to physicians. He believes that utilization review promotes a lesser attendance to patient needs. Choices B and C are headspinners, representing twisted, inverted versions of choice A. Choice D thoroughly ignores the thrust of paragraphs 4, 5, and 6.

CHAPTER 46

UNDERSTANDING THE MCAT ESSAY

46.1 THE ESSAY QUESTION

The third portion of the MCAT requires that you write two essays, each within thirty minutes. Both essays are scored. Taken together, the two scores generate a single score, reported as a letter J-T , where J is low and T is high. Each essay problem provides you with a short statement, the *prompt*, and an instruction that she comment on it. This chapter will show you (a) how the exercises are designed, and (b) how to approach them systematically. Chapter 47 sets forth six sets of simulated MCAT essay problems together with sample answers that would likely receive high scores.

46.1.1 THE PROMPT

As noted, each essay exercise provides you first with a *prompt*. The prompt is a quasi-philosophical statement concerning some aspect of human thought or activity. It might, for example, concern politics, history, art, literature, education, or human relationships.

Following are five simulated prompts, each of which might serve as the basis for an MCAT essay exercise.

1. No person should obey a law that violates his own conscience.

2. Education is ultimately the study of one's own ignorance.

3. Achievements are valuable only to the extent that they are lasting.

4. War is not waged by governments but by people.

5. No two people can form a relationship unless they first trust each other.

46.1.2 THE INSTRUCTIONS

You are instructed to read the statement and then to write a unified essay in which you perform three "tasks." You are to: (1) explain the statement's meaning, (2) describe a situation to which the statement does not apply, and (3) discuss the factors that affect the statement's validity.

46.2 ESSAY GRADES AND GRADING

The test-taker writes two essays. Each is evaluated and graded by two readers, who assign it a tentative raw numerical score on a scale of 1-6. If the two readers reach the same score, then the raw score is final. If the first and second readers reach different scores, the essay is passed to a third reader. The final raw score is then taken as the average of the three tentative scores. The two final raw scores (one for each essay) are then combined and converted to a single final report on the scale J-T.

Unlike other MCAT components, the essay exercise does not allow for objective grading. If a multiple-choice question carries option "D" as the keyed answer, there is little room for dispute as to whether you did or did not select it. Your response is evaluated, by machine, on the basis of the oval you fill in with your pencil, while the essay is evaluated by a human being. And no matter how fair-minded, diligent, detailed, and meticulous a reader may be, there is room, always, for reasonable dispute as to the correctness of an evaluation.

Moreover, AAMC policy requires that essays be read and graded "holistically." Readers are instructed *not* to evaluate an essay in terms of any set of enumerated criteria. Rather they are instructed to view the essay as a "whole" and to award a grade *without* separately considering such matters as clarity, word choice, or sentence structure. Indeed, the graders are encouraged to read and evaluate each essay in less than two minutes. Therefore, the grade an essay receives is going to depend on the *impression* it gives its reader.

46.3 APPROACHING THE MCAT ESSAY SYSTEMATICALLY

Remembering that the essay will be read quickly and "holistically," you should be sure to (a) address the three "tasks" assigned to you, and (b) make it *absolutely clear* that you have done so. The essay should begin with a sentence that addresses the first of the assigned tasks, which is to "explain what the above statement means." The first sentence, therefore, should include the word "means," and you should even underline the word. Consider the sample prompts:

1. No person should obey a law that violates his own conscience.

2. Education is ultimately the study of one's own ignorance.

3. Achievements are valuable only to the extent that they are lasting.

4. War is not waged by governments but by people.

5. No two people can form a relationship unless they first trust each other.

The first essay might begin like this:

> "I think the statement <u>means</u> that each of us owes a greater loyalty to his own conscience than to the laws of the society or social order to which he belongs."

The second essay might begin like this:

> "To me, the statement <u>means</u> that the acquisition of knowledge and understanding perpetually expands the individual's appreciation for the vastness of the ideas and phenomena that he has not mastered and

cannot master."

The third essay might begin like this:

> "In my opinion, the statement <u>means</u> that human attainment is meaningful only if and to the degree that it has a constructive effect on the progress of civilization."

The fourth essay might begin like this:

> "I take the statement to <u>mean</u> that a government cannot wage war without the participation of its people; that if people refuse to fight, war cannot proceed."

The fifth essay might begin like this:

> "The statement most likely <u>means</u> that meaningful human interaction requires that each participant have such confidence in the other as to be willing to open and expose him or herself in whatever manner may be appropriate to the nature of the interaction. "

Regardless of its quality in any other respect, each of the sentences clearly informs the reader that you are addressing the first of the three assigned tasks. Remember that the grader will be reading a great many essays, one after another, and that he will devote less than two minutes to each. The first sentence should *not* begin with some introductory remark that deals generally with the subject matter of the prompt, as that will probably irritate the reader.

Essays should *not* begin like the following examples:

> "The conflict between conscience and duty—between the individual and the group—manifests as a theme throughout the course of human history and, indeed, throughout every great work of literature it has produced."

> "Education and ignorance assume a variety of forms and there are perhaps as many forms of education and ignorance as there are persons to educate."

> "There can be no doubt that some achievements have longer and more wide-reaching effects than do others."

> "Whether war is waged by governments or by people, its repeated arrival on the human stage marks the longest running of human tragedies."

> "Trust is, perhaps, the scarcest of all commodities."

After devoting two to three sentences to the first of the three assigned tasks, you should move to the second. You should begin a *new paragraph* and, once again, signal the reader that you have begun to address the second of the assigned tasks. That paragraph should begin with sentences like these:

> "There is at least one <u>specific situation</u> to which the

statement does not sensibly apply."

"I believe that there are <u>situations in which war is waged more by government</u> than by people."

You should devote one to three paragraphs to the second task and then, when beginning to address the third, start a new paragraph signaling the grader that you have completed the second and are moving to the third.

46.3.1 TASK 1: DESCRIBING THE STATEMENT'S MEANING

The first task is, by nature, somewhat peculiar. If a statement is well-worded, its meaning should be self-evident. In asking you to describe the "meaning" of the statement the test writers are asking you to elaborate on the statement's meaning.

Consider, for example, this prompt:

> The death of one innocent person is as great a tragedy as the deaths of one thousand.

You should begin the essay with a sentence that (a) includes the word "means", and (b) restates the prompt with detail and specificity:

> "I think the statement <u>means</u> that there can be no greater moral injustice than the death of an innocent person, that any one person can die only once, and that the deaths of two, three, or three thousand innocent persons presents no greater a wrong than does the death of one."

With another few sentences you might elaborate on your view of the statement's meaning by illustrating the point.

> "I think the statement <u>means</u> that there can be no greater moral injustice than the death of an innocent person, that any one person can die only once, and that the deaths of two, three, or three thousand innocent persons present no greater a wrong than does the death of one. The author probably believes that a flood, earthquake, famine, epidemic, or war is tragic not because it kills in large numbers, but because it kills the innocent. He would regard as equally tragic an epidemic that kills 10,000 and a murder that kills one."

46.3.2 TASK 2: FINDING PIVOTAL AMBIGUITIES

Having written two or three sentences that address the first task, you should begin a new paragraph and address yourself to the second. As already noted, the paragraph should flag its purpose; it should plainly advise the reader that you have moved on to task #2. Because the reader will not pay scrupulous attention to your ideas, it is not terribly important that the ideas be finely, carefully, and thoroughly reasoned.

Rather, it *is* important that you (a) write something that does in some way *address* the second task, and (b) *announce* that you are doing so. If, on the other hand, you are "stuck" for an idea, you can always make use of this fact: *the prompts invariably pivot on words whose meanings are inherently ambiguous.*

Consider again the five prompts given as illustrations:

1. No person should obey a law that violates his own conscience.

2. Education is ultimately the study of one's own ignorance.

3. Achievements are valuable only to the extent that they are lasting.

4. War is not waged by governments but by people.

5. No two people can form a relationship unless they first trust each other.

Although it may not seem so at first, each prompt features words that are open to diverse interpretation. With reference to the first prompt, for example, one might spend a lifetime attempting to define the words "law" and "conscience." With reference to the second prompt, the words "education" and "ignorance" make ready fuel for philosophical debate. What, after all, is "education?" What is "ignorance?" Does "education" refer to formal schooling? Does "education" denote memorization of fact? Does it refer to one who is widely read about times and cultures remote from his own or does it, instead, refer to one who has acquired the abilities and skills necessary to cope with his own environment?

With reference to the third, fourth, and fifth statements you might note that the words "achievement," "lasting," "government," "people," "relationship," and "trust" are all inherently ambiguous. Does "government" refer to the people who administer a nation, or does it refer to the system *by which* they administer it? Does the word "people" refer to the individuals who compose a group or to the group itself?

Knowing that each prompt embodies at least one word whose meaning is readily debatable, you can easily identify a situation to which it does not apply. Consider, for example, the second sample prompt:

> Education is ultimately the study of one's own igno-
> rance.

You can identify a "specific situation" to which the statement does not apply by noting first that the word "education" is subject to interpretation. If education is taken to mean conventional schooling, the statement has little application. The pupil who masters the distributive principle of multiplication—that $(7 \times 9) = (9 \times 7)$—undertakes no study of his own ignorance. Similarly the student who memorizes the names of the fifty states' capitals probably does not probe deeply the recesses of his own ignorance.

Consider, in this regard, the fifth sample prompt:

> No two people can form a relationship unless they
> first trust each other.

You can identify a "specific situation" to which the statement does not apply by noting that the words "relationship" and "trust" offer diverse meanings. In some sense a relationship is formed with a postal clerk when someone steps up to the counter and asks that his package be weighed. He must, after all, *relate* to the worker and the worker must *relate* to him. If "trust" is taken to mean some abiding confidence in another person's integrity and values, then the statement does not apply to such a situation. In order to relate to a postal clerk, a police officer, or even a neighbor in some casual setting, one need not invest a deep-seated reliance in his or her integrity, honesty, or system of values.

We draw attention to the ambiguities inherent in MCAT essay prompts in order to assist you who, on test day, find yourself at a loss to address the second of the tasks assigned to you. We do not suggest that the essay *necessarily* draw on ambiguities within the prompt but rather note that they *can* be—that in some manner you can always find a situation to which the prompt does not apply by noting that its meaning is open to question.

If you do address the second task by resorting to the prompt's inherent ambiguity, you readily establish a basis on which to address the third task. You need only observe, *in your own words*, that the applicability of the statement depends on the meaning one attaches to its words. Consider once again, for example, the fifth prompt:

> No two people can form a relationship unless they first trust each other.

After having addressed the second task by observing that the words "relationship" and "trust" are ambiguous, you might complete the third task with a paragraph like this:

> "The worth, meaning, and legitimacy of the statement depend on the interpretation one affords its words. Any ongoing, long-lasting relationship that addresses complex and serious issues surely requires that each participant (a) have confidence in the other's integrity, and (b) share with the other a set of values. In that sense then, a relationship requires trust. If, on the other hand, "relationship" refers to any and every interaction that one person may have with another, and "trust" denotes a deep-rooted confidence and kinship, it cannot fairly be asserted that a relationship requires trust. "

46.4 EXPLOITING YOUR RESOURCES

You should use every tool at your disposal to enhance the reader's impression of your essay. If you have a flair for writing you should exploit it. Consider these two phrases:

1. "In order to make a relationship that will exist for an extended period of time..."

2. "In order to forge an enduring relationship..."

The second phrase is better than the first. The word "forge" is more expressive than "make," and the word "enduring" is more precise than the phrase "that will exist for an extended period of time."

Consider these two sentences:

1. No one can fully predict that which will happen in his life and one's life is generally accompanied by the appearance, at times, of difficulty and problems that are unforeseen.

2. Life is full of surprises; vicissitude is its frequent visitor.

The second sentence is better than the first. Its message is conveyed clearly.

If in writing your essays, you meaningfully cite a well-regarded authority, you can only improve your grades. Relevant references to Confucius, the Bible, William Shakespeare, Thomas Moore, Abraham Lincoln, Thurgood Marshall, John Fitzgerald Kennedy, or Martin

Luther King Jr., for example, will likely improve your score. Consider, for example, these paragraphs:

> 1. "In a great many cases wars are fought in order to protect and defend special interests of only a minority of a country's citizens. The interests of the majority of the people are not taken into account. In all probability the peoples that find themselves at war have very little dispute with one another. To a considerable degree they share common goals and objectives and would profit more from cooperation than from fighting."

> 2. "War generally serves the interest not of the many but of the few. In the most vital of their needs, warring populations have more of commonality than of difference. As President Kennedy proclaimed, "We all inhabit this small planet; we all breathe the same air; we all cherish our children's futures and, finally, we are all mortal.""

The second paragraph is better than the first. It employs a relatively tight, engaging style and refers to the words of a highly regarded figure. If you can work an authoritative quotation into your essay you should do so.

46.5 LENGTH AND APPEARANCE

Because the MCAT essay is graded by human beings, you should make the reader's job easier by using your very best handwriting and making sure that the essay is neither too long nor too short. The test booklet provides three pages for each exercise. Try to use at least half the space, but do not use it all. Regardless of its quality, an essay that is only two-thirds of a page in length gives the appearance of a writer who (a) fails to take the assignment seriously or, (b) has little thought to share. A writer who uses all of the space available to him appears as one who has not carefully designed his essay, but rather has written aimlessly until all available space is consumed.

It is difficult to construct a *well ordered* essay in thirty minutes, particularly if the topic is not of your own choosing. You give the *appearance* of organization, however, if you avoid long paragraphs and clearly mark the point at which new ones begin. You should see that no paragraph is longer than eight lines (nor shorter than four) and that each paragraph is clearly marked by a skipped line and a pronounced indentation.

CHAPTER 47

SIX ESSAY EXERCISES

47.1 ESSAY EXERCISE I

Consider this statement:

Without suffering, human beings can experience no real joy.

Write a unified essay in which you perform the following tasks. Explain what you think the above statement means. Describe a specific situation in which human beings can experience joy without suffering. Discuss what you think determines whether human beings can or cannot experience joy without suffering.

Good Response:

I believe this statement means that human beings can appreciate a feeling of profound happiness and well-being in their lives only if they have previously passed through times of distress and anguish with which to compare it. Anyone who is unable or unwilling to experience the emotional depths of life will have experienced only a truncated version of the lower range of human feeling, and so will be unable to take the total measure of its upper range. The statement further implies that human emotions, in general, are truly understandable only in relation to their opposites.

To describe a specific situation in which human joy can be experienced in the absence of suffering, it is necessary first to explore the meaning of the words "suffering" and "real joy." The statement is devoid of meaning without those words, and its validity requires a clear understanding of them.

The word "suffering" is subject to a wide variability of significance. For one person, suffering might entail nothing more than going without food for a day, or having to walk three miles to town because the car broke down. For others, suffering implies the kind of misery and anguish associated with having loved ones away for prolonged periods in situations of adversity and substantial danger, such as war. Still others might relate the word to harsh experiences undergone in extreme situations, such as those experienced at the hands of a brutal and desperate enemy by actual prisoners of war.

"Real joy" is a concept subject to interpretation. When a war is over, and the combatants have signed peace accords and made known their intentions to release prisoners to their respective sides, no doubt a sense of joy is felt by nearly everyone. To say that the joy felt at such a time by the mother or wife or son of a captured soldier is not the same as that felt by the soldier him or herself, is probably true. To say, however, that the soldier's joy is somehow more real, more genuine, more true, or more profound than that felt by his or her family is open to question. One does not have to experience physical agony to experience real joy at the termination of such horrors. Even individuals who have no personal involvement with such a tragic situation may feel a real sense of joy on learning that other human beings have been released from a situation of inhumane treatment.

To further explore the applicability of the statement, let us consider the situation of a person standing on a mountaintop. First, he or she looks down the north side of the mountain into a deep valley below; then, the person looks down the south side of the mountain onto a plains land. In all probability, while looking down into the valley the person will experience a greater sense of altitude than while looking down onto the plains. Similarly, it may be the case that for a given individual, experiences of tribulation and affliction add a dimension to previous or subsequent feelings of joy; and measured according to that extra dimension, the person's sense of joy may be, in some regard, more "real" than it might be without the added scale.

Thus, the relevance of the statement varies according to the interpretation and the context of its terminology. If one limits one's consideration of the statement to the case of a single individual, the statement seems to have meaning. If, however, one attempts to compare different individuals in diverse circumstances who have varying notions of "joy" and "suffering," the meaning appears to offer less in the way of universal truth.

47.2 ESSAY EXERCISE II

Consider this statement:

One who has no committed belief has no meaningful purpose in life.

Write a unified essay in which you perform the following tasks. Explain what you think the above statement means. Describe a specific situation in which a person may have a meaningful purpose in life without a committed belief. Discuss what you think determines whether a person can have a meaningful purpose in life without having a committed belief.

Good Response:

In my view, this statement means that one who does not adhere firmly to a guiding principle or set of principles will find no objective of any true significance in life. The statement indicates that to have substance, a person's ambition must be rooted in a fundamental conviction which the person holds strongly. Furthermore, in the absence of such conviction, a person's life will be devoid of vital goals.

In order to describe a situation in which the statement does not apply, it is necessary to examine the meaning of the words contained in the statement. Without a lucid comprehension of "committed belief" and "meaningful purpose," it is impossible to evaluate the essence of the statement.

A committed belief may mean to some people a conviction that is absolute and inflexible, regardless of the situational ethics that may be involved. Thus, the injunction "Thou shalt not kill" is primary in Western law and religion. Nevertheless, a state legislator, a governor, an attorney general, a judge, a jury, and an executioner who support, sign, endorse, sentence, enforce and enact a death penalty for a capital crime may believe that in so doing they are not violating their commitment to the First Commandment. Moreover, they all may assure themselves that they are, each in his or her respective roles, fulfilling an important purpose.

The concept of "meaningful purpose" might also vary according to an individual's perception of it. Activity which may seem trivial and shallow to some may offer significance and purpose to another. In certain cases, it may be that activity itself, devoid of conviction or import, can offer a meaning and an objective to an individual who otherwise would face the gloom and exasperation of inertia.

On the other hand, it may well be true that some individuals who feel no deep or abiding convictions may find their ambitions in life hollow and superficial. A writer, for example, may find little or no significance in completing a "hack" assignment merely for money. Indeed, the task, even though well remunerated, may present itself as pure drudgery. That same writer, though, might be willing and eager to spend hours upon hours creating a work whose themes have special and vital relevance to his or her life, but which no one is willing to buy.

The truth of this statement, then, varies with the situation to which it is applied, and the interpretation by which it is understood. In some circumstances, a committed belief endows an otherwise empty existence with profoundly significant goals. In other situations, genuine purpose can be found even in the absence of such conviction.

47.3 ESSAY EXERCISE III

Consider this statement:

Human nature ultimately overcomes tyrannical government.

Write a unified essay in which you perform the following tasks. Explain what you think the above statement means. Describe a specific situation in which human nature does not overcome tyrannical government. Discuss what you think determines whether human nature does or does not overcome tyrannical government.

Good Response:

The meaning of this statement is that regardless of the oppressive nature of any given governmental regime, the will, intelligence and humanity of its subjects will ultimately succeed in overcoming it and installing a more representative form of rule. Human beings will not tolerate despotism forever, and eventually their resentment of and resistance to arbitrary and unreasonable limitations on their personal freedoms will lead them to oppose actively such unconscionable restrictions. As Robert Frost once wrote, "Something there is that doesn't love a wall, and wants it down."

Nevertheless, there may be some specific situations in which the idea expressed by this statement does not hold true. There are some societies that have never known anything other than autocratic rule. In these nations, whether by force of habit or lack of awareness of any other political tradition, the people have suffered through centuries of one form of dictatorship or another.

Witness Russia, for example. Prior to the establishment of a repressive Communist regime in the 1920s, that country suffered under generations of harsh, authoritarian rule by the Czars. Even since the overthrow of the communists, Russian society has experienced great difficulty establishing a truly democratic system. Instead of representative rule through legislators elected by popular will, the country is apparently currently run by cartels of organized crime, corrupt military officials, and former party apparatchiks. Instead of rule by constitutional law, the system functions on the basis of terror, bribery, cultism and personal whim. Tyranny by any other name will smell as rank.

Circumstances which determine whether the statement will hold true include the level of education of the people, the degree to which the people have access to a means of political control, and even, perhaps, the genetic makeup of the population. A citizenry with little or no education in history, political and social science, or philosophy, will have less basis upon which to formulate a popular movement against authority than one whose educational horizons are broad and diverse. Similarly, people who have no effective access either to military weapons, mass media outlets, or the secular or religious educational podiums, will have little ability to establish an effective political organization. It may also be true, that the "human nature" of some humans is genetically different from that of other humans, and that part of the difference may be expressed in a predisposition to accept illegitimate authority, or, conversely, in a willfulness to personal liberty and social freedom.

The more recent course of human history, by and large, and certainly in the western countries, has been one of evolution from societies run by minority, central authority, with little or no regard for individual rights, to systems in which the preservation and extension of individual freedom constitutes an important social priority. In societies where, whether by governmental edict, social tradition, or plain ignorance, the people have historically been denied open communication and interchange with the rest of the world, the human push towards liberty has been more easily constrained. However, wherever a citizenry has available to them the means of education and/or military clout, tyranny will not long be tolerated.

47.4 ESSAY EXERCISE IV

Consider this statement:

It is more difficult to relate to people one knows well than to those one knows casually.

Write a unified essay in which you perform the following tasks. Explain what you think the above statement means. Describe a specific situation in which it is easier to relate to people one knows well than to those one knows casually. Discuss what you think determines whether it is more difficult to relate to people one knows well than to those one knows casually.

Good Response:

In my opinion, this statement means that it is easier for a person to be open and honest with strangers than to be so with close friends. Indeed, we often keep our most guarded secrets from those who know us best. Conversely, the very fact of distance between two people can sometimes unlock the gates of intimacy.

There are specific situations in which this dictum might not apply. The circumstance of being arrested for an alleged crime represents one such situation. Confronted with the apparatus of the criminal justice system, an individual would probably relate more easily to a friend or family member than to a stranger. Thus, whereas an agent of the police or the district attorney's office might encounter only silence and suspicion from an accused suspect, a family member or trusted friend might be able to engage the individual in frank conversation. In a context where a person feels threatened and powerless, and must reach out to others for assistance, it is usually to those familiar and trusted, rather than to those unknown, that he or she will relate more readily.

In more everyday settings, however, when dealing with people we know well, numerous factors enter into our consideration which play much less of a role in our relations with casual acquaintances. For one thing, we know a lot more about our close friends than we do about casual acquaintances. Because we understand the issues that our friends are sensitive about or proud of, we might tailor our conversations and relations with them in the light of that understanding. With casual acquaintances, on the other hand, we might brazenly stumble around the conversational turf like bulls in a china shop, not realizing the value to the acquaintance's life of certain issues, or even what those issues might be.

By the same token, if we do unintentionally step on the toes of a close friend, we regret it more deeply than if we offend a casual acquaintance. The emotional stakes are higher when friends, rather than acquaintances, are involved. Even though close friends might be more willing than a casual acquaintance to forgive an offense, we still feel the remorse more deeply if it's a friend we've wounded.

Nonetheless, and seemingly paradoxically, we might be more willing to open ourselves up to a casual acquaintance—such as a therapist we've met for the first time, or even a stranger at a party or a bar in a strange city—than to a close friend or colleague from the office. With people we know well there is often a tendency to project our best self forward, to hide our faults and minimize our weaknesses, so that in our everyday dealings we will not feel ourselves to be at a disadvantage. In the company of people we know less well, in relationship with whom we have little or nothing to lose, and whose opinions mean less to us than do those of our friends, we often feel more able to "let our hair down" and let it "all hang out."

The applicability of the statement, then, depends on the context in which it is considered. In extreme situations of threat or terror, we would probably feel more comfortable relating with people we know well. In other circumstances, though, under certain conditions, it might well be easier to relate to casual acquaintances.

47.5 ESSAY EXERCISE V

Consider this statement:

No work constitutes art unless it appeals to some person other than its creator.

Write a unified essay in which you perform the following tasks. Explain what you think the above statement means. Describe a specific situation in which a work might constitute art even though it appeals only to its creator. Discuss what you think determines whether a creation can constitute art if it appeals to no one other than its creator.

Good Response:

I believe this statement means that in order for any given creative endeavor to be called art, it must, on some level, stimulate in a positive way the aesthetic senses of at least one person other than the one who created it. If someone writes a book or choreographs a dance, or stages a play, or paints a portrait, and the finished product does not excite or tantalize or stir a single other human being, the author of the work has not produced art. By the same measure, even if a creative work engages or interests no more than one person other than its maker, it has, indeed, earned the name of art.

A specific situation to which this statement might not pertain would be a particular work created intentionally to repel the aesthetic senses of its audience. That is, if an artist conceived a project whose objective was to create a feeling of disgust or repulsion or apathy in the audience, and if, in the presentation of the work the artist successfully achieved that objective, then one might fairly say that the work in question was, indeed, art. In such a circumstance, the artist, by creation and/or performance of a purely artificial construct, would have stirred in the audience a genuine human emotion. Thus, even if the emotion generated in the audience was a wholly negative one, and even if the piece could not be said to have "appealed" to anyone, the artist, through the art, would have accomplished his or her artistic purpose.

Normally, one supposes, if a particular work does not appeal to anyone, then it will not serve as a vehicle for communication of its creator's perceptions, or values, or vision. If a creative work refuses in this way to communicate to its audience, perhaps it cannot, justly, be called art. "If a tree falls in the forest, and there's no one near to hear it, does it make a sound?" If an artist, for example, intending to portray all the furious beauty and dazzling energy of life, puts brush to canvas, and if everyone who views the finished product can see only a muddy chaos of meaningless lines and senseless forms, then perhaps the painter has only filled the empty space with paint and has not made art. If there is absolutely no appeal to an audience, and there is absolutely no communication, then perhaps there is no art either.

Therefore, the statement's aptness depends on the context in which it is proposed. Certain works of art, whose very purpose might be to alienate or confuse or repel its audience, might achieve their objectives through the very act of negating their own aesthetic appeal. More generally, however, if a creative work finds no audience, and thus communicates nothing and entertains no one, perhaps it surrenders the right to the title of art.

47.6 ESSAY EXERCISE VI

Consider this statement:

Intelligence and skill are not nearly so valuable as stability and persistence.

Write a unified essay in which you perform the following tasks. Explain what you think the above statement means. Describe a specific situation in which intelligence and skill are more valuable than stability and persistence. Discuss what you think determines whether intelligence and skill are as valuable as stability and persistence.

Good Response:

In my opinion, this statement means that the traits of evenness of temperament, and "stick-to-it-iveness" of habit, are more important to a successful life than are brilliance of mind and technique. Like the famous fable of the tortoise and the hare, the slow and steady often appear more effective than the meteoric and inconsistent. As one wit put it, "Inspiration is ninety-nine percent hard work."

This statement might not apply in the specific situation of someone who is a true genius, and whose endeavors are overly constrained in an educational and social system designed for the average. Albert Einstein, it is widely reported, failed his high school mathematics courses. The material was not too difficult for him to master, it was simply too boring. He preferred not to waste his time or intellectual energy on concepts he deemed elemental and tedious. Because he could not bring himself to squander his hours doing the simple algebra exercises, or learning the trigonometry tables, he failed the course.

Nevertheless, later years proved his genius despite his high school transcripts. Would the world have been better off had Einstein not possessed the genius of intellect which led him to his revolutionary insights, and had he, instead, been an individual of ordinary mental ability and mathematical skill who diligently completed every high school homework assignment? There might be honest debate on that question, but surely his genius and ability are more valuable, in the general sense, than the more stable persistence, however admirable, of his classmates.

On the other hand, it must be acknowledged that a person equipped with all the intelligence and the skill in the world will never accomplish anything until and unless he or she sets a goal and then sets out to pursue it. A very intelligent person might imagine a revolutionary design for, say, a spaceship; without the pluck and tenacity necessary to transform the imaginative act into a form that can be understood by engineers and technicians, the design will never be brought to fruition. A writer, blessed with insight and skill, can not even begin to express his or her vision and ideas if he or she is unwilling to sit down at the word processor, or typewriter, or blank sheet of paper, and put the words down for others to read.

It goes without saying that individuals of average intelligence and only moderate abilities make important contributions day in and day out, and they do so by virtue of steadiness of habit and perseverance of labor. The basketball player who plays twenty minutes every game, scoring ten points with five rebounds, can be counted on for a consistent, nightly contribution to the team effort. The superstar, conversely, who might possess sufficient skill to score fifty points on a given night, but whose unstable temperament causes him or her to lose control and be ejected from the game, might prove less valuable to the team's success in the long run than the journeyman player.

The truth of the statement, therefore, greatly depends on the situation to which it is applied. Intelligence and skill count for a great deal, and in some cases may be more important than steadiness and consistency. In many contexts, though, stability and persistence will prove to be the more valuable characteristics.

REVIEW OF BASIC ARITHMETIC, ALGEBRA, AND GEOMETRY

This appendix provides an overview of fundamental terms, processes, and principles pertaining to basic arithmetic, algebra, and geometry. This is provided as a review of the basic concepts upon which physics, chemistry, and biology are based.

While much of this material was taught in elementary and secondary grades, some of it may have been forgotten, and it may be helpful to review some of these basic principles.

A.1 ARITHMETIC

A.1.1 TERMS

A. Integer: An integer is a whole number. One, 2, 3, –7, –12, and 1004 are all integers. One-half, $\frac{3}{4}$, $\frac{55}{92}$, 0.56, and 4.29 are not integers.

B. Rational Number: A rational number is one that can be expressed as one integer divided by another. $\frac{100}{3}$ is a rational number even though it gives rise to the repeating decimal number 33.333333333... The numbers $\sqrt{2}$ and π are not rational numbers; they give rise to unending decimal numbers that never repeat.

C. Unreal Numbers: The even-numbered root of any negative number is unreal. The square root, fourth root, sixth root, and eighth root of any negative number are unreal.

D. Absolute Value, Magnitude: A number's absolute value is its distance from zero. The absolute value of –2 is 2. The absolute value of +2 is also 2. The absolute value of –9 is 9 and the absolute value of +13 is 13. The magnitude of a value refers to its absolute value. To assert that a particle has a charge of magnitude 3 coulombs is to assert that its charge is either (–) 3 coulombs or (+) 3 coulombs. To assert that a body moves with an acceleration of magnitude 45 m/s^2 is to assert that its acceleration is either (+) 45 m/s^2 or (–) 45 m/s^2.

E. Factor: A factor of any given number is a number that can be divided evenly into it. Four is a factor of 12. Six is also a factor of 12. Five is a factor of 15. One is a factor of every number, and every number is a factor of itself.

F. Prime Number: A prime number is a number that has no factors except 1 and itself. Thus, 2, 3, 5, 7, 11, 13, 17, 19, 23, and 29 are all prime numbers. It is important to note that 1 is *not* prime.

G. Multiple: A multiple of a number is any number into which the given number can be divided without leaving a remainder. Fifty is a multiple of 25. Seventy-five is also a multiple of 25. Eighteen is a multiple of 6. Sixty is also a multiple of 6. A number is a multiple of itself.

A.1.2 FRACTIONS

A. Fraction: A fraction expresses the ratio of two whole numbers; the upper number is termed the numerator and the lower number is termed the denominator. One-half is a fraction, of which 1 is the numerator and 2 is the denominator. Any whole number can be expressed as a fraction, by placing it as the numerator above a denominator of 1. For example, $3 = \dfrac{3}{1}$.

B. Mixed Numbers: A mixed number is a whole number combined with a fraction. For example, $2\dfrac{1}{3}$ is a mixed number.

C. Improper Fractions: In an improper fraction the numerator exceeds its denominator. For example, $\dfrac{9}{4}$ is an improper fraction.

D. Conversions Between Mixed Numbers and Improper Fractions:

(1) Any mixed number can be converted to a fraction; the resulting fraction will be improper. In order to convert the mixed number $2\dfrac{1}{3}$ to a fraction, multiply the whole number by the denominator ($2 \times 3 = 6$) and add the result to the numerator ($6 + 1 = 7$). Leave the denominator unchanged, to obtain $\dfrac{7}{3}$.

(2) Any improper fraction can be converted to a mixed number (or a whole number if the denominator divides evenly into the numerator). In order to convert $\dfrac{21}{8}$ to a mixed number, divide the denominator into the numerator ($21 \div 8 = 2$, with remainder $= 5$). The quotient (2) becomes the whole number and the remainder (5) becomes the numerator. The denominator is unchanged:

$$\frac{21}{8} = 2\frac{5}{8}$$

E. Multiplication of Fractions: Consider the equation: $\dfrac{5}{9} \times \dfrac{15}{4}$. Multiply the two numerators to obtain the numerator's product, and multiply the two denominators to obtain the denominator's product.

$$\frac{5}{9} \times \frac{15}{4} = \frac{75}{36}$$

The result in this case is an improper fraction which can be converted to $2\dfrac{1}{12}$.

F. Division of Fractions: In order to divide fractions, *multiply* the first fraction by the reciprocal of the second fraction. In order to divide:

$$\frac{3}{5} \div \frac{7}{9}$$

multiply the reciprocal of the second fraction by the first fraction:

$$\frac{3}{5} \times \frac{9}{7} = \frac{27}{35}$$

In order to divide the mixed numbers $3\frac{2}{5} \div 8\frac{3}{4}$, convert both mixed numbers to improper fractions and then multiply the first by the reciprocal of the second.

$$3\frac{2}{5} = \frac{17}{5}; \; 8\frac{3}{4} = \frac{35}{4}$$

$$\frac{17}{5} \div \frac{35}{4} = \frac{17}{5} \times \frac{4}{35} = \frac{68}{175}$$

G. Equivalence of Fractions: Two fractions are equivalent if the numerator and the denominator of one bear the same relationship as do the numerator and the denominator of the other. Hence, $\frac{3}{12}$ is equivalent to $\frac{1}{4}$ because for both fractions the ratio of numerator to denominator is 1:4.

Every fraction has an infinite number of equivalent fractions. A fraction is converted to its equivalent by multiplying or dividing the numerator and the denominator by the same number.

Consider the fraction $\frac{4}{9}$. Multiply the numerator and the denominator by 3. The result is $\frac{12}{27}$, which is equivalent to $\frac{4}{9}$. Multiply the numerator and the denominator by 6. The result is $\frac{24}{54}$, which is also equivalent to $\frac{4}{9}$.

H. Common Denominators: In order to add and subtract fractions that bear different denominators (see item J) one must first convert the fractions to equivalents that have a common denominator. To find a common denominator, examine the two denominators to identify a common multiple. The common multiple becomes the common denominator.

Consider the fractions $\frac{4}{6}$ and $\frac{7}{9}$. A cursory examination reveals that 18 is a multiple of both 6 and 9. Having selected 18 as the common denominator:

(1) Identify the number by which each of the two denominators, 6 and 9, must be multiplied or divided in order to obtain 18.

(2) Multiply or divide both the numerator and denominator by that number.

In order to yield 18, the number 6 must be multiplied by 3. The fraction $\frac{4}{6}$ is thus converted to:

$$\frac{(4 \times 3)}{(6 \times 3)} = \frac{12}{18}$$

In order to yield 18, the number 9 must be multiplied by 2. The fraction $\frac{7}{9}$ is thus converted to:

$$\frac{(7 \times 2)}{(9 \times 2)} = \frac{14}{18}$$

The fractions $\frac{4}{6}$ and $\frac{7}{9}$ yield the equivalent fractions $\frac{12}{18}$ and $\frac{14}{18}$, each now having a common denominator of 18.

I. Reducing and Simplifying Fractions: To reduce a fraction is to convert it to an equivalent with a smaller numerator and denominator. In order to reduce a fraction to its smallest equivalent, choose the largest number that is a factor of both the numerator and denominator and divide it into both. Consider the fraction: $\frac{50}{75}$. The largest number that is a factor of both 50 and 75 is 25. Dividing both numerator and denominator by 25 yields $\frac{2}{3}$.

J. Adding and Subtracting Fractions: If two fractions have the same denominator, they are added or subtracted by adding or subtracting the numerators and leaving the denominators unchanged.

$$\frac{3}{7} + \frac{2}{7} = \frac{5}{7}$$

$$\frac{9}{23} - \frac{3}{23} = \frac{6}{23}$$

If two fractions have different denominators, it is neccessary to convert them to equivalents with a common denominator as shown in (H) above. In order to add:

$$\frac{3}{4} + \frac{5}{6}$$

convert both fractions to equivalents with a common denominator. Since 4 and 6 are both factors of 12 it will serve as common denominator. The common denominator can also be arrived at by multiplying the two denominators. Thus, 24 (4 × 6) can also be used as the common denominator.

$$\frac{9}{12} + \frac{10}{12} = \frac{19}{12} = 1\frac{7}{12}$$

$$\frac{18}{24} + \frac{20}{24} = \frac{38}{24} = \frac{19}{12} = 1\frac{7}{12}$$

Consider the subtraction:

$$\frac{6}{7} - \frac{3}{4}$$

Quick inspection reveals no common multiple other than 7 × 4 = 28. Converting each fraction to an equivalent with a denominator of 28, we obtain:

$$\frac{24}{28} - \frac{21}{28} = \frac{3}{28}$$

K. Complex Fractions: A fraction whose numerator and/or denominator is (are) a fraction(s) is called a complex fraction. To simplify it, divide the numerator by the denominator. Consider the complex fraction in which $\frac{2}{5}$ is the numerator and $\frac{5}{8}$ is the denominator: $\dfrac{\dfrac{2}{5}}{\dfrac{5}{8}}$.

Simplify it by dividing:

$$\frac{2}{5} \div \frac{5}{8} = \frac{2}{5} \times \frac{8}{5} = \frac{16}{25}$$

A.1.3 DECIMAL NUMBERS

A. Decimal Numbers: Decimal numbers (0.5, 0.05, 0.3214) represent fractions, every decimal place indicating a multiple of a positive or negative power of 10. Therefore, the denominator of a decimal number is:

- 10 if the number extends only 1 place to the right of the decimal point.

$$0.5 = \frac{5}{10}$$

- 100 if the number extends 2 places to the right of the decimal point.

$$0.05 = \frac{5}{100}$$

- 1,000 if the number extends 3 places to the right of the decimal point.

$$0.005 = \frac{5}{1,000}$$

- 10,000 if the number extnds 4 places to the right of the decimal point.

$$0.0005 = \frac{5}{10,000}$$

B. Adding and Subtracting Decimals: To add or subtract decimals, align them so that the decimal points are in a single column.

Consider the addition 51.9 + 32.7:

$$
\begin{array}{r}
51.90 \\
32.70 \\
\hline
84.60
\end{array}
$$

Consider the subtraction 102.35 − 17.914:

$$
\begin{array}{r}
102.350 \\
17.914 \\
\hline
84.436
\end{array}
$$

C. Multiplication of Decimals: To multiply decimal numbers:

(1) Write the numbers to be multiplied.

(2) Perform ordinary multiplication, ignoring the decimal points.

(3) After reaching a result, examine the original numbers and count all digits to the right of the decimal points (including zeros).

(4) Take *that* number and count an equal number of places to the left of the result in order to place the decimal point.

Consider the multiplication 25.5 × 4.241:

$$
\begin{array}{r}
4.241 \\
25.5 \\
\hline
21205 \\
212050 \\
848200 \\
\hline
108.1455
\end{array}
$$

Count all digits to the right of the decimal point in the numbers that were multiplied, including any zeros. The digits 241 and 5 all fall to the right of decimal points, for a total of 4 digits. The number 1081455 is then provided a decimal point four places to the left of its end: 108.1455.

D. Division of Decimals: To divide decimal numbers:

(1) Position the numbers for division.

(2) Eliminate the decimal point in the divisor by moving it to the right, making the divisor a whole number.

(3) Move the decimal point in the dividend an equal number of places to the right (adding zeros as necessary).

(4) Place a decimal point for the answer (quotient) just above the new decimal point of the dividend.

(5) Divide as usual, keeping the answer's decimal point where you have just placed it.

E. Converting a Decimal to a Fraction or a Mixed Number: In order to convert the decimal number 0.978 to a fraction:

(1) Observe that the decimal number extends 3 positions to the right of the decimal point. The denominator is therefore 1,000.

(2) Write the fraction $\dfrac{978}{1,000}$.

In order to convert the decimal number 2.2 to a mixed number:

(1) Observe that the decimal number extends 1 place to the right of the decimal point. The denominator is 10.

(2) Write the mixed number $2\frac{2}{10}$.

F. Converting a Fraction or Mixed Number to a Decimal:

(1) *Fraction whose denominator is a multiple of 10*

Consider the fraction $\frac{41}{100}$. The denominator is 100 (a multiple of 10). Therefore, the decimal number extends 2 places to the right of the decimal point.

$$\frac{41}{100} = 0.41$$

Consider the fraction $\frac{512}{10}$.

Since the denominator is 10, the decimal number extends 1 place to the right of the decimal point.

$$\frac{512}{10} = 51.2$$

Consider the mixed number $4\frac{17}{100}$. The whole number (4) is positioned to the left of the decimal point. Since the denominator is 100, the decimal number extends 2 places to the right of the decimal point.

$$4\frac{17}{100} = 4.17$$

(2) *Fraction whose denominator is* <u>not</u> *a multiple of 10*

Divide the numerator by the denominator.

Consider the fraction $\frac{3}{5}$. $\quad 5\overline{)3.00}^{.6} \qquad \frac{3}{5} = .6$

Consider the fraction $\frac{9}{14}$.

Follow the procedure described above:

$$\frac{9}{14} = .643$$

A.1.4 PERCENTAGE

A. Percentage: A percentage expresses a fraction in which the denominator is 100.

$$30\% \text{ means } \frac{30}{100}; \ 50\% \text{ means } \frac{50}{100}; \ 23\% \text{ means } \frac{23}{100}$$

B. Converting a Decimal Number to a Percentage: Move the decimal point two places to the right (which represents multiplication by 100).

$$0.27 = 27\% = \left(\frac{27}{100}\right)$$

$$0.687 = 68.7\% = \left(\frac{68.7}{100}\right)$$

C. Converting a Percentage to a Decimal Number: Move the decimal point two places to the left (which represents division by 100).

$$52\% = 0.52 \qquad 38\% = 0.38 \qquad 83.1\% = 0.831$$

D. Converting a Percentage to a Fraction: A percentage is converted to a fraction by imposing a denominator of 100.

$$35\% = \frac{35}{100}$$

E. Converting a Fraction to a Percentage: First, convert the fraction to a decimal number. Second, convert the decimal number to a percentage by moving the decimal point two places to the right.

Consider the fraction $\frac{3}{12}$:

$$\frac{3}{12} = 0.25 = 25\%$$

F. Finding a Percentage of a Number: To find a percentage ($x\%$) of a given number (y), convert $x\%$ to a decimal number, then multiply the decimal number by y.

If, for example, one wishes to find 2% of 50, first convert 2% to a decimal number by moving the decimal point two places to the left (0.02), then multiply 0.02 by 50 ($0.02 \times 50 = 1$).

G. Expressing a Number as a Percentage of Another Number: To express one number (y) as a percentage of another (x), divide y by x, and convert the result to a percentage.

Consider this question: 20 is what percent of 25? (The number 20 is to be expressed as a percentage of 25.)

First, divide $20 \div 25 = 0.8$. Second, convert to a percentage ($0.8 = 80\%$).

H. Increasing a Number by a Stated Percentage: To state that a number is increased by X% is to state that X% of the number is added to the number. To increase 50 by 2%, add 2% of 50 to 50.

$$2\% \text{ of } 50 = (0.02)(50) = 1 \qquad 50 + 1 = 51$$

I. Decreasing a Number by a Stated Percentage: To state that a number is decreased by $x\%$ is to state that $x\%$ of the number is subtracted from the number. To decrease 80 by 40%, subtract 40% of 80 from 80.

$$40\% \text{ of } 80 = (0.4)(80) = 32 \qquad 80 - 32 = 48$$

A.1.5 NEGATIVE NUMBERS

A. Adding a negative number to any other number is the equivalent of subtracting a positive number:

$$7 + (-5) = 2, \text{ and } 3 + (-5) = -2$$

B. Subtracting a negative number from any other number is equivalent to adding a positive number:

$$7 - (-2) = 9, \text{ and } (-8) - (-2) = -6$$

C. Multiplying or dividing a negative number and a positive number yields a negative number:

$$5 \times (-3) = -15, \text{ and } 60 \div (-20) = -3$$

D. Multiplying or dividing two negative numbers yields a positive number:

$$-3 \times (-15) = +45, \text{ and } -15 \div (-5) = +3$$

E. Items C and D mean that any string of numbers multiplied together yields a positive result if it features (a) no negative numbers, or (b) an even number of negative numbers. It yields a negative result if it features an odd number of negative numbers.

$$(-3)(-5)(-2)(+2) = -60, \text{ and } (-3)(-4)(+3) = +36$$

Therefore, when a negative number is squared or raised to any power that is even (see **A.1.6** below) the result is positive. When a negative number is raised to any power that is odd the result is negative.

$$-4^3 = -64, \text{ and } -4^4 = +256$$

F. Multiplying any number by 0 yields 0. Thus if 0 appears in any string of numbers that are multiplied together, the product is 0. Any fraction whose numerator is 0 is equal to 0. (Division by 0 is said not to exist and will not arise on the MCAT.)

A.1.6 EXPONENTIAL NUMBERS

A. 5^3 means the third power of 5, which means $5 \times 5 \times 5$ (125). 9^2 means the second power of 9, which is also expressed "9 squared," which means 9×9 (81).

B. In the expression 5^3, 5 is called the base and 3 is called the exponent.

C. $\sqrt{4}$ means the square root of 4, which means the number whose second power (square) is equal to 4 (which is 2, because $2^2 = 4$).

$\sqrt[3]{27}$ means the third root (also called cubed root) of 27, which means the number whose third power is equal to 27 (which is equal to 3, because $3^3 = 27$).

$\sqrt[5]{3125}$ means the fifth root of 3,125, which means the number whose fifth power is equal to 3,125 (which is 5, because $5^5 = 3,125$).

D. Finding the Power of a Root Requires Multiplication:

$$6^3 = 6 \times 6 \times 6 = 216$$

$$\left(\frac{3}{4}\right)^3 = \frac{3}{4} \times \frac{3}{4} \times \frac{3}{4} = \frac{27}{64}$$

E. Negative Numbers as Bases, Exponents, and Roots:

- 5^{-2} means the negative second power of 5, which means $\frac{1}{5^2}$, which is equal to $\frac{1}{25}$.

- 2^{-3} means the negative third power of 2, which means $\frac{1}{2^3}$, which is equal to $\frac{1}{8}$.

- $-(5^2)$ means negative the square of 5, which is equal to -25.

- $-(7^3)$ means negative the third power of 7, which is equal to -343.

- $(-5)^2$ means the square of negative 5, which means $(-5) \times (-5)$ which is equal to $+25$.

- $(-5)^3$ means the third power (cube) of negative 5, which means $(-5) \times (-5) \times (-5)$ which is equal to -125.

Note that even-numbered roots of any number (square root, fourth root, sixth root, eighth root), always have two solutions: positive and negative.

$\sqrt{16}$ has two solutions: $(+)\ 4$ and $(-)\ 4$

$\sqrt{4}$ has two solutions: $(+)\ 2$ and $(-)\ 2$

However, unless otherwise indicated, the symbol $\sqrt{\ }$ signifies a positive solution $\left(+\sqrt{\ }\right)$.

F. Multiplying and Dividing Two Exponential Numbers Bearing the Same Exponent: To multiply two exponential numbers bearing the same exponent, multiply the bases and leave the exponent unchanged.

$$3^2 \times 5^2 = (3 \times 5)^2 = 15^2 = 225$$

$$45^2 \div 9^2 = (45 \div 9)^2 = 5^2 = 25$$

G. Multiplying and Dividing Two Exponential Numbers Bearing the Same Base but Different Exponents: To multiply two exponential numbers bearing the same base but different exponents, *add* the exponents together, leaving the base unchanged. To divide two exponential numbers bearing the same base but different exponents, subtract the *second* exponent from the first, leaving the base unchanged.

$$5^4 \times 5^3 = 5^{(4+3)} = 5^7 = 78{,}125$$

$$8^9 \div 8^7 = 8^{(9-7)} = 8^2 = 64$$

H. Working with Fractional Exponents:

$$A^{\frac{b}{c}} \text{ means } \left(\sqrt[c]{A}\right)^b$$

$$16^{\frac{1}{2}} \text{ means } \left(\sqrt{16}\right)^1 = 4$$

$$16^{\frac{2}{4}} \text{ means } \left(\sqrt[4]{16}\right)^2 = (2)^2 = 4$$

I. Simplification of Square Radicals:

$$\sqrt{a \times b} = \sqrt{a} \times \sqrt{b}$$

$$\sqrt{16 \times 2} = \sqrt{16} \times \sqrt{2} = \left(4\sqrt{2}\right)$$

$$\sqrt[3]{27 \times 5} = \sqrt[3]{27} \times \sqrt[3]{5} = \left(3\sqrt[3]{5}\right)$$

$$\sqrt[4]{16 \div 19} = \sqrt[4]{16} \div \sqrt[4]{19} = \left(2\sqrt[4]{19}\right)$$

J. Application of an Exponent:

Apply an exponent only to the number immediately preceding it.

$$15x^2 = 15 \cdot (x^2)$$

If $x = 3$:

$$15x^2 = (15)(3^2) = 15 \cdot 9 = 135$$

On the other hand, $(15x)^2$ signifies that the entire value $(15x)$ is to be squared.

If $x = 3$:

$$(15x)^2 = (15 \cdot 3)^2 = 45^2 = 2,205$$

A.2 ALGEBRA

A.2.1 PARENTHETICAL EXPRESSIONS

Within an algebraic expression, any matter inside parenthesis is treated as *one number*. Thus, $10 - (2 + 5) = 10 - 7$, which is equal to 3.

$10 - (2 + 5)$ does *not* mean $10 - 2 + 5$, which is equal to 13.

$15 + (2x + 3x)$ is equal to $15 + 5x$

A.2.2 SIMPLIFYING PARENTHETICAL EXPRESSIONS:

Suppose one wishes to eliminate the parentheses in this expression:

$$6(3x + 2x + 10) + 4(2x + x + 6) - 2(14x + 14)$$

(1) Look at the items within the parentheses and perform those operations that allow the combination of like terms. In the first set, $3x + 2x$ can be added to give $5x$. In the second set, $2x + x$ can be added to yield $3x$. In the third set no operation can be performed because $14x$ and 14 are not like terms.

The result is:

$$6(5x + 10) + 4(3x + 6) - 2(14x + 14)$$

(2) Determine whether any set of parentheses is to be multiplied by some number or variable and perform such multiplication by distribution. In this case, all sets of parentheses are multiplied. The first set is multiplied by 6, the second by 4, and the third by –2. To perform the first multiplication, distribute the 6:

$$6(5x + 10) = 6(5x) + 6(10) = 30x + 60$$

To perform the second multiplication, distribute the 4:

$$4(3x + 6) = 4(3x) + 4(6) = 12x + 24$$

To perform the third multiplication distribute the –2:

(*Remember, when parenthetical matter is subtracted, the negative sign must be distributed when the parentheses are removed as shown in this example: $10 - (5 + 2) = 10 - 5 - 2$.*)

$$-2(14x + 14) = -28x - 28$$

Result:

$$30x + 60 + 12x + 24 - 28x - 28 = 14x - 56$$

A.2.3 ADDING TWO ALGEBRAIC EXPRESSIONS

To add:

$$(4x + 5y - xy) + (9x + 3y + 3x(2x - 2y))$$

Remove the internal parentheses in the second expression by multiplying it out:

$$3x(2x - 2y) = 6x^2 - 6xy$$

That leaves:

$$(4x + 5y - xy) + (9x + 3y + 6x^2 - 6xy)$$

Second: remove all parentheses. Because there is no (–) sign between the two expressions, there is no negative sign to be distributed across the second expression:

$$4x + 5y - xy + 9x + 3y + 6x^2 - 6xy$$

A.2.4 SUBTRACTING TWO ALGEBRAIC EXPRESSIONS

To subtract $(2x + 3y - 2xy) - (7x - 2(x - y))$:

(1) As in **A.2.3**, remove the internal parentheses by performing the indicated operation. *The expression $-2(x-y)$ requires the distribution of a (–) sign:*

$$-2(x - y) = -2x + -2(-y) = -2x + 2y = 2y - 2x$$

(2) Remove all parentheses, but remember to distribute the (–) sign between the two expressions.

$$(2x + 3y - 2xy) - (7x + 2y - 2x) = 2x + 3y - 2xy - 7x - 2y + 2x = y - 2xy - 3x$$

A.2.5 MULTIPLYING TWO ALGEBRAIC EXPRESSIONS

To multiply two algebraic expressions together, multiply every term of the first by every term of the second.

To multiply $(x - 3)(x + 7)$:

(1) Multiply the first term of the first expression by each term of the second:

$$x(x+7) = x^2 + 7x$$

(2) Multiply the second term of the first expression by each term of the second expression:

$$-3(x + 7) = -3x + (-21) = -3x - 21$$

The result is:
$$x^2 + 7x - 3x - 21$$

To multiply $(2x^2 + 3x + 7) (x^2 + 5x)$:

(1) Multiply the first term of the first expression by every term of the second:

$$2x^2 (x^2 + 5x) = 2x^4 + 10x^3$$

(2) Multiply the second term of the first expression by every term of the second:

$$3x (x^2 + 5x) = 3x^3 + 15x^2$$

(3) Multiply the third term of the first expression by every term of the second:

$$7 (x^2 + 5x) = 7x^2 + 35x$$

The result is:
$$2x^4 + 10x^3 + 3x^3 + 15x^2 + 7x^2 + 35x$$

A.2.6 DIVIDING ONE ALGEBRAIC EXPRESSION INTO ANOTHER

To divide an expression of several terms by an expression of one term, divide the one term into each of the several, and add the results.

Consider the division:
$$(4x^2 + 3x + 5) \div x$$

(1) Divide the first term of the longer expression by the second expression:

$$\frac{4x^2}{x} = 4x$$

(2) Divide the second term of the longer expression by the second expression:

$$\frac{3x}{x} = 3$$

(3) Divide the third term of the longer expression by the second expression:

$$\frac{5}{x} = \frac{5}{x}$$

(4) Add the results:

$$4x + 3 = \frac{5}{x}$$

To divide an expression of more than one term by another expression of more than one term, search for common factors to cancel.

Consider the division:

$$(4x^2 - 4x) \div (x - 1) = \frac{4x^2 - 4x}{x - 1}$$

Observe that $4x$ can be factored from the first expression to leave: $\dfrac{4x(x - 1)}{x - 1}$

Notice that the numerator and the denominator can be divided by $(x - 1)$, to leave: $4x$.

A.2.7 REARRANGING EQUATIONS

Equations are unaltered in their accuracy when identical processes are performed on each side of the (=) sign. One may add, subtract, multiply, or divide on each side of the equation and maintain the equation's integrity.

Consider the equation:

$$x = 2 + 5$$

One may *add* 3 to both sides of the equation to obtain:

$$3 + x = 2 + 5 + 3$$

One may *subtract* 5 from both sides of the equation to obtain:

$$x - 5 = 2 + 5 - 5$$

One may *divide* both sides of the equation by 2 to obtain:

$$\frac{x}{2} = \frac{2 + 5}{2}$$

One may *multiply* both sides of the equation by 9 to obtain:

$$9x = 9(2 + 5)$$

In every case the equation's integrity is maintained and $x = 7$.

Consider the equation $5x + 2 = 10x - 8$. To solve for x, rearrange the equation so that x is alone on one side of the equation:

(1) Subtract 2 from each side of the equation to obtain: $5x = 10x - 8 - 2$.

(2) Subtract $10x$ from each side of the equation to obtain:

$$5x - 10x = -8 - 2; \qquad -5x = -10$$

(3) Divide both sides of the equation by -5 so that x is isolated on the left side of the equation: $x = 2$.

Recognize that fractions are eliminated from an equation if both sides of the equation are multiplied by the fraction's denominator or by a multiple of the denominator. Consider this equation with a mind toward solving for x:

$$\frac{5}{3}x = \frac{6}{9}x + 2$$

To eliminate both fractions, multiply by a common multiple of both denominators. In this case, 9 is a common multiple of 3 and of 9. Multiplying both sides of the equation by 9 we obtain $15x = 6x + 18$.

To solve for x, subtract $6x$ from both sides to obtain $9x = 18$.

Divide both sides of the equation by 9 and obtain $x = 2$.

A.2.8 SOLVING FOR VARIABLES RELATED IN TWO SEPARATE EQUATIONS

When presented with two different relationships between two variables, one can solve for both variables. Consider these two relationships between x and y:

(1) $2x = 3y$

(2) $x - 10 = y$

One solves for x and y in four steps.

(1) Choose one of the relationships (equations) and solve for one of the variables in terms of the other. In other words, write an equation that puts one variable alone on one side ($x = \ldots$ or $y = \ldots$).

Let us choose the first equation and solve for x in terms of y.

$$2x = 3y$$

Divide both sides of the equation by 2 to obtain $x = \frac{3}{2}y$

(2) With x now defined in terms of y, address the second equation and substitute $\frac{3}{2}y$ for x each time it appears:

$$\frac{3}{2}y - 10 = y$$

(3) Solve this new equation for y:

$$\frac{3}{2}y - 10 = y \qquad \frac{3}{2}y - y = 10 \qquad \frac{1}{2}y = 10 \qquad y = 20$$

(4) Knowing now that y = 20, substitute 20 for y in either equation and solve for x.

Let us choose the second equation: $x - 10 = y$.

$$x - 10 = 20 \qquad x = 20 - (-10) \qquad x = 20 + 10 \qquad x = 30$$

To verify, substitute 30 for x and 20 for y in both equations:

$$2(30) = 3(20) \text{ (true)} \qquad 30 - 10 = 20 \text{ (true)}$$

A.2.9 PROPORTIONS

If (and only if) two sets of numbers bear the same proportional relationship, the product of the *means* equals the product of the *extremes*.

Consider the two sets of numbers: 10/2 and 60/12. 10 bears the same relation to 2 as does 60 to 12. Therefore, the product of the means (2 × 60) = the product of the extremes (12 × 10).

If one is told that (1) Body A moves with velocity of magnitude V_a = 18 m/s, (2) Body B moves with velocity of magnitude V_b = 12 m/s, (3) Body C moves with velocity of magnitude V_c = 21 m/s, and (4) Body D moves with a velocity whose magnitude V_d bears the same relationship to V_c as does V_b to V_a, he concludes that:

$$\frac{V_a}{V_b} = \frac{V_c}{V_d} \qquad \frac{18}{12} = \frac{21}{V_d} \qquad 18(V_d) = (21)(12)$$

$$18(V_d) = 252 \qquad V_d = \frac{252}{18} \qquad V_d = 14 \text{ m/s}$$

A.2.9.1 Direct Proportionality

If one quantity (Q_1) is *directly proportional* to another quantity (Q_2) then the multiplication or division of either quantity by any factor requires the multiplication or division of the other by that same factor.

If, for example, one is told that the pressure of a gas is directly proportional to its temperature, then:

- doubling the temperature will double the pressure and, conversely, doubling the pressure will double the temperature.

- tripling the temperature will triple the pressure and, conversely, tripling the pressure will triple the temperature.

- reducing the temperature by a factor of 2 (cutting it in half) will reduce the pressure by a factor of 2 and, conversely, reducing the pressure by a factor of 2 will reduce the temperature by a factor of 2.

If one is told that pressure is 2 torr when temperature is 300K, then pressure is 4 torr when temperature is 600K, pressure is 6 torr when temperature is 900K, and pressure is 8 torr when temperature is 1200K.

If two quantities (Q_1 and Q_2) are said to be equal and one of them (Q_2) is the product of two or more quantities, then Q_1 is directly proportional to each of the quantities that compose the product. Within the realm of physics, for example, it is known that:

$$(force) = (mass)\,(acceleration)$$

$$f = ma$$

That means that force is directly proportional to mass and, separately, that force is directly proportional to acceleration. If one is told that a force of 3 newtons causes Body A of mass m to move with acceleration a, she can conclude that:

- a force of 9 newtons will cause Body A to move with acceleration = $(3)(a)$.

- if a second body, Body B, of mass $(6)(m)$ is to move with acceleration a, it will require a force of 6×9 newtons.

When two quantities (Q_1 and Q_2) are said to be equal, and one of them (Q_2) is a fraction, then Q_1 is directly proportional to the numerator of Q_2. The universal law of gravitation provides that the gravitational force between any two objects is:

$$F_g = \frac{(G)(M_1)(M_2)}{r^2}$$

where:

F_g = force due to gravity exerted on one object by the other

G = gravitational constant

M_1 = mass of object 1

M_2 = mass of object 2

r = distance between the center of masses of the two objects

Among other implications, the equation indicates that F_g is directly proportional to M_1 and directly proportional to M_2. Tripling the mass of either object will triple F_g. (Tripling the mass of both objects will multiply F_g by a factor of $3 \times 3 = 9$.)

A.2.9.2 Inverse Proportionality

If one quantity (Q_1) is *inversely proportional* to another (Q_2), then the multiplication of either quantity by any factor occasions the *division* of the other by that same factor; the division of either quantity by some factor occasions the *multiplication* of the other by that same factor.

If, for example, one is told that the pressure of a gas is inversely proportional to its volume, he concludes that:

- doubling the volume will reduce the pressure by a factor of 2 (cut it in half) and, conversely, doubling the pressure will reduce the temperature by a factor of 2.

- tripling the volume will reduce the pressure by a factor of 3 and, conversely, tripling the pressure will reduce the volume by a factor of 3.

- reducing the volume by a factor of 2 will double the pressure and, conversely, reducing the pressure by a factor of 2 will double the volume.

- reducing the volume by a factor of 3 will triple the pressure and, conversely, reducing the pressure by a factor of 3 will triple the volume.

If two quantities (Q_1 and Q_2) are said to be equal, and one or both of them are the product of two or more quantities, then each quantity within a product is inversely proportional to every other. Consider again the equation:

$$(\text{force}) = (\text{mass}) \times (\text{acceleration})$$

$$f = ma$$

We conclude that mass and acceleration are inversely proportional to one another. If you are told that a force of 3 newtons causes Body A of mass m to move with acceleration a, you can conclude that if force is held constant:

- increasing the mass of the body to $2(m)$ will reduce the acceleration to $0.5(a)$.

- decreasing the mass of the body to $\frac{4}{10}(m) = (0.4)(m)$ will increase the acceleration to:

$$\frac{10}{4}(a) = (2.5)(a)$$

If a second body moves with acceleration of $5(a)$ when subjected to a force of 3 newtons, its mass is $\frac{1}{5}(m) = (0.2)(m)$.

You can also conclude that if some second body moves with acceleration $\frac{3}{4}(a) = (0.75)(a)$ its mass is $\frac{4}{3}(m) = 1.33(m)$.

When two quantities (Q_1 and Q_2) are said to be equal, and one of them (Q_2) is a fraction, then Q_1 is inversely proportional to the denominator of Q_2. (If the denominator is the product of two or more quantities, then Q_1 is inversely proportional to each and every quantity that composes the product.)

For example:

$$\text{centripetal acceleration} = \frac{(\text{instantaneous velocity}^2)}{(\text{radius of circular travel})}$$

$$a = \frac{v^2}{r}$$

The equation indicates that centripetal acceleration is inversely proportional to the radius of circular travel (r). Knowing this, one concludes that if velocity is held constant:

- doubling the radius of circular travel will reduce the centripetal acceleration by a factor of 2, and, conversely, doubling the centripetal acceleration will reduce the radius of circular travel by a factor of 2.

- tripling the radius of circular travel will reduce centripetal acceleration by a factor of 3 and, conversely, tripling the centripetal acceleration will reduce the radius of circular travel by a factor of 3.

If you are told that a body moves with centripetal acceleration a at a velocity of constant magnitude v in a circle with radius of r, then you can conclude that if magnitude of velocity is held constant:

- increasing the radius to $2(r)$ will reduce the centripetal acceleration to $0.5(a)$.

- decreasing the radius to $\dfrac{6}{10}(r) = (0.6)(r)$ will increase the centripetal acceleration to:

$$\frac{10}{6}(a) = (1.67)(a)$$

You can further conclude that if a second body moves with centripetal acceleration of $7(a)$ at a velocity of magnitude v, the radius about which it moves is $\dfrac{1}{7}(r) = (0.14)(r)$.

A.2.9.3 Proportionality and Exponential Factors

If one quantity (Q_1) is *directly proportional to the square of another quantity* (Q_2), meaning that Q_1 is directly proportional to $(Q_2)^2$, then multiplying or dividing Q_2 by any factor occasions the multiplication or division of Q_1 by the square of that same factor.

If Q_1 is directly proportional to $(Q_2)^2$, then doubling Q_2 means multiplying Q_1 by 4; tripling Q_2 means multiplying Q_1 by 9; quadrupling Q_2 means multiplying Q_1 by 16.

Consider, again, the formula for centripetal acceleration: $a = \dfrac{v^2}{r}$, which indicates that a is directly proportional to v^2. If you are told that a body travels with centripetal acceleration (a) at a velocity of magnitude (v) in a circle of radius r, then you conclude that if r is held constant:

- raising the magnitude of velocity to $2v$ will raise centripetal acceleration to $4(a)$.

- raising the magnitude of velocity to $3v$ will raise centripetal acceleration to $9(a)$.

- raising the magnitude of velocity to $5v$ will raise centripetal acceleration to $25(a)$.

If one quantity (Q_1) is *inversely proportional to the square of another quantity* (Q_2), meaning that Q_1 is inversely proportional to $(Q_2)^2$, then multiplying Q_2 by any factor occasions the division of Q_1 by the square of that same factor, and dividing Q_2 by any factor occasions the multiplication of Q_1 by the square of that same factor.

If Q_1 is inversely proportional to $(Q_2)^2$, then doubling Q_2 means dividing Q_1 by 4; tripling Q_2 means dividing Q_1 by 9; quadrupling Q_2 means dividing Q_1 by 16.

Consider again the universal law of gravitation $F_g = \dfrac{(G)(M_1)(M_2)}{r^2}$, which indicates that F_g is inversely proportional to r^2. If you are told that two particles separated by a distance r experience a gravitational attraction equal to F_g, you can conclude that in relation to the same bodies:

- increasing the distance to $2(r)$ will decrease the gravitational attraction to $\dfrac{1}{4}(F_g)$.

- increasing the distance to $6(r)$ will decrease the gravitational attraction to $\dfrac{1}{36}(F_g)$.

- decreasing the distance to $\frac{1}{4}(r)$ will increase the gravitational attraction to $16(F_g)$.

- decreasing the distance to $\frac{1}{7}(r)$ will increase the gravitational attraction to $49(F_g)$.

A.3 GEOMETRY

A.3.1 ANGLES

A. A right angle = 90°.

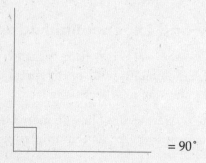

$= 90°$

B. An acute angle is any angle less than 90°.

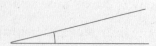

C. An obtuse angle is any angle greater than 90°.

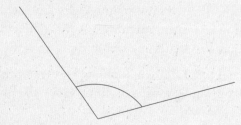

D. A straight line = 180°.

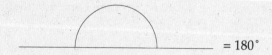

$= 180°$

E. The sum of all angles in a triangle = 180°.

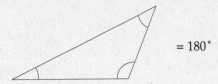

= 180°

F. A circle contains 360°.

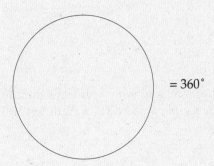

= 360°

A.3.2 CIRCLES

A. The distance between any circle's center and any point on its surface is the **radius** (*r*).

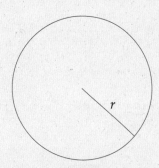

r

B. Any line segment passing through the circle's center and joining two points on its surface is called a **diameter** (*d*). The length of the diameter is twice that of the radius.

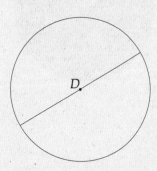

D.

C. A diameter divides the circle into two halves, or semicircles, each of which contains 180°.

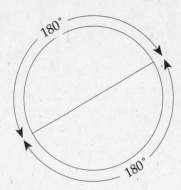

Any angle whose vertex is on the circle and whose sides terminate at opposite ends of a diameter is an angle inscribed in a semicircle and is a right angle (90°).

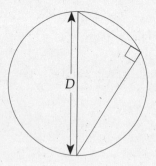

D. The area inside a circle is equal to $\pi \times (\text{radius})^2 = \pi r^2$; π is an irrational number with value equal to approx. $22/7$ = approx. 3.14.

E. The distance around a circle is the circumference and is equal to

(2) × (π) × (*r*) = 2π*r* which is equal also to (π) × (diameter) = π*d*.

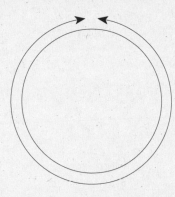

F. Any angle whose vertex is at the circle's center and whose sides terminate on its surface defines a sector of the circle. If the angle defining the sector = ø , then the area of the

sector = $\dfrac{ø}{360}$ ×2 π *r*².

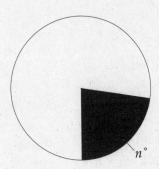

The portion of a circle that borders a sector is termed an arc. Its length = $\dfrac{ø}{360}$ × 2 π *r*.

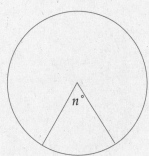

Consider this circle with center C and radius of 5 cm.

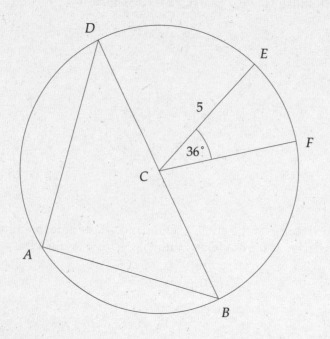

Area of the circle:

$$\pi r^2 = \pi (5^2) = 25\pi = \text{approx. } (25)(3.14) \text{ cm}^2 = 78.5 \text{ cm}^2$$

Circumference of the circle:

$$2\pi r = 2(\pi)(5) = 10\pi = \text{approx. } 31.4 \text{ cm}$$

Size of angle $DAB = 90°$, because angle DAB is an angle inscribed in a semicircle.

The length of arc EF:

$$\frac{36}{360} \times (2\pi r) = \frac{2\pi r}{10} = \frac{\pi r}{5} = \text{approx. } \frac{(3.14)(5)}{5} = 3.14 \text{ cm.}$$

The area of sector ECF:

$$\frac{36}{360} \times (\pi r^2) = \frac{\pi r^2}{10} = \frac{r^2}{5} = \frac{25\pi}{10} = \text{approx. } \frac{(25)(3.14)}{10} = 7.85 \text{ cm}^2$$

G. A cylinder is an elongate structure of circular shape throughout its length. The volume of a cylinder is equal to its height (h) times the area of the circle that comprises its base (πr^2); volume = ($\pi r^2 h$). Consider a cylinder with radius of 2 inches and length of 8 inches.

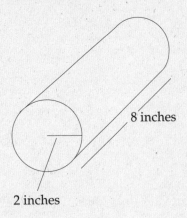

8 inches

2 inches

Volume:

$$\pi(r^2h) = \pi(2^2)(8) = 32\pi \ \text{in}^2 = \text{approx. } 100.5 \ \text{in}^3$$

A.3.3 TRIANGLES

A. In any triangle the sum of the three angles is 180°.

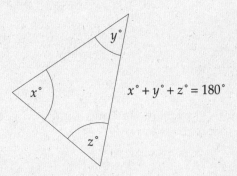

$$x° + y° + z° = 180°$$

B. If one angle of a triangle is 90°, the triangle is a right triangle.

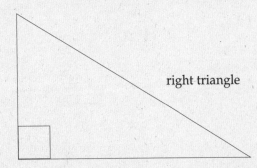

right triangle

C. In a right triangle, the side opposite the right angle is the hypotenuse (*h*), and the other two sides are the legs.

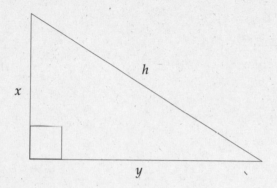

D. The Pythagorean theorem provides that the square of the hypotenuse is equal to the sum of the squares of the legs.

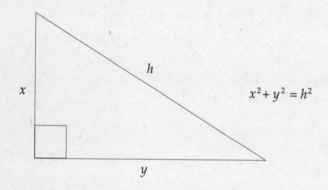

$$x^2 + y^2 = h^2$$

If, for example, the legs of a right triangle are 3 and 4 units long, then *h* is computed according to the Pythagorean theorem:

$$3^2 + 4^2 = h^2$$

$$9 + 16 = h^2$$

$$h^2 = 25$$

$$h = 5$$

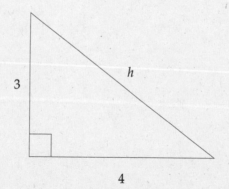

If, for **example**, a hypotenuse is given as 7 units in length, and one leg is known to have length = $\sqrt{5}$, the length of the other leg (l) is computed according to the Pythagorean Theorem:

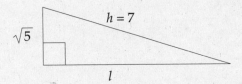

$$l^2 + \left(\sqrt{5}\right)^2 = 7^2 \qquad l^2 + 5 = 49 \qquad l^2 = 49 - 5 = 44 \qquad l = \sqrt{44}$$

E.   In any right triangle, if the two legs are equal, then the hypotenuse is equal to (leg length) × (square root of 2). If, for example, a right triangle's two legs have length = 6, its hypotenuse has length $6\sqrt{2}$.

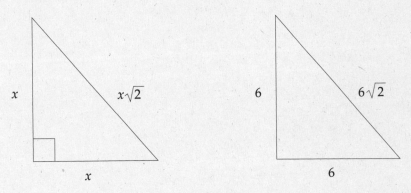

F.   If two sides of any angle are equal, then the angles opposite those sides are equal as well. Conversely, if two angles of a triangle are equal, then the sides opposite the angles are equal as well.

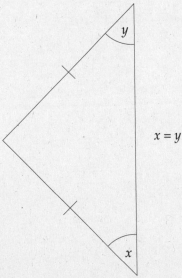

If all of the angles of a triangle are equal, then all of the sides are equal too. If all of the sides of a triangle are equal, then all of the angles are equal as well. Triangles in which all angles are equal and all sides are equal are termed "equilateral." The angles of any equilateral triangle are equal to 60° each. Although all angles of an equilateral triangle are equal to 60°, and all sides of any given equilateral triangle are equal, *two* separate equilateral triangles may have sides of different length.

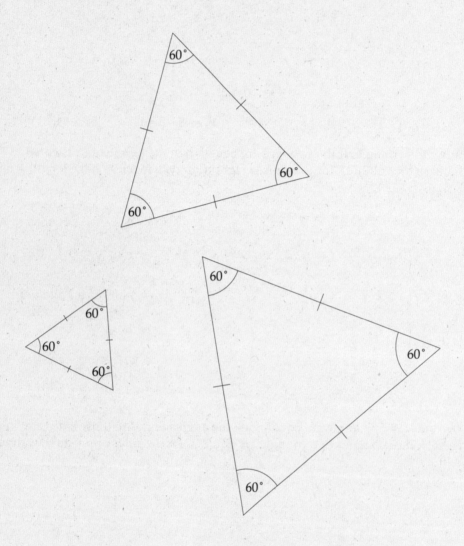

G. If in any triangle, angle x is larger than angle y, then the side opposite angle x is larger than the side opposite angle y. Conversely, if in any triangle, side A is larger than side B, the angle opposite side A is larger than the angle opposite side B.

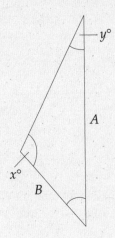

H. Two triangles are congruent if they have identical sides and angles. Congruent triangles are geometric "twins."

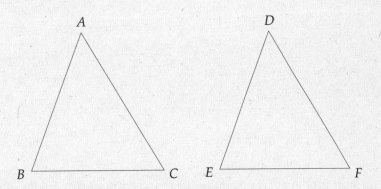

I. **Side-Angle-Side Rule of Congruence**: One may conclude that two triangles are congruent if two pairs of corresponding sides are equal, and the angles between the two sides are equal as well.

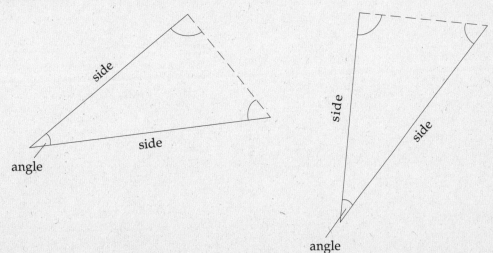

If one knows, for example, that two triangles have in common a side of 3, a side of 5, and an angle between those two sides of 40°, then he knows the two triangles are congruent, and that all other corresponding pairs of sides and angles are equal.

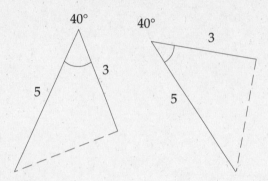

J. **Angle-Side-Angle Rule of Congruence**: One may conclude that two triangles are congruent if two pairs of corresponding angles are equal and the sides between them are also equal.

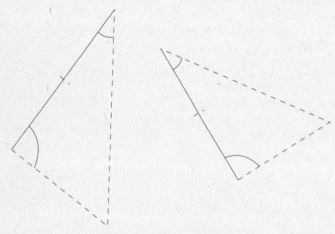

If one knows, for example, that two triangles have in common two angles of 25° and 50°, and a side between these angles of 4, then he knows that the two triangles are congruent and that all other corresponding pairs of sides and angles are equal as well.

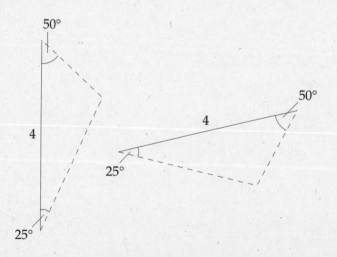

K.   Side-Side-Side Rule of Congruence: One may conclude that two triangles are congruent if all three pairs of corresponding sides are equal.

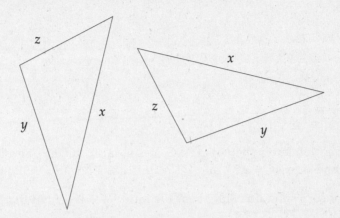

If you know, for example, that two triangles have in common a side of length 4, a side of length 6, and a side of length 7, then you know the two triangles are congruent, and that all pairs of corresponding angles are therefore equal.

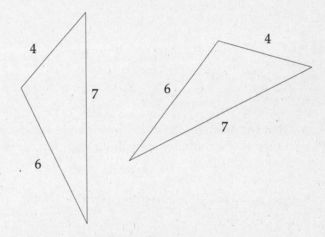

L.   Similar Triangles: Two triangles are similar if all three pairs of corresponding angles are equal. *Two similar triangles need not be congruent; corresponding pairs of sides need not be equal.*

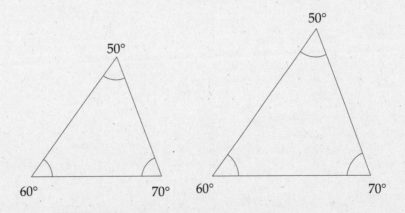

M. When two triangles are similar, corresponding pairs of sides are proportional.

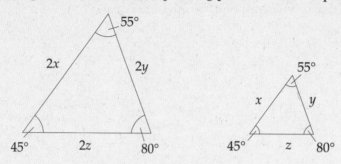

N. If, for example, you know that (1) $\triangle ABC$ is similar to $\triangle DEF$, and (2) $\triangle ABC$ has side $AB = 1$, side $BC = 2$, and side $AC = 2.25$, and (3) $\triangle DEF$ has side $DE = 1.5$, then you know that

the other two pairs of corresponding sides bear the ratio $\dfrac{1.5}{1} = \dfrac{3}{2}$, and that (a) side DF is

therefore $2.25 \times \dfrac{3}{2} = 3.375$, and (b) side EF is therefore $2 \times \dfrac{3}{2} = 3$.

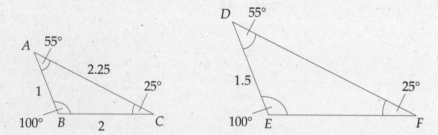

Conversely, if you know that two triangles have all three pairs of corresponding sides in one proportion, then you know that the triangles are similar and that corresponding pairs of angles are equal.

O. The area of a triangle is equal to $\dfrac{1}{2}$(the base)(the height) $= \dfrac{1}{2}(b)(h)$

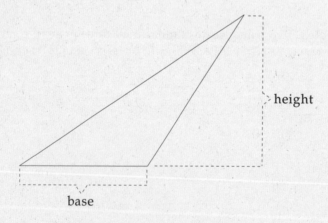

In calculating the area of a triangle one may designate any side as the base. The height is then represented by a line segment perpendicular to the base running as high as the vertex of the angle opposite the base.

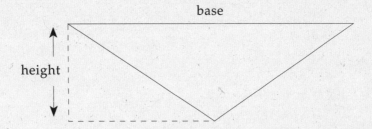

If, in triangle *ABC* below, *BC* is called the base, then the height is represented by the indicated dotted line. If the base and height are 4 and 3, as shown, the area of the triangle is $\frac{1}{2}(4)(3) = 6$.

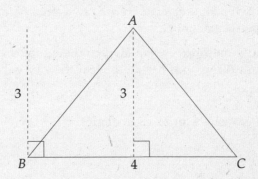

In a right triangle the two *legs* (the sides surrounding the right angle) may be taken as the base and height. In the right triangle below, the area is $\frac{1}{2}(12)(5) = 30$.

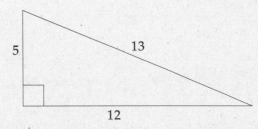

A.3.4 QUADRILATERALS

A.   Parallelograms: If a four-sided figure has any one of the following features, then it has all of them and it is a parallelogram:

(1) Opposite sides are equal and parallel.

(2) Opposite angles are equal.

(3) One diagonal divides the figure into two congruent triangles.

(4) Two diagonals *bisect* each other ("meet" each other halfway along their lengths).

Suppose one is shown this figure and told that angle *BAD* = angle *BCD* and angle ABC = angle ADC.

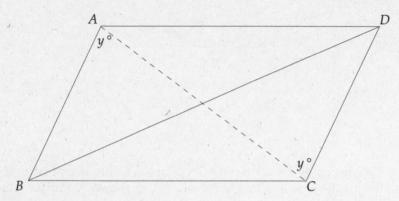

From this data alone you can conclude that the figure is a parallelogram because opposite angles are equal. You can further conclude, that (1) *AD = BC* , (2) *AB = DC* , (3) Δ *ABD* is congruent to Δ *BCD*, and (4) if a line segment were drawn from point A to point C, it would bisect and be bisected by line segment *BD*.

If, in a parallelogram, adjacent sides are equal, then the figure is an equilateral parallelogram or a rhombus. A rhombus has all the features of a parallelogram plus two more:

(1) All sides are equal in length.

(2) The intersection of diagonals forms right angles.

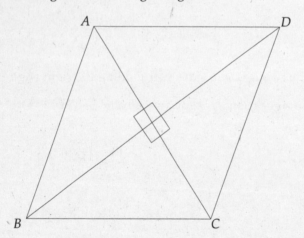

B.   Rectangles: Any four-sided figure whose angles are all right angles is a rectangle. A rectangle has all of the features of a parallelogram (and therefore *is* a parallelgram) plus two more:

(1) All angles are right angles.

(2) The diagonals are equal in length.

When bisected by a diagonal, a rectangle generates two right triangles whose dimensions may be ascertained through the Pythagorean theorem.

Consider this rectangle:

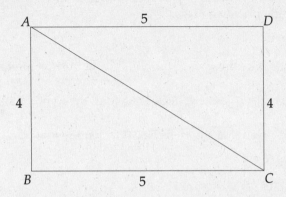

In order to determine the length of diagonal *AC* (to which the length of diagonal *BD* would be equal), apply the Pythagorean theorem recognizing that diagonal *AC* forms the hypotenuse of a right triangle:

$$AC^2 = 4^2 + 5^2 = 16 + 25 = 41$$

$$AC = \sqrt{41}$$

The area of a rectangle is equal to (base × height) which for the rectangle shown above = 5 × 4 = 20.

C. Squares: Any four-sided figure whose angles are all right angles and whose sides are all equal is a square. All squares are also parallelograms, rhombi, and rectangles. A square has every feature of a rectangle plus two more:

(1) All sides are equal.

(2) The two diagonals (like those of a rhombus) meet at right angles.

Since for any right triangle whose two legs are equal, the hypotenuse $= (\text{leg}) \times \sqrt{2}$,

the diagonal that runs through a square is equal to $\left[(\text{side}) \times \sqrt{2} \right]$:

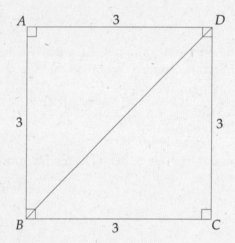

In the illustration above, the diagonal constitutes the hypotenuse of two right triangles, each of which has both its legs equal to 3. The diagonal, therefore, has length $= 3\sqrt{2}$.

The area of a square = (base)(height) = (side)^2.

A.3.5 PARALLEL LINES CROSSED BY A TRANSVERSAL

When two parallel lines are crossed by a transversal (a line segment), eight angles are formed. Four are acute and four are obtuse. The following relations apply:

(1) All of the acute angles are equal.

(2) All of the obtuse angles are equal.

(3) The sum of any acute angle and any obtuse angle is equal to 180°.

Conversely, if two lines are crossed by a transversal and one knows the foregoing relations to apply, he can deduce whether the two lines are parallel.

Consider this figure:

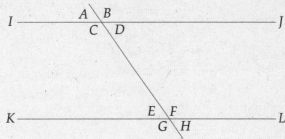

If you are told that line segments *IJ* and *KL* are parallel, you know:

(1) Angles *A*, *E*, *D*, and *H* are all acute and equal.

(2) Angles *C*, *G*, *B*, and *F* are all obtuse and equal.

(3) The sum: (any angle in the first group) + (any angle in the second group) = 180°.

Conversely, if you are told that angles *A* and *H* are equal, or that the sum (angle *A*) + (angle *F*) = 180°, you can conclude that the two line segments *IJ* and *KL* are parallel. The rule is more formally expressed thus:

When two parallel lines are crossed by a transversal:

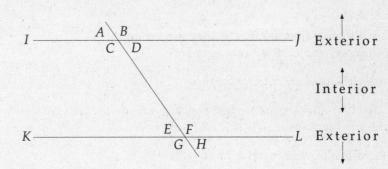

(1) Corresponding angles are equal.

(2) Alternate interior angles are equal.

(3) Alternate exterior angles are equal.

(4) Interior angles on the same side of the transversal are supplementary (meaning their sum is 180°).

(5) Exterior angles on the same side of the transversal are supplementary.

Consider this figure:

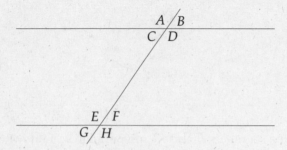

- *A* and *E* are corresponding angles: each is above its line, and to the left of the transversal; *A* and *E* are equal.

- *B* and *F* are corresponding angles; each is above its line and to the right of the transversal.

- *C* and *G* are corresponding angles; each is below its line and to the left of the transversal.

- *D* and *H* are corresponding angles; each is below the line, and to the right of the transversal.

- *C* and *F* are alternate interior angles; they are inside the parallel lines and on opposite sides of the transversal. *C* and *F* are equal.

- *D* and *E* are also alternate interior angles.

- *A* and *H* are alternate exterior angles; they are outside the two parallel lines and on opposite sides of the transversal. *A* and *H* are equal.

- *B* and *G* are also alternate exterior angles.

- *C* and *E* are interior angles on the same side of the transversal. Their sum is 180°.

- *D* and *F* are also interior angles on the same side of the transversal.

- *A* and *G* are exterior angles on the same side of the transversal. They are supplementary; their sum is 180°.

- *B* and *H* are also exterior angles on the same side of the transversal.

hydrogen bonding in, 766-67
hydrolysis, 788
nomenclature of, 765-66
sample passage and questions, 777-81
structure of, 763-67
synthesis of, 769-72
tricarboxylic acids, 764
Carboxylic carbon, 764
Cardiac muscle, 580, 584
Carnivores, 514
Cartesian coordinate system (CCS)
acceleration on, 47-51
graphs, 18-20
speed, 41
vectors, 37-40
Cartilaginous joints, 580
Cartilaginous rings, 551
Catalysts, 280-83, 313, 523
chemical reaction rates, 280-81
Cartesian plane, 17
Catecholamines, 607
Catechol-O-methyl transferase (COMT), 630
Cathode, 405, 414, 415
CCS. See Cartesian coordinate system
Cell diagrams, 410
Cell emf, 408
Cell membrane, 423-25, 505
Cellobiose, 811
Cells
biochemical pathways of, 523-48
blood, 567
concentration, 415-16
electrolytic, 413-14
and endocrine system, 601
energy production in, 528-41
enzymatic facilitation of cellular reactions, 523-28
eukaryotic, 423-42
lymphocytes, 570
reproduction by mitosis, 468-73
sample passage and questions, 542-48
smooth muscle, 548
stomach, 573
See also DNA
Cellular adhesions, 433
Cell wall, 423, 505
Celsius scale, 339-40
Center of mass, 87-88
Central nervous system, 616-19
Centrifugation, 567
Centriole, 436
Centripetal acceleration, 53-55
Centromere, 443, 469, 475, 478
Cerebellum, 617-18
Cerebral cortex, 608, 617-18
Cerebrospinal fluid (CSF), 617
Cerebrum, 617
"Chair" ring conformation, 719-21
Charge, of atom, 232
Charge, electrical
contact, 128-31
and Coulomb's law, 135-38

induction, 133-35
Charles's Law, 343-44
Chemical digestion, 570
Chemical equilibrium, defined, 285
Chemical reactions, fundamental phenomena, 265-83
balanced equations and limiting reagents, 268-71
equilibrium dynamics, 285-97
kinetics and thermodynamic reaction energetics, 304
oxidation-reduction reactions, 271-75
reaction kinetics, 275-81
reactions classes, 265-67
sample passages and questions, 282-83
See also Equilibrium dynamics; Thermodynamics
Chemistry
acid-base, 377-401
electrochemistry, 403-22
hydrocarbons, 721-25
nuclear, 242-43
stereochemistry, 691-712
See also Chemical reactions, fundamental phenomena; Organic compounds, separation and identification of
Chemoreceptors, 632
Chiasma, 473-474
Chief cells, 573
Chirality, 694-97
of amino acids, 786-87
Chiral center, 694-97
Chitin, 511
Chlorophyll, 435
Chloroplasts, 435
Cholinesterase, 630
Chromatid, 469, 470, 474, 476, 478
Chromatography, 822-23
Chromosomes, 436
bacteria, 505
DNA, 443
reproduction, 451-54
sex-linked traits, 650-52
See also Reproduction, bacterial; Reproduction, biological
Chyme, 573
Chymotrypsin, 574
Cilia, 552
Ciliary muscle, 634
Circular motion, 53-56
Circulation
arterial, 557
definition, 563
pulmonary, 561-64
venous, 558
Cis configurations, 691-93
Cis isomer, 723
Citric acid cycle, 532
Class (taxonomic organization), 664
Cleavage, 493, 495
Cleavage furrow, 471, 476

Feedback inhibition, 527
Fermentation, 529, 530-31
Fertilization, 486
F (fertility) factor, 507
Fibrous joints, 580
Filaments
    thick, 582
    thin, 582
Fischer projections, 806-7
Fission, 512
Flagella, 436
Flagellum, 482
Flow, 121-23
    fluid viscosity, 124
Fluid mosaic model, cell membrane, 423-24
Fluids
    buoyancy, 119-21
    density and specific gravity, 118
    flow, 121-23
    pressure, 118-19
Focal length, 213-15, 219
Focal point, 213-14, 219
Focal power, 224
Follicle, 486
Follicle stimulating hormone (FSH), 612, 614
Follicular phase, menstrual cycle, 612
Force per unit area, 340
Force(s)
    definition of, 69
    net, 73-90
    Newton's laws of motion, 69-70, 74-75
    Newton's law of universal gravitation, 72-73
    sample passage and questions, 91-94
    simple harmonic motion, 199-202
    summation of, 73-74
    vertical and horizontal, 78-79
    weight as, 70-72
Forebrain, 617
Formylmethionyl-tRNA, 458-60
Founder effect, 663
Fractional distillation, 817, 819-20
Free energy of activation, 310
Free energy of a system, 307
Free fall motion, 55-58
Freezing, 360
Freezing point depression, 331-32
Frequency, 188
Friction, 84-87
Fructofuranose, 808
Fructose, 807, 808, 811
FSH (follicle stimulating hormone), 612, 614
Fungi, 511-13
    features of, 511-12
    reproduction of, 512-14
Furanose, 808

G

G_1 (gap) phase, 468
G_2 phase, 468
Gall bladder, 575-76

Galvanic cells, 410-13
    comparison with electrolytic cells, 415
Galvanometer, 411
Gametes, 480, 493, 494
Gametogenesis, 473, 480-85
Gamma carbon, 747
Ganglia, 621
Gap junctions, 433
Gap phase, 468
Gas chromatography, 822
Gases, 120, 339-57
    deviations from ideality, 348-49
    diffusion and effusion of, 352-53
    gas laws, 342-47, 349-53
    kinetic molecular theory, 341-42
    mixtures of, 349-51
    noble, 241
    phase changes, 359-76
    pressure, 340-41
    sample passage and questions, 354-57
    solubility of, 322
    STP, 341
    temperature, 339-40
Gas exchange (respiratory system), 549-56
    at alveolar surface, 555-56
    blood gas levels, 555-56
    expiration, 550-51
    inspiration, 549-50
    respiratory tract, structural features of, 551-55
    surface tension of alveoli, 554
    surfactant, role of, 554-5
Gastrointestinal tract, 571
Gastrula, 493, 494, 495
Gay-Lussac's law, 343-44
Gene pool, 657-59
Genes, 641-43
    dominant vs. recessive, 645
Genetic code, 457-58
Genetic drift, 662-63
Genetic recombination, 473, 647-50
Genetics
    DNA, 443-66
    heredity, 641-55
Genetic variability, 647-652
Genome, 469
Genotype, 643-44
Genus, 664
Geometric isomers, 691
Geometry
    molecular and VSEPR model, 258-61
    review of, 944-62
Germ cell layers, 495, 496, 498-99
Germ cells, 467, 495
Gibbs free-energy of a system, 307
Glomerular capillaries, 596
Glomerular filtrate, 596
Glomerulus, 592-93, 595, 596
Glucocorticoids, 607
Gluconeogenesis, 604
Glucopyranose, 808
Glucose, 603-5, 806, 807, 808, 809

Uracil, 454
Urea, 576
Ureter, 594
Urethra, 482, 599, 603
Urinary bladder, 591, 592, 594
Urinary space, 592
Urinary system. *See* Renal system
Urine, 596, 599, 600
Uterus, 486

V

Vacuoles, 435
Vacuum distillation, 820-21
Vagus nerve, 573, 620
Valence electrons, 234
Valence Shell Electron Pair Repulsion (VSEPR), 258-61
Valence shells, 234
    and molecular geometry, 258-61
Valves, heart, 558-59
van der Waal's equation, 348-49
Vaporization, 360, 361, 365
Vapor pressure, 329-30, 350
Variable portion of amino acids, 785
Variable section (DNA), 445, 446
Vas deferens, 480, 482, 483
Vasopressin, 611
Vector(s), 27-40
    addition and subtraction, 28-32
    on Cartesian coordinate system, 37-40
    component, 33-36
    sum, 75
    vector quantities vs. scalar quantities, 27
Vegetative functions, 620
Veins, 558
Velocity, 15, 42
    gases, 340
    Newton's first law, 71
    relative, 43-46
    vs. time, 47-49
    See also Acceleration
Venous circulation, 558
Ventricles, 556
Ventricular contraction, 564
Venules, 558
Verbal reasoning, 2, 4
Vesicle, 431, 432, 434, 435
Vestibular apparatus, 632-33
Vestibular nerve, 633
Vestibular system, 632-33
Virtual images, 215
Viruses, 508-10
    features of, 508
    reproduction of, 509
    and transduction, 507
Visible light, 207
Vision. *See* Visual system
Visual sense, 632
Visual system, 634
Vitreous humor, 634

Voltage, 406, 408
Voltage drop, 174-77
Voltage-gated channels, 625
Voltage-gated sodium channels, 625
Voltaic cell. *See* Galvanic cells
Volume
    deviations in gases, 348
    effect on equilibrium, 292-93
VSEPR (Valence Shell Electron Pair Repulsion), 258-861

W

Water
    dehydration, 577
    dehydration reaction, 733-35
    dehydration synthesis, 795
    ionization of, 377
    phase diagram of, 370
    retention, hormonal regulation of, 599-600
Watt, 104, 164
Wavelength, 190-91
    of light, 207-208
Wave(s)
    dynamics of, 187-91
    longitudinal compression, 191-93
    sample passage and questions, 203-206
    simple harmonic motion, 200
    See also Sound waves
Weight, as force, 70-72
White blood cells, 573
White light, 207
White matter, 619, 620
Work, 97-98
    as function of kinetic and gravitational potential energy, 100-101
    sample passage and questions, 108-110
Writing sample, 3, 4

X

X-ray diffraction, 450, 451

Y

Yeasts, 450, 451
Yellow bone marrow, 578
Young's modulus, 116-118

Z

Z isomer, 723
Z lines, 581-82
Zona pellucida, 486
Zwitterion (dipolar ion), 790
Zygote, 480, 486, 493-94
Zymogens, 574

INSTALLING AND USING YOUR REVIEWARE™ COMPUTER DIAGNOSTIC SOFTWARE

SYSTEM REQUIREMENTS

WINDOWS™ VERSION
- IBM PC or compatible (486 DX or better)
- MS Windows 3.1, 3.11, or '95
- VGA or higher resolution graphics card
- CD-ROM Drive
- Microsoft compatible mouse
- Local Hard Disk with 10 MB free
- 8 MB RAM

MACINTOSH® VERSION
- A Macintosh Computer with System 7 or later
- CD-ROM Drive
- 8 MB RAM
- Local Hard Disk with 10 MB free

ADDITIONAL REQUIREMENTS FOR MSN
- Microsoft Windows 95
- 14.4 kbps Modem (faster modem recommended for optimum performance)
- 16 MB RAM
- 50 MB additional hard disk space
- Sound card recommended

INSTALLATION

WINDOWS '95
1. Insert CD-ROM into CD-ROM drive
2. Choose Run from the Start Menu
3. Type d:\setup.exe in the Command Line box that appears
4. Click OK
5. Follow the directions on the screen

MSN Instructions (For users of Windows '95 operating system only):
Your MSN registration number is 1794. Please write this number down, you will need to input it during the MSN setup process.

1. Turn on your computer and start Microsoft Windows '95 operating system.
2. Insert CD-ROM into your CD-ROM drive
3. Choose Run from the Start Menu
4. Type d:\msn\startup.exe in the Command Line box that appears
5. Should you require assistance, double click on Get Help Connecting to MSN or contact MSN Technical Support at (206) 635-7019 in the U.S. and Canada

WIN 3.1
1. Insert CD-ROM into CD-ROM drive
2. Choose Run from the Program Manager File menu
3. Type d:\setup.exe in the Command Line box that appears
4. Click OK
5. Follow the directions on the screen

MACINTOSH
1. Insert CD-ROM into CD-ROM drive
2. Double click on the GRE Installer icon
3. Follow the directions on the screen

During the installation you will be able to choose which test you would like to install. Each test is meant to be taken once. After taking a test, you should use the drill mode to practice on the questions in that pool. To install a second test, repeat the installation instructions above and choose a different test.

If you have any questions about installing RevieWare Computer Diagnostics, please call (800) 546-2102.

USING REVIEWARE DIAGNOSTICS

GETTING STARTED

WIN '95
1. Choose Programs from the Start Menu
2. Select The Princeton Review program group and select the test you wish to take

MACINTOSH AND WIN 3.1
1. Open The Princeton Review program group
2. Double click on the test you wish to take

The Main Menu contains three sections: Take a Test, Take a Drill, and Review a Test. Click the "Begin" button in any section to start working. It is recommended that you take the diagnostic tests first and then use the drills to work on your weak points.

Take a Test: When you begin a test, you should make sure you have enough time to finish. Computer Adaptive tests can not be suspended. During a test click the "?" button on the bottom of the screen if you need more help on a topic.

Take a Drill: You can choose the number of questions in the drill before you begin. Drills questions are marked as soon as you answer. Your total score will be given at the end.

Review a Test: After you complete an exam it will appear in the Review a Test box. Click on the test title to select it (the title will turn red when it is selected). Then click "Begin."

NOTES:

NOTES:

NOTES:

NOTES:

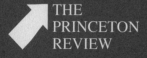
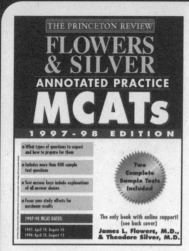
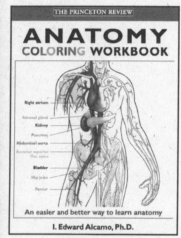
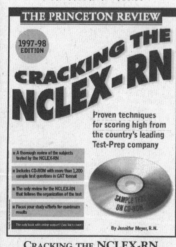

FIND US...

International

Hong Kong
4/F Sun Hung Kai Centre
30 Harbour Road, Wan Chai,
Hong Kong
Tel: (011)85-2-517-3016

Japan
Fuji Building 40, 15-14
Sakuragaokacho, Shibuya Ku,
Tokyo 150, Japan
Tel: (011)81-3-3463-1343

Korea
Tae Young Bldg, 944-24,
Daechi- Dong, Kangnam-Ku
The Princeton Review- ANC
Seoul, Korea 135-280,
South Korea
Tel: (011)82-2-554-7763

Mexico City
PR Mex S De RL De Cv
Guanajuato 228 Col. Roma
06700 Mexico D.F., Mexico
Tel: 525-564-9468

Montreal
666 Sherbrooke St.
West, Suite 202
Montreal, QC H3A 1E7 Canada
Tel: (514) 499-0870

Pakistan
1 Bawa Park - 90 Upper Mall
Lahore, Pakistan
Tel: (011)92-42-571-2315

Spain
Pza. Castilla, 3 - 5° A, 28046
Madrid, Spain
Tel: (011)341-323-4212

Taiwan
155 Chung Hsiao East Road
Section 4 - 4th Floor,
Taipei R.O.C., Taiwan
Tel: (011)886-2-751-1243

Thailand
Building One, 99 Wireless Road
Bangkok, Thailand 10330
Tel: (662) 256-7080

Toronto
1240 Bay Street, Suite 300
Toronto M5R 2A7 Canada
Tel: (800) 495-7737
Tel: (716) 839-4391

Vancouver
4212 University Way NE,
Suite 204
Seattle, WA 98105
Tel: (206) 548-1100

National (U.S.)
We have over 60 offices around the U.S. and
run courses in over 400 sites. For courses and locations
within the U.S. call 1 (800) 2/Review and you will be
routed to the nearest office.

www.review.com

Expert Advice

Talk About It

Pop Surveys

Paying for it

www.review.com

THE
PRINCETON
REVIEW

Getting in

Word du Jour

Find-O-Rama School & Career Search

www.review.com

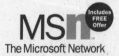
MSn
Includes FREE Offer
The Microsoft Network

Finding it

Best Schools

Free!

Did you know that The Microsoft Network gives you one free month?

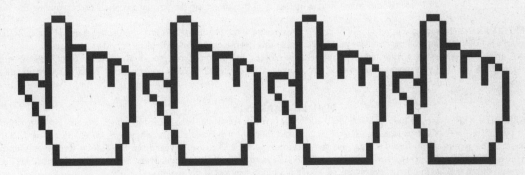

Pop the enclosed CD into your computer and start exploring the World Wide Web for one month, free. Exchange e-mail with your family and friends. Play games, book airline tickets, handle finances, go car shopping, explore old hobbies and discover new ones. There's one big, useful online world out there. And for one month, it's a free world.

If for some reason the CD is missing, call us at **1-800-FREE MSN**, Dept. 3197, for offer details or visit us at **www.msn.com**. Some restrictions apply.

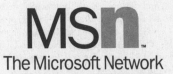

Microsoft Where do you want to go today?®

MSN.
The Microsoft Network

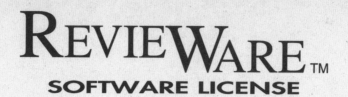

REVIEWARE™
SOFTWARE LICENSE

This License Agreement is your proof of license. Please treat it as valuable property.

REVIEWARE® LICENSE AGREEMENT

This is a legal agreement between you (either an individual or an entity), the end user, and Princeton Review Publishing, L.L.C., ("TPRP"). By using the software enclosed, you and any transferees and/or multiple licensees hereunder agree to be bound by the terms of this RevieWare® License Agreement. If you do not agree to its terms, promptly return the disk package and accompanying items (including written materials and binders or other containers) to the place you obtained them for a full refund.

REVIEWARE® SOFTWARE LICENSE

1. GRANT OF LICENSE This RevieWare® License Agreement ("License") permits you to use one copy of the specified version of the RevieWare software product identified above ("SOFTWARE") on any single computer, provided the SOFTWARE is in use on only one computer at any time. If you have multiple Licenses for the SOFTWARE, then at any time you may have as many copies of the SOFTWARE in use as you have Licenses. The SOFTWARE is "in use" on a computer when it is loaded into the temporary memory (i.e., RAM) or installed into the permanent memory (e.g., hard disk, CD-ROM, or other storage device) of that computer, except that a copy installed on a network server for the sole purpose of distribution to other computers is not "in use." If the anticipated number of users of the SOFTWARE will exceed the number of applicable Licenses, then you must have a reasonable mechanism or process in place to ensure that the number of persons using the SOFTWARE concurrently does not exceed the number of Licenses. If the SOFTWARE is permanently installed on the hard disk or other storage device of a computer (other than a network server) and one person uses that computer more than 80% of the time it is in use, then that person may also use the SOFTWARE on a portable or home computer.

2. COPYRIGHT The SOFTWARE is owned by TPRP or its suppliers and is protected by United States copyright laws and international treaty provisions. Therefore, you must treat the SOFTWARE like any other copyrighted material (e.g., a book or musical recording) except that you may either (a) make one copy of the SOFTWARE solely for backup or archival purposes, or (b) transfer the SOFTWARE to a single hard disk provided you keep the original solely for backup or archival purposes. You may not copy the written materials accompanying the SOFTWARE.

3. OTHER RESTRICTIONS This License is your proof of license to exercise the rights granted herein and must be retained by you. You may not rent or lease the SOFTWARE, but you may transfer your rights under this License on a permanent basis provided you transfer this License, the SOFTWARE, and all accompanying written materials and retain no copies, and the recipient agrees to the terms of this License. You may not reverse engineer, decompile, or disassemble the SOFTWARE. Any transfer of the SOFTWARE must include the most recent update and all prior versions.

LIMITED WARRANTY

LIMITED WARRANTY. TPRP warrants that (a) The SOFTWARE will perform substantially in accordance with the accompanying written materials for a period of ninety (90) days from the date of receipt; and (b) any hardware accompanying the SOFTWARE will be free from defects in materials and workmanship under normal use and service for a period of one (1) year from the date of receipt. Any implied warranties on the SOFTWARE and hardware are limited to ninety (90) days and one (1) year, respectively. Some states or jurisdictions do not allow limitations on duration of an implied warranty, so the above limitation may not apply to you.

CUSTOMER REMEDIES. TPRP's entire liability and your exclusive remedy shall be at TPRP's option, either (a) return of the price paid or (b) repair or replacement of the SOFTWARE or hardware that does not meet TPRP's Limited Warranty and that is returned to TPRP with a copy of your receipt. This Limited Warranty is void if failure of the SOFTWARE or hardware has resulted from accident, abuse, or misapplication. Any replacement SOFTWARE will be warranted for the remainder of the original warranty period or thirty (30) days, whichever is longer. These remedies are **not** available outside the United States of America.

NO OTHER WARRANTIES. TPRP disclaims all other warranties, either express or implied, including but not limited to implied warranties of merchantability and fitness for a particular purpose with respect to the SOFTWARE, the accompanying written materials, and any accompanying hardware. This limited warranty gives you specific legal rights. You may have others, which vary from state or jurisdiction to state or jurisdiction.

NO LIABILITY FOR CONSEQUENTIAL DAMAGES. In no event shall TPRP or its suppliers be liable for any damages whatsoever (including, without limitation, damages for loss of business profits, business interruption, loss or business information, or other pecuniary loss) arising out of the use or inability to use this TPRP product, even if TPRP has been advised of the possibility of such damages. Because some states or jurisdictions do not allow the exclusion or limitation of liability for consequential or incidental damages, the above limitation may not apply to you.

U.S. GOVERNMENT RESTRICTED RIGHTS

The SOFTWARE and documentation are provided with RESTRICTED RIGHTS. Use, duplication, or disclosure by the Government is subject to restrictions as set forth in subparagraph (c)(1)(ii) of the Rights in Technical Data and Computer Software clause at DFARS 252.227-7013 or subparagraphs (c)(1) and (2) of the Commercial Computer Software—Restricted Rights at 48 CFR 52.227-19, as applicable. Contractor manufacturer is TPRP/2315 Broadway/New York, 10024. This Agreement is governed by the laws of the State of New York. For more information about TPRP's licensing policies, please call RevieWare Customer Service at (800) 546-2102, or write: RevieWare Customer Sales and Service/2315 Broadway/New York, NY 10024.

DETAILS OF MSN OFFER

FOR USERS OF WINDOWS 95 OPERATING SYSTEM ONLY. Includes MSN client software only. Internet access providers for Mac and Windows 3.1 users are also included. You must additionally subscribe to MSN™, the Microsoft Network, to access the service. One month free unlimited trial is available to new members of MSN in the 50 United States, the District of Columbia, and Canada only. A credit card is required. MSN premium charges, access charges (if access is purchased from a provider other than MSN) and local phone and/or long distance toll charges may apply. Access availability may be affected by local market network activity and capacity. Offer expires July 31, 1998. Microsoft and MSN are either registered trademarks or trademarks of Microsoft Corporation in the U.S. and/or other countries.